Drug-Induced Ocular Side Effects

Drug-Induced Ocular Side Effects

FOURTH EDITION

F. T. FRAUNFELDER, M.D.

Professor and Chairman
Casey Eye Institute
Department of Ophthalmology
Oregon Health Sciences University
Portland, Oregon

ASSOCIATE EDITOR

JOAN A. GROVE

Associate Director
National Registry of Drug-Induced
   Ocular Side Effects
Casey Eye Institute
Oregon Health Sciences University
Portland, Oregon

Williams & Wilkins

BALTIMORE • PHILADELPHIA • HONG KONG
LONDON • MUNICH • SYDNEY • TOKYO

A WAVERLY COMPANY

1996

Executive Editor: Darlene B. Cooke
Developmental Editor: Francis Klass
Production Manager: Laurie Forsyth
Project Editor: Susan Rockwell

Copyright © 1996
Williams & Wilkins
Rose Tree Corporate Center
1400 North Providence Road
Building II, Suite 5025
Media, PA 19063-2043 USA

Accurate indications, adverse reactions, and dosage schedules for drugs are provided in this book, but it is possible they may change. The reader is urged to review the package information data of the manufacturers of the medications mentioned.

Printed in the United States of America

ISBN 0-683-03356-5

The Publishers have made every effort to trace the copyright holders for borrowed material. If they have inadvertantly overlooked any, they will be pleased to make the necessary arrangements at the first opportunity.

95 96 97 98 99
1 2 3 4 5 6 7 8 9 10

Reprints of chapters may be purchased from Williams & Wilkins in quantities of 100 or more. Call Isabella Wise, Special Sales Department, (800) 358-3583.

To
Yvonne, Yvette, Helene Jean,
Nina, Rick, and Nick

Kevin, Bing, Scott, Wendee

Matthew, Kara, Courtney

———

To

Eric, Jenni, Dani, and Kevin

Preface

When a medical text or reference book makes it to a fourth edition, it probably fills a need. Today's clinician is overwhelmed by the volume of ocular toxicology and needs a "quick" reference book that "boils it down." The basic problem is that very little scientific data are available on the side effects of drugs in general, and on the eye in particular. There are many variables in assessing a cause-and-effect relationship and very few research dollars available for such studies. Peer review journals have difficulty in accepting papers on visual side effects of drugs, since causation is difficult to prove by scientific parameters. Ten + percent of the information in this book may be incorrect; my problem is I don't know which 10 + percent. This book is intended as a guide to help the physician decide whether a visual problem is drug related. The physician's past experience and previous reports on the drug help in making an informed decision. The clinician knows that there is no active drug which is without an undesirable side effect, in part based on the immune system, past drug exposure, interaction with other drugs, the volume of the drug taken, etc. It is the intent of this book to compile and organize "previous reports" into a format that the busy clinician may find useful.

This fourth edition has incorporated the most recent data from the Federal Drug Administration, Rockville, MD, World Health Organization, Uppsala, Sweden, and the National Registry of Drug-Induced Ocular Side Effects, Casey Eye Institute, Oregon Health Sciences University, Portland, Oregon. The Registry contains cases received from many countries and the world literature as its data base. Data in this book have been accumulated from innumerable physicians and scientists who have suspected adverse drug reactions and reported their suspicions to FDA, WHO, or the National Registry. At least 44 drugs not covered in the 3rd edition have been added. Owing to the nature of this book and the volume of material covered, errors, omissions and misemphasis are inevitable. We welcome your comments and hope this book helps you in your medical decision making.

Portland, Oregon   *F. T. Fraunfelder, M.D.*

Instructions to Users

The basic format used in each chapter for each drug or group of drugs in this book is described below.

Class: The general category of the primary action of the drug is given.

Generic Name: The United States National Formulary name of each drug is listed. (A name in parentheses following the National Formulary name is the international generic name if it differs from the one used in the United States);

Proprietary Name: The more common trade names are given. (In a group of drugs, the number before a generic names corresponds to the number preceding the proprietary drug. This is true for both the systemic and ophthalmic forms of the drug. If a proprietary drug is made in the United States, the name will appear in bold type, with the other countries in which that proprietary drug is made in parentheses. Combination drugs are seldom included);

Primary Use: The type of drug and its current use in the management of various conditions are listed.

Ocular Side Effects

Systemic Administration: Ocular side effects as reported from oral, nasal, intravenous, intramuscular, or intrathecal administration.

Local Ophthalmic Use or Exposure: Ocular side effects as reported from topical ocular application, subconjunctival, retrobulbar, or intracameral injection.

Inadvertent Ocular Exposure: Ocular side effects as reported due to accidental ocular exposure from any form of the drug.

Inadvertent Systemic Exposure: Ocular side effects as reported due to accidental systemic exposure exposure from topical ophthalmic medications.

Systemic Absorption from Topical Application to the Skin: Ocular side effects as reported secondary to topical dermatologic application.

The ocular side effects are listed in probable order or importance. The determination of importance is based on incidence of significance of the side effect. The name of a drug in parentheses adjacent to an adverse reaction indicates that this is the only agent in the group reported to have caused this side effect.

Systemic Side Effects
Systemic Administration: Systemic side effects as reported from ophthalmic medications administered by an oral, intravenous or intramuscular route.

Local Ophthalmic Use or Exposure: Systemic side effects as reported from topical ocular application or subconjunctival or retrobulbar injection.

The systemic side effects are listed in probable order of importance. The determination of importance is based on incidence of significance of the side effect. Side effects of inadequate documentation or current debate are followed by (?). The name of a drug in parentheses adjacent to an adverse reaction indicates that this is the only agent in the group reported to have caused this side effect.

Clinical Significance: A concise overview of the general importance of the ocular side effects produced is given to the clinician.

References: References have been limited to either the best articles, the most current, or those with the most complete bibliography.

Index of Side Effects: The lists of adverse ocular side effects due to drugs are intended in part to be indexes in themselves. The adverse ocular reactions are not separated in this index as to route of administration; however, this can be obtained by going to the text.

Index: The index includes the drugs' generic and proprietary names. In addition, classification group names have been added. The index is the primary source of entry into this book. This is a necessity because many drugs are in groups and would otherwise be missed.

In the following section, the services of the National Registry of Drug-Induced Ocular Side Effects are outlined. The intent of this Registry is to make available data of possible drug-induced ocular side effects and to provide a central agency where possible adverse ocular drug reactions can be reported.

National Registry of Drug-Induced Ocular Side Effects

Rationale

In a specialized area such as ophthalmology, seldom does a practitioner or even a group of practitioners see the patient volume necessary to make a correlation between possible cause and effect of drug-related or drug induced ocular disease. A national registry to correlate this type of data may be of value because this task would be difficult to accomplish by any other method. If a number of these "possible" associations are found with a particular drug, then definitive controlled studies could be undertaken to obtain valid data. It is hoped that future editions of this book will present data with greater scientific significance, in part due to the reports of possible drug-induced ocular side effects which physicians will send to the Registry.

Objectives

• To establish a national center where possible drug-induced ocular side effects can be accumulated.

• To review possible drug-induced ocular side effect data collected through the Food and Drug Administration (FDA) (Rockville, MD) and the World Health Organization (WHO) (Uppsala, Sweden).

• To compile the data in the world literature on reports of possible drug-induced ocular side effects.

• To make available this data to physicians who feel they have a possible drug-induced ocular side effect.

Format

The cases of primary interest are those adverse ocular reactions not previously recognized or those that are rare, severe, serious, or unusual. To be of value data should be complete and follow the basic format shown below.

Age:

Sex:

Suspected drug:

Suspected reaction—date of onset:

Route, dose and when drug started:

Improvement after suspected drug stopped-if restarted, did adverse reaction recur:

Other drugs taken at time of suspected adverse reaction:

Comments—optional: Your opinion if drug-induced, probably related, possibly related, or unrelated.)

Your name and address—optional:

We are expanding the Registry from only drugs to include chemicals and other substances which may have potential ocular toxicology. We welcome all case reports and any impressons even without specific cases.

Send to:

Joan Grove, Associate Director
National Registry of Drug-Induced Ocular Side Effects
Casey Eye Institute
Oregon Health Sciences University
3375 S.W. Terwilliger Blvd.
Portland, Oregon 97201-4197
(503)494-5686

Abbreviations

Alg.	Algeria	Ital.	Italy
Arg.	Argentina	Jap.	Japan
Austral.	Australia	Lux.	Luxemburg
Aust.	Austria	Mon.	Monaco
Belg.	Belgium	Mor.	Morocco
Braz.	Brazil	Neth.	Netherlands
Canad.	Canada	Norw.	Norway
Cz.	Czechoslovakia	N.Z.	New Zealand
Denm.	Denmark	Pol.	Poland
Fin.	Finland	Port.	Portugal
Fr.	France	Rus.	Russia
G.B.	Great Britain	S. Afr.	South Africa
Germ.	Germany	Scand.	Scandinavia
Gr.	Greece	Span.	Spain
Hung.	Hungary	Swed.	Sweden
Ind.	India	Switz.	Switzerland
Ire.	Ireland	Tun.	Tunisia
Isr.	Israel		

Contents

V. Gastrointestinal Agents

VI. Cardiac, Vascular, and Renal Agents

VII. Hormones and Agents Affecting Hormonal Mechanisms

VIII. Agents Affecting Blood Formation and Coagulability

IX. Homeostatic and Nutrient Agents

Contents

Anti-infectives

Class: AIDS-related Agents

Generic Name: Didanosine

Proprietary Name: Videx

Primary Use: A purine analogue with antiretrovirus activity.

Ocular Side Effects:
- A. Systemic Administration
    1. Retina—choroid
        a. Retinal pigment epithelium mottling
        b. Retinal pigment epithelium atrophy
        c. Retinal pigment epithelium hypertrophy
        d. Abnormality of neurosensory retina
        e. Loss of choriocapillaris
    2. Electro-oculograms—reduced Arden ratio
    3. Visual field defects
        a. Scotoma
        b. Constriction

Clinical Significance: Whitcup, et al. have described retinal lesions that first appear as patches of retinal pigment epithelium mottling and atrophy in the midperiphery of the fundi in patients taking didanosine. In time, these lesions become more circumscribed and develop a border of retinal pigment epithelium hypertrophy. If didanosine therapy is continued, progression occurs; progression decreases once the drug is stopped. Although the midperiphery is the area first involved, lesions may well encroach on the posterior pole if the drug is continued at high dosage. To date, central visual acuity has been preserved. Didanosine's toxic effects on the retina appear related both to peak dosage and accumulated dosage. These changes were first described in children, but a few adult cases have also been reported. Patients

1

taking this drug should be monitored for the development and progression of retinal lesions.

References:

Nguyen, B.Y., et al.: A pilot study of sequential therapy with zidovudine plus acyclovir, dideoxyinosine, and dideoxycytidine in patients with severe human immunodeficiency virus infection. J. Infect. Dis. *168*:810–817, 1993.

Whitcup, S.M., et al.: Retinal toxicity in human immunodeficiency virus-infected children treated with 2′, 3′-dideoxyinosine. Am. J. Ophthalmol. *113*:1–7, 1992.

Whitcup, S.M., et al.: A clinicopathologic report of the retinal lesions associated with didanosine. Arch. Ophthalmol. *112*:1594–1598, 1994.

Generic Name: Dideoxyinosine

Proprietary Name: Hivid

Primary Use: A synthetic pyrimidine nucleoside with virustatic activity against the retroviruses. It is commonly used in combination with zidovudine.

Ocular Side Effects:
   A. Systemic Administration—Oral
      1. Neuropathy
         a. Optic neuritis
         b. Optic atrophy
      2. Decreased vision
         a. Amblyopia
         b. Blindness
      3. Diplopia
      4. Visual field defects—scotomas

Clinical Significance: Dideoxyinosine has caused peripheral neuropathy in up to one-third of patients, but only a few reports of adverse effects on the optic nerve are in the literature and the Registry. Therefore, the above side effects are only possible and have not been proven. Peripheral neuropathy has been well documented with dideoxyinosine and appears to be dose related, usually occurring within the first 6 months of therapy, and is reversible when the drug is discontinued. The optic neuropathy cases seem to occur early after drug exposure, i.e., within a few days to weeks after drug exposure. Symptomatology includes sensation of bright lights, a mottling of visual effect, and multiple blind spots. If the drug is continued, there are cases of marked visual deterioration.

References:

Lafeuillade, A., et al.: Optic neuritis associated with dideoxyinosine. Lancet *1*:615–616, 1991.

Generic Name: Zidovudine

Proprietary Name: Retrovir

Primary Use: Zidovudine remains the mainstay for patients infected with human immunodeficiency virus.

Ocular Side Effects:
A. Systemic Administration
 1. Cystoid macular edema
 2. Hypertrichosis
 3. Eyelids
  a. Urticaria
  b. Rashes
  c. Vasculitis
 4. Hyperpigmentation of the eyelids and conjunctiva
 5. Diplopia
 6. Visual hallucinations
 7. Nystagmus (overdose)

Clinical Significance: In a disease such as HIV, which is usually treated with many agents, it is often difficult to find a cause-and-effect relationship between a drug and an ocular side effect. However, there have been a number of reports of cystoid macular edema while taking this agent that have resolved when the drug was discontinued. Clearly, hypertrichosis can occur as well as skin rashes. Hyperpigmentation of the eyelids, conjunctiva, fingernails, etc., especially in heavily pigmented people, has been reported. Diplopia may occur secondary to a generalized myopathy. Nystagmus has only been reported in overdose situations.

References:

Geier, S.A., et al.: Impairment of tritan colour vision after initiation of treatment with zidovudine in patients with HIV disease or AIDS. Br. J. Ophthalmol. 77:315–316, 1993.

Klutman, N.E., and Hinthorn, D.R.: Excessive growth of eyelashes in a patient with AIDS being treated with zidovudine. N. Engl. J. Med. 324(26):1896, 1991.

Lalonde, R.G., Deschênes, J.G., and Seamone, C.: Zidovudine-induced macular edema. Ann. Intern. Med. 114(4):297–298, 1991.

Merenich, J.A., et al.: Azidothymidine-induced hyperpigmentation mimicking primary adrenal insufficiency. Am. J. Med. 86:469–470, 1989.

Spear, J.B., et al.: Zidovudine overdose. First report of ataxia and nystagmus: case report. Ann. Intern. Med. 109:76–77, 1988.

Strominger, M.B., Sachs, R., and Engel, H.M.: Macular edema from zidovudine? Ann. Intern. Med. 115(1):67, 1991.

Wilde, M.I., and Langtry, H.D.: Zidovudine: An update of its pharmacodynamic and pharmacokinetic properties, and therapeutic efficacy. Drugs 46(3):515–578, 1993.

Class: Amebicides

Generic Name: 1. Amodiaquine; 2. Chloroquine; 3. Hydroxychloroquine. See under *Class: Antimalarial Agents.*

Generic Name: 1. Broxyquinoline; 2. Iodochlorhydroxyquin; 3.Iodoquinol (Diiodohydroxyquinoline)

Proprietary Name: 1. Available in multi-ingredient preparations only; 2. Linola-sept (Germ.), Silic C (Austral.), **Vioform** (Austral., Canad.); 3. Dioboquin (Canad.), Direxiode (Fr.), Floraquin (Austral., S. Afr., Span.), Ovoquinol (Canad.), **Yodoxin** (Canad.)

Primary Use: These amebicidal agents are effective against *Entamoeba histolytica.*

Ocular Side Effects:
   A. Systemic Administration
      1. Decreased vision
      2. Optic atrophy
      3. Optic neuritis—Subacute myelo-optic neuropathy (SMON)
      4. Nystagmus
      5. Toxic amblyopia
      6. Macular edema
      7. Macular degeneration
      8. Diplopia
      9. Absence of foveal reflex
      10. Problems with color vision
          a. Color vision defect
          b. Purple spots on white background

Clinical Significance: Major toxic ocular effects may occur with long-term oral administration of these amebicidal agents, especially in children. Since these agents are given orally for *Entamoeba histolytica*, most reports are from the Far East. Data suggest that these amebicides may cause subacute myelo-optic neuropathy (SMON). This neurologic disease has a 19% incidence of decreased vision and a 2.5% incidence of toxic amblyopia. Possibly, iodoquinol causes fewer side effects because less is absorbed through the gastrointestinal tract than with iodochlorhydroxyquin. It has been suggested that in patients being treated for acrodermatitis enteropathica, a disease of inherited zinc deficiency, optic atrophy may be secondary to zinc deficiency instead of iodochlorhydroxyquin or iodoquinol. Since long-term quinolone exposure has been shown to result in accumulation of the drug in pigmented tissues, retinal degenerative changes may be observed.

References:

Baumgartner, G., et al.: Neurotoxicity of halogenated hydroxyquinolines: Clinical analysis of cases reported outside Japan. J. Neurol. Neurosurg. Psychiatry *42*:1073, 1979.

Committee on Drugs, 1989–1990: Clioquinol (iodochlorhydroxyquin, vioform) and iodquinol (diiodohydroxyquin): Blindness and neuropathy. Pediatrics *86(5)*: 797–798, 1990.

Guy-Grand, B., Basdevant, A., and Soffer, M.: Oxyquinoline neurotoxicity. Lancet *1*: 993, 1983.

Hanakago, R., and Uono, M.: Clioquinol intoxication occurring in the treatment of acrodermatitis enteropathica with reference to SMON outside of Japan. Clin. Toxicol. *18*:1427, 1981.

Hansson, O., and Herxheimer, A.: Neurotoxicity of oxyquinolines. Lancet 2:1253, 1980.

Kauffman, E.R., et al.: Clioquinol (iodochlorhydroxyquin, vioform) and iodoquinol (diiodohydroxyquin): Blindness and neuropathy. Pediatrics 86:978–979, 1990.

Kono, R.: Review of subacute myelo-optic neuropathy (SMON) and studies done by the SMON research commission. Jpn. J. Med. Sci. Biol. *28*(Suppl):1–21, 1975.

Oakley, G.P.: The neurotoxicity of the halogenated hydroxyquinolines. JAMA *225*: 395–397, 1973.

Ricoy, J.R., Ortega, A., and Cabello, A.: Subacute myelo-optic neuropathy (SMON): First neuro-pathological report outside Japan. J. Neurol. Sci. *53*:241, 1982.

Rose, F.C., and Gawel, M.: Clioquinol neurotoxicity: An overview. Acta. Neurol. Scand. *70*(Suppl. 100):137–145, 1984.

Shibasaki, H., et al.: Peripheral and central nerve conduction in subacute myelo-optic neuropathy. Neurology *32*:1186, 1982.

Shigematsu, I.: Subacute myelo-optic neuropathy (SMON) and clioquinol. Jpn. J. Med. Sci. Biol. *28*(Suppl):35–55, 1975.

Sturtevant, F.M.: Zinc deficiency: Acrodermatitis enteropathica, optic atrophy, SMON, and 5, 7-dihalo-8-quinolinols. Pediatrics *65*:610, 1980.

Tjalve, H.: The aetiology of SMON may involve an interaction between clioquinol and environmental metals. Med. Hypotheses *15*:293, 1984.

Generic Name: Emetine

Proprietary Name: Emetine (also available in multi-ingredient preparations.)

Primary Use: This alkaloid is effective in the treatment of acute amebic dysentery, amebic hepatitis, and amebic abscesses.

Ocular Side Effects:

   A. Systemic Administration
      1. Nonspecific ocular irritation
         a. Lacrimation
         b. Hyperemia
         c. Photophobia

    2. Pupils
      a. Mydriasis
      b. Absence of reaction to light
    3. Paralysis of accommodation
    4. Decreased vision
    5. Eyelids or conjunctiva
      a. Urticaria
      b. Purpura
      c. Eczema
    6. Visual fields
      a. Scotomas—central
      b. Constriction
  B. Inadvertent Ocular Exposure
    1. Irritation
      a. Lacrimation
      b. Hyperemia
      c. Photophobia
    2. Eyelids or conjunctiva
      a. Allergic reactions
      b. Conjunctivitis—nonspecific
      c. Edema
      d. Blepharospasm
    3. Keratitis
    4. Corneal ulceration
    5. Iritis
    6. Corneal opacities

Clinical Significance: Systemic emetine occasionally causes adverse ocular effects; however, discontinuation of the drug returns the eyes to normal within a few days to weeks. Inadvertent topical ocular exposure may cause a severe irritative response lasting from 24 to 48 hours. Typically, this ocular discomfort does not occur until 4 to 10 hours after the initial contact. To our knowledge, only one case of permanent blindness secondary to corneal opacities has been reported from inadvertent ocular exposure of emetine.

References:

Blue, J.B.: Emetin: A warning. (Correspondence). JAMA 65:1297, 1915.

Duke-Elder, S.: Systems of Ophthalmology. St. Louis, C.V. Mosby, Vol. XIV, Part 2, 1972, p. 1187.

Jacovides: Troubles visuels a la suite d'injections fortes d'emetine. Arch. Ophthalmol. (Paris) 40:657, 1923.

Lasky, M.A.: Corneal response to emetine hydrochloride. Arch. Ophthalmol. 44:47, 1950.

Porges, N.: Tragedy in compounding. (Letter). J. Am. Pharm. Assoc. Pract. Pharm. 9: 593, 1948.

Reynolds, J.E.F. (Ed.): Martindale: The Extra Pharmacopoeia. 28th Ed., London, Pharmaceutical Press, 1982, pp. 978–979.
Torres Estrada, A.: Ocular lesions caused by emetine. Bol. Hosp. Oftal. NS Luz. (Mex.) 2:145, 1944 (Am. J. Ophthalmol. 28:1060, 1945).

Class: Anthelmintics

Generic Name: Diethylcarbamazine

Proprietary Name: Filarcidan (Span.), Hetrazan (Austral., Canad., G.B., Germ.), Notézine (Fr.)

Primary Use: This antifilarial agent is particularly effective against *W. bancrofti, W. malayi, O. volvulus,* and *Loa loa.*

Ocular Side Effects:
A. Systemic Administration
1. Eyelids or conjunctiva
   a. Allergic reactions
   b. Conjunctivitis—nonspecific
   c. Edema
   d. Urticaria
   e. Nodules
2. Uveitis
3. Punctate keratitis
4. Corneal opacities
5. Chorioretinitis
6. Visual field defects
7. Retinal pigmentary changes
8. Loss of eyelashes or eyebrows
9. Toxic amblyopia
B. Local Ophthalmic Use or Exposure—Topical Application
1. Eyelids or conjunctiva
   a. Allergic reactions
   b. Erythema
   c. Edema
2. Irritation
   a. Lacrimation
   b. Hyperemia
   c. Photophobia
   d. Ocular pain
3. Corneal opacities
4. Uveitis

Clinical Significance: Adverse ocular reactions to diethylcarbamazine may occur but are often difficult to differentiate from the drug-induced death of the filaria with resultant allergic reactions due to the release of foreign protein. Nodules may form in the area of the dead worm with a resultant inflammatory reaction. This reaction in the eye may be so marked that toxic amblyopia follows. The use of diethylcarbamazine eye drops for treatment of ocular onchocerciasis produces dose-related inflammatory reactions similar to those seen with systemic use of the drug. Local ocular effects may include globular limbal infiltrates, severe vasculitis, itching, and erythema.

References:

Bird, A.C., et al: Changes in visual function and in the posterior segment of the eye during treatment of onchocerciasis with diethylcarbamazine citrate. Br. J. Ophthalmol. 64:191, 1980.

Bird, A.C., et al.: Visual loss during oral diethylcarbamazine treatment for onchocerciasis. Br. Med. J. 2:46, 1979.

Dukes, M.N.G. (Ed.): Meyler's Side Effects of Drugs. Amsterdam, Excerpta Medica, Vol. X, 1984, pp. 592–593.

Jones, B.R., Anderson J., and Fuglsang, H.: Effects of various concentrations of diethylcarbamazine citrate applied as eye drops in ocular onchocerciasis, and the possibilities of improved therapy from continuous non-pulsed delivery. Br. J. Ophthalmol. 62:428, 1978.

Taylor, H.R., and Greene, B.M.: Ocular changes with oral and transepidermal diethylcarbamazine therapy of onchocerciasis. Br. J. Ophthalmol. 65:494, 1981.

Generic Name: Piperazine

Proprietary Name: Adelmintex (Span.), Antepar (Ire.), Anticucs (Span.), Ascarient (S. Afr.), Citrazine (Ire.), Citropiperazina (Ital.), Ectodyne (G.B.), Entacyl (Canad.), Pap-A-Ray (S. Afr.), Pipralen (S. Afr.), Uvilon (Ital.), Vermi (Span.), Wormelix (S. Afr.), Wormex (G.B.)

Primary Use: This anthelmintic agent is used in the treatment of ascariasis and enterobiasis.

Ocular Side Effects:

A. Systemic Administration
   1. Decreased vision
   2. Problems with color vision—color vision defect
   3. Paralysis of accommodation
   4. Miosis
   5. Nystagmus
   6. Visual hallucinations
   7. Paralysis of extraocular muscles
   8. Visual sensations
      a. Flashing lights
      b. Entopic light flashes
   9. Eyelids or conjunctiva

    a. Allergic reactions
    b. Edema
    c. Photosensitivity
    d. Urticaria
    e. Purpura
    f. Erythema multiforme
    g. Eczema
10. Lacrimation
11. Subconjunctival or retinal hemorrhages secondary to drug-induced anemia

Clinical Significance: While a number of ocular side effects have been attributed to piperazine, they are rare, reversible, and usually of little clinical importance. Adverse ocular reactions generally occur only in instances of overdose or in cases of impaired renal function. Only a few cases of well-documented extraocular muscle paralysis have been reported. There is some data on the cataractogenic potential of this drug, but these are unproven; however, there is data to suggest that photosensitizing drugs may have this potential.

References:
Bomb, B.S., and Bebi, H.K.: Neurotoxic side-effects of piperazine. Trans. R. Soc. Trop. Med. Hyg. 70:358, 1976.
Brown, H.W., Chan, K.F., and Hussey, K.L.: Treatment of enterobiasis and ascariasis with piperazine. JAMA 161:515, 1956.
Combes, B., Damon, A., Gottfried, E.: Piperazine (Antepar) neurotoxicity: Report of a case probably due to renal insufficiency. N. Engl. J. Med. 254:223, 1956.
Mezey, P.: The role of piperazine derivates in the pathogenesis of cataract. Klin. Monatsbl. Augenheilkd. 151:885, 1967.
Walsh, F.B., and Hoyt, W.F.: Clinical Neuro-Ophthalmology. 3rd Ed., Baltimore, Williams & Wilkins, Vol. III, 1969, pp. 2637–2638.

Generic Name: Quinacrine (Mepacrine)

Proprietary Name: Atabrine (Canad.), **Atabrine Hydrochloride**

Primary Use: This methoxyacridine agent is effective in the treatment of tapeworm infestations and in the prophylaxis and treatment of malaria.

Ocular Side Effects:
A. Systemic Administration
    1. Decreased vision
    2. Visual fields
      a. Scotomas
      b. Enlarged blind spot

    3. Optic neuritis
    4. Cornea
       a. Corneal edema
       b. Superficial punctate keratitis
    5. Yellow, white, clear, brown, blue, or grey punctate deposits
       a. Conjunctiva
       b. Cornea
       c. Nasolacrimal system
    6. Problems with color vision
       a. Color vision defect
       b. Objects have yellow, green, blue, or violet tinge
       c. Colored haloes around lights—mainly blue
    7. Subconjunctival or retinal hemorrhages secondary to drug-induced anemia
    8. Eyelids or conjunctiva
       a. Blue-black hyperpigmentation
       b. Yellow discoloration
       c. Urticaria
       d. Exfoliative dermatitis
       e. Eczema
    9. Photophobia
   10. Visual hallucinations
  B. Inadvertent Direct Ocular Exposure
    1. Blue haloes around lights
    2. Eyelids, conjunctiva, or cornea
       a. Edema
       b. Yellow discoloration
    3. Irritation
       a. Lacrimation
       b. Ocular pain

Clinical Significance: Adverse ocular reactions due to quinacrine are common but seldom of major clinical significance. Nearly all are reversible and fairly asymptomatic. Scotomas, enlarged blind spots, and hallucinations are only found at high dosages and are reversible. Drug-induced corneal edema may be precipitated in sensitive individuals who will most often, in time, show hepatic dysfunction. This can occur with dosages as low as 0.10 g/day and takes several weeks to occur. If the drug is discontinued, this will resolve; but if the drug is restarted, the edema occurs again in a few days. Drug-related corneal deposits will disappear with time once the drug is discontinued; skin pigmentation will likewise diminish and often disappears. The sclera remains uninvolved. Topical ocular application has been used for self-inflicted ocular damage; however, permanent ocular damage has not been reported. There is only one published report of retinal toxicity (Carr).

References:

Ansdell, V.E., and Common, J.D.: Corneal changes induced by mepacrine. J. Trop. Med. Hyg. *82*:206–207. 1979.

Carr, R.E., et al.: Ocular toxicity of antimalarial drugs: Long term follow-up. Am. J. Ophthalmol. *66*:738–744, 1968.

Chamberlain, W.P., and Boles, D.J.: Edema of cornea precipitated by quinacrine (Atabrine). Arch. Ophthalmol. *35*:120–134, 1946.

Evans, R.L., et al.: Antimalarial psychosis revisited. Arch. Dermatol. *120*:765, 1984.

Granstein, R.D., and Sober, A.J.: Drug- and heavy metal-induced hyperpigmentation. J. Am. Acad. Dermatol. *5*:1, 1981.

Koranda, F.C.: Antimalarials. J. Am. Acad. Dermatol. *4*:650, 1981.

Sokol, R.J., Lichenstein, P.K., and Farrell, M.K.: Quinacrine hydrochloride yellow discoloration of the skin in children. Pediatrics *69*:232, 1982.

Generic Name: Suramin. See under *Class: Antiprotozoal Agents.*

Generic Name: Thiabendazole

Proprietary Name: Mintezol (Austral., G.B., S. Afr.), Triasox (Span.)

Primary Use: This benzimidazole compound is used in the treatment of enterobiasis, strongyloidiasis, ascariasis, uncinariasis, trichuriasis, and cutaneous larva migrans. It has been advocated as an antimycotic in corneal ulcers.

Ocular Side Effects:
    A. Systemic Administration
        1. Decreased vision
        2. Problems with color vision
            a. Color vision defect
            b. Objects have yellow tinge
        3. Abnormal visual sensations
        4. Eyelids or conjunctiva
            a. Allergic reactions
            b. Hyperemia
            c. Angioneurotic edema
            d. Erythema multiforme
            e. Stevens-Johnson syndrome
            f. Exfoliative dermatitis
            g. Lyell's syndrome
            h. Urticaria
        5. Visual hallucinations
        6. Subconjunctival or retinal hemorrhages secondary to drug-induced anemia
        7. Keratoconjunctivitis sicca

Clinical Significance: While thiabendazole is a potent therapeutic agent, it has surprisingly few reported ocular or systemic toxic side effects. Ocular side effects that may occur are transitory, reversible, and seldom of clinical importance. However, a mother and daughter developed keratoconjunctivitis sicca, xerostomia, cholangiostatic hepatitis, and pancreatic dysfunction after only a few doses. This may have been an immunologic reaction, and the drug possibly acted as a hapten.

References:

Drugs for parasitic infections. Med. Lett. Drugs Ther. *24*:12, 1982.

Fink, A.I., MacKay, C.J., and Cutler, S.S.: Sicca complex and cholestatic jaundice in two members of a family caused by thiabendazole. Trans. Am. Ophthalmol. Soc. *76*:108, 1978.

Fraunfelder, F.T.: Interim report: National Registry of Drug-Induced Ocular Side Effects. Ophthalmology *86*:126, 1979.

Gilman, A.G., Goodman, L.S., and Gilman, A. (Eds.): The Pharmacological Basis of Therapeutics. 8th Ed., New York, Macmillan, 1990, pp. 970–971.

Class: Antibiotics

Generic Name: Amikacin

Proprietary Name: Amicasil (Ital.), **Amikin** (Austral., Canad., G.B., Ire., S.Afr.), Amikine (Switz.), Amiklin (Fr.), Amukin (Neth.), Biclin (Span.), Biklin (Germ., Swed.), Chemacin (Ital.), Kanbine (Span.), Likacin (Ital.), Lukadin (Ital.), Migracin (Ital.), Mikavir (Ital.), Pierami (Ital.), Sifamic (Ital.)

Primary Use: This systemically administered aminoglycoside is primarily used for Gram-negative infections.

Ocular Side Effects:
    A. Systemic Administration
        1. Decreased vision
        2. Eyelids or conjunctiva
            a. Urticaria
            b. Purpura
    B. Local Ophthalmic Use or Exposure—Intravitreal Injection
        1. Macular infarcts

Clinical Significance: Systemic amikacin rarely causes ocular side effects of any consequence; there is seldom reason to stop the medication. However, a recent report by Campochiaro and Lim emphasizes the potential hazards of the intravitreal use of amikacin, as with other aminoglycosides. They emphasize that a localized increase in concentration of these drugs, especially in the dependent areas of the retina, may play a role in retinal toxicity. If some of the parafoveal capillaries are not involved, retention of central vision is possible. These authors described eight patients who suffered macular infarcts after intravitreal injections of 0.2 or 0.4 mg of amikacin sulfate. Eiferman and Stagner have shown that amikacin will bind to ocular pigments.

References:

Campochiaro, P.A., and Lim, J.I.: Aminoglycoside toxicity in the treatment of endophthalmitis. Arch. Ophthalmol. *112*:48–53, 1994.

Doft, B.H., and Barza, M.: Ceftazidime or amikacin: Choice of intravitreal antimicrobials in the treatment of postoperative endophthalmitis. Arch. Ophthalmol. *112*:17–18, 1994.

Eiferman, R.A., and Stagner, J.I.: Intraocular penetration of amikacin: iris binding and bioavailability. Arch. Ophthalmol. *100*:1817–1819, 1982.

Woo, F.L., et al.: Gentamicin, tobramycin, amikacin and netilmicin levels in tears following intravenous administration. Arch. Ophthalmol. *103*:216–218, 1985.

Generic Name: 1. Amoxicillin; 2. Ampicillin; 3. Azlocillin; 4. Bacampicillin; 5. Carbenicillin; 6. Cloxacillin; 7. Cyclacillin; 8. Dicloxacillin; 9. Hetacillin; 10. Methicillin; 11. Mezlocillin; 12. Nafcillin; 13. Oxacillin; 14. Piperacillin; 15. Ticarcillin

Proprietary Name: 1. Actimoxi (Span.), Agerpen (Span.), A-Gram (Fr.), A-Gram I.M.(Fr.), Alfamox (Ital.), Almodan (G.B., Ire.), Alphamox (Austral.), AM 73 (Ital.), Amagesan (Germ.), Amitron (Span.), Amix (G.B.), Amocillin (S. Afr.), Amodex (Fr.), Amoflamisan (Span.), Amoflux (Ital.), Amopen (G.B.), Amoram (G.B.), Amox (Ital., Span.), Amoxaren (Span.), Amoxi Gobens (Span.), Amoxibacter (Span.), Amoxi-Basan (Germ.), Amoxibiotic (Ital.), Amoxidel (Span.), Amoxihexal (Germ.), **Amoxil** (Austral., Canad., G.B., Ire., S. Afr.), Amoxillat (Germ.), Amoxillin (Ital.), Amoxi-Mépha (Switz.), Amoximedical (Span.), Amoximex (Switz.), Amoxina (Ital.), Amoxine (Fr.), Amoxipen (Ital., Span.), Amoxi-Tablinen (Germ.), Amoxi-Wolff (Germ.), Amoxy-Diolan (Germ.), Amoxypen (Germ.), Amrit (G.B.), AMX (S. Afr.), Antiotic (Switz.), Apamox (Span.), Apo-Amoxi (Canad.), Arcanacillin (S. Afr.), Ardine (Span.), Aspenil (Ital.), Azilline (Switz.), Becabil (Span.), Betamox (S. Afr.), Bimoxi (Span.), Bioxidona (Span.), Bolchipen (Span.), Borbalan (Span.), Bristamox (Fr., Swed.), Brondix (Span.), Cabermox (Ital.), Cabermox 1000 (Ital.), Cidanamox (Span.), Cilamox (Austral.), Clamoxyl (Fr., Germ., Neth., Span., Switz.), Clonamox (Ire.), C-Mox (S.Afr.), Co Amoxin (Span.), Cuxacillin (Germ.), Dacala (Span.), Damoxicil (Span.), Dobriciclin (Span.), dura AX (Germ.), Edoxil (Span.), Eupen (Span.), Flemoxin (G.B. Neth.), Galenamox (G.B.), Glassatan (Germ.), Gramidil (Fr.), Halitol (Span.), Helvamox (Switz.), Hiconcil (Fr., Ire., Neth.), Hosboral (Span.), Ibiamox (Austral., Ital., S. Afr.), Imacillin

(Swed.), Inexbron (Span.), Isimoxin (Ital.), **Larotid**, Majorpen (Ital.), Maxcil (S. Afr.), Maxiampil (Span.), Mediamox (Span.), Metifarma (Span.), Mopen (Ital.), Morgenxil (Span.), Moxacin (Austral., Ital.), Moxan (S. Afr.), Moxipin (Span.), Moxypen (S. Afr.), Neo-Ampiplus (Ital.), Neotetranase (Ital.), Norimox (S. Afr.), Novagcilina (Span.), Novamoxin (Canad.), Oramox (Ire.), Pädiamox (Germ.), Pamocil (Ital.), Penimox (Switz.), Pinamox (Ire.), Piramox (Ital.), **Polymox** (S. Afr.), Precopen (Span.), Raudopen (Span.), Recefril (Span.), Reloxyl (Span.), Remisan (Span.), Rimoxallin (G.B.), Riotapen (Span.), Rocillin (S. Afr.), Salvapen (Span.), Sigamopen (Germ., Switz.), Simoxil (Ital.), Simplamox (Ital.), Sintopen (Ital.), Spectroxyl (Switz.), Suamoxil (Span.), Superpeni (Span.), Supramox (Switz.), Tolodina (Span.), **Trimox**, Ultramox (S. Afr.), Velamox (Ital.), **Wymox**, Zamocillin (Ital.), Zamocilline (Fr.), Zimox (Ital.); 2. Alphacin (Austral.), Amblosin (Germ.), Amfipen (G.B., Neth.), Ampen (Ital.), Ampensaar (Germ.), Ampi Oral (Span.), Ampicillat (Germ.), Ampicin (Canad.), Ampicur (Span.), Ampicyn (Austral., S. Afr.), Ampikel (Span.), Ampilan (Ital.), Ampilean (Canad.), Ampilisa (Ital.), Ampilux (Ital.), Ampipen (S. Afr.), Ampiplus (Ital., Span.), Ampiplus Simplex (Ital.), Ampi-Rol (S. Afr.), Ampisint (Ital.), Ampi-Tablinen (Germ.), Ampi-Zoja (Ital.), Amplipenyl (Ital.), Amplital (Ital.), Amplizer (Ital.), Antibiopen (Span.), Apo-Ampi (Canad.), Austrapen (Austral.), Be-Ampicil (S. Afr.), Binotal (Germ.), Britapen (Span.), Ciarbiot (Span.), Cimexillin (Switz.), Citicil (Ital.), Clonamp (Ire.), Co-Cillin (S. Afr.), Doktacillin (Swed.), Electopen (Span.), Espectral (Span.), Gobemicina (Span.), Gramcillina (Ital.), Herpen (Jap.), Ibimicyn (Ital.), Lampocillina (Ital.), Maxicilina (Span.), Negmapen (Fr.), Novapen (Ire.), Nu-Ampi (Canad.), Nuvapen (Span.), **Omnipen, Omnipen-N**, Pénicline (Fr.), Penampil (Ital.), Pen-Bristol (Germ.), Penbritin (Austral., Canad., G.B., Ire., Neth., S. Afr.), Penrite (S. Afr.), Pentrex (S. Afr.), Pentrexil (Ital.), Pentrexyl (Ire., Neth., Swed.), Petercillin (S. Afr.), Platocillina (Ital.), **Polycillin, Principen** (Ital.), Radiocillina (Ital.), Rimacillin (G.B.), Rosampline (Fr.), Sesquicillina (Ital.), Spectracil (S. Afr.), Statcillin (S. Afr.), Togram (Span.), **Totacillin,** Totalciclina (Ital.), Totapen (Fr.), Ukapen (Fr.), Ultrabion (Span.), Urebion (Span.), Vidopen (G.B., Ire.); 3. Securopen (Austral., Fr., Germ., G.B., Ire., Ital., Span.); 4. Albaxin (Ital.), Ambacamp (Germ.), Ambaxin (G.B., Ire.), Ambaxino (Span.), Amplibac (Ital.), Bacacil (Ital., Switz.), Bacampicin (Neth., Switz.), Bacampicine (Fr.), Penglobe (Canad., Fr., Germ., Ital., Neth., Span., Swed.), **Spectrobid**, Velbacil (Span.); 5. Carbapen (Austral.), Geopen (Ital.), Pyopen (Canad., G.B.); 6. Alclox (Austral.), Anaclosil (Span.), Apo-Cloxi (Canad.), Austrastaph (Austral.), Bactopen (Canad.), Clocillin (S. Afr.), **Cloxapen**, Cloxin (S. Afr.), Cloxypen (Fr.), Ekvacillin (Swed.), Landerclox (Span.), Novocloxin (Canad.), Nu-Cloxi (Canad.), Orbenin (Austral., Canad., G.B., Ire., Neth., S. Afr., Span.), Orbénine (Fr.), **Tegopen** (Canad.); 8. Ampiplus (Ital.), Diamplicil (Ital.), Duplamox (Ital.), Duplexcillina (Ital.), Velamox D (Ital.); 9. Etaciland (Span.); 10. Celbenin (G.B., Neth.), Metin (Austral.), Staficyn

(Ital.), **Staphcillin**; 11. Baypen (Fr., Germ., Ital., Span.), **Mezlin**; 12. **Nafcil**, **Unipen** (Canad.); 13. **Bactocill**, Bristopen (Fr.), Penstapho (Ital.), **Prostaphlin**, Stapenor (Germ.); 14. Avocin (Ital.), Ivacin (Swed.), Picillin (Ital.), Pipcil (Neth.), Pipérilline (Fr.), Piperzam (Span.), **Pipracil** (Canad.), Pipril (Austral., G.B., Germ., S. Afr., Span., Switz.); 15. Tarcil (Austral.), **Ticar** (Canad., G.B.), Ticarpen (Fr., Neth., Span.), Ticillin (Austral.)

Primary Use: Semisynthetic penicillins are primarily effective against staphylococci, streptococci, pneumococci, and various other Gram-positive and Gram-negative bacteria.

Ocular Side Effects:
   A. Systemic Administration
      1. Eyelids or conjunctiva
         a. Allergic reactions
         b. Blepharoconjunctivitis
         c. Edema
         d. Photosensitivity
         e. Angioneurotic edema
         f. Urticaria
         g. Erythema multiforme
         h. Stevens-Johnson syndrome
         i. Exfoliative dermatitis
         j. Lyell's syndrome
      2. Subconjunctival or retinal hemorrhages secondary to drug-induced anemia
      3. Myasthenic neuromuscular blocking effect
         a. Paralysis of extraocular muscles
         b. Ptosis
         c. Diplopia
   B. Local Ophthalmic Use or Exposure—Topical Application or Subconjunctival Injection
      1. Irritation—primarily with subconjunctival injection
         a. Hyperemia
         b. Ocular pain
         c. Edema
      2. Eyelids or conjunctiva
         a. Allergic reactions
         b. Angioneurotic edema
      3. Overgrowth of nonsusceptible organisms
      4. Corneal opacities (cloxacillin)—primarily with subconjunctival injection
      5. Conjunctival necrosis (nafcillin)—primarily with subconjunctival injection
   C. Local Ophthalmic Use or Exposure—Intracameral Injection

1. Uveitis (methicillin)
2. Corneal edema (methicillin)
3. Lens damage (methicillin)

Clinical Significance: Surprisingly few ocular side effects other than derma-
tologic- or hematologic-related conditions have been reported with the semisynthetic penicillins. The incidence of allergic skin reactions due to ampicillin, however, is quite high. Ampicillin may unmask or aggravate ocular
signs of myasthenia gravis. Nafcillin has been reported to cause conjunctival
necrosis with subconjunctival injections. Many, and maybe all, of these
agents can be found in the tears in therapeutic levels and can cause local
reactions if sensitive to the drug.

References:

Argov Z., et al.: Ampicillin may aggravate clinical and experimental myasthenia gravis.
    Arch. Neurol. *43*:255, 1986.
Brick, D.C., West, C., and Ostler, H.B.: Ocular toxicity of subconjunctival nafcillin.
    Invest. Ophthalmol. Vis. Sci. *18*(Suppl):132, 1979.
Drug Evaluations. 6th Ed., Chicago, American Medical Association, 1986, pp.
    1312–1328.
Ellis, P.P.: Handbook of Ocular Therapeutics and Pharmacology. 6th Ed., St. Louis,
    C.V. Mosby, 1981, pp. 42–45, 165–169.
Kaeser, H.E.: Drug-induced myasthenic syndromes. Acta Neurol. Scand. *70*(Suppl.
    100):39, 1984.
Johnson, A.P., et al.: Azlocillin levels in human tears and aqueous humor. Am. J.
    Ophthalmol. *99*:469–472, 1985

Generic Name: Bacitracin

Proprietary Name: *Systemic*: **Baci-IM** *Ophthalmic*: Bacitin (Canad.) *Topical*: Baciguent (Canad.)

Primary Use: This polypeptide bactericidal agent is primarily effective
against Gram-positive cocci, *Neisseria*, and organisms causing gas gangrene.

Ocular Side Effects:
   A. Systemic Administration
       1. Myasthenic neuromuscular blocking effect
           a. Paralysis of extraocular muscles
           b. Ptosis
       2. Decreased vision
       3. Diplopia
       4. Eyelids or conjunctiva
           a. Allergic reactions

        b. Angioneurotic edema
        c. Urticaria
   B. Local Ophthalmic Use or Exposure—Topical Application or Subconjunctival Injection
     1. Irritation
     2. Eyelids or conjunctiva
        a. Allergic reactions
        b. Blepharoconjunctivitis
        c. Edema
        d. Urticaria
     3. Keratitis
     4. Overgrowth of nonsusceptible organisms
     5. Delayed corneal wound healing—toxic states
   C. Local Ophthalmic Use or Exposure—Intracameral Injection
     1. Uveitis
     2. Corneal edema
     3. Lens damage

Clinical Significance: Ocular side effects from either systemic or ocular administration of bacitracin are rare. However, with increasing use of "fortified" bacitracin solution (10,000 units/mL), marked conjunctival irritation and keratitis may occur, especially if the solutions are used frequently. The potential of decreased wound healing with prolonged use is real. The myasthenic neuromuscular blocking effect is more commonly seen if systemic bacitracin is used in combination with neomycin, kanamycin, polymyxin, or colistin. Severe ocular or periocular allergic reactions, while rare, have been seen due to topical ophthalmic bacitracin application. An anaphylactic reaction was reported after the use of bacitracin ointment.

References:

Fisher, A.A., and Adams, R.M.: Anaphylaxis following the use of bacitracin ointment. Am. Acad. Dermatol. *16*:1057, 1987.

Kaeser, H.E.: Drug-induced myasthenic syndromes. Acta Neurol. Scand. *70*(Suppl. 100):39, 1984.

McQuillen, M.P., Cantor, H.E., and O'Rourke, J.R.: Myasthenic syndrome associated with antibiotics. Arch. Neurol. *18*:402, 1968.

Petroutsos, G., et al.: Antibiotics and corneal epithelial wound healing. Arch. Ophthalmol. *101*:1775, 1983.

Reynolds, J.E.F. (Ed.): Martindale: The Extra Pharmacopoeia. 28th Ed., London, Pharmaceutical Press, 1982, p. 1100.

Small, G.A.: Respiratory paralysis after a large dose of intraperitoneal polymyxin B and bacitracin. Anesth. Analg. *43*:137, 1964.

Walsh, F.B., and Hoyt, W.F.: Clinical Neuro-Ophthalmology. 3rd Ed., Baltimore, Williams & Wilkins, Vol. III, 1969, p. 2680.

Generic Name: 1. Benzathine Penicillin G; 2. Hydrabamine Penicillin V; 3. Potassium Penicillin G (Benzylpenicillin Potassium); 4. Potassium Penicillin V (Phenoxymethylpenicillin Potassium); 5. Potassium Phenethicillin; 6. Procaine Penicillin G

Proprietary Name: 1. Benzetacil (Span.), **Bicillin L-A** (Austral., Canad., S. Afr.), Cepacilina (Span.), Diaminocillina (Ital.), Extencilline (Fr.), Megacillin (Canad.), Penadur (Switz.), Penidural (G.B., Ire., Neth.), Penilente-LA (S. Afr.), Peniroger Retard (Span.), Provipen Benzatina (Span.), Stabillicine (Switz.), Wycillina (Ital.); 3. Benzatec (S. Afr.), Cilina (Span.), Cilipen (Span.), Coliriocilina (Span.), Crystapen (Austral., Canad., G.B., Ire.), Megacillin (Canad.), Novopen (S. Afr.), Novopen-G (Canad.), Penibiot (Span.), Penilevel (Span.), Peniroger (Span.), **Pentids, Pfizerpen**, Sodiopen (Span.), Spécilline G (Fr.), Unicilina (Span.); 4. Abbocillin-VK (Austral.), Abbopen (Swed.), Acipen-V (Neth.), Antibiocin (Germ.), Apo-Pen-VK (Canad.), Apsin VK (G.B.), Arcasin (Germ., Switz.), **Beepen-VK**, Betacillin VK (S. Afr.), Betapen (S. Afr.), **Betapen VK**, Brunocilline (Switz.), Calciopen (Swed.), Calvepen (Ire.), Cilicaine VK (Austral.), Cliacil (Switz.), Copen (S. Afr.), Darocillin (S. Afr.), Deltacillin (S. Afr.), Distaquaine V-K (G.B.), durapenicillin (Germ.), Fenospen (Ital.), Fenoxypen (Swed., Switz.), Isocillin (Germ.), Ispenoral (Germ.), Kåvepenin (Swed.), Ledercilin VK (Canad.), Len V.K. (S. Afr.), LPV (Austral.), Megacillin oral (Germ.), Mégacilline (Switz.), Monocilline (Switz.), Nadopen-V (Canad.), Novo V-K (S. Afr.), Novopen-VK (Canad.), Nu-Pen-VK (Canad.), Oracillin VK (S. Afr.), Oracilline (Fr.), Ospen (Fr., Germ., Switz.), Penadur VK Mega (Switz.), Pen-Hexal (Germ.), Penicillat (Germ.), Penilevel (Span.), pen-V-basan (Germ.), Pen-Vee (Canad.), **Pen-Vee K**, Phenocilline (Switz.), P-Mega-Tablinen (Germ.), PVFK (Canad.), PVK (Austral.), Rimapen (G.B.), Roscopenin (Swed.), Stabillicine (Switz.), Stabillin V-K (G.B.), V-Cil-K (Ire., S. Afr.), **V-Cillin K** (Canad.), VC-K (Canad.), **Veetids**; 5. Bendralan (Span.), Broxil (Neth.), Drastina (Span.), Pensig (Austral.); 6. Aqucilina (Span.), Ayercillin (Canad.), Cilicaine Syringe (Austral.), Cilina 900 (Span.), Farmaproina (Span.), Fradicilina (Span.), Novocillin (S. Afr.), **Pfizerpen-AS**, Procillin (S. Afr.), Provipen Procaina (Span.), Quick-Cillin (S. Afr.), **Wycillin** (Canad.)

Primary Use: These bactericidal penicillins are effective against streptococci, *S. aureus*, gonococci, meningococci, pneumococci, *T. pallidum, Clostridium, B. anthracis, C. diphtheriae*, and several species of *Actinomyces*.

Ocular Side Effects:
   A. Systemic Administration
      1. Mydriasis
      2. Decreased accommodation
      3. Diplopia
      4. Papilledema secondary to pseudotumor cerebri
      5. Decreased vision

      6. Visual hallucinations
      7. Visual agnosia
      8. Eyelids or conjunctiva
        a. Allergic reactions
        b. Erythema
        c. Blepharoconjunctivitis
        d. Edema
        e. Angioneurotic edema
        f. Urticaria
        g. Lupoid syndrome
        h. Stevens-Johnson syndrome
        i. Lyell's syndrome
      9. Subconjunctival or retinal hemorrhages secondary to drug-induced anemia
    B. Local Ophthalmic Use or Exposure—Topical Application or Subconjunctival Injection
      1. Irritation
      2. Eyelids or conjunctiva—allergic reactions
      3. Overgrowth of nonsusceptible organisms
    C. Local Ophthalmic Use or Exposure—Intracameral Injection
      1. Uveitis
      2. Corneal edema
      3. Lens damage

Clinical Significance: Systemic administration of penicillin only rarely causes ocular side effects. The most serious adverse reaction is papilledema secondary to elevated intracranial pressure. The incidence of allergic reactions is greater in patients with Sjögren's syncrome or rheumatoid arthritis than in other individuals. Most other ocular side effects due to penicillin are transient and reversible. Topical ocular administration results in a high incidence of allergic reactions.

References:

Alarcón-Segovia, D.: Drug-induced antinuclear antibodies and lupus syndromes. Drugs *12*:69, 1976.

Crews, S.J.: Ocular adverse reactions to drugs. Practitioner *219*:72, 1977.

Katzman, B., et al.: Pseudotumor cerebri: An observation and review. Ann. Ophthalmol. *13*:887, 1981.

Leopold, I.H., and Wong, E.K., Jr.: The eye: Local irritation and topical toxicity. *In* Drill, V.A., and Lazar, P. (Eds.): Cutaneous Toxicity. New York, Raven Press, 1984, pp. 99–103.

Robertson, C.R., Jr.: Hallucinations after penicillin injection. Am. J. Dis. Child. *139*: 1074, 1985.

Snavely, S.R., and Hodges, G.R.: The neurotoxicity of antibacterial agents. Ann. Intern. Med. *101*:92, 1984.

Tseng, S.C.G., et al.: Topical retinoid treatment for various dry-eye disorders. Ophthalmology 92:717, 1985.

Generic Name: 1. Cefaclor; 2. Cefadroxil; 3. Cefamandole; 4. Cefazolin; 5. Cefonicid; 6. Cefoperazone; 7. Ceforanide; 8. Cefotaxime; 9. Cefotetan; 10. Cefoxitin; 11. Cefsulodin; 12. Ceftazidime; 13. Ceftizoxime; 14. Ceftriaxone; 15. Cefuroxime; 16. Cephalexin; 17. Cephaloridine; 18. Cephalothin; 19. Cephapirin; 20. Cephradine; 21. Moxalactam

Proprietary Name: 1. Alfatil (Fr.), **Ceclor** (Austral., Canad., Neth., S. Afr., Span., Switz.), Distaclor (G.B.), Kefolor (Swed.), Panacef (Ital.), Panoral (Germ.); 2. Baxan (G.B.), Bidocef (Germ.), Cefadril (Ital.), Cefadrox (S. Afr.), Cefamox (Swed.), Cefroxil (Span.), Ceoxil (Ital.), Cephos (Ital.), Crenodyn (Ital.), Droxicef (Ital.), Duracef (S. Afr., Span., Switz.), **Duricef** (Canad.), Ibidroxil (Ital.), Kefroxil (Ital.), Moxacef (Ital., Neth.), Oracefal (Fr.), Oradroxil (Ital.), Sedral (Jap.), **Ultracef** (Ire.); 3. Cedol (Ital.), Cefam (Ital.), Cefamen (Ital.), Cefaseptolo (Ital.), Cefiran (Ital.), Cemado (Ital.), Fado (Ital.), Ibiman (Ital.), Kéfandol (Fr.), Kefadol (G.B.), Lampomandol (Ital.), Mancef (Ital.), Mandokef (Germ., Ital., S. Afr., Span., Switz.), **Mandol** (Austral., Canad., Neth.), Mandolsan (Ital.), Septomandolo (Ital.); 4. Acef (Ital.), **Ancef** (Canad.), Areuzolin (Span.), Biazolina (Ital.), Bor-Cefazol (Ital.), Brizolina (Span.) Caricef (Span.), Céfacidal (Fr.), Cefabiozim (Ital.), Cefacidal (Neth.), Cefakes (Span.), Cefamezin (Austral., Ital., Jap., Span.), Cefazil (Ital.), Cefazina (Ital.), Cromezin (Ital.), Dacovo (Span.), Elzogram (Germ.), Fazoplex (Span.), Firmacef (Ital.), Gramaxin (Germ.), Kefol (Span.), **Kefzol** (Austral., Canad., Fr., G.B., Ire., Neth., S. Afr., Switz.), Kurgan (Span.), Lampocef (Ital.), Recef (Ital.), Sicef (Ital.), Tasep (Span.), Totacef (Ital.), **Zolicef**, Zolin (Ital.), Zolisint (Ital.), Zolival (Span.); 5. Cefodie (Ital.), **Monocid** (Ital., Span.), Praticef (Ital.); 6. Bioperazone (Ital.), **Cefobid** (Canad., Ital., Span.), Céfobis (Fr., Switz.), Cefazone (Ital.), Cefobis (Germ.), Cefogram (Ital.), Cefoneg (Ital.), Cefoper (Ital.), Cefosint (Ital.), Dardum (Ital.), Farecef (Ital.), Ipazone (Ital.), Kefazon (Ital.), Mediper (Ital.), Novobiocyl (Ital.), Perocef (Ital.), Prontokef (Ital.), Tomabef (Ital.), Zoncef (Ital.); 7. **Precef**; 8. Cefacron (Span.), **Claforan** (Austral., Canad., Fr., G.B., Germ., Ire., Ital., Neth., S. Afr., Span., Swed., Switz.), Primafen (Span.), Zariviz (Ital.); 9. Apacef (Fr.), Apatef (Germ., Ital.), **Cefotan**, Cepan (Ital.), Darvilen (Ital.), Yamatetan (Jap.); 10. Betacef (Ital.), Cefaxicina (Span.), Cefociclin (Ital.), Méfoxin (Fr.), **Mefoxin** (Austral., Canad., G.B., Ital., Neth., S. Afr.), Mefoxitin (Germ., Span., Swed., Switz.), Stovaren (Ital.), Tifox (Ital.); 11. Monaspor (G.B., Neth.), Pseudocef (Germ.), Pyocéfal (Fr.), Takesulin (Jap.); 12. Ceftim (Ital.), **Ceptaz**, Fortam (Span., Switz.), **Fortaz** (Canad.), Fortum (Austral., Fr., G.B., Germ., Ire., Neth., S. Afr., Swed.), Glazidim (Ital.), Kefamin (Span.), Kefzim (S. Afr.), Panzid (Ital.), Potendal (Span.), Spectrum (Ital.), Starcef (Ital.), **Tazicef**, **Tazidime**; 13. **Cefizox** (Canad., Fr., G.B., Ire., Span.), Ceftix (Germ.), Epo-

celin (Jap., Span.), Eposerin (Ital.); 14. Rocefalin (Span.), Rocefin (Ital.),
Rocephin (Austral., Canad., Germ., Ire., Neth., S. Afr.), Rocéphine (Fr.,
Switz.); 15. Biociclin (Ital.), Biofurex (Ital.), Bioxima (Ital.), Cépazine (Fr.),
Cefamar (Ital.), Cefoprim (Ital.), **Ceftin**, Cefumax (Ital.), Cefur (Ital.), Cef-
urex (Ital.), Cefurin (Ital.), Colifossim (Ital.), Curoxim (Ital.), Curoxima
(Span.), Curoxime (Fr.), Deltacef (Ital.), Duxima (Ital.), Elobact (Germ.),
Gibicef (Ital.), Ipacef (Ital.), Itorex (Ital.), Kefox (Ital.), **Kefurox**, Kesint
(Ital.), Lafurex (Ital.), Lamposporin (Ital.), Medoxim (Ital.), Polixima (Ital.),
Supero (Ital.), Ultroxim (Ital.), **Zinacef** (Canad., G.B., Germ., Ire., Neth.,
S. Afr., Swed., Switz.), Zinat (Switz.), Zinnat (Fr., G.B., Germ., Ire., Neth.,
S. Afr., Span.); 16. Abiocef (Ital.), Apo-Cephalex (Canad.), Bioporina
(Span.), Céporexine (Fr.), Cefadina (Span.), Cefadros (Ital.), Cefaleh Ina
(Span.), Cefalexgobens (Span.), Cefalorex (Span.), Cefamiso (Span.), **Cefa-
nex**, Ceferran (Span.), Cefibacter (Span.), Ceporex (Austral., Canad., G.B.,
Ire., Ital., Neth., S. Afr., Switz.), Ceporexin (Germ.), Cerexin (S. Afr.),
Cilicef (Span.), Coliceflor (Ital.), Defaxina (Span.), Domucef (Ital.), Efem-
ida (Span.), Erifalecin (Span.), Ibilex (Austral., Ital.), Karilexina (Span.),
Keflet, **Keflex** (Austral., Canad., G.B., Ire., S. Afr., Swed., Switz.), Keflori-
dina (Span.), Keforal (Fr., Ital., Neth.), **Keftab**, Lafarin (Ital.), Latoral (Ital.),
Lenocef (S. Afr.), Lerporina (Span.), Lexincef (Span.), Lorexina (Ital.),
Novolexin (Canad.), Oracef (Germ.), Sintolexyn (Ital.), Sporol (Span.), Sul-
quipen (Span.), Torlasporin (Span.), Ultralexin (Span.), Valesporin (Span.),
Zetacef (Ital.); 17. Ceporin (Ital.), Céporine (Fr.), Dinasint (Ital.), Faredina
(Ital.), Floridin (Ital.), Keflodin (Ital.), Latorex (Ital.), Lauridin (Ital.); 18.
Ceporacin (Austral., Canad., Neth.), Cepovenin (Germ.), Keflin (Canad.,
Fr., Ire., Ital., Neth., S. Afr., Span., Swed.), Keflin N (Switz.), Keflin Neutral
(Austral.); 19. Brisfirina (Span.), **Cefadyl**, Céfaloject (Fr.), Piricef (Ital.);
20. **Anspor**, Cefamid (Ital.), Cefrabiotic (Ital.), Cefrasol (Ital.), Cefril (S.
Afr.), Celex (Ital.), Cesporan (Ital.), Citicef (Ital.), Ecosporina (Ital.), Eska-
cef (Fr.), Lenzacef (Ital.), Lisacef (Ital.), Maxisporin (Neth.), Samedrin
(Ital.), Sefril (Germ., Switz.), Septacef (Span.), Velocef (Ital., Span.), **Velo-
sef** (Canad., G.B., Fr., Ire., Neth.); 21. Baxal (Ital.), Betalactam (Ital.), Festa-
moxin (Germ.), Latoxacef (Ital.), Mactam (Ital.), Moxacef (Ital.), Moxalactam (Austral., Fr., Germ., Span.), Moxatres (Ital.), Oxacef (Ital.), Polimoxal
(Ital.), Priolatt (Ital.), Sectam (Ital.), Shiomarin (Jap.)

Primary Use: Cephalosporins are effective against streptococci, staphylococci, pneumococci, and strains of *E. coli, P. mirabilis,* and *Klebsiella.*

Ocular Side Effects:
   A. Systemic Administration
      1. Eyelids or Conjunctiva
      2. Nystagmus
         a. Allergic reactions
         b. Erythema

   c. Conjunctivitis—nonspecific
   d. Edema
   e. Angioneurotic edema
   f. Urticaria
   g. Erythema multiforme
   h. Stevens-Johnson syndrome
   i. Exfoliative dermatitis
  3. Subconjunctival or retinal hemorrhages secondary to drug-induced anemia
  4. Visual hallucinations
  5. Diplopia (cephaloridine)
  6. Problems with color vision—color vision defect (cephaloridine)
  7. Corneal edema—peripheral (cefaclor)
 B. Local Ophthalmic Use or Exposure—Topical Application or Subconjunctival Injection
  1. Irritation
   a. Hyperemia
   b. Ocular pain
   c. Edema
  2. Eyelids or conjunctiva
   a. Allergic reactions
   b. Angioneurotic edema
   c. Urticaria
  3. Overgrowth of nonsusceptible organisms

Clinical Significance: Rarely does this group of drugs given systemically cause ocular side effects; however, if they occur, they are usually associated with a generalized allergic event. Type III hypersensitivity, including reversible limbal hyperemia, mild conjunctivitis, and peripheral corneal edema, has been reported with cefaclor therapy. All reported ocular side effects appear to be transitory if the drug is discontinued. These agents are having increasing popularity with local ocular use. A single subconjunctival injection of cefuroxime given after cataract surgery was shown to be less toxic than gentamicin. Intravitreal injections of these agents have caused retinal toxicity; however, lower dosages appear to be safe.

References:
Campochiaro, P.A., and Green, R.: Toxicity of intravitreous ceftazidime in primate retina. Arch. Ophthalmol. *110*:1625–1629, 1992.

Green, S.T., Natarajan, S., and Campbell, J.C.: Erythema multiforme following cefotaxime therapy. Postgrad. Med. J. *62*:415, 1986.

Jenkins, C.D.G., McDonnell, P.J., and Spalton, D.J.: Randomized single blind trial to compare the toxicity of subconjunctival gentamicin and cefuroxime in cataract surgery. Br. J. Ophthalmol. *74*:734, 1990.

Kannangara, D.W., Smith, B., and Cohen, K.: Exfoliative dermatitis during cefoxitin therapy. Arch. Intern. Med. *142*:1031, 1982.

Murray, D.L., et al.: Cefaclor-A cluster of adverse reactions. N. Engl. J. Med. *303*: 1003, 1980.

Okumoto, M., et al.: In vitro and in vivo studies on cefoperazone. Cornea 2:35, 1983.

Platt, L.W.: Bilateral peripheral corneal edema after cefaclor therapy. Arch. Ophthalmol. *108*:175, 1990.

Taylor, R., et al.: Cephaloridine encephalopathy. Br. Med. J. *283*:409, 1981.

Richards, D.M., et al.: Ceftriaxone: A review of its antibacterial activity, pharmacological properties and therapeutic use. Drugs 27:469, 1984.

Van Klingeren, B.: Penicillins, cephalosporins and tetracyclines. *In* Dukes, M.N.G. (Ed.): Side Effects of Drugs. Annual 4, Amsterdam, Excerpta Medica, 1980, p. 188.

Generic Name: Chloramphenicol

Proprietary Name: *Systemic*: **AK-Chlor** (Canad.), Aquamycetin (Germ)., Cébénicol (Fr.), Chemicetina (Ital., Span.), Chloramex (S. Afr.), Chloramsaar N (Germ.), Chlorcol (S. Afr.), **Chloromycetin** (Austral., Canad., G.B., Ire., Ital., S. Afr., Span., Swed., Switz.), **Chloromycetin Palmitate** (Ire.), Chloromycetin Palmitato (Span.), **Chloromycetin Sodium Succinate**, Chloromycetin Succinate (Ire.), Chloromycetin Succinato (Span.), Chloromycetin-succinat (Swed.), Chloroptic (Austral., Canad., Germ., Ire., S. Afr.), Chlorphen (S. Afr.), Chlorsig (Austral.), Cloramfen (Ital.), Cloramplast (Span.), Cloranf Succi (Span.), Cloranfen (Span.), Cloranfenico (Span.), Clorofenicina (Span.), Fenicol (Canad., S. Afr.), Globenicol (Neth.), Isopto Fenicol (Span., Swed.), Kemicetine (G.B.), Lennacol (S. Afr.), Micoclorina (Ital.), Micoclorina Glicinato (Ital.), Micodry (Ital.), Mycetin (Ital.), Normofenicol (Span.), Novochlorocap (Canad.), Oleomycetin (Germ.), Ophtaphénicol (Fr.), Ophtho-Chloram (Canad.), Pantofenicol (Span.), Paraxin (Germ.), Pentamycetin (Canad.), Plastodermo (Span.), Sificetina (Ital.), Sno Phenicol (G.B., Ire.), Sopamycetin (Canad.), Spersanicol (Canad., S. Afr., Switz.), Thilocanfol C (Germ.), Tifomycine (Fr.), Tramina (Span.), Troymycetin (S. Afr.), Vitamfenicolo (Ital.) *Ophthalmic*: **AK-Chlor** (Canad.), **Antibiopto, Chloramphenicol, Chlorofair, Chloromycetin, Chloroptic** (Austral.), **Chloroptic S.O.P.**, Chlorsig (Austral.), **Cloroptic, Econochlor**, Kemicetin (Span.), **Ocu-Chlor, Ophthochlor**

Primary Use: This bacteriostatic dichloracetic acid derivative is particularly effective against *Salmonella typhi, H. influenzae meningitis*, rickettsia, the lymphogranuloma-psittacosis group, and is useful in the management of cystic fibrosis.

Ocular Side Effects:
  A. Systemic Administration
     1. Decreased vision
     2. Visual fields

         a. Scotomas
         b. Constriction
    3. Retrobulbar or optic neuritis
    4. Optic atrophy
    5. Toxic amblyopia
    6. Problems with color vision
         a. Color vision defect
         b. Objects have yellow tinge
    7. Eyelids or conjunctiva
         a. Allergic reactions
         b. Conjunctivitis—nonspecific
         c. Angioneurotic edema
         d. Urticaria
    8. Paralysis of accommodation
    9. Pupils
         a. Mydriasis
         b. Absence of reaction to light
   10. Retinal pigmentary changes
   11. Retinal edema
   12. Subconjunctival or retinal hemorrhages secondary to drug-induced anemia
  B. Local Ophthalmic Use or Exposure—Topical Application or Subconjunctival Injection
    1. Irritation
    2. Eyelids or conjunctiva
         a. Allergic reactions
         b. Conjunctivitis—nonspecific
         c. Depigmentation
         d. Anaphylactic reaction
    3. Keratitis
    4. Overgrowth of nonsusceptible organisms
  C. Local Ophthalmic Use or Exposure—Intracameral Injection
    1. Uveitis
    2. Corneal edema
    3. Lens damage

Systemic Side Effects:
  A. Local Ophthalmic Use or Exposure
    1. Aplastic anemia
    2. Various blood dyscrasias

Clinical Significance: Ocular side effects from systemic chloramphenicol administration are uncommon in adults but may occur more frequently in children, especially if the total dose exceeds 100 g or if therapy lasts more than 6 weeks. Topical ophthalmic application causes infrequent ocular side effects. Although chloramphenicol has fewer allergic reactions than neomycin, those due to chloramphenicol are often more severe. Like other antibiotics, this agent may cause latent hypersensitivity that may last for many years. Topical ocular chloramphenicol probably has fewer toxic effects on the corneal epithelium than other antibiotics. Twenty-three cases of significant blood dyscrasia or aplastic anemia following topical ocular chloramphenicol have been reported in the literature and to the Registry, with 12 fatalities. Whether there is a cause-and-effect relationship is unknown. Oral chloramphenicol is the drug most commonly associated with aplastic anemia. The risk of developing pancytopenia or aplastic anemia after oral chloramphenicol treatment is 13 times greater than the risk of idiopathic aplastic anemia in the general population. Two forms of hemopoietic abnormalities, idiosyncratic and dose-related, may occur following systemic chloramphenicol. Although the latter response is unlikely from topical ophthalmic use of the drug, the incidence of the idiosyncratic response is unknown and indeed a controversial topic at this time. Each physician must weigh the evidence and decide if there is a specific reason for topical ophthalmic use of chloramphenicol. It seems unlikely that medical data will provide an answer to this question in the near future, and each physician will have to decide individually the benefit-risk ratio. In some physicians' opinions, the only indication for the topical ocular use of this drug is if the organism is resistant to all other antibiotics.

References:

Abrams, S.M., Degnan, T.J., and Vinciguerra, V.: Marrow aplasia following topical application of chloramphenicol eye ointment. Arch. Intern. Med. *140*:576, 1980.

Brodsky, E., et al.: Topical application of chloramphenicol eye ointment followed by fatal bone marrow aplasia. Isr. J. Med. Sci. *25*:54, 1989.

Bron, A.J., et al.: Ofloxacin compared with chloramphenicol in the management of external ocular infection. Br. J. Ophthalmol. *75*(11):675–679, 1991.

Chalfin, J., and Putterman, A.M.: Eyelid skin depigmentation. Ophthalmic Surg. *11*: 194, 1980.

De Sevilla, T.F., et al.: Adult pure red cell aplasia following topical ocular chloramphenicol. Br. J. Ophthalmol. *74*:640, 1990.

Fraunfelder, F.T., Bagby, G.C., Jr., and Kelly, D.J.: Fatal aplastic anemia following topical administration of ophthalmic chloramphenicol. Am. J. Ophthalmol. *93*:356, 1982.

Fraunfelder, F.T., Morgan, R.L., and Yunis, A.A.: Blood dyscrasias and topical ophthalmic chloramphenicol. Am. J. Ophthalmol. *115(6)*:812–813, 1993.

Godel, V., Nemet, P., and Lazar, M.: Chloramphenicol optic neuropathy. Arch. Ophthalmol. *98*:1417, 1980.

Issaragrisil, S. and Piankijagum, A.: Aplastic anemia following administration of ophthalmic chloramphenicol: Report of a case and review of the literature. J. Med. Assoc. Thai. *68*:309, 1985.

Lamda, P.A., Sood, N.N., and Moorthy, S.S.: Retinopathy due to chloramphenicol. Scott. Med. J. *13*:166, 1968.

Liphshitz, I., and Loewenstein, A.: Anaphylactic reaction following application of chloramphenicol eye ointment. Br. J. Ophthalmol. *75*:64, 1991.
McGuinness, R.: Chloramphenicol eye drops and blood dyscrasia. Med. J. Aust. *140*: 383, 1984.
Wilson, F.M., III: Adverse external ocular effects of topical ophthalmic medications. Surv. Ophthalmol. *24*:57, 1979.
Wilson, W.R., Cockerill, F.R., III: Tetracyclines, chloramphenicol, erythromycin, and clindamycin. Mayo Clin. Proc. *58*:92, 1983.

Generic Name: 1. Chlortetracycline; 2. Demeclocycline; 3. Doxycycline; 4. Methacycline; 5. Minocycline; 6. Oxytetracycline 7. Tetracycline

Proprietary Name: *Systemic*: 1. Aureomicina (Ital., Span.), **Aureomycin** (Austral., Canad., G.B., Germ., Neth., S. Afr., Swed.), Auréomycine (Switz.), Dermosa Cusi Aureomicina (Span.); 2. Bioterciclin (Ital.), Clortetrin (Ital.), **Declomycin** (Canad.), Detravis (Ital.), Fidocin (Ital.), Ledemicina (Ital.), Ledermycin (Austral., G.B., Neth., S.Afr.), Rynabron (Span.); 3. Abadox (Ital.), Apo-Doxy (Canad.), Azudoxat (Germ.), Azudoxat-T (Germ.), Bassado (Ital.), Clinofug (Germ.), Cyclidox (Austral., S. Afr.), Dagracycline (Neth.), Demix (G.B.), Diocimex (Switz.), Docostyl (Span.), **Doryx** (Austral.), Dosil (Span.), Doxi Crisol (Span.), Doxi Sergo (Span.), Doxicento (Ital.), Doxiclat (Span.), Doxifin (Ital.), Doxilen (Ital.), Doxina (Ital.), Doxinate (Span.), Doxiten Bio (Span.), Doxivis (Ital.), Doxy (Germ.), Doxy-100 (Fr.), doxy-basan (Germ.), Doxybiocin (Germ.), **Doxy-Caps**, Doxycin (Canad.), Doxyclin (S. Afr.), Doxycline (Switz.), Doxy-Diolan (Germ.), Doxygram (Fr.), Doxyhexal (Germ.), Doxylag (Switz.), Doxylar (G.B.), Doxylets (S. Afr.), Doxylin (Austral.), Doxymycin (Neth., S. Afr.), Doxy-N-Tablinen (Germ.), Doxy-P (Germ.), Doxy-Puren (Germ.), Doxysol (Switz.), Doxy-Tablinen (Germ.), **Doxy-Tabs**, Doxytem (Germ.), Doxy-Wolff (Germ.), Doxy-Wolff Tabs (Germ.), Dumoxin (Neth., S. Afr.), Duradoxal (Germ.), Esadoxi (Ital.), Farmodoxi (Ital.), Germiciclin (Ital.), Ghimadox (Ital.), Gram-Val (Ital.), Granudoxy (Fr.), Ichthraletten Doxy (Germ.), Iclados (Ital.), Idocyklin (Swed.), Mespafin (Germ.), Minidox (Ital.), Miraclin (Ital.), Monocline (Fr.), Monodoxin (Ital.), Neo-Dagracycline (Neth.), Nordox (G.B.), Novelciclina (Span.), Novodoxylin (Canad.), Nymix-cyclin N (Germ.), Philcociclina (Ital.), Radox (Ital.), Ramysis (G.B.), Relociclina (Span.), Remicyclin D (Germ.), Retens (Span.), Samecin (Ital.), Semelciclina (Ital.), Sigacyclat (Germ.), Sigadoxin (Germ., Switz.), Solupen (Span.), Spanor (Fr.), Stamicina (Ital.), Supracyclin (Germ.), Supracycline (Switz.), Tetrasan (Span.), Tolexine (Fr.), Unacil (Ital.), Vibracina (Span.), **Vibramycin** (Austral., Canad., G.B., Germ., Neth., S. Afr., Swed.), Vibramycin N (Germ.), Vibramycin-D (G.B.), Vibramycine (Fr., Switz.), Vibramycine N (Fr.), Vibra-S (Neth.), **Vibra-Tabs** (Austral., Canad.), Vibraveineuse (Fr., Switz.), Vibravenös (Germ.), Vibravenosa (Span)., Ximicina (Ital.), Zadorine (Switz.); 4. Benciclina (Ital.), Esarondil (Ital.), Franciclina

(Ital.), Francomicina (Ital.), Medomycin (Ital.), Metadomus (Ital.), Meta-micina (Ital.), Paveciclina (Ital.), Physiomycine (Fr.), Quickmicina (Ital.), Rondomycin (Austral., Swed.), Rotilen (Ital.), Stafilon (Ital.), Treis-Ciclina (Ital.), Wassermicina (Ital.); 5. Klinomycin (Germ.), Lederderm (Germ.), Mestacine (Fr.), **Minocin** (Canad., G.B., Ital., Neth., Span., Switz.), Mino-mycin (Austral., S. Afr.), Mynocine (Fr.); 6. Aknin (Germ., Switz.), Be-Oxytet (S. Afr.), Berkmycen (G.B., Ire.), Betacycline (S. Afr.), Clinimycin (Ire.), Cotet (S. Afr.), duratetracyclin (Germ.), Imperacin (G.B., Ire.), Maco-cyn (Germ.), 0-4 Cycline (S. Afr.), Oxy (S. Afr.), Oxy-Dumocyclin (Swed.), Oxymycin (G.B., S. Afr.), Oxypan (S. Afr.), Oxytetral (Swed.), Oxytetramix (G.B.), Posicycline (Fr.), Rocap (S. Afr.), Roxy (S. Afr.), Terramicina (Span.), **Terramycin** (Austral., G.B., Germ., S. Afr.), Terramycine (Fr., Switz.), Tetracycletten N (Germ.), Tetramel (S. Afr.), Tetra-Tablinen (Germ.); 7. **Achromycin** (Austral., Canad., G.B., Germ., Swed.), **Achromy-cin V** (Austral., Canad., G.B., S. Afr.), Achromycine (Switz.), Acromicina (Ital.), Akne-Pyodron Kur (Germ.), Akne-Pyocron oral (Germ.), Ambrami-cina (Ital., Span.), Apo-Tetra (Canad.), Arcanacycline (S. Afr.), Austra-mycin V (Austral.), Bristaciclina (Span.), Calociclina (Ital.), Dispatetrin (Germ.), Economycin (G.B.), Hexacycline (Fr.), Hortetracin (Span.), Hosta-cyclin (Germ.), Hostacycline (Ire.), Hostacycline-P (Austral.), Hydracycline (Austral.), Ibicyn (Ital.), Imex (Germ.), Latycin (Austral.), Novotetra (Canad.), Nu-Tetra (Canad.), Panmycin P (Austral.), Quimocyclin N (Germ.), Quimpe Antibiotico (Span.), Rotet (S. Afr.), Sagittacin N (Germ.), Spaciclina (Ital.), Steclin (Germ.), Steclin-V (Austral.), **Sumycin**, Su-pramycin (Germ.), Sustamycin (G.B.), Tefilin (Germ.), Tetra Hubber (Span.), Tetrabakat (Germ.), Tetrabid-Organon (G.B.), Tetrabioptal (Ital.), Tetrablet (Germ.), Tetrachel (G.B. Ire.), Tetractro S (Germ.), Tetracyn (Canad.), Tetrafosammina (Ital.), Tetralen (Span.), Tetralution (Germ.), Tét-ramig (Fr.), Tetramykoin (Austral.), Tetra-Proter (Ital.), Tetrarco (Neth.), Tetraseptin (Switz.), Tetrex (Austral., S. Afr.), Topitetrina (Span.), Tripha-cycline (Switz.) *Ophthalmic:* 1. **Aureomycin** 7. **Achromycin**

Primary Use: These bacteriostatic derivatives of polycyclic naphthacene car-boxamide are effective against a wide range of Gram-negative and Gram-positive organisms, mycoplasm, and members of the lymphogranuloma-psittacosis group.

Ocular Side Effects:
    A. Systemic Administration
        1. Myopia
        2. Papilledema secondary to pseudotumor cerebri
        3. Decreased vision
        4. Photophobia
        5. Diplopia (minocycline, tetracycline)
        6. Problems with color vision (chlortetracycline)

       a. Color vision defect
       b. Objects have yellow tinge
    7. Eyelids or conjunctiva
       a. Erythema
       b. Edema
       c. Yellow discoloration (methacycline, tetracycline)
       d. Hyperpigmentation (doxycycline, methacycline,
          minocycline, tetracycline)
       e. Photosensitivity
       f. Angioneurotic edema
       g. Urticaria
       h. Lupoid syndrome
       i. Erythema multiforme
       j. Stevens-Johnson syndrome
       k. Lyell's syndrome
    8. Myasthenic neuromuscular blocking effect
       a. Paralysis of extraocular muscles
       b. Ptosis
    9. Subconjunctival or retinal hemorrhages secondary to drug-induced anemia
   10. Enlarged blind spot
   11. Visual hallucinations
  B. Local Ophthalmic Use or Exposure—Topical Application or Subconjunctival Injection
    1. Irritation
    2. Eyelids or conjunctiva
       a. Allergic reactions
       b. Conjunctivitis—nonspecific
    3. Overgrowth of nonsusceptible organisms
    4. Keratitis
    5. Yellow-brown corneal discoloration (with drug-soaked hydrophilic lenses)
  C. Local Ophthalmic Use or Exposure—Intracameral Injection
    1. Uveitis
    2. Corneal edema
    3. Lens damage

Clinical Significance: Systemic or ocular use of the tetracyclines rarely causes significant ocular side effects. While a large variety of drug-induced ocular side effects have been attributed to tetracyclines, most are reversible. This group of drugs can cause pseudotumor cerebri. This is most commonly reported with tetracycline and minocycline. Minocycline possibly possesses greater lipid solubility as it passes into cerebral spinal fluid more readily than other polycyclic naphthacene carboxamides. Increased intracranial pressure is not dose related and may occur as early as 4 hours after first taking the drug or after many years of drug usage. Paresis or paralysis of extraocular muscles may occur secondary to pseudotumor cerebri. The tetracyclines have been implicated in aggravating or unmasking myasthenia gravis with its own associated ocular findings. Transient color defects have been reported only with chlortetracycline. Methacycline and tetracycline have caused hyperpigmentation in light-exposed skin and yellow-brown pigmentation of light-exposed conjunctiva after long-term therapy. This occurs in about 3% of patients taking 400 to 1600 g of these agents. No permanent adverse effects are associated with these findings. Yellow-brown discoloration of the cornea, if hydrophilic contact lenses are presoaked in tetracycline before ocular application, can occur. The lowest reported incidence of contact dermatitis due to commonly used antibiotics is with chlortetracycline. All tetracycline agents are photosensitizers and, therefore, may enhance any or all light-induced ocular changes. This group of drugs is secreted in the tear film, most in therapeutic concentrations. Long-term therapy may cause subconjunctival concretions, possibly mixed with breakdown drug products, in intraepithelial cysts, which may take on characteristics of the drug, i.e., yellow color, fluorescence, etc.

References:

Brothers, D.M., and Hidayat, A.A.: Conjunctival pigmentation associated with tetracycline medication. Ophthalmology 88:1212, 1981.

Kaeser, H.E.: Drug-induced myasthenic syndromes. Acta Neurol. Scand. 70(Suppl. 100):39, 1984.

Krejci, L., Brettschneider, I., and Triska, J.: Eye changes due to systemic use of tetracycline in pregnancy. Ophthalmic Res. 12:73, 1980.

Meacock, D.J., and Hewer, R.L.: Tetracycline and benign intracranial hypertension. Br. Med. J. 282:1240, 1981.

Messmer, E., et al.: Pigmented conjunctival cysts following tetracycline/minocycline therapy: Histochemical and electron microscopic observations. Ophthalmology 90: 1462, 1983.

Salamon, S.M.: Tetracycline in ophthalmology. Surv. Ophthalmol. 29:265, 1985.

Shum, D.T., et al.: Unusual skin pigmentation from long-term methacycline and minocycline therapy. Arch. Dermatol. 122:17, 1986.

Tabbara, K. F., and Cooper, H.: Minocycline levels in tears of patients with active trachoma. Arch. Ophthalmol. 107:93–95, 1989.

Walters, B., and Gubbay, S.: Tetracycline and benign intracranial hypertension: Report of five cases. Br. Med. J. 282:19, 1981.

White, S.W., and Besanceney, C.: Systemic pigmentation from tetracycline and minocycline therapy. Arch. Dermatol. 119:1, 1983.

Wilson, F.M., III: Adverse external ocular effects of topical ophthalmic medications. Surv. Ophthalmol. 24:57, 1979.

Generic Name: 1. Ciprofloxacin; 2. Norfloxacin; 3. Ofloxacin

Proprietary Name: *Systemic:* 1. Baycip (Span.), Cetraxal (Span.), Ciflox (Fr., Ital.), **Cipro** (Canad.), Ciprobay (Germ., S. Afr.), Ciproxin (Austral.,

G.B., Ire., Ital., Neth., Swed.), Ciproxine (Switz.), Cunesin (Span.), Floci-
prin (Ital.), Rigoran (Span.), Septocipro (Span.), Velmonit (Span.); 2. Ami-
crobin (Span.), Baccidal (Jap., Span.), Barazan (Germ.), Esclebin (Span.),
Espeden (Span.), Fortimax (Span.), Fulgram (Ital.), Lexinor (Swed.), Nalion
(Span.), **Noroxin** (Austral., Canad., Ital., Neth., S. Afr., Span., Switz.), Nor-
oxine (Fr.), Sebercim (Ital.), Senro (Span.), Uroctal (Span.), Utinor (G.B.),
Vicnas (Span.); 3. Flobacin (Ital.), **Floxin**, Oflocet (Fr.), Oflocin (Ital.),
Tarivid (G.B., Germ., Ire., Jap., Neth., S.Afr., Swed., Switz.) *Ophthalmic*:
1. **Ciloxan**; 2. **Chibroxin**, Chibroxol (Switz.), Noroxin (G.B.); 3. **Ocuflox**

Primary Use: These fluoroquinolone antibacterial agents are used primarily
against most Gram-negative aerobic and many Gram-positive aerobic bacteria.

Ocular Side Effects:
(The following side effects have only been reported with ciprofloxacin
unless otherwise stated.)
  A. Systemic Administration
    1. Eyelids
        a. Hyperpigmentation
        b. Angioneurotic edema
        c. Erythema multiforme
        d. Erythema nodosum
        e. Urticaria
        f. Exfoliative dermatitis
        g. Lyell's syndrome
    2. Exacerbation myasthenia
        a. Paresis of extraocular muscles
        b. Diplopia *(also seen with ofloxacin)*
    3. Visual sensations
        a. Glare phenomenon (overbrightness of lights)
        b. Flashing lights
    4. Photosensitivity *(also seen with ofloxacin)*
    5. Visual hallucinations
    6. Abnormal visual evoked response
    7. Nystagmus *(also seen with ofloxacin)*
    8. Toxic optic neuropathy (reversible)
    9. Papilledema secondary to pseudotumor cerebri

Ocular Side Effects:
(The following side effects have only been reported with ciprofloxacin
unless otherwise stated.)
  B. Local Ophthalmic Use or Exposure—Topical Application
    1. Irritation
        a. Pain

   b. Burning sensation *(also seen with norfloxacin)*
   c. Lacrimation
   d. Foreign body sensation
2. Eyelids
   a. Crusting—crystalline
   b. Edema
   c. Allergic reactions
   d. Itching
3. Cornea
   a. Precipitates—white
   b. Keratitis
   c. Infiltrates
   d. Superficial punctate keratitis
4. Conjunctiva
   a. Hyperemia *(also seen with norfloxacin)*
   b. Chemosis *(also seen with norfloxacin)*
5. Decreased vision
6. Photophobia *(also seen with norfloxacin)*
7. Retrobulbar neuritis *(also seen with ofloxacin)*
8. Poor central color recognition *(also seen with ofloxacin)*
9. Central scotomas *(also seen with ofloxacin)*
C. Systemic reactions from topical ocular medication
   1. Metallic taste *(also seen with norfloxacin)*
   2. Dermatitis
   3. Nausea
   4. Pediatric warning: (under age 12) arthropathy

Clinical Significance: To date, systemically administered fluoroquinolones have rarely caused ocular problems. Because only a few cases have been reported for any of the above side effects, these data must be considered soft. Visual sensations such as increased glare and increased brightness of color or lights have been reported and appear to be well documented. One case, which was partially reversible, of toxic optic neuropathy while taking high-dose oral ciprofloxacin was reported by Vrabec, et al. Pseudotumor was only reported in one case in a 14 year old (Winrow and Supramaniam). Ofloxacin can cause diplopia, photosensitivity, and nystagmus, but there is seldom a need to discontinue the drug. Ophthalmic preparations of norfloxacin and ofloxacin have only recently become available. Therefore, mainly ciprofloxacin data are included here. Ciprofloxacin ophthalmic solutions are generally well tolerated. Transient ocular burning and discomfort, however, occurs in approximately 10% of patients. Seldom does this necessitate the drug being discontinued. The most disturbing side effect is the deposition of the drug as a white crystalline deposit on the abraded epithelium or corneal stroma. This may occur in approximately 20% of treated bacterial corneal ulcers. It may start as early as 24 hours after starting therapy, may resolve while on full therapy, can be irrigated off, or may last a few weeks after the drug is discontinued. This does not appear to inhibit drug activity; in fact, some have claimed enhancement of antibiotic activity. These drug crystals may deposit on the lids and lashes as well. Other than a foreign body sensation, this side effect is usually well tolerated. Other ocular side effects listed above secondary to topical ocular application occur in less than 1% of patients. Systemic reactions may occur from topical ocular ciprofloxacin. The primary one is a metallic or foul taste, which occurs in 5% of patients, and nausea, which occurs in 1%. There is a warning based on animal work to not use this drug in patients 12 years and younger for fear of causing degenerative articular changes in weight-bearing joints. There are no human data to support this.

References:

Cokingtin, C.D., and Hyndiuk, R.A.: Insights from experimental data on ciprofloxacin in the treatment of bacterial keratitis and ocular infections. Am. J. Ophthalmol. *112*: 255–285, 1991.

Kanellopoulos, A.J., Miller, F., and Wittpenn, J.R.: Deposition of topical ciprofloxacin to prevent re-epithelialization of a corneal defect. Am. J. Ophthalmol. *117*:258–259, 1994.

Leibowitz, H.W.: Clinical evaluation of ciprofloxacin 0.3% ophthalmic solution for treatment of bacterial keratitis. Am. J. Ophthalmol. *112*(Suppl):34–47, 1991.

Moore, B., Safani, M., and Keesey, J.: Ciprofloxacin exacerbation of myasthenia gravis?: Case report. Lancet *1*:882, 1988.

Nederost, S.T., and Dijkstra, J.W.E.: Drug-induced photosensitivity reaction. Arch. Dermatol. *125*:433–434, 1989.

Motolese, E., D'Aniello, B., and Addabbo, G.: Toxic optic neuropathy after administration of quinolone derivative. Boll. Oculist. *69*:1011–1013, 1990.

Schacht, P., and Hullmann, R.: Safety of oral ciprofloxacin. Am. J. Med. *87*(Suppl. 5a):98-102, 1989.

Stevens, D., and Samples, J.R.: Fluoroquinolones for the treatment of microbial infections. J. Toxicol. Cut. & Ocular Toxicol. *13(4)*: 275–277, 1994.

Von Rosenstiel, N., and Deiter, A.: Quinolone antibacterials, an update of their pharmacology and therapeutic use. Drugs *47(6)*:872–901, 1994.

Vrabec, T.R., et al: Reversible visual loss in a patient receiving high-dose ciprofloxacin hydrochloride. Ophthalmology *97(6)*:707–710, 1990.

Wilhelmus, K.R., et al: 0.3% Ciprofloxacin ophthalmic ointment in the treatment of bacterial keratitis. Arch. Ophthalmol. *111*:1210–1218, 1993.

Winrow, A.P., and Supramaniam, G.: Benign intracranial hypertension after ciprofloxacin administration. Arch. Dis. Child. *65*:1165–1166, 1990

Generic Name: 1. Clindamycin; 2. Erythromycin; 3. Lincomycin; 4. Vancomycin

Proprietary Name: *Systemic:* 1. **Cleocin HCL, Cleocin Pediatric, Cleocin Phosphate, Cleocin T**, Dalacin (Span., Swed.), Dalacin C (Austral., Canad., G.B., Ire., Ital., Neth., S. Afr., Switz.), Dalacin C Palmitate (Canad.), Dalacin C Phosphate (Austral., Canad., G.B., Ire.), Dalacin T (G.B., Ire., Ital., Neth., S. Afr., Switz.), Dalacine (Fr.), Dalacine T (Fr.), Sobelin (Germ.); 2. Abboticin (Swed.), Abboticine (Fr.), Apo-Erythro Base (Canad.), Apo-Erythro E-C (Canad.), Apo-Erythro-ES (Canad.), Apo-Erythro-S (Canad.), Arcanamycin (S. Afr.), Arpimycin (G.B.), Bio Exazol (Span.), Cimetrin (Switz.), Doranol (Span.), Dreimicina (Span.), Durapaediat (Germ.), Émestid (Fr.), Éry (Fr.), Érythrocine (Fr.), **EES**, (Austral., Canad.), Emu-V (Austral., S. Afr.), **E-Mycin** (Canad.), Endoeritrin (Span.), Erios (Switz.), Eritrobios (Ital.), Eritrocina (Ital.), Eritrogobens (Span.), Eritroveinte (Span.), Eromel (S. Afr.), Eromel-S (S.Afr.), Ery (Switz.), **Eryc**, (Austral., Canad., Neth.), Erycen (G.B., Ire.), Erycocci (Fr.), Ery-Diolan (Germ.), EryHexal (Germ.), Erymax (Ire., S.Afr.), Ery-Max (Swed.), Erymycin AF (S. Afr.), Erymycin P & PF (S. Afr.), **EryPed**, **Ery-Tab**, Erythro-Basan (Germ.), **Erythrocin**, (Austral., Canad., G.B., Germ., Ire. S.Afr.), Erythrocin Neo (Germ.), Erythrocine (Fr., Neth., Switz.), Erythrocine ES (Neth., Switz.), Erythrogenat (Germ.), Erythrogram (Fr.), Erythromid (Canad., G.B., Ire., S. Afr.), Erythroped (G.B., Ire.), Erythroped A (S. Afr.), Erytran (Switz.), Erytrociclin (Ital.), Estomycin (S. Afr.), Ethimycin (S. Afr.), Ilocap (Austral.), **Ilosone** (Austral., Canad., G.B., Ital., S. Afr., Switz.), **Ilotycin**, **Ilotycin Gluceptate** (Canad., Switz.), Inderm (Germ., Neth., Switz.), Infectocin (S. Afr.), Lagarmicin (Span.), Marocid (Ital.), Monomycin (Germ.), Monomycine (Switz.), Neo Iloticina (Span.), Novorythro (Canad.), Paediathrocin (Germ.), Pantomicina (Span.), **PCE** (Canad.), Pharyngocin (Germ.), Praecimycin (Germ.), Primacine (Ire.), Propiocine (Fr., Switz.), Proterytrin (Ital.), Purmycin (S. Afr.), Retcin (G.B.), Rommix (G.B.), Ronmix (G.B.), Rossomicina (Ital.), Roviciclina Enzimatica (Span.), Roxochemil (Ital.), Rubimycin (S. Afr.), Sanasepton (Germ.), Sigapaedil (Germ.), Spectrasone (S. Afr.), Stellamicina (Ital.), Tiprocin (Ire.), Togiren (Germ.), **Wyamycin**; 3. Albiotic (Germ.), Cillimicina (Ital., Span.), **Lincocin** (Austral., Canad., Ire., Ital., Neth., S. Afr., Span., Swed., Switz.), Lincocine (Fr.); 4. Diatracin (Span.), **Lyphocin**, Vancocin (Austral., Canad., G.B., Ire., Neth., S. Afr., Swed., Switz.), **Vancocin HCL**, Vancocina (Ital.), Vancocine (Fr.), Vancoled (Swed.), **Vancor** *Ophthalmic*: 2. **AK-Mycin**, **Erythromycin Ointment**, Eupragin (Germ.), **Ilotycin** (Canad.), **Ilotycin Gluceptate** (Canad., Switz.) *Topical*: 2. Aknefug-EL (Germ.), Aknemycin (Germ., Neth.), Akne-mycin (Switz.), Aknin (Germ.), **A/T/S**, Deripil (Span.), Eboren (Neth.), **Erycette** (S.Afr.), **Eryderm** (Neth., S.Afr., Switz.), Eryfluid (Fr.), **Erygel**, Erythrogel B (Fr.), **ETS-2%**, Iloticina (Span.), Iloticina Anti Acne (Span.), Ilotycin (S.Afr.), Staticin (Canad.), Staticine (Switz.), Stiemycin (G.B.), Stiemycine (Germ., Switz.), Stimycine (Fr.), **Theramycin Z**, **T-Stat**

Primary Use: These bactericidal antibiotics are effective against Gram-positive or Gram-negative organisms.

Ocular Side Effects:
  A. Systemic Administration
      1. Problems with color vision—color vision defect, blue-yellow
         defect (erythromycin)
      2. Eyelids or conjunctiva
          a. Allergic reactions
          b. Hyperemia
          c. Photosensitivity
          d. Angioneurotic edema
          e. Urticaria
          f. Stevens-Johnson syndrome
          g. Exfoliative dermatitis
          h. Lyell's syndrome (erythromycin)
      3. Myasthenic neuromuscular blocking effect (clindamycin,
         erythromycin, lincomycin)
          a. Paralysis of extraocular muscles
          b. Ptosis
          c. Myasthenia gravis-exacerbation (erythromycin)
      4. Subconjunctival or retinal hemorrhages secondary to drug-
         induced anemia
  B. Local Ophthalmic Use or Exposure—Topical Application or
     Subconjunctival Injection
      1. Irritation
          a. Hyperemia
          b. Ocular pain
          c. Edema
      2. Eyelids or conjunctiva
          a. Allergic reactions
          b. Angioneurotic edema
          c. Stevens-Johnson syndrome (erythromycin)
      3. Overgrowth of nonsusceptible organisms
      4. Subconjunctival hemorrhages (lincomycin)
      5. Mydriasis (erythromycin)
  C. Local Ophthalmic Use or Exposure—Intracameral Injection
      1. Uveitis (erythromycin)
      2. Corneal edema (erythromycin)
      3. Lens damage (erythromycin)
  D. Local Ophthalmic Use or Exposure—Retrobulbar or Subtenon
     Injection
      1. Irritation (clindamycin)
      2. Optic neuritis (clindamycin)
      3. Optic atrophy (clindamycin)
      4. Diplopia (clindamycin)

Clinical Significance: Few adverse ocular reactions due to either systemic
or topical ocular use of these antibiotics are seen. Nearly all ocular side

effects are transitory and reversible after the drug is discontinued. Most adverse ocular reactions are secondary to dermatologic or hematologic conditions. A well-documented rechallenged idiosyncratic response to topical ocular application of erythromycin causing mydriasis has been reported to the Registry. An interaction of erythromycin with carbamazepine causing mydriasis and gaze-evoked nystagmus has been reported. A case of Stevens-Johnson syndrome following topical ophthalmic erythromycin ointment has also been received by the Registry.

References:

Birch, J., et al.: Acquired color vision defects. *In* Pokorny, J., et al. (Eds.): Congenital and Acquired Color Vision Defects. New York, Grune & Stratton, 1979, pp. 243–350.

Kaeser, H.E.: Drug-induced myasthenic syndromes. Acta Neurol. Scand. *70*(Suppl. 100):39, 1984.

Lund Kofoed, M., and Oxholm, A.: Toxic epidermal necrolysis due to erythromycin. Contact Dermatitis *13*:273, 1985.

May, E.F., and Calvert, P.C.: Aggravation of myasthenia gravis by erythromycin. Ann. Neurol. *28*:577–579, 1990.

Oral erythromycins. Med. Lett. Drugs Ther. *27*:1, 1985.

Tate, G.W., Jr., and Martin, R.G.: Clindamycin in the treatment of human ocular toxoplasmosis. Can. J. Ophthalmol. *12*:188, 1977.

Zitelli, B.J., et al.: Erythromycin-induced drug interactions. An illustrative case and review of the literature. Clin. Pediatr. *26*:117-119, 1987

Generic Name: 1. Colistimethate; 2. Colistin

Proprietary Name: 1. and 2. Belcomycine (Neth.), Colimicina (Ital., Span.), Colimycine (Fr., Neth.), Colomycin (G.B.), **Coly-Mycin M** (Austral.), **Coly-Mycin S**

Primary Use: These bactericidal polypeptides are effective against *Aerobacter, E. coli, K. pneumoniae, Ps. aeruginosa, Shigella,* and *Salmonella.*

Ocular Side Effects:

A. Systemic Administration
 1. Nystagmus
 2. Myasthenic neuromuscular blocking effect
  a. Paralysis of extraocular muscles
  b. Ptosis
 3. Diplopia
 4. Mydriasis
B. Local Ophthalmic Use or Exposure—Topical Application or Subconjunctival Injection
 1. Irritation

    2. Eyelids or conjunctiva—allergic reactions
    3. Overgrowth of nonsusceptible organisms
  C. Local Ophthalmic Use or Exposure—Intracameral Injection
    1. Uveitis
    2. Corneal edema
    3. Lens damage

Clinical Significance: Only a few cases of ocular side effects from systemic or ocular colistimethate or colistin therapy have been reported. These adverse ocular reactions are usually transitory, reversible, and are of little clinical importance. In bacterial-resistant cases with overgrowth of nonsusceptible organisms, *Proteus* has been the most common bacterial organism found. Unfortunately, Colimycin is also the name given to an antibiotic of the neomycin group available in Russia.

References:

Argov, Z., and Mastaglia, F.L.: Disorders of neuromuscular transmission caused by drugs. N. Engl. J. Med. *301*:409, 1979.
Gold, G.N., and Richardson, A.P.: An unusual case of neuromuscular blockade seen with therapeutic blood levels of colistin methanesulfonate. (Coly-Mycin). Am. J. Med. *41*:316, 1966.
Hudgson, P.: Adverse drug reactions in the neuromuscular apparatus. Adverse Drug React. Acute Poisoning Rev. *1*:35, 1982.
Lane, R.J.M., and Routledge, P.A.: Drug-induced neurological disorders. Drugs *26*: 124, 1983.
Lund, M.H.: Colistin sulfate ophthalmic in the treatment of ocular infections. Arch. Ophthalmol. *81*:4, 1969.
McQuillen, M.P., Cantor, H.E., and O'Rourke, J.R.: Myasthenic syndrome associated with antibiotics. Arch. Neurol. *18*:402, 1968.
Wolinsky, E., and Hines, J.D.: Neurotoxic and nephrotoxic effects of colistin in patients with renal disease. N. Engl. J. Med. *266*:759, 1962.

Generic Name: Cycloserine. See under *Class: Antitubercular Agents*

Generic Name: 1. Framycetin; 2. Neomycin

Proprietary Name: *Systemic*: 1. Sofra-Tüll (Germ.), Sofra-Tulle (Austral., Canad., G.B., Ital., Neth., S. Afr., Swed., Switz.); 2. Bykomycin (Germ.), Endomixin (Ital.), Glycomycin (Germ.), Mycifradin (Austral., Canad., G.B., Ire., S. Afr.), Myciguent (Canad., Ire.), Nebacetin N (Germ.), Neopt (Austral.), Neosulf (Austral.), Nivemycin (G.B.), Siguent Neomycin (Austral.) *Ophthalmic*: 2. **Myciguent**, Nivemycin (G.B.)

Primary Use: These bactericidal aminoglycosidic agents are effective against *Ps. aeruginosa, Aerobacter, K. pneumoniae, P. vulgaris, E. coli, Salmonella, Shigella,* and most strains of *S. aureus.*

Ocular Side Effects:
  A. Systemic Administration—Neomycin
      1. Myasthenic neuromuscular blocking effect
          a. Paralysis of extraocular muscles
          b. Ptosis
      2. Decreased or absent pupillary reaction to light
  B. Local Ophthalmic Use or Exposure—Topical Application or
      Subconjunctival Injection
      1. Irritation
          a. Hyperemia
          b. Ocular pain
          c. Edema
          d. Burning sensation
      2. Eyelids or conjunctiva
          a. Allergic reactions
          b. Erythema
          c. Blepharoconjunctivitis—follicular
          d. Urticaria
      3. Punctate keratitis
      4. Overgrowth of nonsusceptible organisms
  C. Local Ophthalmic Use or Exposure—Intracameral Injection
      1. Uveitis (neomycin)
      2. Corneal edema (neomycin)
      3. Lens damage (neomycin)

Clinical Significance: It is rare for these agents to cause ocular side effects; however, there are well-documented reports of decreased or absent pupillary reactions due to application of neomycin to the pleural or peritoneal cavities during a thoracic or abdominal operation. Topical ocular application of neomycin has been reported to cause allergic conjunctival or lid reactions in 4% of patients using this drug. Elsewhere on the skin, it is from 1% to 6% of patients, since the drug is a potent contact sensitizer. If neomycin is used topically for longer than 7 days on inflammatory dermatosis, the incidence of allergic reaction is increased 13-fold over matched control subjects. Neomycin preparations for minor infections should rarely be used for more than 7 days. Also, if the patient has been previously exposed to neomycin or is currently receiving this therapy for more than 7 days, there is a significantly higher chance of an allergic response. In one study, neomycin was found to be one of the three more common drugs causing periocular allergic contact dermatitis. In addition, some feel that, of the more commonly used antibiotics, topical neomycin has the greatest toxicity to the corneal epithelium. It probably produces plasma membrane injury and cell death, primarily of the superficial cell layers, with chronic exposure. After long-term ocular exposure to framycetin or neomycin, fungi superinfections have been reported. Nystagmus has been reported in a 9-year-old child following topical

treatment of the skin with 1% neomycin in 11% dimethyl sulfoxide ointment.

References:
Baldinger, J., and Weiter, J.J.: Diffuse cutaneous hypersensitivity reaction after dexa-
methasone/polymyxin B/neomycin combination eyedrops. Ann. Ophthalmol. *18*:
95, 1986.
Fisher, A.A.: Topical medications which are common sensitizers. Ann. Allergy *49*:97,
1982.
Fisher, A.A., and Adams, R.M.: Alternative for sensitizing neomycin topical medica-
tions. Cutis *28*:491, 1981.
Kaufman, H.E.: Chemical blepharitis following drug treatment. Am. J. Ophthalmol.
95:703, 1983.
Kaeser, H.E.: Drug-induced myasthenic syndromes. Acta Neurol. Scand. *70*:(Suppl.
100):39, 1984.
Kruyswijk, M.R.J., et al: Contact allergy following administration of eyedrops and eye
ointments. Doc. Ophthalmol. *48*:251, 1979.
Wilson, F.M., II: Adverse external ocular effects of topical ophthalmic medications.
Surv. Ophthalmol. *24*:57, 1979

Generic Name: Gentamicin

Proprietary Name: *Systemic*: Alcomicin (Canad., Span.), Biogen (Span.),
Biomargen (Span.), Cidomycin (Austral., Canad., G.B., Ire., S. Afr.), Coliri-
ocilina Gentam (Span.), Dispagent (Germ.), Duragentam (Germ.), Fer-
mentmycin (S. Afr.), **Garamycin** (Austral., Canad., G.B., Neth., S. Afr.,
Swed., Switz.), Genoptic (Austral., S. Afr., Span.), Gensumycin (Swed.),
Genta Gobens (Span.), **Gentafair**, Gentalline (Fr.), Gentallorens (Span.),
Gentalodina (Span.), Gentalyn (Ital.), Gentamedical (Span.), Gentamen
(Ital.), Gentamin (Span.), Gentamival (Span.), Gentamix (Germ.), Genta-
morgens (Span.), Gentamytrex (Germ., Neth.), Gentibioptal (Ital.), Genticin
(G.B., Ire.), Genticina (Span.), Genticol (Ital.), Gentisum (Span.), Gento-
gram (Fr., Neth.), Gent-Ophtal (Germ.), Gentoptine (Mon.), **Gentrasul**
(Canad.), Gevramicina Crema (Span.), Gevramycin (Span.), **G-Myticin**,
Hosbogen (Span.), Martigenta (Fr.), Megental Pediatrico (Ital.), Ophtagram
(Fr., Switz.), Quintamicina (Span.), Refobacin (Germ.), Rexgenta (Span.),
Ribomicin (Ital.), Sulmycin (Germ.), Supragenta (Span.), Yedoc (Switz.)
Ophthalmic: **Garamycin, Genoptic, Genoptic S.O.P., Gentacidin, Gen-
tak**, Genticin (G.B.)

Primary Use: This aminoglycoside is effective against *Ps. aeruginosa, Aerobacter, E. coli, K. pneumoniae,* and *Proteus.*

Ocular Side Effects:
   A. Systemic Administration
      1. Decreased vision

2. Papilledema secondary to pseudotumor cerebri
3. Loss of eyelashes or eyebrows
4. Subconjunctival or retinal hemorrhages secondary to drug-induced anemia
5. Myasthenic neuromuscular blocking effect
    a. Paralysis of extraocular muscles
    b. Ptosis
6. Eyelids
    a. Photosensitivity
    b. Urticaria
7. Visual hallucinations

B. Local Ophthalmic Use or Exposure—Topical Application or Subconjunctival Injection
    1. Conjunctiva
        a. Hyperemia
        b. Mucopurulent discharge
        c. Chemosis
        d. Ulceration—necrosis
        e. Mild papillary hypertrophy
        f. Delayed healing
        g. Localized pallor
    2. Eyelids
        a. Allergic reactions
        b. Blepharoconjunctivitis
        c. Depigmentation
    3. Cornea
        a. Superficial punctate keratitis
        b. Ulceration
        c. Delayed healing
    4. Overgrowth of nonsusceptible organisms
    5. Extraocular and periocular muscle myopathy

C. Local Ophthalmic Use or Exposure—Intravitreal or Intraocular Injection
    1. Vitreous reaction
    2. Retinal degeneration
    3. Retinal vascular disorders
        a. Retinal edema
        b. Occlusion
        c. Hemorrhages
        d. Ischemia
    4. Optic atrophy

Clinical Significance: Surprisingly few drug-induced ocular side effects from systemic administration of gentamicin have been reported. Pseudotumor cerebri with secondary papilledema and visual loss following systemic use of gentamicin is the most significant. Other adverse ocular effects are reversible and transitory after discontinued use of the drug. Topical ocular gentamicin may cause significant local side effects, the most common being a superficial punctate keratitis. Chronic use can also cause keratinization of the lid margin and blepharitis. Skin depigmentation in blacks, when topical ocular gentamicin was associated with eye pad use, has occurred. Conjunctival necrosis, especially with fortified solutions, may occur. This usually is found in the inferior nasal conjunctiva, starts as a localized area of hyperemia or pallor, and stains with fluorescein. The lesions start after 5 to 7 days of either gentamicin solution or ointment treatment and resolve within 2 weeks after discontinuing the drug. Green, et al. have recently shown that subconjunctival injections of gentamicin can cause myopathy with resultant ocular motility impairment.

Intraocular gentamicin has caused severe retinal ischemia, rubeosis iridis, neovascular glaucoma, optic atrophy, and blindness. A number of cases of inadvertent intraocular injections have been reported in the literature and to the Registry. The degree of ocular damage is primarily dependent on trauma of the inadvertent injection, amount of the injection, location of the injection, and toxicity of the drug. Injections into the anterior chamber are rarely devastating, in part due to the early recognition of the inadvertent injection and the small volume injected (compared to intravitreal); in addition, because this usually occurs immediately after anterior segment surgery, the gentamicin can be irrigated out. These factors are almost the opposite for an inadvertent posterior injection. The volume injected is usually larger and can go unrecognized for some time. The resultant elevated intraocular pressure may cause a central retinal artery occlusion. The trauma of the injection may cause significant intraocular bleeding and a retinal detachment. The amount of direct toxicity of the drug is unclear; however, some feel the degree of vitreous and adjacent retinal reaction suggests direct toxicity as a factor. Regardless, some eyes have been lost after this has occurred.

References:

Awan, K.J.: Mydriasis and conjunctival paresthesia from local gentamicin. Am. J. Ophthalmol. 99:723, 1985.

Chapman, J.M., et al.: Subconjunctival gentamicin induction of extraocular toxic muscle myopathy. Ophthalmic Res. 24:189–196, 1992.

Conway, B.P., and Campochiaro, P.A.: Macular infarction after endophthalmitis treated with vitrectomy and intravitreal gentamicin. Arch. Ophthalmol. 104:367, 1986.

Davison, C.R., Tuft, S.J., and Dart, J.K.G.: Conjunctival necrosis after administration of topical fortified aminoglycosides. Am. J. Ophthalmol. 111:690–693, 1991.

Green, K., Chapman, J.M., and Cheeks, L.: Ocular toxicity of subconjunctival gentamicin. Third Congress International Society of Ocular Toxicity, November 15–19, 1992, Sedona, Arizona.

Kaufman, H.E.: Chemical blepharitis following drug treatment. Am. J. Ophthalmol. *95*:703, 1983.

Kuwajima, I., et al.: A case of allergic blepharokeratoconjunctivitis due to gentamycin ophthalmic solution (Gentacin). Folia Ophthalmol. Jpn. *36*:2153, 1985.

McDonald, H.R., et al.: Retinal toxicity secondary to intraocular gentamicin injection. Ophthalmology *93*:871, 1986.

Nauheim, R., Nauheim, J., and Merrick, N.Y.: Bulbar conjunctival defects associated with gentamicin. Arch. Ophthalmol. *105*:1321, 1987.

Schatz, H., and McDonald, H.R.: Acute ischemic retinopathy due to gentamicin injection. JAMA *256*:1725, 1986.

Stern, G.A., et al.: Effect of topical antibiotic solutions on corneal epithelial wound healing. Arch. Ophthalmol. *101*:644, 1983.

Waltz, K.: Intraocular gentamicin toxicity. Arch. Ophthalmol. *109*:911, 1991

Generic Name: Kanamycin

Proprietary Name: Kamycine (Fr.), Kanacolirio (Span.), Kanamytrex (Germ.), Kanescin (Span.), Kannasyn (G.B., Ire.), **Kantrex** (Span.), Keimicina (Ital.)

Primary Use: This aminoglycoside is effective against Gram-negative organisms and in drug-resistant staphylococcus.

Ocular Side Effects:

    A. Systemic Administration
        1. Decreased vision
        2. Myasthenic neuromuscular blocking effect
            a. Paralysis of extraocular muscles
            b. Ptosis
        3. Eyelids or conjunctiva
            a. Allergic reactions
            b. Lyell's syndrome
    B. Local Ophthalmic Use or Exposure—Subconjunctival Injection
        1. Irritation
        2. Eyelids or conjunctiva—allergic reactions
        3. Overgrowth of nonsusceptible organisms

Clinical Significance: Systemic and ocular side effects due to kanamycin are quite rare, partially due to its poor gastrointestinal absorption. Myasthenic neuromuscular blocking effect occurs more frequently if kanamycin is given in combination with other antibiotics, such as neomycin, gentamicin, polymyxin B, colistin, or streptomycin. Adverse ocular reactions to this agent are reversible, transitory, and seldom have residual complications. While optic neuritis has been reported to be associated with this drug, it has not been proven.

References:
D'Amico, D.J., et al.: Comparative toxicity of intravitreal aminoglycoside antibiotics. Am. J. Ophthalmol. *100*:264, 1985.
Finegold, S.M.: Kanamycin. Arch. Intern. Med. *104*:15, 1959.
Finegold, S.M.: Toxicity of kanamycin in adults. Ann. N.Y. Acad. Sci. *132*:942, 1966.
Freemon, F.R., Parker, R.L., Jr., and Greer, M.: Unusual neurotoxicity of kanamycin. JAMA *200*:410, 1967.
Kaeser, H.E.: Drug-induced myasthenic syndromes. Acta Neurol. Scand. *70*(Suppl. 100):39, 1984.
Walsh, F.B., and Hoyt, W.F.: Clinical Neuro-Ophthalmology. 3rd Ed., Baltimore, Williams & Wilkins, Vol. III, 1969, pp. 2655, 2680

Generic Name: Nalidixic Acid

Proprietary Name: Betaxina (Ital.), Faril (Ital.), Nalicidin (Ital.), Nalidixin (Ital.), Naligram (Ital.), Nalissina (Ital.), Négram (Fr., Switz.), **NegGram** (Canad.), Neg-Gram (Ital.), Negram (Austral., G.B., Ire., Neth., Swed.), Nogram (Germ.), Notricel (Span.), Puromylon (S. Afr.), Uralgin (Ital.), Uriben (G.B.), Uri-Flor (Ital.), Urogram (Ital.), Uropan (Ital.), Winlomylon (S. Afr.), Mintomylon (Span.)

Primary Use: This bactericidal naphthyridine derivative is effective against *E. coli, Aerobacter,* and *Klebsiella;* however, its primary clinical use is against *Proteus.*

Ocular Side Effects:

A. Systemic Administration
   1. Visual sensations
      a. Glare phenomenon
      b. Flashing lights—white or colored
      c. Scintillating scotomas—may be colored
   2. Problems with color vision
      a. Color vision defect
      b. Objects have green, yellow, blue, or violet tinge
   3. Photophobia
   4. Paresis of extraocular muscles
   5. Papilledema secondary to pseudotumor cerebri
   6. Decreased vision
   7. Decreased accommodation
   8. Diplopia
   9. Mydriasis—may precipitate narrow-angle glaucoma
   10. Nystagmus
   11. Eyelids or conjunctiva
       a. Photosensitivity

      b. Angioneurotic edema
      c. Urticaria
      d. Lupoid syndrome
  12. Visual hallucinations
  13. Subconjunctival or retinal hemorrhages secondary to drug-induced anemia

Clinical Significance: Numerous ocular side effects due to nalidixic acid have been reported. The most common adverse ocular reaction is a curious visual disturbance, which includes brightly colored appearances of objects as the main feature. This often appears soon after the drug is taken. Temporary visual loss has also occurred and lasted from 30 minutes to 72 hours. Papilledema secondary to elevated intracranial pressure is probably the most serious ocular reaction. Most of the reports concerning intracranial hypertension deal with children and adolescents, the oldest being 20 years of age. A large series of pseudotumor cerebri occurred in infants younger than 6 months of age who were given 100-150 mg/kg/day for acute bacillary dysentery. Use of nalidixic acid during pregnancy carries the possible prenatal risk of increased intracranial pressure. Most adverse ocular reactions due to nalidixic acid are transitory and reversible if the dosage is decreased or the drug is discontinued.

References:

Birch, J., et al.: Acquired color vision defects. *In* Pokorny, J., et al. (Eds.): Congenital and Acquired Color Vision Defects. New York, Grune & Stratton, 1979, pp. 243–350.

Drugs that cause psychiatric symptoms. Med. Lett. Drugs Ther. *28*:81, 1986.

Gedroyc, W., and Shorvon, S.D.: Acute intracranial hypertension and nalidixic acid therapy. Neurology *32*:212, 1982.

Granstrom, G., and Santesson, B.: Unconsciousness after one therapeutic dose of nalidixic acid. Acta Med. Scand. *216*:237, 1984.

Katzman, B., et al.: Pseudotumor cerebri: An observation and review. Ann. Ophthalmol. *13*:887, 1981.

Kilpatrick, C., and Ebeling, P.: Intracranial hypertension in nalidixic acid therapy. Med. J. Aust. *1*:252, 1982.

Lane, R.J.M., and Routledge, P.A.: Drug-induced neurological disorders. Drugs *26*:124, 1983.

Mukherjee, A., et al.: Benign intracranial hypertension after nalidixic acid overdose in infants. Lancet *335*:1602, 1990.

Rubinstein, A.: LE-like disease caused by nalidixic acid. N. Engl. J. Med. *301*:1288, 1979.

Safety of antimicrobial drugs in pregnancy. Med. Lett. Drugs Ther. *27*:93, 1985

Generic Name: Nitrofurantoin

Proprietary Name: Chemiofurin (Span.), Cistofuran (Ital.), Cystit (Germ.), **Furadantin** (Austral., G.B., Germ., Ire., Ital., S Afr., Swed.), Furadantine

(Fr., Switz.), Furadantine MC (Neth.), Furantoina (Span.), Furedan (Ital.), Furil (Ital.), Furobactina (Span.), Furophen Tc (Neth.), Ituran (Germ.), Macrobid (G.B.), **Macrodantin** (Austral., Canad., G.B, Ire., Ital., S. Afr.), Microdoïne (Fr.), Neo-Furadantin (Ital.), Nephronex (Canad.), Nierofu (Germ.), Nitrofurin G.W. (Ital.), Novofuran (Canad.), Phenurin (Germ.), Trocurine (Switz.), Urantoin (G.B.), Urodil (Germ.), Urolisa (Ital.), Urolong (Germ., Switz.), Uro-Tablinen (Germ.), Uvamine retard (Switz.)

Primary Use: This bactericidal furan derivative is effective against specific organisms that cause urinary tract infections, especially *E. coli,* enterococci, and *S. aureus.*

Ocular Side Effects:
    A. Systemic Administration
        1. Nonspecific ocular irritation
            a. Lacrimation
            b. Burning sensation
        2. Diplopia
        3. Nystagmus
        4. Decreased vision
        5. Paresis or paralysis of extraocular muscles
        6. Eyelids or conjunctiva
            a. Allergic reactions
            b. Photosensitivity
            c. Angioneurotic edema
            d. Urticaria
            e. Lupoid syndrome
            f. Erythema multiforme
            g. Lyell's syndrome
            h. Loss of eyelashes or eyebrows
        7. Papilledema secondary to pseudotumor cerebri
        8. Subconjunctival or retinal hemorrhages secondary to drug-induced anemia
        9. Problems with color vision
            a. Color vision defect
            b. Objects have yellow tinge
        10. Retinal—crystalline retinopathy

Clinical Significance: The most aggravating ocular side effects due to nitrofurantoin are the severe itching, burning, and tearing that may persist long after use of the drug is stopped in some patients. Paralysis of extraocular muscles has been reported in association with nitrofurantoin and may take up to 5 months to resolve once the medication is discontinued. In addition, severe polyneuropathies with demyelination and degeneration of sensory and motor nerves have occurred with long-term use of nitrofurantoin. Pseudotumor cerebri associated with nitrofurantoin therapy is well documented. A recent report by Ibanez, et al. suggests an intraretinal crystalline deposit in both eyes of a 69-year-old man who, for 19 years, received nitrofurantoin daily for a chronic urinary tract infection.

References:
Chapman, J.A.: An unusual nitrofurantoin-induced drug reaction. Ann. Allergy 56:16, 1986.

Delaney, R.A., Miller, D.A., and Gerbino, P.P.: Adverse effects resulting from nitrofurantoin administration. Am. J. Pharm. *149*:26, 1977.

Ibanez, H.E., Williams, D.F., and Boniuk, I.: Crystalline retinopathy associated with long-term nitrofurantoin therapy. Case report. Arch. Ophthalmol. *112*:304–305, 1994.

Mesaros, M.P., Seymour, J., and Sadjadpour, K.: Lateral rectus muscle palsy associated with nitrofurantoin (Macrodantoin). Am. J. Ophthalmol. *94*:816, 1982.

Mushet, G.R.: Pseudotumor and nitrofurantoin therapy. Arch. Neurol. *34*:257, 1977.

Nitrofurantoin. Med. Lett. Drugs. Ther. 22:36, 1980.

Penn, R.G., and Griffin, J.P.: Adverse reactions to nitrofurantoin in the United Kingdom, Sweden, and Holland. Br. Med. J. *284*:1440, 1982.

Sharma, D.B., and James, A.: Benign intracranial hypertension associated with nitrofurantoin therapy. Br. Med. J. *4*:771, 1974.

Young, T.L., et al.: Chronic active hepatitis induced by nitrofurantoin. Cleveland Clinic Quarterly *52*:253, 1985.

Generic Name: Polymyxin B

Proprietary Name: *Systemic*: **Aerosporin** (Canad., G.B., Ire.) *Ophthalmic*: Aerosporin (Canad., G.B.), **Polymyxin B Sulfate**

Primary Use: This bactericidal polypeptide is effective against Gram-negative bacilli, especially *Ps. aeruginosa*.

Ocular Side Effects:
A. Systemic Administration
1. Myasthenic neuromuscular blocking effect
    a. Paralysis of extraocular muscles
    b. Ptosis
2. Decreased vision
3. Diplopia
4. Nystagmus
5. Mydriasis
B. Local Ophthalmic Use or Exposure—Topical Application or Subconjunctival Injection
1. Irritation—ocular pain
2. Eyelids or conjunctiva—allergic reactions
3. Myasthenic neuromuscular blocking effect

a. Paralysis of extraocular muscles
b. Ptosis
4. Overgrowth of nonsusceptible organisms
C. Local Ophthalmic Use or Exposure—Intracameral Injection
1. Uveitis
2. Corneal edema
3. Lens damage

Clinical Significance: Although ocular side effects due to polymyxin B are well documented, they are quite rare and seldom of major clinical importance, except for topical ocular irritative or allergic reactions. There have, however, been rare reports of anaphylactic reactions from topical polymyxin B-bacitracin applications. The clinically important side effects are secondary to intracameral injections where permanent changes to the cornea and lens have occurred.

References:

Baldinger, J., and Weiter, J.J.: Diffuse cutaneous hypersensitivity reaction after dexamethasone/polymyxin B/neomycin combination eyedrops. Ann. Ophthalmol. *18*: 95, 1986.
Francois, J., and Mortiers, P.: The injurious effects of locally and generally applied antibiotics on the eye. T. Geneeskd. *32*:139, 1976.
Hudgson, P.: Adverse drug reactions in the neuromuscular apparatus. Adverse Drug React. Acute Poisoning Rev. *1*:35, 1982.
Kaeser, H.E.: Drug-induced myasthenic syndromes. Acta Neurol. Scand. *70*:(Suppl. 100):39, 1984.
Koenig, A., and Ohrloff, C.: Influence of local application of Isoptomax eyedrops on neuromuscular transmission. Klin. Monatsbl. Augenheilkd. *179*:109, 1981.
Lane, R.J.M., and Routledge, P.A.: Drug-induced neurological disorders. Drugs *26*: 124, 1983.
Stern, G.A., et al.: Effect of topical antibiotic solutions on corneal epithelial wound healing. Arch. Ophthalmol. *101*:644, 1983.

Generic Name: Streptomycin

Proprietary Name: Cidan Est (Span.), Novostrep (S. Afr.), Solustrep (S. Afr.), Streptocol (Ital.), Strepto-Fatol (Germ.)

Primary Use: This bactericidal aminoglycosidic agent is effective against *Brucella, Pasteurella, Mycobacterium,* and *Shigella.*

Ocular Side Effects:
A. Systemic or Intrathecal Administration
1. Nystagmus
2. Decreased vision
3. Toxic amblyopia

4. Myasthenic neuromuscular blocking effect
   a. Paresis or paralysis of extraocular muscles
   b. Ptosis
5. Visual sensations
   a. Visual disturbance during motion
   b. Continuance of image after ocular movement
6. Photophobia
7. Problems with color vision
   a. Color vision defect, blue-green defect
   b. Objects have yellow tinge
8. Decreased accommodation
9. Retrobulbar or optic neuritis
10. Scotomas
11. Optic atrophy
12. Retinal vasospasm
13. Eyelids or conjunctiva
    a. Allergic reactions
    b. Erythema
    c. Conjunctivitis—nonspecific
    d. Edema
    e. Angioneurotic edema
    f. Urticaria
    g. Lupoid syndrome
    h. Exfoliative dermatitis
    i. Lyell's syndrome
14. Subconjunctival or retinal hemorrhages secondary to drug-induced anemia

B. Local Ophthalmic Use or Exposure—Subconjunctival Injection
   1. Irritation
   2. Eyelids or conjunctiva—allergic reactions
   3. Overgrowth of nonsusceptible organisms
C. Local Ophthalmic Use or Exposure—Intracameral Injection
   1. Uveitis
   2. Corneal edema
   3. Lens damage

Clinical Significance: Since more effective aminoglycosidic antibiotics exist, the clinical use of streptomycin is limited. Toxic visual effects are rare, usually transitory, and reversible with systemic administration; however, permanent blindness and optic atrophy have been reported with intrathecal injection. Nystagmus due to streptomycin can be produced without vestibular damage. Skin sensitization is common among medical personnel who handle this drug and may lead to dermatitis frequently associated with periorbital edema and conjunctivitis.

References:

Birch, J., et al.: Acquired color vision defects. *In* Pokorny, J., et al. (Eds.): Congenital and Acquired Color Vision Defects. New York, Grune & Stratton, 1979, pp. 243–350.

Kaeser, H.E.: Drug-induced myasthenic syndromes. Acta Neurol. Scand. *70*(Suppl. 100):39, 1984.

Kushimoto, H., and Aoki, T.: Toxic erythema with generalized follicular pustules caused by streptomycin. Arch. Dermatol. *117*:444, 1981.

Reynolds, J.E.F. (Ed.): Martindale: The Extra Pharmacopoeia. 28th Ed., London, Pharmaceutical Press, 1982, pp. 1212–1215.

Zurcher, K., and Krebs, A.: Cutaneous Side Effects of Systemic Drugs. Basel, S. Karger, 1980, pp. 20–23.

Generic Name: 1. Sulfacetamide; 2. Sulfacytine (Sulfacitine); 3. Sulfadiazine; 4. Sulfadimethoxine; 5. Sulfamerazine; 6. Sulfamethazine (Sulfadimidine); 7. Sulfamethizole; 8. Sulfamethoxazole; 9. Sulfamethoxypyridazine; 10. Sulfanilamide; 11. Sulfapyridine; 12. Sulfasalazine; 13. Sulfathiazole; 14. Sulfisoxazole (Sulfafurazole)

Proprietary Name: *Systemic*: 1. Acetopt (Austral.), Ak-Sulf (Canad.), Albucid (G.B., S. Afr.), Antébor (Fr., Switz.), Balsulph (Canad.), Bleph-10 (Ire., S. Afr.), Bleph-10 Liquifilm (Austral., Canad.), Cetamide (Canad.), Covosulf (S. Afr.), Isopto Cetamide (Canad.), Lersa (Span.), Ophtho-Sulf (Canad.), Optamide (Austral.), Opticet (S. Afr.), Prontamid (Ital.), **Sebizon, Sodium Sulamyd** (Canad.), Spersacet (Switz.), Spersamide (S. Afr.), Sulfableph N Liquifilm (Germ.), Sulfaceta (Span.), Sulfacetam (Span.), Sulfex (Canad.): 3. Adiazine (Fr.); 4. Chemiosalfa (Ital.), Deltin (Ital.), Risulpir (Ital.), Ritarsulfa (Ital.), Sulfadren (Ital.), Sulfastop (Ital.), Sulfathox (S. Afr.); 6. Sulphamezathine (Ire.); 7. Rufol (Fr., Ital.), **Thiosulfil Forte**, Tiosulfan (Span.), Urolucosil (Austral., Switz.); 8. **Gantanol** (Canad.); 9. Sulfalex (Ital.); 10. **AVC** (Canad.), Azol Polvo (Span.), Defonamid (Germ.), Exoseptoplix (Fr.), Pomada Sulfamida Orravan (Span.), Pulvi-Bactéramide (Fr.); 11. Dagenan (Canad.), M & B 693 (Austral.); 12. **Azulfidine** (Germ.), Colo-Pleon (Germ), Salazopyrin (Austral., Canad., G.B., Ital., S. Afr., Swed.), Salazopyrina (Span.), Salazopyrine (Fr., Neth., Switz.), Salisulf Gastroprotetto (Ital.), S.A.S. (Canad.), Sulazine (Austral.), Sulfazine (Ire.), Ulcol (Austral.); 14. **Gantrisin** (Austral.), Novosoxazole (Canad.) *Ophthalmic*: 1. Acetopt (Austral.), **AK-Sulf**, Albucid (G.B., S. Afr.), **Bleph-10, Cetamide, Isopto Cetamide, Ocusulf-10**, Optamide (Austral.), **Sodium Sulamyd, Sulf-10, Sulf-15**, Sulphacetamide (G.B.); 7. Sulfamethizoli (G.B.); 14. **Gantrisin**

Primary Use: The sulfonamides are bacteriostatic agents effective against most Gram-positive and some Gram-negative organisms. Sulfonamides are the agents of choice for treatment of nocardiosis, chancroid, and toxoplasmosis.

Ocular Side Effects:
A. Systemic Administration
   1. Decreased vision
   2. Myopia—with or without astigmatism
   3. Decreased depth perception—with or without decreased adduction at near
   4. Nonspecific ocular irritation
      a. Lacrimation
      b. Photophobia
   5. Keratitis
   6. Problems with color vision
      a. Color vision defect
      b. Objects have yellow or red tinge
   7. Subconjunctival or retinal hemorrhages
   8. Visual fields
      a. Scotomas
      b. Constriction
      c. Blind spot enlargement
   9. Optic neuritis
  10. Myasthenic neuromuscular blocking effect
      a. Paralysis of extraocular muscles
      b. Ptosis
  11. Periorbital edema
  12. Visual hallucinations
  13. Papilledema (pseudotumor cerebri)
  14. Cortical blindness
  15. Vivid light lavender-colored retinal vascular tree
  16. Decreased anterior chamber depth—may precipitate narrow-angle glaucoma
  17. Eyelids or conjunctiva
      a. Allergic reactions
      b. Conjunctivitis—nonspecific
      c. Photosensitivity
      d. Urticaria
      e. Purpura
      f. Lupoid syndrome
      g. Erythema multiforme
      h. Stevens-Johnson syndrome
      i. Exfoliative dermatitis
      j. Lyell's syndrome
      k. Pemphigoid lesion with or without symblepharon
      l. Loss of eyelashes or eyebrows
  18. Contact lenses stained yellow
  19. Uveitis

  B. Local Ophthalmic Use or Exposure—Topical Application
     1. Irritation
     2. Eyelids or conjunctiva
        a. Allergic reactions
        b. Conjunctivitis—follicular
        c. Deposits
        d. Photosensitivity
        e. Lupoid syndrome
        f. Erythema multiforme
        g. Stevens-Johnson syndrome
     3. Overgrowth of nonsusceptible organisms
     4. Delayed corneal wound healing
     5. Cornea—peripheral immune ring

Clinical Significance: While there are numerous reported ocular side effects
from systemic sulfa medication, most are rare and reversible. Probably the
most common ocular side effect seen in patients receiving systemic therapy
is myopia. This is transient, with or without induced astigmatism, usually
bilateral, and may exceed several diopters. This is most likely due to an
increased anterior-posterior lens diameter secondary to ciliary body edema.
Also, sulfa can cause dermatologic problems, associated conjunctivitis, keratitis, and lid problems. Optic neuritis has been reported even in low oral
dosages and is usually reversible with full recovery of vision. Uveitis, usually bilateral, may occur after starting oral sulfa preparations, with or without
other systemic manifestations. This has been proven by rechallenge. The
ophthalmologist should be aware that anaphylactic reactions, Stevens-Johnson syndrome, and exfoliative dermatitis have all been reported, although
rarely, from topical ocular administration of sulfa preparations. Ocular irritation from crystalline sulfa in the tear strip may occur. Recently, Gutt, et
al. reported immune rings in the peripheral cornea, probably secondary to
sulfamethoxazole.

References:

Bovino, J.A., and Marcus, D.F.: The mechanism of transient myopia induced by sulfon-
    amide therapy. Am. J. Ophthalmol. *94*:99, 1982.
Chirls, I.A., and Norris, J.W.: Transient myopia associated with vaginal sulfanilamide
    suppositories. Am. J. Ophthalmol. *98*:120, 1984.
Fajardo, R.V.: Acute bilateral anterior uveitis caused by sulfa drugs. *In* Saari, K.M.
    (Ed.): Uveitis Update. Amsterdam, Excerpta Medica, 1984, pp. 115–118.
Flach, A.J., Peterson, J.S., and Mathias, C.G.T.: Photosensitivity to topically applied
    sulfisoxazole ointment: Evidence for a phototoxic reaction. Arch. Ophthalmol. *100*:
    1286, 1982.
Genvert, G.I., et al.: Erythema multiforme after use of topical sulfacetamide. Am. J.
    Ophthalmol. *99*:465, 1985.
Gutt, L., et al: Corneal ring formation after exposure to sulfamethoxazole. Arch. Oph-
    thalmol. *106*:726–727, 1988.

Hook, S.R., et al.: Transient myopia induced by sulfonamides. Am. J. Ophthalmol. *101*:495, 1986.

Lane, R.J.M., and Routledge, P.A.: Drug-induced neurological disorders. Drugs *26*: 124, 1983.

Mackie, B.S., and Mackie, L.E.: Systemic lupus erythematosus—Dermatomyositis induced by sulphacetamide eyedrops. Aust. J. Dermatol. *20*:49, 1979.

Riley, S.A., Flagg, P.J., and Mandal, B.K.: Contact lens staining due to sulphasalazine. Lancet *1*:972, 1986.

Tilden, M.E., Rosenbaum, J.T., and Fraunfelder, F.T.: Systemic sulfonamides as a cause of bilateral, anterior uveitis. Arch. Ophthalmol. *109*:67–69, 1991.

Vanheule, B.A., and Carswell, F.: Sulphasalazine-induced systemic lupus erythematosus in a child. Eur. J. Pediatr. *140*:66, 1983.

Generic Name: Tobramycin

Proprietary Name: *Systemic*: Gernebcin (Germ.), **Nebcin** (Austral., Canad., G.B., Ire., S. Afr.), Nebcina (Swed.), Nebcine (Fr.), Nebicina (Ital.), Obracin (Neth., Switz.), Tobra Gobens (Span.), Tobra Laf (Span.), Tobradistin (Span.), Tobral (Ital.), Tobralex (G.B.), Tobramaxin (Germ.), **Tobrex** (Austral., Canad., Fr., Ital., Neth., S. Afr., Span., Switz.) *Ophthalmic*: **Tobrex**

Primary Use: This aminoglycoside is effective against many Gram-negative organisms, including *Ps. aeruginosa, E. coli, K. pneumoniae, Proteus* and *Enterobacter,* and some Gram-positive organisms, including staphylococci and streptococci.

Ocular Side Effects:

A. Systemic Administration
   1. Decreased vision
   2. Visual hallucinations
   3. Nystagmus
   4. Myasthenic neuromuscular blocking effect
      a. Paresis or paralysis of extraocular muscles
      b. Ptosis
   5. Problems with color vision—color vision defect
B. Local Ophthalmic Use or Exposure—Topical Application
   1. Irritation
      a. Lacrimation
      b. Hyperemia
      c. Ocular pain
      d. Edema
      e. Burning sensation
   2. Punctate keratitis
   3. Overgrowth of nonsusceptible organisms
   4. Photophobia
   5. Conjunctival necrosis (fortified solutions)

    C. Inadvertent Ocular Exposure—Intraocular Injection
        1. Optic atrophy
        2. Retinal degeneration

Clinical Significance: Few drug-induced ocular side effects from systemic administration of tobramycin have been reported. Topical ophthalmic application of tobramycin may be associated with a significantly lower frequency of local irritative adverse reactions than gentamicin, especially in ointment form. Inadvertent intraocular injection of tobramycin has been followed by retinal degeneration and optic atrophy. Intraocular complication has possibly occurred from subconjunctival injection through the cataract wound. There are two cases in the Registry of abnormal renal function tests in borderline-compromised kidney patients secondary to topical tobramycin, confirmed on rechallenge.

References:

Balian, J.V.: Accidental intraocular tobramycin injection: A case report. Ophthalmic Surg. *14*:353, 1983.

Davison, C.R., Tuft, S.J., and Dart, K.G.: Conjunctival necrosis after administration of topical fortified aminoglycosides. Am. J. Ophthalmol. *111*:690-693, 1991.

Judson, P.H.: Aminoglycoside macular toxicity after subconjunctival injection. Arch. Ophthalmol *107*:1282–1283, 1989.

Kaeser, H.E.: Drug-induced myasthenic syndromes. Acta Neurol. Scand. *70*(Suppl. 100):39, 1984.

Leibowitz, H.M., et al.: Tobramycin in external eye disease: A double-masked study vs. gentamicin. Curr. Eye Res. *1*:259, 1981.

McCartney, C.F., Hatley, L.H., and Kessler, J.M.: Possible tobramycin delirium. JAMA *247*:1319, 1982.

Speirs, C.F.: Tobramycin side effects-International results. Scot. Med. J. *21*:78, 1976.

Wilhelmus, K.R., Gilbert, M.L., and Osato, M.S.: Tobramycin in ophthalmology. Surv. Ophthalmol. *32(2)*:111–122, 1987.

Class: Antifungal Agents

Generic Name: Amphotericin B

Proprietary Name: AmBisome (G.B.), Ampho-Moronal (Germ., Switz.), Funganiline (Span.), Fungilin (Austral., G.B., Ital.), Fungizona (Span.), **Fungizone** (Austral., Canad., Fr., G.B., Ital., Neth., S. Afr., Swed., Switz.)

Primary Use: This polyene fungistatic agent is effective against *Blastomyces, Histoplasma, Cryptococcus, Coccidiomyces, Candida,* and *Aspergillus.*

Ocular Side Effects:
    A. Systemic Administration
        1. Decreased vision

2. Paresis of extraocular muscles
3. Retinal exudates
4. Subconjunctival or retinal hemorrhages secondary to drug-induced anemia
5. Diplopia
B. Local Ophthalmic Use or Exposure—Topical Application or Subconjunctival Injection
  1. Irritation
    a. Ocular pain
    b. Burning sensation
  2. Punctate keratitis
  3. Eyelids or conjunctiva
    a. Allergic reactions
    b. Ulceration
    c. Conjunctivitis—follicular
    d. Necrosis—subconjunctival injection
    e. Nodules—subconjunctival injection
    f. Yellow discoloration—subconjunctival injection
  4. Overgrowth of nonsusceptible organisms
  5. Uveitis
  6. Delayed corneal wound healing
C. Local Ophthalmic Use or Exposure—Intracameral Injection
  1. Uveitis
  2. Corneal edema
  3. Lens damage

Clinical Significance: Seldom are significant ocular side effects seen from systemic administration of amphotericin B, except with intrathecal injections. In general, transitory blurred vision is the most common ocular side effect. Allergic reactions are so rare that it was initially believed that they did not even occur. Topical ocular administration of amphotericin B can be quite irritating, with significant conjunctival and corneal irritative responses. This agent can affect cell membranes and allow increased penetration of other drugs into the cornea. There have been rare reports of marked iridocyclitis with small hyphemas occurring after each reapplication of topical ocular amphotericin B. The formation of salmon-colored raised nodules can occur secondary to subconjunctival injection, especially if the dosage exceeds 5 mg. The injection of this agent subconjunctivally or subcutaneously can cause permanent yellowing. Some clinicians feel that amphotericin B is too toxic to the tissue to be given subconjunctivally, especially since scleral penetration is poor.

References:
Brod, R.D., et al: Endogenous Candida endophthalmitis: Management without intravenous amphotericin B. 97:666–674, 1990.

Doft, B. H., et al.: Amphotericin clearance in vitrectomized versus nonvitrectomized eyes. Ophthalmology *92*:1601, 1985.

Dukes, M.N.G. (Ed.): Meyler's Side Effects of Drugs. Amsterdam, Excerpta Medica, Vol. X, 1984, pp. 517–519.

Foster, C.S., et al.: Ocular toxicity of topical antifungal agents. Arch. Ophthalmol. *99*: 1081, 1981.

Li, P.K.T., and Lai, K.N.: Amphotericin B-induced ocular toxicity in cryptococcal meningitis. Br. J. Ophthalmol. *73*:397–398, 1989.

Lavine, J.B., Binder, P.S., and Wickham, M.G.: Antimicrobials and the corneal endothelium. Ann. Ophthalmol. *11*:1517, 1979.

O'Day, D.M., Smith, R., Stevens, J.B.: Toxicity and pharmacokinetics of subconjunctival amphotericin B. Cornea *10(5)*:411–417, 1991.

O'Day, D.M., et al.: Intraocular penetration of systemically administered antifungal agents. Curr. Eye Res. *4*:131, 1985.

Generic Name: Griseofulvin

Proprietary Name: Delmofulvina (Ital.), Fulcin (Austral., G.B., Ire., Ital., Neth., S. Afr., Span., Swed., Switz.), Fulcin S (Germ.), Fulcine (Fr.), **Fulvicin P/G** (Canad.), **Fulvicin U/F** (Canad.), Fulvicina (Span.), Greosin (Span.), **Grifulvin V**, **Grisactin**, **Grisactin Ultra**, Griséfuline (Fr.), Griseoderm (Ire.), Griseostatin (Austral.), Grisovin (Austral., G.B., S. Afr., Swed., Switz.), Grisovina FP (Ital.), Grisovin-FP (Canad.), **Gris-PEG** (Switz.), Lamoryl (Swed.), Likuden M (Germ.), Microcidal (S. Afr.), Polygris (Germ.), Sulvina (Span.)

Primary Use: This oral antifungal agent is effective against tinea infections of the nails, skin, and hair.

Ocular Side Effects:
  A. Systemic Administration
      1. Decreased vision
      2. Problems with color vision—objects have green tinge
      3. Photosensitivity
      4. Visual hallucinations
      5. Eyelids or conjunctiva
          a. Allergic reactions
          b. Hyperemia
          c. Edema
          d. Photosensitivity
          e. Angioneurotic edema
          f. Urticaria
          g. Lupoid syndrome
          h. Exfoliative dermatitis
      6. Papilledema secondary to pseudotumor cerebri

7. Subconjunctival or retinal hemorrhages secondary to drug-induced anemia

Clinical Significance: Griseofulvin rarely causes ocular side effects. Those of major clinical importance are severe allergic reactions with secondary ocular involvement. Decreased vision rarely occurs and seldom requires stopping the drug except in cases of pseudotumor cerebri. One published case of transient macular edema secondary to this agent is suspect. There is a case of superficial corneal deposits resembling Meesman's corneal dystrophy that was reported to resolve after discontinuation of the drug. This agent is a photosensitizing drug, and increased light exposure increases the prevalence of eyelid and conjunctival reactions.

References:

Alarcón-Segovia, D.: Drug-induced antinuclear antibodies and lupus syndromes. Drugs *12*:69, 1976.

Delman, M., and Leubuscher, K.: Transient macular edema due to griseofulvin. Am. J. Ophthalmol. *56*:658, 1963.

Epstein, J.H., and Wintroub, B.U.: Photosensitivity due to drugs. Drugs *30*:41, 1985.

Madhok, R., et al.: Fatal exacerbation of systemic lupus erythematosus after treatment with griseofulvin. *Br. Med. J.* 291:249, 1985.

Spaeth, G.L., Nelson, L.B., and Beaudoin, A.R.: Ocular teratology. *In* Jakobiec, F.A. (Ed.): Ocular Anatomy, Embryology and Teratology. Philadelphia, J.B. Lippincott, 1982, pp. 955–975.

Generic Name: Nystatin

Proprietary Name: Adiclair (Germ.), Biofanal (Germ.), Candida-Lokalicid (Germ.), Candio-Hermal (Germ., Switz.), Canstat (S. Afr.), Cordes Nystatin Soft (Germ.), Moronal (Germ.), **Mycostatin** (Austral., Canad., Ire., Ital., S. Afr., Span., Swed.), Mycostatine (Fr., Switz.), Mykundex (Germ.), Mykundex mono (Germ.), Nadostine (Canad.), **Nilstat** (Austral., Canad.), Nyaderm (Canad.), Nyspes (G.B.), Nystan (G.B.), Nystatin-Dome (G.B.), **Nystex**

Primary Use: This polyene fungistatic and fungicidal agent is effective against *Candida*.

Ocular Side Effects:

A. Systemic Administration
  1. Optic neuritis
  2. Decreased vision
B. Local Ophthalmic Use or Exposure—Topical Application or Subconjunctival Injection
  1. Irritation
  2. Eyelids or conjunctiva—allergic reactions
  3. Overgrowth of nonsusceptible organisms

Clinical Significance: Ocular side effects from systemic or ocular nystatin administration are unusual. Most adverse ocular reactions due to this agent are reversible and transitory.

References:

Ellis, P.P.: Ocular Therapeutics and Pharmacology. 6th Ed., St. Louis, C.V. Mosby, 1981, p. 255.
Havener, W.H.: Ocular Pharmacology. 5th Ed., St. Louis, C.V. Mosby, 1983, pp. 161–164.
Saraux, H.: La nevrite optique par intoxication medicamenteuse. Communication Soc. Med. Milit. December 17, 1970.
Wasilewski, C.: Allergic contact dermatitis from nystatin. Arch Dermatol. *102*:216, 1970.

Generic Name: Thiabendazole. See under *Class: Anthelmintics.*

Class: Antileprosy Agents

Generic Name: Amithiozone. See under *Class: Antitubercular Agents.*

Generic Name: Clofazimine

Proprietary Name: Lamprène (Switz.), Lampren (Neth., Span.), **Lamprene** (Austral., G.B., Ire., S. Afr.)

Primary Use: This phenazine derivative is used in the treatment of leprosy and also as an anti-inflammatory in psoriasis, discoid lupus, and pyoderma gangrenosum.

Ocular Side Effects:
   A. Systemic Administration
      1. Ocular irritation
      2. Decreased vision
      3. Eyelids or conjunctiva
         a. Pigmentation (red-brown)
         b. Discoloration of lashes
         c. Perilimbal crystalline deposits
      4. Tears
         a. Discoloration
         b. Crystalline deposits
         c. Aggravation of keratoconjunctivitis sicca
      5. Cornea—polychromatic crystalline deposits
      6. Photosensitivity

Clinical Significance: This phenazine derivative can cause a dose-related reversible reddish pigmentation of the skin, conjunctiva, and cornea similar to that seen with chloroquine. These polychromatic crystals have been found in the tear film and have colored tears. Findings include fine brownish subepithelial lines and perilimbal crystalline deposits seen on biomicroscopy. This rarely interferes with vision, and the crystalline deposits on the surface of the eye can disappear within a few months to years after clofazimine has been discontinued. It is unclear if this drug can cause keratoconjunctivitis sicca; more likely, the crystals act as an aggravation in patients with already compromised tear production. These crystals may give a foreign body sensation and symptomatology consistent with a sicca-like syndrome. In one series, up to 50% of patients had some form of conjunctival pigmentation, 12% had variable changes in their perception of their vision, 25% had ocular irritation, and 32% had crystals in their tears. Retinal changes have been published in one case and were believed to be roughly the same as seen with chloroquine, i.e., starting as a fine pigmentary macular change and progressing to bull's-eye retinopathy. There are no other reports of retinal changes with this agent in the literature or in the Registry.

References:

Craythorn, J.M., Swartz, M. and Creel, D.J.: Clofazimine-induced bull's-eye retinopathy. Retina 6:50, 1986.

Davies, D.M. (Ed.): Textbook of Adverse Drug Reactions. New York, Oxford University Press, 1977, p. 297.

Granstein, R.D., and Sober, A.J.: Drug and heavy metal-induced hyperpigmentation. J. Am. Acad. Dermatol. 5:1, 1981.

Kaur, I., et al.: Effect of clofazimine on eye in multibacillary leprosy. Indian J. Lepr. 62(1):87-90, 1990.

Moore, V.J.: A review of side effects experienced by patients taking clofazimine. Lepr. Rev. 54:327–335, 1983.

Ohman, L., and Wahlberg, I.: Ocular side effects of clofazimine. Lancet 2:933, 1975.

Font, R.L., Sobol, W., and Matoba, A.: Polychromatic corneal and conjunctival crystals secondary to clofazimine therapy in a leper. Ophthalmology 96(3):311–315, 1989.

Reynolds, J.E.F, (Ed.): Martindale: The Extra Pharmacopoeia. 28th Ed., London, Pharmaceutical Press, 1982, pp. 1488–1489.

Walinder, P.E., Gip, L., and Stempa, M.: Corneal changes in patients treated with clofazimine. Br. J. Ophthalmol. 60:526, 1976.

Generic Name: Dapsone

Proprietary Name: Avlosulfon (Canad.), Sulfona (Span.)

Primary Use: This sulfone is used in the treatment of all forms of leprosy.

Ocular Side Effects:

    A. Systemic Administration
        1. Decreased vision
        2. Eyelids or conjunctiva

    a. Edema
    b. Hyperpigmentation
    c. Urticaria
    d. Purpura
    e. Erythema multiforme
    f. Exfoliative dermatitis
    g. Lyell's syndrome
3. Visual hallucinations
4. Optic nerve—toxic states
    a. Optic neuritis
    b. Optic atrophy
5. Photosensitivity
6. Subconjunctival or retinal hemorrhages secondary to drug-induced anemia

Clinical Significance: This sulfone has been reported to cause optic neuritis, optic atrophy, and massive bilateral retinal necrosis with permanent blindness. These cases have occurred only when patients were given massive doses. Otherwise, other adverse ocular reactions are seldom of clinical importance. Darkening of skin color may be due to iatrogenic cyanosis, as a slate gray discoloration is characteristic of drug-induced methemoglobinemia. Some patients under treatment with dapsone for leprosy have been known to develop lagophthalmos and posterior synechiae, but these effects are probably due to the disease rather than to the drug.

References:
Brandt, F., Adiga, R.B., and Pradhan, H.: Lagophthalmos and posterior synechias during treatment of leprosy with diaminodiphenylsulfone. Klin. Monatsbl. Augenheilkd. *184*:28, 1984.
Daneshmend, T.K., and Homeida, M.: Dapsone-induced optic atrophy and motor neuropathy. Br. Med. J. *283*:311, 1981.
Foucauld, J., Uphouse, W., and Berenberg, J.: Dapsone and aplastic anemia. Ann. Intern. Med. *102*:139, 1985.
Homeida, M., Babikr, A., and Daneshmend, T. K.: Dapsone-induced optic atrophy and motor neuropathy. Br. Med. J. *281*:1180, 1980.
Kenner, D.J., et al.: Permanent retinal damage following massive dapsone overdose. Br. J. Ophthalmol. *64*:741, 1980.
Leonard, J.N., et al.: Dapsone and the retina. Lancet *1*:453, 1982.
Ree, G.H., and Kame, P.: Skin reactions to dapsone. Papua New Guinea Med. J. *24*:57, 1981.

Class: Antimalarial Agents

Generic Name: 1. Amodiaquine; 2. Chloroquine; 3. Hydroxychloroquine

Proprietary Name: 1. Flavoquine (Fr.); 2. Aralen (Canad.), **Aralen Hydrochloride**, **Aralen Phosphate**, Avloclor (G.B., Ire.), Chlorquin (Austral.),

Cidanchin (Span.), Dichinalex (Ital.), Malaviron (G.B.), Nivaquine (Austral., G.B., Ire., Fr., Neth., S. Afr., Switz.), Resochin (Germ., Span.), Résochine (Switz.), Weimerquin (Germ.); 3. Plaquenil (Austral., Fr., G.B., Ire., Ital., Neth., Swed., Switz.), **Plaquenil Sulfate** (Canad.), Quensyl (Germ.)

Primary Use: These aminoquinolines are used in the treatment of malaria, extraintestinal amebiasis, rheumatoid arthritis, and lupus erythematosus.

Ocular Side Effects:
 A. Systemic Administration
    1. Decreased vision
    2. Cornea
       a. Whirl-like deposits
       b. Hudson-Stähli lines
       c. Punctate to lineal opacities
       d. Edema—transient
       e. Decreased sensitivity
       f. Aggravation of keratoconjunctivitis sicca
    3. Retinal or macular
       a. Pigmentary changes—pigmentary retinopathy, bull's eye, doughnut
       b. Vasoconstriction
       c. Decreased or absent foveal reflex
       d. Edema
       e. Abnormal ERG or EOG
       f. Degeneration—toxic states
       g. Abnormal critical flicker fusion
       h. Increased macular recovery time
       i. Attenuation of retinal arterioles
       j. Peripheral fine granular pigmentary changes
       k. Prominent choroidal pattern
       l. Decreased dark adaptation
    4. Visual fields
       a. Scotomas—annular, central, paracentral
       b. Constriction
       c. Hemianopsia
    5. Problems with color vision
       a. Color vision defect
       b. Objects have yellow, green, or blue tinge
       c. Colored haloes around lights
    6. Nystagmus
    7. Visual hallucinations
    8. Myasthenic neuromuscular blocking effect
       a. Paralysis of extraocular muscles

      b. Ptosis
      c. Diplopia
  9. Eyelids or conjunctiva
      a. Allergic reactions
      b. Photosensitivity
      c. Poliosis
      d. Yellow discoloration
      e. Hyperpigmentation
      f. Hypopigmentation
      g. Depigmentation
      h. Blepharoclonus
      i. Blepharospasm
      j. Erythema multiforme
      k. Stevens-Johnson syndrome
      l. Exfoliative dermatitis
      m. Loss of eyelashes or eyebrows
10. Decreased accommodation
11. Oculogyric crises
12. Optic atrophy
13. Subconjunctival or retinal hemorrhages secondary to drug-induced anemia

Clinical Significance: Significant ocular side effects, including blindness, have occurred due to these drugs. It is becoming increasingly apparent that hydroxychloroquine in daily dosages not exceeding 400 mg is a much safer drug compared with chloroquine as far as ocular side effects are concerned. Chloroquine alone appears to have more ocular side effects than if given with hydroxychloroquine. Although the incidence of hydroxychloroquine side effects seems significantly less compared with chloroquine, all side effects seen with chloroquine can also be seen with hydroxychloroquine. Since amodiaquine is used comparatively infrequently, not enough data are available to make generalizations for this agent. In the United States, chloroquine is still used because some rheumatologists believe that it is a more effective arthritic agent. In dosages below 250 mg per day (3.5 to 4.0 mg/kg) and cumulative less than 300 g, chloroquine seldom causes significant ocular side effects. These guidelines are not hard and fast since significant retinal changes have occurred in rare instances at lower dosages, especially in patients with renal disease and those with low body weight. Reversible chloroquine corneal deposition has no direct relationship to posterior segment disease and may be seen as early as 3 weeks. With chloroquine, corneal changes may first appear as a Hudson-Stähli line or an increase in a pre-existing Hudson-Stähli line. Probably more common is a whirl-like pattern known as "cornea verticillata." It is known that a number of drugs and diseases can cause this pattern, which morphologically, histologically, and electron microscopically are identical. "Amphophilic" drugs, such as chloroquine, amiodarone, and chlorpromazine, form complexes with cellular phospholipids, which cannot be metabolized by lysosomal phospholipases. Therefore, these intracellular deposits occur and are visible in the superficial portion of the cornea. Corneal deposits due to hydroxychloroquine, however, are of major clinical importance. These are best seen with a dilated pupil and retroillumination. These deposits are finer and less extensive than with chloroquine. Easterbrook has found these corneal deposits to be an indicator of possible hydroxychloroquine macular toxicity. Hydroxychloroquine crystals have been found in the tear film which may aggravate some sicca patients.

Toxic maculopathy is usually reversible only in its earliest phases. If these drugs have caused skin, eyelid, corneal (hydroxychloroquine), or hair changes, this may be an indicator of possible drug-induced retinopathy. Since the aminoquinolines are concentrated in pigmented tissue, macular changes have been thought to progress long after the drug is stopped. (This is now being questioned by some investigators for hydroxychloroquine.) The bull's-eye macula is not diagnostic for aminoquinoline-induced disease since a number of other entities can cause this same clinical picture. While retinal toxicity occurs in patients taking hydroxychloroquine, the incidence is lower than with chloroquine.

How to detect early toxic changes is still the subject of debate. Easterbrook has published extensively on chloroquine and hydroxychloroquine retinal toxicity. His current method of examination includes seeing the patient every 6 months and obtaining best corrected vision, examining the cornea with the pupil dilated with retroillumination, and performing an Amsler examination. (He has his patients test themselves every few weeks at home with an Amsler grid.) If the results of the Amsler grid examination are abnormal, a Humphrey field with the 10-2 red and white program is performed. If color vision is deficient on Ishihara testing or there is any question of a patient's reliability in terms of visual field assessment, fluorescein angiography is done as well. According to Easterbrook, electroretinographic and electro-oculogram studies are either too variable or are abnormal only in late signs of chloroquine retinopathy, so their usefulness is suspect. Color testing is more useful in elderly patients where coincidental age-related macular changes occur. Easterbrook also feels that early retinopathy (i.e., small paracentral relative scotomas) does not appear to progress, at least in the short term. Patients who present with absolute scotomas and positive fluorescein angiography should be warned that their retinopathy may progress even if the chloroquine therapy is discontinued. There are numerous instances of progression of macular and optic nerve damage even years after these drugs are discontinued. This may not be as true for hydroxychloroquine since the progression of the maculopathy may be significantly less than with chloroquine once the drug is stopped.

Some patients wish to continue taking these drugs even with the visual side effects because only these drugs improve their quality of life. If reproducible abnormalities of the Amsler grids occur in this group of patients, kinetic and static perimetry are obtained. If field defects are confirmed, consultation with the rheumatologist concerning discontinuation of the drug is advised. If the patient is reluctant, one may consider halving the usual dosages and following the patient every 3-4 months even with relative paracentral scotomas with serial fields. If however, there is any progression, the recommendation is to stop the drug.

Decreased vision may initially be due to a direct effect of these aminoquinolines on the ciliary body decreasing accommodation. This effect is variable and reversible. A neuromuscular blockade can occur causing abnormal extraocular muscle responses. A myasthenia gravis-like syndrome can result. There are numerous reports of eyelid changes, which are reversible, and a few reports of lens changes attributed to chloroquine therapy that have not been fully substantiated.

References:

Beebe, W.E., Abbott, R.L., and Fung, W.E.: Hydroxychloroquine crystals in the tear film of a patient with rheumatoid arthritis. Am. J. Ophthalmol. *101*:377, 1986.

Bernstein, H.N.: Ophthalmologic considerations and testing in patients receiving long-term antimalarial therapy. Am. J. Med. *75*:25, 1983.

Easterbrook, M.: The use of Amsler grids in early chloroquine retinopathy. Ophthalmology *91*:1368, 1984.

Easterbrook, M.: Ocular effects and safety of antimalarial agents. Am. J. Med. *85*(Suppl 4A):23–29, 1988.

Easterbrook, M.: Is corneal deposition of antimalarial any indication of retinal toxicity? Can. J. Ophthalmol. *25(5)*:249–251, 1990.

Ehrenfeld, M., Nesher, R., and Merin, S.: Delayed-onset chloroquine retinopathy. Br. J. Ophthalmol. *70*:281, 1986.

Finbloom, D.S., et al.: Comparison of hydroxychloroquine and chloroquine use and the development of retinal toxicity. J. Rheumatol. *12*:692, 1985.

Hart, W.M., et al.: Static perimetry in chloroquine retinopathy. Perifoveal patterns of visual field depression. Arch. Ophthalmol. *102*:377, 1984.

Johnson, M.W., and Vine, A.K.: Hydroxychloroquine therapy in massive total doses without retinal toxicity. Am. J. Ophthalmol. *104*:139, 1987.

Khamis, A.R.A., and Easterbrook, M.: Critical flicker fusion frequency in early chloroquine retinopathy. Can. J. Ophthalmol. *18*:217, 1983.

Marks, J.S.: Chloroquine retinopathy: Is there a safe daily dose? Ann. Rheum. Dis. *41*:52, 1982.

Portnoy, J.Z., and Callen, J.P.: Ophthalmologic aspects of chloroquine and hydroxychloroquine therapy. Int. J. Dermatol. *22*:273, 1983.

Robertson, J.E., and Fraunfelder, F.T.: Hydroxychloroquine retinopathy. JAMA *255*: 403, 1986.

Rynes, R.I.: Ophthalmologic safety of long-term hydroxychloroquine sulfate treatment. Am. J. Med. *75*:35, 1983.

Sassani, J.W., et al.: Progressive chloroquine retinopathy. Ann. Ophthalmol. *15*:19, 1983.

Tobin, D.R., Krohel, G.B., and Rynes, R.I.: Hydroxychloroquine. Seven-year experience. Arch. Ophthalmol. *100*:81, 1982.

Weiner, A., et al: Hydroxychloroquine retinopathy. Am. J. Ophthalmol. *112*:528–534, 1991.

Generic Name: Quinine

Proprietary Name: Adaquir (Austral.), Bi-Chinine (Austral.), Biquin (Austral.), Biquinate (Austral.), Bisulquin (Austral.), Chinine (Austral.), **Legatrin**, Myoquin (Austral.), **Quinamm**, Quinate (Austral, Canad.), Quinbisan (Austral.), Quinbisul (Austral.), **Quindan**, Quinoctal (Austral.), Quinsan (Austral.), Quinsul (Austral.), Sulquin (Austral.)

Primary Use: This alkaloid is effective in the management of nocturnal leg cramps, myotonia congenita, and in resistant *P. falciparum*. It is also used in attempted abortions. Ophthalmologically, it is useful in the treatment of eyelid myokymia.

Ocular Side Effects:
A. Systemic Administration
   1. Decreased vision—all gradations of visual loss including toxic amblyopia
   2. Pupils
      a. Mydriasis
      b. Decreased or absent reaction to light
   3. Retinal or macular
      a. Edema
      b. Degeneration
      c. Pigmentary changes
      d. Exudates
      e. Vasodilatation followed by vasoconstriction
      f. Absence of foveal reflex
      g. Abnormal ERG, EOG, VEP or critical flicker fusion
   4. Visual sensations
      a. Distortion due to flashing lights
      b. Distortion of images secondary to sensations of wave
   5. Optic nerve
      a. Papilledema
      b. Atrophy
   6. Problems with color vision
      a. Color vision defect, red-green or blue-yellow defect
      b. Objects have red or green tinge
   7. Visual fields

      a. Scotomas
      b. Constriction
  8. Iris atrophy
  9. Eyelids or conjunctiva
      a. Allergic reactions
      b. Edema
      c. Photosensitivity
      d. Angioneurotic edema
      e. Purpura
      f. Urticaria
      g. Erythema multiforme
      h. Stevens-Johnson syndrome
10. Ocular teratogenic effects—optic nerve hypoplasia
11. Night blindness
12. Visual hallucinations
13. Vertical nystagmus
14. Subconjunctival or retinal hemorrhages secondary to drug-induced anemia
15. Myasthenic neuromuscular blocking effect
      a. Paralysis of extraocular muscles
      b. Ptosis
      c. Diplopia
16. Photophobia
17. Myopia

Clinical Significance: The use of quinine with the resultant adverse ocular side effects is on the rise. It has become increasingly used as a diluent for many of the "street drugs" and as a possible method to terminate a pregnancy. In general, quinine seldom causes ocular side effects except in overdose situations. In cases of massive exposure, visual loss may be sudden or progressive over a number of hours or days. In the worst cases, retinal arteriolar constriction, venous congestion, and retinal and papillary edema are pronounced. Complete loss of vision may occur, but most patients have some return of vision. Mild cases may only show minimal macular changes by Amsler grid, blurred vision, or some constriction of the visual field. According to the evidence currently available, the etiology of the toxic effect of quinine seems to involve not only an early effect on the outer layers of the retina and pigment epithelium, but also probably a direct effect on retinal ganglion cells and optic nerve fibers. Therapy for this entity is also controversial. Suggested treatment includes stellate ganglion blocks, vasodilators, anterior chamber paracentesis, corticosteroids, vitamin B, and iodides. It is difficult to prove that any of these have significant clinical effects, since the drug may have a direct toxic effect on the retina. It is apparent that quinine can cause optic nerve hypoplasia and decreased vision, including blindness, in the offspring secondary to prenatal maternal ingestion, if taken in toxic doses. While the primary adverse reactions are dose related and usually occur only with massive amounts, a few idiosyncratic reactions, as well as chronic low dosage exposure, may on rare occasions cause an ocular side effect.

References:

Birch, J., et al.: Acquired color vision defects. *In* Pokorny, J., et al. (Eds.): Congenital and Acquired Color Vision Defects. New York, Grune & Stratton, 1979, pp. 243–350.

Brinton, G.S., et al.: Ocular quinine toxicity. Am. J. Ophthalmol. *90*:403, 1980.

Dyson, E.H., et al.: Death and blindness due to overdose of quinine. Br. Med. J. *291*: 31, 1985.

Dyson, E.H., Proudfoot, A.T., and Bateman, D.N.: Quinine amblyopia: Is current management appropriate? Clin. Toxicol. *23*:571, 1985–1986.

Fisher, C.M.: Visual disturbances associated with quinidine and quinine. Neurology *31*:1569, 1981.

Fong, L.P., Kaufman, D.V., and Galbraith, J.E.K.: Ocular toxicity of quinine. Med. J. Aust. *141*:528, 1984.

Friedman, L., Rothkoff, L., and Zaks, U.: Clinical observations on quinine toxicity. Ann. Ophthalmol. *12*:641, 1980.

Gangitano, J.L., and Keltner, J.L.: Abnormalities of the pupil and visual-evoked potential in quinine amblyopia. Am. J. Ophthalmol. *89*:425, 1980.

Kaeser, H.E.: Drug-induced myasthenic syndromes. Acta Neurol. Scand. *70*(Suppl. 100):39, 1984.

Rheeder, P., and Sieling, W.L.: Acute, persistent quinine-induced blindness. A case report. S. Afr. Med. J. *79*:563–564, 1991.

Segal, A., Aisemberg, A., and Ducasse, A.: Quinine transitory myopia, and angle-closure glaucoma. Bull. Soc. Ophtalmol. Fr. *83*:247, 1983.

Zahn, J.R., Brinton, G.F., and Norton, E.: Ocular quinine toxicity followed by electro-retinogram, electro-oculogram, and pattern visually evoked potential. Am. J. Optom. Physiol. Optics *58*:492, 1981.

Generic Name: Mefloquine

Proprietary Name: Lariam (Austral., Fr., G.B., Germ., Ire., Neth., Swed., Switz.), Méphaquine (Switz.)

Primary Use: This agent is primarily used in the treatment of malaria.

Ocular Side Effects:

A. Systemic Administration
1. Blurred vision
2. Diplopia
3. Eyelids
   a. Urticaria
   b. Rash
   c. Pruritus
   d. Stevens-Johnson syndrome
4. Visual hallucinations

Clinical Significance: This agent was developed for resistant malaria and does not cause deposits in the cornea and retina, etc., that are seen with other commonly used antimalarial agents. This agent seldom causes ocular side effects, and few effects are serious.

References:
Ekue, J.M.K., et al.: A double-blind comparative clinical trial of mefloquine and chloroquine in symptomatic falciparum malaria. Bull. World Health Organ. *61*:713–718, 1983.

Harinasuta, T., Bunnag, D., and Wernsdorfer, W.H.: A phase II clinical trial of mefloquine in patients with chloroquine-resistant falciparum malaria in Thailand. Bull. World Health Organ. *61*:299–305, 1983.

Lobel, H.O, et al.: Effectiveness and tolerance of long-term malaria prophylaxis with mefloquine. J. Am. Med. Assoc. *3*:361–364, 1991.

Palmer, K.J., Holliday, S.M., and Brogden, R.N.: Mefloquine: A review of its antimalarial activity, pharmacokinetic properties and therapeutic efficacy. Drugs *45(3)*: 430–475, 1993.

Shlim, D.R.: Severe facial rash associated with mefloquine. (Correspondence). J. Am. Med. Assoc. *13*:2560, 1991.

Suriyamongkol, V., Timsaad, S., and Shanks, G.D.: Mefloquine chemoprophylaxis of soldiers on the Thai-Cambodian border. Southeast Asian J. Trop. Med. Public Health *22*:515–518, 1991.

Class: Antiprotozoal Agents

Generic Name: Metronidazole

Proprietary Name: Abbonidazole (S. Afr.), Amotein (Span.), Anaerobyl (S. Afr.), Anaeromet (Neth.), Arilin (Germ., Switz.), Bemetrazole (S. Afr.), Berazole (S. Afr.), Clont (Germ.), Deflamon (Ital.), Elyzol (Swed., Switz.), **Flagyl** (Austral., Canad., Fr., Germ., G.B., Ire., Ital., Neth., S. Afr., Span., Swed., Switz.), **Flagyl I.V. RTU**, Fossyol (Germ.), Gineflavir (Ital.), Medamet (S. Afr.), Metrazole (S. Afr.), **Metric**, Metrizol (Switz.), **Metro**, Metrogel (G.B.), Metrogyl (Austral.), Metrolag (Switz.), Metrolyl (G.B.), Metronide (Ire.), Metrostat (S. Afr.), Metrotop (G.B.), Metrozine (Austral.), Metrozol (G.B.), Metryl (S. Afr.), Narobic (S. Afr.), Neo-Metric (Canad.), Novonidazol (Canad.), **Protostat** (Austral.), Rathimed (Germ.), Rathimed N (Germ.), Rosalox (Switz.), Trichazole (S. Afr.), Tricho Cordes (Germ.), Trichozole (Austral.), Tricowas B (Span.), Trikacide (Canad.), Vagilen (Ital.), Vaginyl (G.B.), Zadstat (G.B.), Zolerol (S. Afr.)

Primary Use: This nitroimidazole derivative is an antibacterial and antiprotozoal agent effective in the treatment of trichomoniasis, amebiasis, giardiasis, and anaerobic bacterial infections.

Ocular Side Effects:
   A. Systemic Administration
      1. Decreased vision
      2. Photophobia
      3. Retrobulbar or optic neuritis
      4. Myopia
      5. Eyelids or conjunctiva
         a. Erythema
         b. Conjunctivitis—nonspecific
         c. Edema
         d. Photosensitivity
         e. Angioneurotic edema
         f. Urticaria
      6. Visual hallucinations
      7. Oculogyric crises
      8. Diplopia
      9. Subconjunctival or retinal hemorrhages secondary to drug-induced anemia

Clinical Significance: Ocular side effects from systemic use of metronidazole are unusual and most are reversible on discontinuation of treatment. In all probability, metronidazole can cause optic neuritis. This is associated with color vision defects, decreased vision, and various scotomas. This may be unilateral initially, but most are bilateral. A well-documented case with rechallenge shows this agent can cause a reversible myopia. Oculogyric crises have been reported in one patient who also experienced limb tremors. A midline facial defect, including telecanthus, has been reported following maternal use of this drug during the first trimester.

References:

Cantu, J.M., and Garcia-Cruz, D.: Midline facial defect as a teratogenic effect of metronidazole. Birth Defects *18*:85, 1982.

Dunn, P.M., Stewart-Brown, S., and Peel, R.: Metronidazole and the fetal alcohol syndrome. Lancet 2:144, 1979.

Grinbaum, A., et al: Transient myopia following metronidazole treatment for trichomonas vaginallis. JAMA *267(4)*:511–512, 1992.

Kirkham, G., and Gott, J.: Oculogyric crisis associated with metronidazole. Br. Med. J. *292*:174, 1986.

Metronidazole hydrochloride (Flagyl I. V.). Med. Lett. Drugs Ther. *23*:13, 1981.

Putnam, D., Fraunfelder, F.T., and Dreis, M.: Metronidazole and optic neuritis. Am. J. Ophthalmol. *112(6)*:737.

Schentag, J.J., et al.: Mental confusion in a patient treated with metronidazole-A concentration-related effect? Pharmacotherapy 2:384, 1982.

Snavely, S.R., and Hodges, G.R.: The neurotoxicity of antibacterial agents. Ann. Intern. Med. *101*:92, 1984.

Generic Name: Suramin

Proprietary Name: Suramin (S. Afr.)

Primary Use: This nonmetallic polyanion is effective in the treatment of trypanosomiasis and used as adjunctive therapy in onchocerciasis and acquired immune deficiency syndrome.

Ocular Side Effects:
   A. Systemic Administration
       1. Nonspecific ocular irritation
           a. Lacrimation
           b. Photophobia
       2. Eyelids or conjunctiva
           a. Edema
           b. Urticaria
       3. Cornea
           a. Whorl-like deposits
           b. Keratitis
       4. Iritis
       5. Optic atrophy
       6. Subconjunctival or retinal hemorrhages secondary to drug-induced anemia

Clinical Significance: Suramin can cause a variety of untoward reactions that vary in intensity and frequency with the nutritional status of the patient and reach rather serious proportions among the malnourished. Most of these adverse ocular reactions occur within 24 hours after drug administration. Suramin has been associated with a diffuse subepithelial vortex keratopathy similar to that in Fabry's disease or chloroquine keratopathy. It is postulated that the suramin-induced keratitis may be produced by lysosomal enzyme inhibition, and optic atrophy occurs secondary to an inflammatory response in the optic nerve from the dead microfilariae.

References:
Adverse effects of antiparasitic drugs. Med. Lett. Drugs Ther. *24*:12, 1982.
Holland, E.J., et al.: Suramin Keratopathy. Am. J. Ophthalmol. *106*:216–220, 1988.
Reynolds, J.E.F. (Ed.): Martindale: The Extra Pharmacopoeia. 28th Ed., London, Pharmaceutical Press, 1982, pp. 983–984.
Teich, S.A., et al.: Toxic keratopathy associated with suramin therapy. N. Engl. J. Med. *314*:1455, 1986.
Thylefors, B., and Rolland, A.: The risk of optic atrophy following suramin treatment of ocular onchocerciasis. Bull. World Health Organ. *57*:479, 1979.

Generic Name: Tryparsamide

Proprietary Name: Tryparson (G.B.)

Primary Use: This organic arsenical is used in the treatment of trypanosomiasis (African sleeping sickness).

Ocular Side Effects:
A. Systemic Administration
   1. Constriction of visual fields
   2. Decreased vision
   3. Visual sensations
      a. Smokeless fog
      b. Shimmering effect
   4. Optic neuritis
   5. Optic atrophy
   6. Toxic amblyopia

Clinical Significance: The most serious and common adverse drug reactions due to tryparsamide involve the eye. Incidence of ocular side effects vary from 3% to 20% of cases, with constriction of visual fields followed by decreased vision as the characteristic sequence. Almost 10% of individuals taking tryparsamide experience visual changes consisting of ''shimmering'' or ''dazzling,'' which may persist for days or even weeks. If the medication is not immediately discontinued following these visual changes, the pathologic condition of the optic nerve may become irreversible and progress to blindness. Due to the severity of side effects of this drug on the optic nerve, it has generally been replaced by melarsoprol.

References:
Doull, J., Klaassen, C.D., and Amdur, M.O. (Eds.): Casarett and Doull's Toxicology. The Basic Science of Poisons. 2nd Ed., New York, Macmillan, 1980, pp. 301–302.
LeJeune, J.R.: Les oligo-elements et chelateurs. Bull. Soc. Belge Ophtalmol. *160*:241, 1972.
Potts, A.M.: Duality of the optic nerve in toxicology. *In* Merigan, W.H., and Weiss, B. (Eds.): Neurotoxicity of the Visual System. New York, Raven Press, 1980, pp. 1–15.
Walsh, F.B., and Hoyt, W.F.: Clinical Neuro-Ophthalmology. 3rd Ed., Baltimore, Williams & Wilkins, Vol. III, 1969, pp. 2594–2596.

Class: Antitubercular Agents

Generic Name: Amithiozone (Thiacetazone)

Proprietary Name: None

Primary Use: This tuberculostatic agent is effective against *M. tuberculosis* and *M. leprae*.

Ocular Side Effects:
   A. Systemic Administration
      1. Decreased vision
      2. Nonspecific ocular irritation
         a. Photophobia
         b. Ocular pain
         c. Burning sensation
      3. Eyelids or conjunctiva
         a. Allergic reactions
         b. Hyperemia
         c. Blepharoconjunctivitis
         d. Erythema multiforme
         e. Stevens-Johnson syndrome
         f. Exfoliative dermatitis
         g. Hypertrichosis
      4. Retinal edema
      5. Subconjunctival or retinal hemorrhages secondary to drug-
         induced anemia

Clinical Significance: Numerous adverse ocular reactions due to amithiozone have been seen. Skin manifestations have been the most frequent.
Nearly all ocular side effects are reversible and of minor clinical significance. One instance of toxic amblyopia has been reported; however, the
patient was also receiving aminosalicylic acid.

References:
Ravindran, P., and Joshi, M.: Dermatological hypersensitivity to thiacetazone. Indian
   J. Chest. Dis. *16*:58, 1974.
Reynolds, J.E.F. (Ed.): Martindale: The ExtraPharmacopoeia. 30th Ed., London, Phar-
   maceutical Press, 1993, pp. 216–217.
Sahi, S.P., and Chandra, K.: Thiacetazone-induced Stevens-Johnson syndrome: A case
   report. Indian J. Chest Dis. *16*:124, 1974.
Sarma, O.A.: Reactions to thiacetazone. Indian J. Chest Dis. *18*:51, 1976.

Generic Name: Capreomycin

Proprietary Name: Capastat (G.B., Span.), **Capastat Sulfate**, Ogostal
(Germ.)

Primary Use: This polypeptide tuberculostatic antibiotic is effective against
M. tuberculosis. It is used when less-toxic antitubercular agents have been
ineffective.

Ocular Side Effects:
   A. Systemic Administration
      1. Visual sensations

      a. Flickering vision

      b. Flashing lights

  2. Problems with color vision—objects have white tinge

  3. Eyelids or conjunctiva

      a. Angioneurotic edema

      b. Urticaria

  4. Decreased vision

Clinical Significance: Adverse ocular reactions due to capreomycin are not common, and all ocular side effects are transitory and reversible. Decreased vision is usually of short duration and reversible.

References:

Davidson, S.I.: Reports of ocular adverse reactions. Trans. Ophthalmol. Soc. U.K. *93*: 495, 1973.

Lane, R.J.M., and Routledge, P.A.: Drug-induced neurological disorders. Drugs *26*: 124, 1983.

Reynolds,J.E.F. (Ed.): Martindale: The Extra Pharmacopoeia. 28th Ed., London, Pharmaceutical Press, 1982, pp. 1568–1569.

Generic Name: Cycloserine

Proprietary Name: Closina (Austral.), Cycloserine (G.B.), **Seromycin**

Primary Use: This isoxazolidone is effective against certain Gram-negative and Gram-positive bacteria and *M. tuberculosis*.

Ocular Side Effects:

  A. Systemic Administration

    1. Decreased vision

    2. Eyelids or conjunctiva

      a. Allergic reactions

      b. Conjunctivitis—nonspecific

      c. Photosensitivity

    3. Visual hallucinations

    4. Flickering vision

    5. Subconjunctival or retinal hemorrhages secondary to drug-induced anemia

    6. Eyelashes—increased

    7. Decreased accommodation

Clinical Significance: Although ocular complications due to cycloserine are quite rare, this drug is primarily used in combination with other drugs; therefore, pinpointing cause-and-effect for an ocular side effect is most difficult. An increased number of eyelashes (hypertrichosis) has been reported and may prompt the clinical suspicion of an immune system abnormality. Optic nerve damage (including optic neuritis and atrophy) has been reported, but these data are not conclusive.

References:

Drug Evaluations. 6th Ed., Chicago, American Medical Association, 1986, pp. 1539–1540.
Drugs that cause psychiatric symptoms. Med. Lett. Drugs Ther. *28*:81, 1986.
Gilman, A.G., Goodman, L.S., and Gilman, A. (Eds.): The Pharmacological Basis of Therapeutics. 6th Ed., New York, Macmillan, 1980, pp. 1210–1211.
Grant, W.M.: Toxicology of the Eye. 3rd Ed., Springfield, Charles C Thomas, 1986, p. 300.
Walsh, F.B., and Hoyt, W.F.: Clinical Neuro-Ophthalmology. 3rd Ed. Baltimore, Williams & Wilkins, Vol. III, 1969, p. 2680.
Weaver, D.T., Bartley, G.B.: Cyclosporine-induced trichomegaly. Am. J. Ophthalmol. *109(2)*:239, 1990.

Generic Name: Ethambutol

Proprietary Name: Cidanbutol (Span.), Dexambutol (Fr.), EMB (Germ.), Etapiam (Ital.), Etibi (Canad., Ital.), Inagen (Span.), Miambutol (Ital.), **Myambutol** (Austral., Canad., Fr., G.B., Germ., Neth., Span., Swed., Switz.), Mycrol (S. Afr.)

Primary Use: Ethambutol is a tuberculostatic agent that is effective against *M. tuberculosis.*

Ocular Side Effects:

A. Systemic Administration
   1. Decreased vision
   2. Visual fields
      a. Scotomas—annular, central, or centrocecal
      b. Constriction
      c. Hemianopsia
      d. Enlarged blind spot
   3. Optic nerve
      a. Retrobulbar or optic neuritis
      b. Papilledema
      c. Peripapillary atrophy
   4. Photophobia
   5. Problems with color vision—color vision defect, red-green or blue-yellow defect
   6. Retinal or macular
      a. Vascular
         (1) Hemorrhages

      (2) Dilatation
      (3) Spasms
    b. Edema
    c. Pigmentary changes
  7. Paresis of extraocular muscles
  8. Eyelids or conjunctiva-Lyell's syndrome
  9. Toxic amblyopia
 10. Abnormal VEP

Clinical Significance: A large number of adverse ocular responses due to ethambutol are reversible, but there are some well-documented irreversible changes, including blindness. The "D" isomer of ethambutol is the form currently in use, since the "L" isomer caused significant toxic optic nerve effects. In general the side effects of ethambutol are dose related, although occasionally an adverse ocular response may occur after only a few days or weeks of therapy. There are histologic data in primates and in humans that this drug can cause chiasmal demyelinization. Although between 1% and 2% of patients taking 25 mg/kg or more of ethambutol will have a significant adverse ocular effect, the ethambutol daily dosage range of 15 mg/kg appears to be comparatively free from adverse ocular effects. While the onset of most adverse ocular reactions is abrupt, they may occasionally be insidious.

There are two types of optic neuritis, axial and periaxial. The axial type is associated with a macular degeneration, decreased visual acuity, and decreased color perception. The periaxial type is more often associated with visual field defects, paracentral scotomas with normal vision, and normal color perception. With axial involvement, green color vision testing loss is more common than red loss. Symptoms of optic neuritis generally first become evident 3 to 6 months after starting the drug. The use of visual evoked cortical responses and color discrimination as potential means to detect subclinical optic toxic effects secondary to ethambutol has been confirmed, while the use of electroretinographic findings remains controversial.

The management of patients already receiving or about to receive ethambutol therapy should include the following: an ocular examination before starting therapy and informed patient consent if there is a history of optic atrophy or optic neuritis. Patients with renal disease have a much higher incidence of optic nerve toxicity because blood levels of ethambutol are elevated due to the inability of the body to rid itself of the drug. Patients should be instructed in home testing for visual acuity and color vision. If the dosage exceeds 15 mg/kg, screening the patient on 2- to 4-week intervals is recommended. If there is any change in the patient's vision, he or she should be instructed to stop the drug and seek an ocular examination. Visual recovery is variable but usually occurs within 3 to 12 months, although in some instances no recovery is obtained. There are data to suggest that cases of optic nerve toxicity should be treated with 100 to 250 mg of oral zinc sulfate three times daily. When the vision does not improve 10 to 15 weeks after ethambutol discontinuation, parenteral administration of 40 mg of hydroxocobalamin daily over a 10- to 28-week period has been suggested as a possible treatment.

References:
Arruga, J.: Test of subjective desaturation of color in diagnosis of effect of ethambutol on anterior optic pathway. Bull. Soc. Ophtalmol. Fr. *82*:182, 1982.

Chatterjee, V.K.K., et al.: Ocular toxicity following ethambutol in standard dosage. Br. J. Dis. Chest *80*:288, 1986.

Chaulet, P.: Toxicity of modern tuberculosis chemotherapy regimens. Drugs Exp. Clin. Res. *8*:443, 1982.

Gigon, S., and de Haller, R.: Retinal lesions due to ethambutol and serum levels of zinc and vitamin A. Klin. Monatsbl. Augenheilkd. *182*:469, 1983.

Hennekes, R.: Clinical ERG findings in ethambutol intoxication. Graefes Arch. Clin. Exp. Ophthalmol. *218*:319, 1982.

Joubert, P.H., et al.: Subclinical impairment of colour vision in patients receiving ethambutol. Br. J. Clin. Pharmacol. *21*:213, 1986.

Karnik, A.M., Al-Shamali, M.A., and Fenech, F.F.: A case of ocular toxicity to ethambutol—An idiosyncratic reaction? Postgrad. Med. J. *61*:719, 1985.

Trau, R., et al.: Early diagnosis of Myambutol (ethambutol) ocular toxicity by electrophysiological examination. Bull. Soc. Belge Ophtalmol. *193*:201, 1981.

Yiannikas, C., Walsh, J.C., and McLeod, J.G.: Visual evoked potentials in the detection of subclinical optic toxic effects secondary to ethambutol. Arch. Neurol. *40*:645, 1983.

Generic Name: Ethionamide

Proprietary Name: Ethatyl (S. Afr.), Etiocidan (Span.), Trécator (Fr.), **Trecator**

Primary Use: This isonicotinic acid derivative is effective against *M. tuberculosis* and *M. leprae*. It is indicated in the treatment of patients when resistance to primary tuberculostatic drugs has developed.

Ocular Side Effects:
A. Systemic Administration
1. Decreased vision
2. Diplopia
3. Eyelids or conjunctiva
   a. Allergic reactions
   b. Erythema
   c. Photosensitivity
   d. Urticaria
   e. Exfoliative dermatitis

4. Photophobia
5. Problems with color vision
   a. Color vision defect
   b. Heightened color perception
6. Visual hallucinations

Clinical Significance: The incidence of adverse ocular effects due to ethionamide is quite small and seldom of clinical significance. While certain adverse effects occur at low dosage levels, they usually do not continue even if the dosage is increased. Optic neuritis has been reported, but in so few cases that it is difficult to pinpoint a cause-and-effect relationship.

References:

Argov, Z., Mastaglia, F.L.: Drug-induced peripheral neuropathies. Br. Med. J. *1*: 663–666, 1979.

Drugs that cause psychiatric symptoms. Med. Lett. Drugs Ther. *28*:81, 1986.

Fox, W., et al.: A study of acute intolerance to ethionamide, including a comparison with prothionamide, and of the influence of a vitamin B-complex additive in prophylaxis. Tubercule *50*:125, 1969.

Michiels, J. (Ed.): Noxious effects of systemic medications on the visual apparatus. Bull. Soc. Belge. Ophtalmol. *160*:5-516, 1972. (French)

Reynolds, J.E.F. (Ed.): Martindale: The Extra Pharmacopoeia. 30th Ed., London, Pharmaceutical Press, 1993, pp. 166.

Zurcher, K., and Krebs, A.: Cutaneous Side Effects of Systemic Drugs. Basel, S. Karger, 1980, pp. 18–19.

Generic Name: Isoniazid

Proprietary Name: Anidrasona (Span.), Cemidon (Span.), Cin (Ital.), Isotamine (Canad.), Isozid (Germ.), **Laniazid Syrup**, Nicazide (Ital.), Nicizina (Ital.), Nicozid (Ital.), Pyreazid (Span.), Rimifon (Fr., G.B., Switz.), tebesium-s (Germ.), Tibinide (Swed.)

Primary Use: This hydrazide of isonicotinic acid is effective against *M. tuberculosis.*

Ocular Side Effects:

A. Systemic Administration
   1. Decreased vision
   2. Retrobulbar or optic neuritis
   3. Optic atrophy
   4. Visual fields
      a. Scotomas
      b. Constriction
      c. Hemianopsia

5. Papilledema
6. Problems with color vision—color vision defect, red-green defect
7. Eyelids or conjunctiva
    a. Allergic reactions
    b. Angioneurotic edema
    c. Urticaria
    d. Lupoid syndrome
    e. Erythema multiforme
    f. Stevens-Johnson syndrome
    g. Exfoliative dermatitis
    h. Lyell's syndrome
8. Pupils
    a. Mydriasis
    b. Absence of reaction to light
9. Paralysis of accommodation
10. Diplopia
11. Paresis of extraocular muscles
12. Keratitis
13. Nystagmus
14. Subconjunctival or retinal hemorrhages secondary to drug-induced anemia
15. Toxic amblyopia
16. Photophobia
17. Visual hallucinations

Clinical Significance: The true incidence or significance of isoniazid-induced ocular side effects is difficult to evaluate since they are seen most commonly in malnourished, chronic alcoholics and in individuals who are characteristically taking multiple drugs. Diabetics and patients with hepatic insufficiency, hyperthyroidism, and epilepsy are more prone to display adverse reactions to isoniazid. Many, if not almost all, of the neurologic side effects can be prevented by the daily administration of pyridoxine. Under current guidelines of therapy for this drug, one would not expect to see any of the above ocular side effects. Signs and symptoms other than the neuro-ophthalmic complications are usually insignificant and reversible. It has been shown that isoniazid can cause an antinuclear antibody in the majority of patients taking this drug; however, only a small percentage develop the lupus syndrome.

References:
Alarcón-Segovia, A.: Drug-induced antinuclear antibodies and lupus syndromes. Drugs *12*:69, 1976.
Birch, J., et al.: Acquired color vision defects. *In* Pokorny, J., et al. (Eds.): Congenital

and Acquired Color Vision Defects. New York, Grune & Stratton, 1979, pp. 243–350.

Bomb, B.S,, Purohit, S.D., and Bedi, H.K.: Stevens-Johnson syndrome caused by isoniazid. Tubercle 57:229, 1976.

Karmon, G., et al.: Bilateral optic neuropathy due to combined ethambutol and isoniazid treatment. Ann. Ophthalmol. 11:1013, 1979.

Kiyosawa, M., and Ishikawa, S.: A case of isoniazid-induced optic neuropathy. Neuro-Ophthalmology 2:67, 1981.

Nair, K.G.: Optic neuritis due to INH complicating tuberculous meningitis. J. Assoc. Physicians India 24:263, 1976.

Neff, T.A.: Isoniazid toxicity—lactic acidosis and keratopathy. Chest 59:245, 1971.

Renard, G., and Morax, P.V.: Optic neuritis in the course of treatment of tuberculosis. Ann. Oculist 210:53, 1977.

Stratton, M.A.: Drug-induced systemic lupus erythematosus. Clin. Pharm. 4:657, 1985.

Zurcher, K, and Krebs, A.: Cutaneous Side Effects of Systemic Drugs. Basel, S. Karger, 1980, pp. 18–21.

Generic Name: Rifabutin

Proprietary Names: Mycobutin

Primary Use: This agent is used in the treatment of *Mycobacterium avium*, leprosy, tuberculosis, staphylococcal infections, brucellosis, HIV, and legionnaires' disease. It is also used in the prophylaxis of haemophilus, meningococcal meningitis, and *Mycobacterium avium*.

Ocular Side Effects:
   A. Systemic Administration
      1. Iridocyclitis
      2. Hypopyon
      3. Blurred vision
      4. Pain
      5. Posterior uveitis
      6. Eyelids
         a. Contact dermatitis
         b. Rashes
         c. Orange-tan discoloration
      7. Conjunctival-retinal micro-hemorrhages

Clinical Significance: An anterior uveitis is commonly seen in AIDS patients and can be a diagnostic and therapeutic challenge. However, there has been a large series of well-documented cases where a fulminating unilateral or bilateral anterior uveitis with or without hypopyon, with or without a vitritis, has been reported in AIDS patients taking rifabutin. The fulminating nature of this response with associated hypopyon and a rapid clearing with intensive topical ocular steroids sets this apart from the infectious forms of uveitis in patients with AIDS. This ocular inflammatory response clears on topical ocular steroids with or without reduction of rifabutin's therapy. The etiology of this uveitis is unknown, and Jacobs, et al. postulate the possibility of interaction of multiple drugs, an altered immune system, underlying infections, or drug-related factors contributing to the development of this uveitis syndrome. High doses of rifabutin also have been associated with an orange-tan discoloration of the skin that may also involve the sclera and oral mucosa.

References:

Brogden, R.N., and Fitton, A.: Rifabutin: A review of its antimicrobial activity, pharmacokinetic properties and therapeutic efficacy. Drugs 47(6):983–1009, 1994.

Frank, M.O., Graham, M.B., and Wispelway, B.: Rifabutin and uveitis. To the Editor. N. Engl. J. Med.:868, 1994.

Jacobs, D.S., et al.: Acute uveitis associated with rifabutin use in patients with human immunodeficiency virus infection. Am. J. Ophthalmol. 118:716–722, 1994.

Saran, B.R., et al.: Hypopyon uveitis in patients with acquired immunodeficiency syndrome treated for systemic Mycobacterium avium complex infection with rifabutin. Arch. Ophthalmol. 112:1159–1165, 1994.

Shafran, S.D., et al. Uveitis and pseudojaundice during a regimen of clarithromycin, rifabutin, and ethambutol. N. Engl. J. Med. 330:438, 1994.

Generic Name: Rifampin (Rifampicin)

Proprietary Name: *Systemic*: Diabacil (Span.), Dinoldin (Span.), Eremfat (Germ.), Rifa (Germ.), **Rifadin** (Austral., Canad., G.B., Ital., Neth., S. Afr., Swed.), Rifadine (Fr.), Rifagen (Span.), Rifaldin (Span.), Rifapiam (Ital.), Rifaprodin (Span.), Rifcin (S. Afr.), Rifoldine (Switz.), Rimactan (Fr., Germ., Ital., Neth., Span., Swed., Switz.), **Rimactane** (Canad., G.B., Ire., S. Afr.), Rimycin (Austral.), Rofact (Canad.) *Ophthalmic*: **Rifampin**

Primary Use: *Systemic:* This bactericidal as well as bacteriostatic agent is effective against *Mycobacterium,* many Gram-positive cocci, and some Gram-negative cocci, including *Neisseria* species and *Hemophilus influenzae. Ophthalmic:* This agent is used for treatment of ocular chlamydia infections.

Ocular Side Effects:
A. Systemic Administration
1. Decreased vision
2. Eyelids or conjunctiva
   a. Hyperemia
   b. Erythema
   c. Blepharoconjunctivitis
   d. Edema

      e. Yellow or red discoloration
      f. Angioneurotic edema
      g. Urticaria
      h. Purpura
      i. Lupoid syndrome
      j. Stevens-Johnson syndrome
      k. Exfoliative dermatitis
      l. Pemphigoid lesion
   3. Lacrimation
   4. Problems with color vision—color vision defect, red-green defect
   5. Tears and/or contact lenses stained orange
   6. Uveitis
   7. Subconjunctival or retinal hemorrhages secondary to drug-induced anemia
  B. Local Ophthalmic Use or Exposure
   1. Irritation
      a. Lacrimation
      b. Hyperemia
      c. Ocular pain
      d. Edema

Clinical Significance: Ocular side effects from rifampin may occur in 5% to 15% of patients, depending on the frequency and amount of this drug. Reactions vary from conjunctival hyperemia, to a mild blepharoconjunctivitis, to a painful severe exudative conjunctivitis. The latter includes tender, markedly congested palpebral and bulbar conjunctiva with thick white exudates. Although not all patients secrete this drug or a byproduct in their tears, the Registry has received reports of orange staining of contact lenses and the inability to wear lenses while taking this drug. In general, these ocular side effects appear to occur more frequently during intermittent treatment than during daily treatment and have been reversible when the drug has been discontinued. Topical ocular use of 1% rifampin ointment has been reported to cause approximately a 10% incidence of adverse effects, which are primarily due to irritation and include discomfort, tearing, lid edema, and conjunctival hyperemia. The irritation, discomfort, and tearing usually last only 10 to 50 minutes after the application of the ointment.

References:

Birch, J., et al.: Acquired color vision defects. *In* Pokorny, J., et al. (Eds.): Congenital and Acquired Color Vision Defects. New York, Grune & Stratton, 1979, pp. 243–350.

Bolan, G., Laurie, R.E., and Broome, C.V.: Red man syndrome: Inadvertent administration of an excessive dose of rifampin to children in a day-care center. Pediatrics 77:633, 1986.

Darougar, S., et al.: Topical therapy of hyperendemic trachoma with rifampicin, oxytetracycline, or spiramycin eye ointments. Br. J. Ophthalmol. *64*:37, 1980.

Fraunfelder F.T.: Orange tears. Am. J. Ophthalmol. *89*:752, 1980.

Girling, D.J.: Ocular toxicity due to rifampicin. Br. Med. J. *1*:585, 1976.

Grosset, J. and Leventis, S.: Adverse effects of rifampin. Rev. Infect. Dis. *5*(Suppl.
3):440, 1983.

Lyons, R.W.: Orange contact lenses from rifampin. N. Engl. J. Med. *300*:372, 1979.

Mangi, R.J.: Reactions to rifampin. N. Engl. J. Med. *294*:113, 1976.

Nyirenda, R., and Gill, G.V.: Stevens-Johnson syndrome due to rifampicin. Br. Med.
J. *2*:1189, 1977.

Ruocco, V. and Pisani, M.: Induced pemphigus. Arch. Dermatol. Res. *274*:123, 1982.

Stewart, W.M.: Pemphigus et pemphigoide. Dermatologica *160*:217, 1980.

Generic Name Streptomycin. See under *Class: Antibiotics.*

II Agents Affecting the Central Nervous System

Class: Analeptics

Generic Name: Lamotrigine

Proprietary Name: Lamictal (G.B.)

Primary Use: This is an antiepileptic drug believed to suppress seizures by inhibiting the release of excitatory neurotransmitters.

Ocular Side Effects:
  A. Systemic Administration
    1. Diplopia
    2. Blurred vision
    3. Nystagmus
    4. Angioneurotic edema
    5. Stevens-Johnson syndrome

Clinical Significance: In a controlled trial, as many as 33% of patients taking this agent developed diplopia and 24% had blurred vision compared with those taking a placebo. About 9% of patients could not tolerate the drug, in part for the above reasons, but also because of rash, increased frequency of seizures, nausea, and vomiting. In less than 5% of patients taking this drug nystagmus would occur, but if the dosage of lamotrigine was decreased, this side effect usually abated.

References:
Betts, T., et al.: Human safety of lamotrigine. Epilepsia *32*(Suppl. 1):17–21, 1991.
Goa, K.L., Ross, S.R., and Chrisp, P.: Lamotrigine. Drugs *46(1)*:152–176, 1993.
Schachter, S.C.: A multicenter, placebo-controlled evaluation of the safety of lamotrigine (Lamictal®) as add-on therapy in out-patients with partial seizures. Presented at the 1992 Annual Meeting of the American Epilepsy Society, Seattle, December 4–10, 1992.

Class: Anorexiants

Generic Name: 1. Amphetamine; 2. Dextroamphetamine (Dexamphetamine); 3. Methamphetamine; 4. Phenmetrazine

Proprietary Name: 1. Centramina (Span.); 2. Dexedrina (Span.), **Dexedrine** (Canad., G.B.); 3. **Desoxyn**; 4. **Preludin Endurets**

Street Name: 1-3. Crank, Rx Diet Pills, Speed, Uppers, Ups

Primary Use: These sympathomimetic amines are used in the management of exogenous obesity. Amphetamine, dextroamphetamine, and methamphetamine are also effective in narcolepsy and in the management of minimal brain dysfunction in children.

Ocular Side Effects:
 A. Systemic Administration
  1. Decreased vision
  2. Pupils
   a. Mydriasis—may precipitate narrow-angle glaucoma
   b. Decreased reaction to light
  3. Widening of palpebral fissure
  4. Decreased accommodation
  5. Decreased convergence
  6. Visual hallucinations
  7. Problems with color vision—objects have blue tinge (amphetamine)
  8. Blepharospasm
  9. Retina—toxic states (phenmetrazine)
   a. Venous thrombosis
   b. Intraretinal hemorrhage (methamphetamine)
  10. Posterior subcapsular cataracts—toxic states (phenmetrazine)
  11. Ocular teratogenic effects (methamphetamine)

Clinical Significance: Ocular side effects due to these sympathomimetic amines are seldom of consequence and are mainly seen in overdose situations. Possible posterior subcapsular cataracts were seen in two young females taking phenmetrazine who were on a massive weight-reduction program and whose vision decreased enough to require cataract extraction. Retinal venous thrombosis can occur with massive dosages of phenmetrazine. Blurred vision and intraretinal hemorrhages have been reported in a case of intranasal methamphetamine abuse. Septic submacular choroidal embolus has been associated with heroin and phenmetrazine abuse.

References:

Acute drug abuse reactions. Med. Lett. Drugs Ther. *27*:77, 1985.

D'Souza, T., and Shraberg, D.: Intracranial hemorrhage associated with amphetamine use. Neurology *31*:922, 1981.

Gualtieri, C.T., and Evans, R.W.: Carbamazepine-induced tics. Dev. Med. Child Neurol. *26*:546, 1984.

Lien, E.J., and Koda, R.T.: Structure-side effect sorting of drugs: V. Glaucoma and cataracts associated with drugs and chemicals. Drug Intell. Clin. Pharm. *15*:434, 1981.

Limaye, S.R., and Goldberg, M.H.: Septic submacular choroidal embolus associated with intravenous drug abuse. Ann. Ophthalmol. *14*:518, 1982.

Lowe, T., et al.: Stimulant medications precipitate Tourette's syndrome. JAMA *247*: 1729, 1982.

Spaeth, G.L., Nelson, L.B., and Beaudoin, A.R.: Ocular teratology. *In* Jakobiec, F.A. (Ed.): Ocular Anatomy, Embryology and Teratology. Philadelphia, J.B. Lippincott, 1982, pp. 955–975.

Vesterhauge, S., and Peitersen, E.: The effects of some drugs on the caloric induced nystagmus. Adv. Otorhinolaryngol. *25*:173, 1979.

Wallace, R.T., et al.: Sudden retinal manifestations of intranasal cocaine and methamphetamine abuse. Am. J. Ophthalmol. *114*:158–160, 1992.

Generic Name: 1. Benzphetamine; 2. Chlorphentermine; 3. Diethylpropion (Amfepramone); 4. Fenfluramine; 5. Phendimetrazine; 6. Phentermine

Proprietary Name: 1. **Didrex;** 2. Pre-Sate (Canad. Fr.); 3. Anorex (Fr.), Delgamer (Span.), Linea (Ital.), Modératan Diffucap (Fr.), Nobesine (Canad.), Préfamone Chronules (Fr., Switz.), Regenon (Germ., Switz.), **Tenuate** (Canad.), **Tenuate Dospan** (Fr., G.B.,, Ital., S. Afr.), Tenuate Retard (Germ., Switz.), **Tepanil;** 4. Dima-Fen (Ital.), Fenured (S. Afr.), Pesos (Ital.), Pondéral (Fr.), Ponderal (Canad., Ital., Neth., Span.), Ponderax (Austral., G.B., Germ., Ire., S. Afr.), **Pondimin** (Canad.), Ponflural (Switz.); 5. **Adipost, Bontril, Dital,** Obesan-X (S. Afr.), Obex-LA (S. Afr.), **Phenazine, Plegine** (Ital.), **Prelu-2, Rexigen Forte, Trimstat, Wehless-105 Timecelles, X-trozine;** 6. **Adipex-P,** Duromine (Austral., G.B., S. Afr.), **Fastin** (Canad.), **Ionamin** (Canad., G.B.), Ionamine (Switz.), Minobese (S. Afr.), Normaform (Switz.), **Oby-Trim 30, T-Diet, Teramine, Zantryl**

Primary Use: These sympathomimetic amines are used in the treatment of exogenous obesity.

Ocular Side Effects:

    A. Systemic Administration

        1. Decreased vision

        2. Pupils

            a. Mydriasis—may precipitate narrow-angle glaucoma

            b. Absence of reaction to light (fenfluramine)—toxic states

3. Rotary nystagmus (fenfluramine)—toxic states
4. Decreased accommodation
5. Diplopia
6. Visual hallucinations
7. Nonspecific ocular irritation
   a. Photophobia
   b. Ocular pain
   c. Burning sensation
8. Eyelids or conjunctiva
   a. Allergic reactions
   b. Erythema
   c. Urticaria
9. Subconjunctival or retinal hemorrhages secondary to drug-induced anemia (fenfluramine)

Clinical Significance: Ocular side effects due to these sympathomimetic amines are rare and seldom of clinical significance. Nystagmus and dilated nonreactive pupils can occur in fenfluramine overdose. Posterior subcapsular cataracts have been reported in patients receiving phentermine or diethylpropion, but a cause-and-effect relationship has not been proven.

References:
Campbell, D.B.: Signs and symptoms of fenfluramine overdosage and its treatment—The question of drug interactions. S. Afr. Med. J. *45*(Suppl.) 51, 1971.
Riley, I., et al.: Fenfluramine overdosage. Lancet 2:1162, 1969.
Veltri, J.C., and Temple, A.R.: Fenfluramine poisoning. J. Pediatr. *87*:119, 1975.

Generic Name: Phenylpropanolamine

Proprietary Name: Acutrim Late Day, **Amfed TD**, Dexatrim (Switz), **Diet-Aid**, Fugoa N (Switz.), Kontexin Retard (Switz.), Monydrin (Swed.), Procol (G.B.), **Propagest**, Rinexin (Swed.), **Stay Trim**

Street Name: Black Beauty, Pink Lady, Speckled Pup

Primary Use: This sympathomimetic agent is used in the symptomatic treatment of hay fever and allergic rhinitis and for short-term treatment of exogenous obesity. Phenylpropanolamine has been mistaken for "look-alike" illicit amphetamines.

Ocular Side Effects:
A. Systemic Administration
   1. Decreased vision
   2. Pupils
      a. Mydriasis—may precipitate narrow-angle glaucoma

      b. Anisocoria—toxic states
      c. Absence of reaction to light—toxic states
   3. Visual hallucinations
   4. Retinal vascular disorders
      a. Thrombosis
      b. Hemorrhage
      c. Spasm
   5. Papilledema secondary to pseudotumor cerebri
   6. Optokinetic nystagmus
   7. May aggravate hyperthyroidism

Clinical Significance: The incidence of adverse effects in patients receiving therapeutic doses of phenylpropanolamine is low. Excessive doses of phenylpropanolamine may produce pupillary disorders and acute psychotic reactions, including colored hallucinations. Numerous reports to the Registry include retinal vascular abnormalities, pseudotumor cerebri, and optokinetic nystagmus; however, these are all with excessive phenylpropanolamine use.

References:

Bale, J.F., Jr., Fountain, M.T., and Shaddy, R.: Phenylpropanolamine-associated CNS complications in children and adolescents. Am. J. Dis. Child. *138*:683, 1984.

Fallis, R.J., and Fisher, M.: Cerebral vasculitis and hemorrhage associated with phenylpropanolamine. Neurology *35*:405, 1985.

Gillmer, G., et al.: Over-the-counter phenylpropanolamine: A possible cause of central retinal vein occlusion. Arch. Ophthalmol. *104*:642, 1986.

Kase, C.S., et al.: Intracerebral hemorrhage and phenylpropanolamine use. Neurology *37*:399, 1987.

McDowell, J.R., and LeBlanc, H.J.: Phenylpropanolamine and cerebral hemorrhage. West. J. Med. *142*:688, 1985.

Mueller, S.: Neurologic complications of phenylpropanolamine use. Neurology *33*: 650, 1983.

Class: Antianxiety Agents

Generic Name: 1. Alprazolam; 2. Chlordiazepoxide; 3. Clonazepam; 4. Clorazepate; 5. Diazepam; 6. Flurazepam; 7. Halazepam; 8. Lorazepam; 9. Midazolam; 10. Nitrazepam; 11. Oxazepam; 12. Prazepam; 13. Temazepam; 14. Triazolam

Proprietary Name: 1. Tafil (Germ.), Trankimazin (Span.), Valeans (Ital.), **Xanax** (Austral., Canad., Fr., G.B., Ire., Ital., Switz.), Xanor (S. Afr., Swed.); 2. Benzodiapin (Ital.), Huberplex (Span.), **Libritabs**, **Librium** (Austral., Canad., Fr., G.B., Germ., Ire., Ital., Neth., S. Afr., Span., Swed., Switz.), Medilium (Canad.), Multum (Germ.), Normide (Span.), Novopoxide (Canad.), Omnalio (Span.), Psicofar (Ital.), Psicoterina (Ital.), Reliberan

(Ital.), Seren (Ital.), Solium (Canad.), Tropium (G.B.); 3. Iktorivil (Swed.), **Klonopin**, Rivotril (Austral., Canad., Fr., G.B., Germ., Ire., Ital., Neth., S. Afr., Span., Switz.); 4. **Clorazecaps**, **Clorazetabs**, **Gen-Xene**, Nansius (Span.), Novoclopate (Canad.), Transene (Ital.), Tranxène (Fr., Neth.), **Tranxene** (Austral., Canad., G.B., S. Afr.), Tranxilen (Swed.), Tranxilium (Germ., Span., Switz.); 5. Aliseum (Ital.), Ansiolin (Ital.), Antenex (Austral.), Anxicalm (Ire.), Apozepam (Swed.), Atensine (G.B., Ire.), Benzopin (S. Afr.), Betapam (S. Afr.), Calmigen (Ire.), Diaceplex (Span.), Dialar (G.B.), Diaquel (S. Afr.), Diazemuls (Austral., Canad., G.B., Germ., Ire., Neth.), Doval (S. Afr.), Drenian (Span.), Ducene (Austral.), Eridan (Ital.), Ethipam (S. Afr.), Lamra (Germ.), Mandro-Zep (Germ.), Meval (Canad.), Neurolytril (Germ.), Noan (Ital.), Novazam (Fr.), Novodipam (Canad.), Paceum (Switz.), Pax (S. Afr.), Pro-Pam (Austral.), Psychopax (Switz.), Rima-pam (G.B.), Scriptopam (S. Afr.), Sico Relax (Span.), Solis (G.B.), Stesolid (G.B., Neth., Span., Swed., Switz.), Tensium (G.B.), **T-Quil**, Tranquase (Germ.), Tranquirit (Ital.), Tranquo (Germ.), Valaxona (Germ.), Valiquid (Germ.), Valitran (Ital.), **Valium** (Austral., Canad., Fr., G.B., Germ., Ire., Ital., Neth., S. Afr., Span., Swed., Switz.), **Valrelease**, Vatran (Ital.), Vivol (Canad.); 6. Dalmadorm (Germ., Ital., Neth., S. Afr., Switz.), **Dalmane** (Austral., Canad., G.B., Ire.), Dormodor (Span.), Felison (Ital.), Flunox (Ital.), Irdal (Ire.), Midorm A.R. (Ital.), Novoflupam (Canad.), Remdue (Ital.), Somnol (Canad.), Valdorm (Ital.); 7. Alapryl (Span.), Pacinone (Neth.), **Paxipam** (Ital.); 8. Almazine (G.B.), **Ativan** (Austral., Canad., G.B., Ire., S. Afr.), Control (Ital.), Donix (Span.), Duralozam (Germ.), Idalprem (Span.), Laubeel (Germ.), Lorans (Ital.), **Loraz**, Novolorazem (Canad.), Orfidal (Span.), Pro Dorm (Germ.), Punktyl (Germ.), Sedizepan (Span.), Somagerol (Germ.), Tavor (Germ., Ital.), Témesta (Fr.), Temesta (Neth, Swed., Switz.), Tolid (Germ.), Tran-Qil (S. Afr.), Tranqipam (S. Afr.); 9. Dormicum (Germ., Neth., S. Afr., Span., Swed., Switz.), Hypnovel (Austral., Fr., G.B.), **Versed** (Canad.); 10. Alodorm (Austral.), Apodorm (Swed.), Arem (S. Afr.), Dormigen (Ire.), Dormo-Puren (Germ.), Eatan N (Germ.), Imeson (Germ.), Imeson (Switz.), Insoma (Austral.), Ipersed (Ital.), Mitidin (Ital.), Mogadan (Germ.), Mogadon (Austral., Canad., Fr., G.B., Ire., Ital., Neth., S. Afr., Span., Swed., Switz.), Nitrados (Ire.), Nitrazepan (Span.), Novanox (Germ.), Ormodon (S. Afr.), Paxadorm (S. Afr.), Pelson (Span.), Remnos (G.B.), Somnibel N (Germ.), Somnipar (S. Afr.), Somnite (G.B.), Surem (G.B.), Tri (Ital.), Unisomnia (G.B.); 11. Adumbran (Germ., Ital., Span.), Alepam (Austral.), Alopam (Swed.), Anxiolit (Switz.), Aplakil (Span.), Azutranquil (Germ.), Benzotran (Austral.), durazepam (Germ.), Limbial (Ital.), Murelax (Austral.), Noctazepam (Germ.), Norkotral N (Germ.), Novoxapam (Canad.), Oxaline (S. Afr.), Oxa-Puren (Germ.), Praxiten (Germ.), Psiquiwas (Span.), Purata (S. Afr.), Quilibrex (Ital.), **Serax** (Canad.), Serepax (Austral., S. Afr., Swed.), Séresta (Fr.), Seresta (Neth., Switz.), Serpax (Ital.), Sigacalm (Germ.), Sobile (Span.), Sobril (Swed.), Uskan (Germ., Switz.), Zapex (Canad.), **Zaxopam**; 12. **Centrax** (Ire.), Demetrin (Germ., S. Afr., Span., Switz.), Lysanxia (Fr.), Mono-Demetrin (Germ.), Prazene (Ital.), Reapam (Neth.), Trepidan (Ital.); 13. Euhypnos (Austral., G.B., S. Afr.), Levanxol (S. Afr.), Normison (Austral., Fr., G.B., Ire., Neth., S. Afr., Switz.), Planum (Germ., Switz.), Remestan (Germ.), **Restoril** (Canad.), **Temaz**, Temaze (Austral.), Tenso (Span.), Z-Pam (S. Afr.); 14. Apo-Triazo (Canad.), Dumozolam (Swed.), **Halcion** (Canad., Fr., Germ., Ire., Ital., Neth., S. Afr., Span., Swed., Switz.), Novodorm (Span.), Songar (Ital.)

Primary Use: These benzodiazepine derivatives are effective in the management of psychoneurotic states manifested by anxiety, tension, or agitation. They are also used as adjunctive therapy in the relief of skeletal muscle spasms and as preoperative medications.

Ocular Side Effects:
  A. Systemic Administration
    1. Decreased vision
    2. Eyelids or conjunctiva
      a. Allergic reactions
      b. Erythema
      c. Conjunctivitis—nonspecific
      d. Photosensitivity
      e. Angioneurotic edema
      f. Urticaria
      g. Purpura
      h. Erythema multiforme
      i. Blepharospasm (lorazepam)
    3. Decreased corneal reflex (clorazepate, diazepam)
    4. Extraocular muscles
      a. Oculogyric crises
      b. Decreased spontaneous movements
      c. Abnormal conjugate deviations
      d. Jerky pursuit movements
      e. Decreased saccadic movements
      f. Nystagmus—horizontal or gaze evoked
      g. Paralysis
    5. Decreased accommodation
    6. Decreased depth perception (chlordiazepoxide)
    7. Diplopia
    8. Visual hallucinations
    9. Pupils
      a. Mydriasis—may precipitate narrow-angle glaucoma
      b. Miosis (midazolam)
      c. Decreased reaction to light

10. Problems with color vision—color vision defect (lorazepam,
    nitrazepam, oxazepam)
11. Nonspecific ocular irritation
    a. Photophobia
    b. Lacrimation
    c. Burning sensation
    d. Ocular pain
12. Abnormal EOG (diazepam)
13. Subconjunctival or retinal hemorrhages secondary to drug-
    induced anemia
14. Ocular teratogenic effects
    a. Increased incidences strabismus (diazepam)
    b. Epicanthal folds (oxazepam, diazepam)
    c. "Slant eyes" (oxazepam, diazepam)
15. Loss of eyelashes or eyebrows (clonazepam)

Clinical Significance: Significant ocular side effects due to these benzodiazepine derivatives are rare and reversible. Most reports are secondary to diazepam since, at one time, this was the largest selling prescription drug in the
world. At therapeutic dosage levels, these agents may cause decreased corneal reflex, decreased accommodation, decreased depth perception, and abnormal extraocular muscle movements. Abnormal extraocular muscle
movements and decreased accommodation may be enhanced with the concomitant use of alcohol. These drugs can cause an allergic conjunctivitis.
All can cross-react because they have the common metabolite desmethyldi-
azepam, which is the primary antigen and probable cause of the conjunctivitis. This may give a type I immune reaction. Typically, the allergic conjunctivitis occurs within 30 minutes after taking these drugs, with the peak
reaction occurring within 4 hours and subsiding in 1 to 2 days. Symptoms
include blurred vision, burning, tearing, and a foreign body sensation. Contact lens wearers have confused this adverse drug effect with poorly fitted
lenses. To what degree these benzodiazepine derivatives cause pupillary
dilatation is uncertain; however, there are cases in the literature and Registry
of patients who probably were predisposed to narrow-angle glaucoma precipitated by a narrow-angle attack after receiving one of these drugs. It has
been reported that diazepam may cause brownish lens deposits, but these
data have not been confirmed.

References:
Berlin, R.M., and Conell, L.J.: Withdrawal symptoms after long-term treatment with
    therapeutic doses of flurazepam: A case report. Am. J. Psychiatry *140*:488, 1983.
Cunningham, T.A.: Adverse reaction to flurazepam. Can. Med. Assoc. J. *112*:805,
    1975.
Eckerskorn, U., and Hockwin, O.: The human eye: Initial and manifestation organ of
    drug-induced side effects. Concepts Toxicol. *4*:15–20, 1987.

Einarson, T.R., and Yoder, E.S.: Triazolam psychosis—A syndrome? Drug Intell. Clin. Pharm. *16*:330, 1982.

Laegreid, L., et al.: Teratogenic effects of benzodiazepine use during pregnancy. J. Pediatr. *114*:126–131, 1989.

Laroche, J., Laroche, C.: Modification of colour vision. Annales Pharmaceutiques Francaises. *35*:5–6;173–179, 1977.

Levy, A.B.: Delirium and seizures due to abrupt alprazolam withdrawal: Case report. J. Clin. Psychiatry *45*:38, 1984.

Lutz, E.G.: Allergic conjunctivitis due to diazepam. Am. J. Psychiatry *132(5)*:548, 1975.

Marttila, J. K., et al.: Potential untoward effects of long-term use of flurazepam in geriatric patients. J. Am. Pharmaceut. Assoc. *17*:692, 1977.

Nelson, L.B., et al: Occurrence of strabismus in infants born to drug-dependent women. Am J Dis Children *141*:175–178, 1987.

Noyes, R., et al.: A withdrawal syndrome after abrupt discontinuation of alprazolam. Am. J. Psychiatry *142*:114, 1985.

Sandyk, R.: Orofacial dyskinesia associated with lorazepam therapy. Clin. Pharm. *5*: 419, 1986.

Tien, A.Y., and Gujavarty, K.S.: Seizure following withdrawal from triazolam. Am. J. Psychiatry *142*:1516, 1985.

Tyrer, P. J., and Seivewright, N.: Identification and management of benzodiazepine dependence Postgrad. Med. J. *60*(Suppl. 2):41, 1984.

Vital-Herne, J., et al.: Another case of alprazolam withdrawal syndrome. Am. J. Psychiatry *142*:1515, 1985.

Generic Name: 1. Carisoprodol; 2. Meprobamate

Proprietary Name: 1. Carisoma (G.B.), Flexartal (Fr.), **Rela**, Sanoma (Germ.), **Soma** (Canad.), Somadril (Swed.); 2. Ansiowas (Span.), Dapaz (Span.), Équanil (Fr.), **Equanil** (Austral., Canad., G.B., Ire., S. Afr.), Exphobin N (Germ.), Meditran (Canad.), Meprate (G.B.), Meprepose (S. Afr.), Meprodil (Switz.), **Meprospan** (Span.), Miltown (Span.), **Miltown-200**, Novomepro (Canad.), Oasil Simes (Span.), Procalmadiol (Fr.), Quanil (Ital.), Restenil (Swed.), Stensolo (Ital.), Urbilat (Germ.), Visano N (Germ.)

Primary Use: These agents are used to treat skeletal muscle spasms. In addition, meprobamate is used as a psychotherapeutic sedative in the treatment of nervous tension, anxiety, and simple insomnia.

Ocular Side Effects:
A. Systemic Administration
   1. Decreased accommodation
   2. Decreased vision
   3. Diplopia
   4. Paralysis of extraocular muscles
   5. Decreased corneal reflex

    6. Constriction of visual fields
    7. Eyelids or conjunctiva
      a. Allergic reactions
      b. Angioneurotic edema
      c. Urticaria
      d. Erythema multiforme
      e. Stevens-Johnson syndrome
      f. Exfoliative dermatitis
    8. Nonspecific ocular irritation
      a. Edema
      b. Burning sensation
    9. Pupils
      a. Mydriasis
      b. Miosis
      c. Decreased or absent reaction to light
   10. Nystagmus
   11. Subconjunctival or retinal hemorrhages secondary to drug-induced anemia
   12. Random ocular movements

Clinical Significance: Significant ocular side effects due to these drugs are uncommon and transitory. At normal dosage levels, decreased accommodation, diplopia, and paralysis of extraocular muscles may be found. Pupillary responses are variable, even in drug-induced coma.

References:

Barret, L.G., et al.: Internuclear ophthalmoplegia in patients with toxic coma. Frequency, prognostic value, diagnostic significance. J. Toxicol. Clin. Toxicol. *20*:373, 1983.

Edwards, J.G.: Adverse effects of antianxiety drugs. Drugs *22*:495, 1981.

Hermans, G.: Les Psychotropes. Bull. Soc. Belge Ophtalmol. *160*:15, 1972.

McEvoy, G.K. (Ed.): American Hospital Formulary Service Drug Information 87. Bethesda, American Society of Hospital Pharmacists, 1987, pp. 1024–1026, 1146–1153.

Walsh, F.B., and Hoyt, W.F.: Clinical Neuro-Ophthalmology. 3rd Ed., Baltimore, Williams & Wilkins, Vol. III, 1969, pp. 2633–2634.

Generic Name: Doxepin. See under *Class: Antidepressants.*

Class: Anticonvulsants

Generic Name: 1. Divalproex Sodium; 2. Valproate Sodium; 3. Valproic Acid

Proprietary Name: Convulex (Germ., Neth., S. Afr., Switz.), **Depa, Depakene** (Canad.), Depakin (Ital.), Dépakine (Fr., Switz.), Depakine (Neth.,

Span.), Depakine Zuur (Neth.), **Depakote**, Dépamide (Fr.), Depamide (Ital., Span.), **Deproic**, Epicon (Ital.), Epilim (Austral., G.B., S. Afr.), Epival (Canad.), Ergenyl (Germ., Swed.), Leptilan (Germ.), Leptilen (Swed.), Myl-proin (Germ.), Orfilept (Swed.), Orfiril (Germ., Switz.), Orlept (G.B.), Val-cote (Austral.)

Primary Use: Valproic acid is a carboxylic acid derivative, and valproate sodium is the sodium salt of valproic acid. Divalproex sodium is a compound comprised of valproate sodium and valproic acid. These antiepileptic agents are used in the prophylactic management of petit mal seizures.

Ocular Side Effects:
  A. Systemic Administration
    1. Diplopia
    2. Nystagmus
    3. Oscillopsia
    4. Visual hallucinations

Clinical Significance: Ocular side effects due to these drugs are rare and seldom of clinical significance. There is, however, an idiosyncratic suscepti-bility in some patients characterized by various forms of diplopia, oscillop-sia, impaired vergence mechanisms, vertical nystagmus, or abnormalities of the vestibular-ocular reflex. Other ocular motor abnormalities may include pursuit and gaze holding patterns. It has been suggested that this group of drugs may have some effect on the retinal pigment epithelium; this is based on animal work, theoretical implications, and one 14-year-old who showed retinal pigment epithelial changes while taking valproic. The authors felt that abnormal tissue, i.e., from retinitis pigmentosa or benzodiazepines, has more susceptibility for increased problems. These data have not been confirmed.

References:
Bellman, M.H., and Ross, E.M.: Side effects of sodium valproate. Br. Med. J. *1*:1662, 1977.
Chadwick, D.W., et al.: Acute intoxication with sodium valproate. Ann. Neurol. *6*: 552, 1979.
Hassan, M.N., Laljee, H.C.K., and Parsonage, M.J.: Sodium valproate in the treatment of resistant epilepsy. Acta Neurol. Scand. *54*:209, 1976.
McEvoy, G.K. (Ed.): American Hospital Formulary Service Drug Information 87. Bethesda, American Society of Hospital Pharmacists, 1987, pp. 1042–1045.
Remler, B.F., Leigh, R.J., Osorio, I., et al: The characteristics and mechanisms of visual disturbance associated with anticonvulsant therapy. Neurology *40*:791–796, 1990.
Scullica, L., Trombetta, C.J., Tuccari, G.: Toxic effect of valproic acid on the retina. Clinical and experimental investigation. Blodi, F. et al. (Eds.): Acta XXV Concilium Ophthalmologicum. Proceedings of the XXVth International Congress of Ophthal-

mology, held in Rome, Italy, May 4–10, 1986. Kugler & Ghedini Publishers, Vol. 2, 1988.

Generic Name: 1. Ethosuximide; 2. Methsuximide; 3. Phensuximide

Proprietary Name: 1. Emeside (G.B.), Pétinamid (Switz.), Petnidan (Germ.), Pyknolepsinum (Germ.), Simatin (Span.), Suxinutin (Germ., Swed., Switz.), **Zarontin** (Austral., Canad., Fr., G.B., Ire., Ital., Neth., S. Afr., Span.); 2. **Celontin** (Austral., Canad., Neth., S. Afr.), Petinutin (Germ.); 3. **Milontin** (Austral.)

Primary Use: These succinimides are effective in the management of petit mal seizures.

Ocular Side Effects:
    A. Systemic Administration
        1. Decreased vision
        2. Diplopia
        3. Photophobia
        4. Myopia
        5. Periorbital edema or hyperemia
        6. Subconjunctival or retinal hemorrhages secondary to drug-induced anemia
        7. Eyelids or conjunctiva
            a. Allergic reactions
            b. Angioneurotic edema
            c. Lupoid syndrome
            d. Erythema multiforme
            e. Stevens-Johnson syndrome
            f. Exfoliative dermatitis
        8. Visual hallucinations

Clinical Significance: Methsuximide induces ocular side effects more frequently than ethosuximide or phensuximide. All adverse ocular reactions other than those due to anemias or dermatologic conditions are reversible after discontinuation of the drug. This group of drugs can trigger systemic lupus erythematosus by producing antinuclear antibodies.

References:
Alarcón-Segovia, D.: Drug-induced antinuclear antibodies and lupus syndrome. Drugs *12*:69, 1976.
Beghi, E., DiMascio, R., and Tognoni, G.: Adverse effects of anticonvulsant drugs—A critical review. Adverse Drug React. Acute Poisoning Rev. *5*:63, 1986.
Drug Evaluations. 6th Ed., Chicago, American Medical Association, 1986, pp. 172, 187.

Drugs for epilepsy. Med. Lett. Drugs Ther. *25*:83, 1983.

Millichap, J.G.: Anticonvulsant drugs. Clinical and electroencephalographic indications, efficacy and toxicity. Postgrad. Med. *37*:22, 1965.

Taaffe, A., and O'Brien, C.: A case of Stevens-Johnson syndrome associated with the anti-convulsants sulthiame and ethosuximide. Br. Dent. J. *138*:172, 1975.

Walsh, F.B., and Hoyt, W.F.: Clinical Neuro-Ophthalmology. 3rd Ed., Baltimore, Williams & Wilkins, Vol. III, 1969, p. 2645.

Generic Name: 1. **Ethotoin**; 2. **Mephenytoin**

Proprietary Name: 1. **Peganone**; 2. **Mesantoin** (Canad.)

Primary Use: These hydantoins are effective in the management of psycho-motor and grand mal seizures.

Ocular Side Effects:

A. Systemic Administration
1. Nystagmus
2. Diplopia
3. Photophobia
4. Eyelids or conjunctiva
   a. Allergic reactions
   b. Conjunctivitis—nonspecific
   c. Angioneurotic edema
   d. Urticaria
   e. Lupoid syndrome
   f. Erythema multiforme
   g. Stevens-Johnson syndrome
   h. Exfoliative dermatitis
   i. Lyell's syndrome
5. Subconjunctival or retinal hemorrhages secondary to drug-induced anemia

Clinical Significance: These hydantoin agents have fewer adverse ocular reactions than phenytoin. Ocular side effects are seen more frequently with mephenytoin than with ethotoin and are reversible either by decreasing the dosage or discontinuing use of the drug. As with phenytoin, nystagmus may persist for some time after the drug is stopped. Mephenytoin has been implicated in inducing systemic lupus erythematosus by producing antinuclear antibodies. While in many instances these antibodies are produced, only a small number produce lupus syndromes. Corneal or lens opacities and myasthenic neuromuscular blocking effect have been reported in only one series.

References:

Alarcón-Segovia, D.: Drug-induced antinuclear antibodies and lupus syndromes. Drugs *12*:69, 1976.

Gilman, A.G., Goodman, L.S., and Gilman, A. (Eds.): The Pharmacological Basis of Therapeutics. 6th Ed., New York, Macmillan, 1980, pp. 455–456.
Hermans, G.: Les anticonvulsivants. Bull. Soc. Belge Ophtalmol. *160*:89, 1972.
Livingston, S.: Drug Therapy for Epilepsy. Springfield, Charles C. Thomas, 1966.
Walsh, F.B., and Hoyt, W.F.: Clinical Neuro-Ophthalmology. 3rd Ed., Baltimore, Williams & Wilkins, Vol. III, 1969, p. 2644.

Generic Name: 1. Paramethadione; 2. Trimethadione

Proprietary Name: 1. **Paradione**; 2. **Tridione** (Germ.)

Primary Use: These oxazolidinediones are used primarily in the treatment of refractory petit mal seizures and myoclonic contractions.

Ocular Side Effects:
   A. Systemic Administration
      1. Glare phenomenon—objects appear covered with snow
      2. Photophobia
      3. Night blindness
      4. Gaze evoked nystagmus
      5. Problems with color vision
         a. Color vision defect, red-green or yellow-blue defect
         b. Objects have dazzling white tinge
         c. Colored haloes around lights—mainly white
         d. Colors appear faded
      6. Scotomas
      7. Eyelids or conjunctiva
         a. Allergic reactions
         b. Photosensitivity
         c. Angioneurotic edema
         d. Lupoid syndrome
         e. Erythema multiforme
         f. Stevens-Johnson syndrome
         g. Exfoliative dermatitis
         h. Lyell's syndrome
      8. Subconjunctival or retinal hemorrhages secondary to drug-induced anemia
      9. Ocular teratogenic effects (fetal trimethadione syndrome)
         a. "V"-shaped eyebrows
         b. Epicanthus
         c. Strabismus
         d. Hypertelorism
         e. Myopia
     10. Myasthenic neuromuscular blocking effect
         a. Paralysis of extraocular muscles

    b. Ptosis

    c. Diplopia

Clinical Significance: The oxazolidinediones have the unusual side effect of causing a prolonged "dazzle effect" when the eyes are exposed to light. This includes decreased vision, momentary loss of vision, loss of color perception, and illuminated objects appear to be covered by snow. This toxic effect seems to be specific for retinal cones and in all but two instances has been reversible. In general, this phenomenon ceases to occur even if therapy is restarted after a few months. Symptoms last from a few days to a few weeks after use of the drug is discontinued. These drugs can produce antinuclear antibodies; however, lupus erythematosus is rarely precipitated. Paramethadione has significantly fewer and less-prolonged ocular side effects than trimethadione. Trimethadione is said to be teratogenic and to cause a typical phenotype-fetal trimethadione syndrome.

References:

Alarcón-Segovia, D.: Drug-induced antinuclear antibodies and lupus syndromes. Drugs *12*:69, 1976.

Argov, Z., and Mastaglia, F.L.: Disorders of neuromuscular transmission caused by drugs. N. Engl. J. Med. *301*:409, 1979.

Dekking, H.M.: Visual disturbances due to Tridione. Acta Cong. Ophthalmol. *1*:465, 1950.

Gilman, A.G., Goodman, L.S., and Gilman, A. (Eds.): The Pharmacological Basis of Therapeutics. 6th Ed., New York, Macmillan, 1980, pp. 465–466.

Gordon, N.: Fetal drug syndrome. Postgrad. Med. J. *54*:796, 1978.

Kaeser, H.E.: Drug-induced myasthenic syndromes. Acta Neurol. Scand. *70*(Suppl. 100):39, 1984.

Lee, S.L., Rivero, I., and Siegel, M.: Activation of systemic lupus erythematosus by drugs. Arch. Intern. Med. *117*:620, 1966.

Peterson, H. deC.: Association of trimethadione therapy and myasthenia gravis. N. Engl. J. Med. *274*:506, 1966.

Sloan, L.L., and Gilger, A.P.: Visual effects of Tridione. Am. J. Ophthalmol. *30*:1387, 1947.

Weisbecker, C.A.: Ophthalmic side effects of systemic medications. Hosp. Form. *12*:709, 1977.

Generic Name: Phenytoin

Proprietary Name: Aleviatin (Jap.), Antisacer (Switz.), Di-Hydan (Fr.), **Dilantin** (Austral., Canad.), Dintoina (Ital.), Epanutin (G.B., Germ., Ire., Neth., S. Afr., Span., Swed., Switz.), Epilantine (Switz.), Fenantoin (Swed.), Lehydan (Swed.), Muldis (Neth.), Neosidantoina (Span.), Phenhydan (Germ., Switz.), Pyorédol (Fr.), Zentropil (Germ.)

Primary Use: This hydantoin is effective in the prophylaxis and treatment of chronic epilepsy.

Ocular Side Effects:
  A. Systemic Administration
    1. Nystagmus—downbeat, horizontal, or vertical
    2. Decreased vision
    3. Pupils
       a. Mydriasis
       b. Decreased reaction to light
    4. Myasthenic neuromuscular blocking effect
       a. Paralysis of extraocular muscles
       b. Ptosis
       c. Diplopia
    5. Decreased accommodation
    6. Decreased convergence
    7. Visual hallucinations
    8. Visual sensations
       a. Glare phenomenon—objects appear covered with snow
       b. Flashing lights
       c. Oscillopsia
       d. Photophobia
    9. Orbital or periorbital pain
   10. Problems with color vision
       a. Objects have white tinge
       b. Colors appear faded
       c. Color vision abnormalities
   11. Eyelids or conjunctiva
       a. Allergic reactions
       b. Ulceration
       c. Purpura
       d. Lupoid syndrome
       e. Erythema multiforme
       f. Stevens-Johnson syndrome
       g. Exfoliative dermatitis
       h. Lyell's syndrome
   12. Ocular teratogenic effects (fetal hydantoin syndrome)
       a. Hypertelorism
       b. Ptosis
       c. Epicanthus
       d. Strabismus
       e. Glaucoma
       f. Optic nerve or iris hypoplasia
       g. Retinal coloboma
       h. Retinoschisis
       i. Trichomegaly
   13. Subconjunctival or retinal hemorrhages secondary to drug-induced anemia

14. Papilledema secondary to pseudotumor cerebri
15. Cataracts

Clinical Significance: Nearly all ocular side effects due to phenytoin are reversible after discontinuation of the drug. The first sign of systemic phenytoin toxicity is nystagmus and is directly related to the blood levels of the drug. Instances of nystagmus persisting for 20 months or longer after discontinued use of phenytoin have been reported. Fine nystagmus may occur even at therapeutic dosages, but coarse nystagmus is indicative of toxic states. Downbeat and unidirectional gaze paretic nystagmus has even been reported due to phenytoin. Paralysis of extraocular muscles is uncommon, reversible, and primarily found in toxic states. Remler, et al. have reported that patients taking carbamazepine and phenytoin have increased incidences of vertical and horizontal diplopia with or without oscillopsia. This appears to be a central effect on the vergence centers and/or the vestibulo-ocular reflex. A prodrome of ocular or systemic "discomfort" frequently occurred before the onset of the above. The authors believed that this was an idiosyncratic response. Color vision changes are complex, with various manifestations including frosting or white tinges on objects, decreased brightness, or specific loss especially in the tritan/tetartan axis. Color loss may be due to cones as well as disturbances in the receptoral mechanism itself. Glare sensitivity is also increased by this drug. Although the fetal hydantoin syndrome is well accepted in the pediatric literature, there is some disagreement in the ophthalmic community as to a true cause-and-effect relationship. However, an increasing number of cases in the literature tends to support the fact that the maternal ingestion of hydantoins can produce congenital abnormalities. Ocular abnormalities are quite common in this syndrome. Benign intracranial hypertension in a patient with a seizure disorder has been confirmed with phenytoin rechallenge. A few cases of presenile cataracts have been reported in patients receiving prolonged hydantoin therapy, with toxic levels of phenytoin or with concomitant phenobarbital ingestion.

References:
Bar, S., Feller, N., and Savir, N.: Presenile cataracts in phenytoin-treated epileptic patients. Arch. Ophthalmol. *101*:422, 1983.
Bartoshesky, L.E., et al.: Severe cardiac and ophthalmologic malformations in an infant exposed to diphenylhydantoin in utero. Pediatrics *69*:202, 1982.
Bayer, A., Zrenner, E., Thiel, H.J., et al: Retinal disorders induced by anticonvulsant drugs. Third Congress. International Society of Ocular Toxicology. November 15–19, 1992, Sedona, Arizona. p. 11.
Boles, D.M.: Phenytoin ophthalmoplegia. S. Afr. Med. J. *65*:546, 1984.
Burge, S.M., and Dawber, R.P.: Stevens-Johnson syndrome and toxic epidermal necrolysis in a patient with systemic lupus erythematosus. J. Am. Acad. Dermatol. *13*: 665, 1985.

Herishanu, Y., Osimani, A., and Louzoun, Z.: Unidirectional gaze paretic nystagmus induced by phenytoin intoxication. Am. J. Ophthalmol. *94*:122, 1982.

Kalanie, H., et al.: Phenytoin-induced intracranial hypertension. Neurology *36*:443, 1986.

Mathers, W., et al.: Development of presenile cataracts in association with high serum levels of phenytoin. Ann. Ophthalmol. *19*:291, 1987.

Remler, B.F., et al.: The characteristics and mechanisms of visual disturbance associated with anticonvulsant therapy. Neurology *40*:791–796, 1990.

Rizzo, M., and Corbett, J.: Bilateral internuclear ophthalmoplegia reversed by naloxone. Arch. Neurol. *40*:242, 1983.

Spaeth, G.L., Nelson, L.B., and Beaudoin, A.R.: Ocular teratology. *In* Jakobiec, F.A. (Ed.): Ocular Anatomy, Embryology and Teratology. Philadelphia, J.B. Lippincott, 1982, pp. 955–981.

Generic Name: Sulthiame (Sultiame)

Proprietary Name: Ospolot (Austral., Germ., Ital., Span.)

Primary Use: This sulfonamide congener is a carbonic anhydrase inhibitor and is used in the treatment of psychomotor epilepsy.

Ocular Side Effects:
  A. Systemic Administration
    1. Decreased vision
    2. Diplopia
    3. Problems with color vision
      a. Color vision defect
      b. Objects have red tinge
    4. Eyelids or conjunctiva
      a. Edema
      b. Stevens-Johnson syndrome
      c. Ptosis
    5. Papilledema

Clinical Significance: This anticonvulsant has infrequently caused ocular side effects. These adverse ocular reactions are reversible upon discontinuance of the drug. One patient, after ingesting sulthiame for 2 weeks, developed papilledema and transient subjective changes in color vision. Within 2 weeks after the drug was stopped, the papilledema receded. It is possible that these signs and symptoms represented a toxic reaction to sulthiame, but this is unproven.

References:
Dukes, M.N.G. (Ed.): Meyler's Side Effects of Drugs. Amsterdam, Excerpta Medica, Vol. IX, 1980, pp. 92, 100.

Engelmeirer, M.P.: On clinical evaluation of anti-epileptic drugs with special attention to Opsolot. Deutsch. Med. Wschr. *85*:2207–2211, 1960.

Garland, H., and Summer, D.: Sulthiame in treatment of epilepsy. Br. Med. J. *1*:474, 1964.

Liske, E., and Forster, F.M.: Clinical evaluation of the anticonvulsant effects of sulthiame. J. New Drugs *3*:32, 1963.

Reynolds, J.E.F. (Ed.): Martindale: The Extra Pharmacopoeia. 28th Ed., London, Pharmaceutical Press, 1982, pp. 1254–1255.

Taaffe, A., and O'Brien, C.: A case of Stevens-Johnson syndrome associated with the anti-convulsants sulthiame and ethosuximide. Br. Dent. J. *138*:172, 1975.

Class: Antidepressants

Generic Name: 1. Amitriptyline; 2. Desipramine; 3. Imipramine; 4. Nortriptyline; 5. Protriptyline

Proprietary Name: 1. Adepril (Ital.), Amilit-IFI (Ital.), Amineurin (Germ.), Amitrip (Austral.), Amyline (Ire.), Domical (G.B., Ire.), Élavil (Fr.), **Elavil** (Canad., G.B.), **Endep** (Austral., S. Afr.), Euplit (Germ.), Laroxyl (Austral., Fr., Germ., Ire., Ital.), Lentizol (G.B., Ire.), Levate (Canad.), Novotriptyn (Canad.), Saroten (Austral., Germ., S. Afr., Swed., Switz.), Sarotex (Neth.), Sylvemid (Germ.), Trepiline (S. Afr.), Triptizol (Ital.), Tryptanol (Austral., S. Afr.), Tryptizol (G.B., Neth., Span., Swed., Switz.); 2. **Norpramin** (Canad.), Nortimil (Ital.), Pertofran (Austral., Fr., G.B., Germ., Ire., Neth., S. Afr., Switz.), **Pertofrane** (Canad.); 3. Ethipramine (S. Afr.), Imiprin (Austral.), Impril (Canad.), **Janimine Filmtab.** Medipramine (S. Afr.), Novopramine (Canad.), Surplix (Ital.), **Tofranil** (Austral., Canad., Fr., G.B., Germ., Ire., Ital., Neth., S. Afr., Span., Swed., Switz.), Tofranil Pamoato (Span.), **Tofranil-PM**; 4. Allegron (Austral., G.B.), Aventyl (Canad., G.B., Ire., S. Afr.), **Aventyl HCL**, Martimil (Span.), Noritren (Ital., Swed.), Nortab (Austral.), Nortrilen (Germ., Neth., Switz.), **Pamelor**, Paxtibi (Span.), Sensaval (Swed.), Vividyl (Ital.); 5. Concordin (G.B., Swed.), Triptil (Canad.), **Vivactil**

Primary Use: These tricyclic antidepressants are effective in the relief of symptoms of mental depression. Imipramine is also used in the management of enuresis.

Ocular Side Effects:
    A. Systemic Administration
        1. Decreased or blurred vision
        2. Decrease or paralysis of accommodation
        3. Pupils
            a. Mydriasis—may precipitate narrow-angle glaucoma
            b. Decreased or absent reaction to light

    4. Diplopia
    5. Photophobia
    6. Visual hallucinations
    7. Extraocular muscles
       a. Paresis or paralysis—primarily lateral rectus
       b. Oculogyric crises
       c. Decreased spontaneous movements
       d. Abnormal conjugate deviations
       e. Jerky pursuit movements
       f. Blepharospasm
       g. Nystagmus
    8. Decreased lacrimation
    9. Decreased corneal reflex
  10. Retrobulbar or optic neuritis
  11. Eyelids or conjunctiva
       a. Erythema
       b. Edema
       c. Photosensitivity
       d. Urticaria
       e. Purpura
       f. Increased blink rate
  12. Toxic amblyopia
  13. Subconjunctival or retinal hemorrhages secondary to drug-induced anemia
  B. Local Ophthalmic Use or Exposure—Protriptyline
    1. Decreased intraocular pressure—especially if in combination with sympathomimetics
    2. Mydriasis—may precipitate narrow-angle glaucoma
    3. Corneal opacities

Clinical Significance: Adverse ocular reactions due to these tricyclic antidepressants are reversible, transitory, and in most cases, of little clinical significance. The most common ocular side effects include decreased vision, decreased accommodation, mydriasis, and cycloplegia. A number of cases of narrow-angle glaucoma precipitated by amitriptyline and imipramine have been reported to the Registry. However, this is indeed a rare finding compared to the number of patients taking these drugs. These agents probably cause few ocular sicca problems in normal tear producers. In patients with an already compromised tear production, these drugs may have the potential to aggravate latent or manifested keratoconjunctivitis sicca. This may be due to an initial, probably transitory (a few months), decrease in tear production and an increased frequency of blinking. The clinician needs to be aware always of the interaction between the tricyclic antidepressants and the epinephrine preparations. Deaths have been attributed to the combination use of these drugs. All of these agents are potent photosensitizers, although their peak absorption would be blocked by the cornea. Topical ocular protriptyline has been used as an antiglaucoma agent, but it has not been marketed since it can cause corneal opacities of unknown composition.

References:

Beal, M.F.: Amitriptyline ophthalmoplegia. Neurology *32*:1409, 1982.

Blackwell, B., et al.: Anticholinergic activity of two tricyclic antidepressants. Am. J. Psychiatry *135*:722, 1978.

Delaney, P., and Light, R.: Gaze paresis in amitriptyline overdose. Ann. Neurol. *9*: 513, 1981.

Hotson, J.R., and Sachdev, H.S.: Amitriptyline: Another cause of internuclear ophthalmoplegia with coma. Ann. Neurol. *12*:62, 1982.

Karson, C.N.: Oculomotor signs in a psychiatric population: A preliminary report. Am. J. Psychiatry *136*:1057, 1979.

Pulst, S.M., and Lombroso, C.T.: External ophthalmoplegia, alpha and spindle coma in imipramine overdose: Case report and review of the literature. Ann. Neurol. *14*: 587, 1983.

Spector, R.H., and Schnapper, R.: Amitriptyline-induced ophthalmoplegia. Neurology *31*:1188, 1981.

von Knorring, L.: Changes in saliva secretion and accommodation width during short-term administration of imipramine and zimelidine in healthy volunteers. Int. Pharmacopsychiatry *16*:69, 1981.

Vonvoigtlander, P.F., Kolaja, G.J., and Block, E.M.: Corneal lesions induced by antidepressants: A selective effect upon young Fischer 344 rats. J. Pharmacol. Exp. Ther. *222*:282, 1982.

Walter-Ryan, W.G., et al.: Persistent photoaggravated cutaneous eruption induced by imipramine. JAMA *254*:357, 1985.

Generic Name: 1. Amoxapine; 2. Clomipramine; 3. Doxepin; 4. Trimipramine

Proprietary Name: 1. **Asendin** (Canad.), Asendis (G.B.), Défanyl (Fr.), Demolox (Span.); 2. **Anafranil** (Austral., Canad., Fr., G.B., Germ., Ire., Ital., Neth., S.Afr., Span., Swed., Switz.); 3. Aponal (Germ.), Deptran (Austral.), Sinéquan (Fr.), **Sinequan** (Austral., Canad., G.B., Neth., Span.), Sinquan (Germ.), Sinquane (Switz.), Triadapin (Canad.); 4. Apo-Trimip (Canad.), Rhotrimine (Canad.), Stangyl (Germ.), **Surmontil** (Austral., Canad., Fr., G.B., Ire., Ital., Neth., S. Afr., Span., Swed., Switz.), Tydamine (S. Afr.)

Primary Use: These tricyclic antidepressants are used in the treatment of psychoneurotic anxiety or depressive reactions.

Ocular Side Effects:

A. Systemic Administration
1. Decreased vision
2. Pupils

        a. Mydriasis—may precipitate narrow-angle glaucoma
        b. Decreased or absent reaction to light—toxic states
    3. Decrease or paralysis of accommodation
    4. Eyelids or conjunctiva
        a. Erythema
        b. Edema
        c. Photosensitivity
        d. Urticaria
        e. Pigmentation
        f. Blepharospasm
        g. Lyell's syndrome
    5. Extraocular muscles
        a. Nystagmus—horizontal or rotary—toxic states
        b. Oculogyric crises (doxepin)
        c. Paresis or paralysis—toxic states
        d. Abnormal conjugate deviations (amoxapine)
    6. Visual hallucinations

Clinical Significance: Adverse ocular reactions due to these tricyclic antidepressants are seldom of major clinical importance. Anticholinergic effects are the most frequent and include blurred vision, disturbance of accommodation, and mydriasis. There have been reports to the Registry of keratoconjunctivitis sicca associated with the use of doxepin, but this has not been proven. There is a question whether an increase in the blink rate is due to the drug, an associated sicca, or normally found with mental stress. Since these tricyclic antidepressants may be bound to ocular melanin, there is a potential for retinal damage. A few cases of retinal pigment abnormalities have been reported to the Registry, but no definitive relationship has been established.

References:

Barnes, F.F.: Precipitation of mania and visual hallucinations by amoxapine hydrochloride. Compr. Psychiatry 23:590, 1982.

Botter, P.A., and Sunier, A.: The treatment of depression in geriatrics with Anafranil. J. Int. Med. Res. 3:345, 1975.

D'Arcy, P.F.: Disorders of the eye. In D'Arcy, P.F., and Griffin, J.P.: Iatrogenic Diseases. 2nd Ed., Oxford, Oxford University Press, 1983, pp. 162–168.

Donhowe, S.P.: Bilateral internuclear ophthalmoplegia from doxepin over-dose. Neurology 34:259, 1984.

Horstl, H., Pohlmann-Eden, B.: Amplitudes of somatosensory evoked potentials reflect cortical hyperexcitability in antidepressant-induced myoclonus. Neurology 40:924-926, 1990.

Hughes, I.W.: Adverse reactions in perspective, with special reference to gastrointestinal side-effects of clomipramine (Anafranil). J. Int. Med. Res. 1:440, 1973.

LeWitt, P.A.: Transient ophthalmoparesis with doxepin overdosage. Ann. Neurol. 9: 618, 1981.

Litovitz, T.L., and Troutman, W.G.: Amoxapine overdose. Seizures and fatalities. JAMA *250*:1069, 1983.

Micev, V., and Marshall, W.K.: Undesired effects in slow intravenous infusion of clomipramine (Anafranil). J. Int. Med. Res. *1*:451, 1973.

Steele, T.E.: Adverse reactions suggesting amoxapine-induced dopamine blockade. Am. J. Psychiatry *139*:1500, 1982.

Generic Name: Carbamazepine

Proprietary Name: Carpaz (S. Afr.), Degranol (S. Afr.), **Epitol**, Hermolepsin (Swed.), Mazepine (Canad.), Novocarbamaz (Canad.), Sirtal (Germ.), Tegretal (Germ.), Tégrétol (Fr., Switz.), **Tegretol** (Austral., Canad., G.B., Ire., Ital., Neth., S. Afr., Span., Swed.), Teril (Austral.), Timonil (Germ., Switz.)

Primary Use: This iminostilbene derivative is used in the treatment of pain associated with trigeminal neuralgia.

Ocular Side Effects:
  A. Systemic Administration
      1. Extraocular muscles
          a. Paralysis—toxic states
          b. Diplopia
          c. Downbeat nystagmus
          d. Oculogyric crises—toxic states
          e. Decreased spontaneous movements
      2. Decreased vision
      3. Visual hallucinations
      4. Eyelids or conjunctiva
          a. Allergic reactions
          b. Conjunctivitis—nonspecific
          c. Edema
          d. Photosensitivity
          e. Urticaria
          f. Blepharoclonus
          g. Purpura
          h. Lupoid syndrome
          i. Erythema multiforme
          j. Stevens-Johnson syndrome
          k. Exfoliative dermatitis
          l. Lyell's syndrome
      5. Mydriasis—may precipitate narrow-angle glaucoma—toxic states
      6. Decreased accommodation
      7. Subconjunctival or retinal hemorrhages secondary to drug-induced anemia

    8. Papilledema—toxic states

    9. Retinal pigmentary changes

Clinical Significance: Probably the most common side effects due to carbamazepine are ocular, with diplopia being the most frequent followed by blurred vision and a "heavy feeling in the eyes." Ocular adverse reactions will occur in most patients when the dosage exceeds 1.2 g and usually disappear as the dosage is decreased. Most ocular side effects are reversible and may spontaneously clear even without reduction of the drug dosage. About 25% of patients receiving this drug develop neurologic or hematopoietic reactions, some of which are associated with eye abnormalities. The most common drug-related neurologic state is the toxic ataxia syndrome. This may occur as an acute phenomenon with carbamazepine usage and may include downbeat nystagmus, confusion, drowsiness, and ataxia. The cataractogenic potential of this agent is still open to debate. Toxic reactions in overdosage situations can cause dilated, sluggish, or nonreactive pupils and papilledema. This drug can also cause the ocular effects of lupus erythematosus. Carbamazepine can be recovered in the tears; this method has been advocated as a noninvasive technique to test for blood levels in the pediatric age group. Neilsen and Syversen reported two patients with retinotoxicity attributed to therapeutic use of carbamazepine. We have some cases as well in the Registry, but to date this is not a proven association. There are reports of ocular abnormalities seen as a teratogenic effect; however, this is still debatable.

References:

Breathnach, S.M., et al.: Carbamazepine ('Tegretol') and toxic epidermal necrolysis: Report of three cases with histopathological observations. Clin. Exp. Dermatol. *7*: 585, 1982.

Chrousos, G.A., et al.: Two cases of downbeat nystagmus and oscillopsia associated with carbamazepine. Am. J. Ophthalmol. *103*:221, 1987.

Delafuente, J.C.: Drug-induced erythema multiforme: A possible immunologic pathogenesis. Drug Intell. Clin. Pharm. *19*:114, 1985.

Gualtieri, C.T., and Evans, R.W.: Carbamazepine-induced tics. Dev. Med. Child Neurol. *26*:546, 1984.

Mullally, W.J.: Carbamazepine-induced ophthalmoplegia. Arch. Neurol. *39*:64, 1982.

Neilsen, N., and Syversen, K.: Possible retinotoxic effect of carbamazepine. Acta Ophthalmol. *64*:287, 1986.

Noda, S., and Umezaki, H.: Carbamazepine-induced ophthalmoplegia. Neurology *32*: 1320, 1982.

Silverstein, F.S., Parrish, M.A., and Johnston, M.V.: Adverse behavioral reactions in children treated with carbamazepine (Tegretol). J. Pediatr. *101*:785, 1982.

Smith, H., and Newton, R.: Adverse reactions to carbamazepine managed by desensitization. Lancet *1*:785, 1985.

Sullivan, J.B., Rumack, B.H., and Peterson, R.G.: Acute carbamazepine toxicity resulting from overdose. Neurology *31*:621, 1981.

Tedeschi, G., et al: Neuro-ocular side effects of carbamazepine and phenobarbital in epileptic patients as measured by saccadic eye movements analysis. Epilepsia. *30(1)*: 62–66, 1989.

West, J., Burke, J.P., and Stachan, I.: Carbamazepine, epilepsy, and optic nerve hypoplasia. Br. J. Ophthalmol. *74*:511, 1990.

Wheller, S.D., Ramsey, R.E., and Weiss, J.: Drug-induced downbeat nystagmus. Ann. Neurol. *12*:227, 1982

Generic Name: 1. Fluoxetine Hydrochloride; 2. Fluvoxamine Maleate

Proprietary Name: 1. Adofen (Span.), Fluctin (Germ.), Fluctine (Switz.), Fluoxeren (Ital.), **Prozac** (Canad., G.B., Ital., Neth., S. Afr., Span.), Reneuron (Span.); 2. Dumirox (Span.), Faverin (G.B., Ire.), Fevarin (Germ., Neth., Swed.), Floxyfral (Fr., Switz.), Maveral (Ital.).

Primary Use: These selective inhibitors of serotonin re-uptake are used as antidepressants. They are chemically unrelated to tricyclic, tetracyclic, or other available antidepressant agents and are reported to cause fewer antimuscarinic side effects than tricyclic antidepressants. Their mode of action in depression is not fully understood.

Ocular Side Effects:

A. Systemic Administration
   1. Blurred vision
   2. Mydriasis
   3. Narrow-angle glaucoma
   4. Photophobia
   5. Diplopia—transitory
   6. Ptosis—unilateral
   7. Eyelids
      a. Tics
      b. Rash
      c. Urticaria
      d. Angioedema
   8. Ocular pain

Clinical Significance: More than 6 million people have taken fluoxetine, which makes it the most prescribed antidepressant in the world. For practical purposes, ocular side effects are rare and reversible. In rare instances, however, mydriasis (three cases of anisocoria in the Registry—all unproven) may possibly precipitate narrow-angle glaucoma. Blurred vision may occur but is seldom of significance. Diplopia, ptosis, and nystagmus have been reported, but are primarily associated with the concomitant use of other agents, such as lithium, carbamazepine, diazepam, etc. There are two cases of possible fluoxetine-induced myopia of up to 3.0 diopters. While it is well documented that fluoxetine can cause dry mouth, sicca is as yet to be documented. A series of three cases of reactivation of genital herpes has been attributed to fluoxetine; however, no cases of reactivation of ocular herpes have been reported to the Registry. Concomitant use with phenytoin (Dilantin) can cause elevated plasma phenytoin . . . *see ocular signs of phenytoin*. To date, few adverse ocular reactions have been reported due to fluvoxamine.

References:

Ahmad, S.: Fluoxetine and glaucoma. DICP, Ann. Pharmacother. *25*:436, 1991.

Cunningham, M., Cunningham, K., Lydiard, R.B.: Eye tics and subjective hearing impairment during fluoxetine therapy. Am. J. Psychiat. *147*:947–948, 1990.

FDA Medical Bulletin, Alerts and Recalls: Fluoxetine-Phenytoin Interaction, pp. 3–4, May, 1994.

Pearson, H.J.: Interaction of fluoxetine with carbamazepine. J. Clin. Psychiat. *51*:126, 1990.

Physicians Desk Reference, Medical Economics Company, Montvale, NJ, 48th Ed., pp. 877–880, 1994.

Reed, S.M. and Glick, G.W.: Fluoxetine and reactivation of the herpes simplex virus. Am. J. Psychiat. *148*:949–950, 1991.

Sternback, H.: Danger of MAOI therapy after fluoxetine withdrawal. Lancet 2: 850–851, 1988.

Generic Name: 1. Isocarboxazid; 2. Nialamide; 3. Phenelzine; 4. Tranylcypromine

Proprietary Name: 1. **Marplan** (Austral., Canad., G.B., Ire., Ital.); 2. Niamide (Fr.); 3. Nardelzine (Span.), **Nardil** (Austral., Canad., G.B., Ire.); 4. **Parnate** (Austral., Canad., G.B., Germ., Ire., S. Afr., Span.)

Primary Use: These monoamine oxidase inhibitors are used in the symptomatic relief of reactive or endogenous depression.

Ocular Side Effects:

A. Systemic Administration
1. Decreased vision
2. Pupils—toxic states
    a. Mydriasis—may precipitate narrow-angle glaucoma
    b. Miosis
    c. Anisocoria
    d. Absence of reaction to light
3. Extraocular muscles
    a. Diplopia
    b. Nystagmus (phenelzine, tranylcypromine)
    c. Strabismus

4. Myasthenic neuromuscular blocking effect
   a. Paralysis of extraocular muscles
   b. Ptosis
5. Photophobia
6. Problems with color vision—color vision defect, red-green defect
7. Eyelids
   a. Photosensitivity
   b. Lupoid syndrome
8. Visual hallucinations (nialamide, phenelzine)
9. Visual field defects (tranylcypromine)
10. Subconjunctival or retinal hemorrhages secondary to drug-induced anemia

Clinical Significance: Most ocular side effects due to these monoamine oxidase inhibitors are reversible and insignificant. Pupillary reactions occur primarily in overdose situations. Nystagmus may be induced by phenelzine or tranylcypromine, and visual hallucinations by nialamide or phenelzine therapy, but these symptoms have not been reported due to any other monoamine oxidase inhibitors.

References:
Drugs for psychiatric disorders. Med. Lett. Drugs Ther. *25*:45, 1983.
Drugs that cause photosensitivity. Med. Lett. Drugs Ther. *28*:51, 1986.
Kaeser, H.E.: Drug-induced myasthenic syndromes. Acta Neurol. Scand. *70*(Suppl. 100):39, 1984.
Kaplan, R.F., et al.: Phenelzine overdose treated with dantrolene sodium. JAMA *255*: 642, 1986.
Thomann, P., and Hess, R.: Toxicology of antidepressant drugs. Handb. Exp. Pharmacol. *55*:527, 1980.
Weaver, K.E.C.: Amoxapine overdose. J. Clin. Psychiatry *46*:545, 1985.
Zaratzian, V.L.: Psychotropic drugs-neurotoxicity. Clin. Toxicol. *17*:231, 1980.

Generic Name: 1. Maprotiline; 2. Mianserin

Proprietary Name: 1. Aneural (Germ.), Delgian (Germ.), Depressase (Germ.), Deprilept (Germ.), Kanopan (Germ.), **Ludiomil** (Canad., Fr., G.BB., Germ., Ire., Ital., Neth., S. Afr., Span., Swed., Switz.), Mapro-Gry (Germ.), Maprolit (Ital.), Maprolu (Germ.), Mapro-Tablinen (Germ.), Mirpan (Germ.), Psymion (Germ.); 2. Athymil (Fr.), Bolvidon (G.B.), Lantanon (Ital., S. Afr., Span.), Norval (G.B.), Tolvin (Germ.), Tolvon (Austral., Neth., Swed., Switz.)

Primary Use: These tetracyclic antidepressants are used in the treatment of depression.

Ocular Side Effects:
  A. Systemic Administration
    1. Decreased vision
    2. Decreased accommodation
    3. Eyelids or conjunctiva
      a. Erythema
      b. Conjunctivitis—nonspecific
      c. Edema
      d. Photosensitivity
      e. Angioneurotic edema
      f. Erythema multiforme
      g. Urticaria
    4. Visual hallucinations
    5. Mydriasis—may precipitate narrow-angle glaucoma (maprotiline)
    6. Subconjunctival or retinal hemorrhages secondary to drug-induced anemia

Clinical Significance: Adverse ocular reactions due to these tetracyclic antidepressants are seldom of major clinical significance. Anticholinergic effects are the most frequent and include blurred vision, disturbance of accommodation, and mydriasis. Several instances of increased intraocular pressure have been reported to the Registry following pupillary dilatation in patients taking maprotiline. Visual hallucinations are usually associated with drug overdosage. Myoclonus can be seen in other muscles, so one can expect to see this in periocular muscles as well.

References:
Albala, A.A., Weinberg, N., and Allen, S.M.: Maprotiline-induced hypnopompic hallucinations. J. Clin. Psychiatry *44*:149, 1983.

Forstl, H., Pohlmann-Eden, B.: Amplitudes of somatosensory evoked potentials reflect cortical hyperexcitability in antidepressant-induced myoclonus. Neurology *40*: 924–926, 1990.

Oakley, A.M.M., and Hodge, L.: Cutaneous vasculitis from maprotiline. Aust. NZ J. Med. *15*:256,1985.

Park, J., and Proudfoot, A.T.: Acute poisoning with maprotiline hydrochloride. Br. Med. J. *1*:1573, 1977.

Quraishy, E.: Erythema multiforme during treatment with mianserin-A case report. Br. J. Dermatol. *104*:481, 1981.

Generic Name: Methylphenidate

Proprietary Name: Ritalin (Austral., Canad., Germ., Neth., S. Afr.), Ritaline (Switz.), Rubifen (Span.)

Primary Use: This piperidine derivative is used in the treatment of mild depression and in the management of children with the hyperkinetic syndrome.

Ocular Side Effects:
    A. Systemic Administration—Oral
        1. Eyelids or conjunctiva
           a. Urticaria
           b. Erythema multiforme
           c. Stevens-Johnson syndrome
           d. Exfoliative dermatitis
        2. Visual hallucinations—toxic states
        3. Mydriasis—toxic states
        4. Blepharoclonus
        5. Subconjunctival or retinal hemorrhages secondary to drug-induced anemia
    B. Systemic Administration—Intravenous
        1. Talc retinopathy
           a. Small yellow-white emboli
           b. Neovascularization—late
           c. Retinal hemorrhages
        2. Decreased vision
        3. Tractional retinal detachment

Clinical Significance: Ocular side effects due to methylphenidate are rare, reversible, and seldom clinically significant. Mydriasis rarely occurs except in overdose situations. Methylphenidate tablets intended for oral use have been popular among drug addicts who crush the tablets and inject the drug intravenously. The filler in the tablet is insoluble talc, cornstarch, or various binders and lodges in the retina and other tissues as emboli. These glistening refractile particles in the retina that are fairly stationary may cause visual symptoms, and neovascularization may form in time.

References:
Acute drug abuse reactions. Med. Lett. Drugs Ther. *27*:77. 1985.

Atlee, W.E., Jr.: Talc and cornstarch emboli in eyes of drug abusers. JAMA *219*:49, 1972.

Bluth, L.L., and Hanscom, T.A.: Retinal detachment and vitreous hemorrhages due to talc emboli. JAMA *246*:980, 1981.

Dukes, M.N.G. (Ed.): Meyler's Side Effects of Drugs. Amsterdam, Excerpta Medica, Vol. X, 1984, pp. 14–15.

Gualtieri, C.T., and Evans, R.W.: Carbamazepine-induced tics. Dev. Med. Child Neurol. *26*:546, 1984.

Gunby, P.: Methylphenidate abuse produces retinopathy. JAMA *241*:546, 1979.

Lederer, C.M., Jr., and Sabates, F.N.: Ocular findings in the intravenous drug abuser. Ann. Ophthalmol. *14*:436, 1982.

McEvoy, G.K. (Ed.): American Hospital Formulary Service Drug Information 87. Bethesda, American Society of Hospital Pharmacists, 1987, pp. 1115–1117.

Methylphenidate (Ritalin) and other drugs for treatment of hyperactive children. Med. Lett. Drugs Ther. *19*:53, 1977.

Tse, D.T., and Ober, R.R.: Talc retinopathy. Am. J. Ophthalmol. *90*:624, 1980.

Generic Name: Pemoline

Proprietary Name: Cylert (Canad.), Dynalert (S. Afr.), Senior (Germ.), Tradon (Germ.), Volital (G.B.)

Primary Use: This oxazolidinone derivative is used as an adjunct to attention deficit disorders.

Ocular Side Effects:
A. Systemic Administration
1. Extraocular muscles
a. Diplopia
b. Nystagmus
c. Oculogyric crises
d. Strabismus
2. Decreased vision
3. Visual hallucinations
4. May aggravate Tourette's syndrome

Clinical Significance: Reversible abnormal oculogyric function, diplopia, and strabismus related to pemoline administration have been reported to the Registry. Hallucinations are commonly seen in overdosage situations. Rarely, motor tics associated with Tourette's syndrome may develop in patients treated with this agent, and eyelid blinking may persist after the stimulant is withdrawn.

References:
Bachman, D.: Pemoline-induced Tourette's disorder: A case report. Am. J. Psychiatry *138*:1116, 1981.

Lowe, T., et al.: Stimulant medications precipitate Tourette's syndrome. JAMA *247*: 1729, 1982.

Polchert, S.E., and Morse, R.M.: Pemoline abuse. JAMA *254*:946, 1985.

Generic Name: Trazodone

Proprietary Name: Deprax (Span.), **Desyrel** (Canad.), Molipaxin (G.B., Ire., S. Afr.), Pragmarel (Fr.), Thombran (Germ.), Trazolan (Neth.), **Trialodine**, Trittico (Ital., Switz.)

Primary Use: This triazolopyridine derivative is used in the treatment of depression.

Ocular Side Effects:
A. Systemic Administration
   1. Decreased vision
   2. Visual image
      a. Objects have sheen, metallic ghost images, bright shiny lights
   3. Visual hallucinations
   4. Nonspecific ocular irritation
      a. Hyperemia
      b. Photophobia
      c. Ocular pain
      d. Burning sensation
   5. Eyelids or conjunctiva
      a. Allergic reactions
      b. Erythema
      c. Blepharoconjunctivitis
      d. Photosensitivity
      e. Erythema multiforme
   6. Diplopia
   7. Subconjunctival or retinal hemorrhages secondary to drug-induced anemia
   8. Increased blink rate
   9. Mydriasis—toxic states

Clinical Significance: Ocular side effects due to trazodone occur only occasionally and are reversible with decreased dosage or discontinued drug use. Palinopsia, the persistence or reappearance of an image of a recently viewed object, has been well documented. Other patients complain of a sheen on objects, etc. There is one well-documented report in the literature of this drug causing an increased blink rate. The Registry has cases of changes in refraction, transient problems with accommodation, central or paracentral scotomas, and optic neuritis. A cause-and-effect relationship of these findings and this drug has not been established.

References:
Ban, T.A., et al.: Comprehensive clinical studies with trazodone. Curr. Ther. Res. *15*: 540, 1973.
Damlouji, N.F., and Ferguson, J.M.: Trazodone-induced delirium in bulemic patients. Am. J. Psychiatry *141*:434, 1984.
Ford, N.E., Jenike, M.A.: Erythema multiforme associated with trazodone therapy: Case report. J. Clin. Psychiatry *46*:294, 1985.
Hassan, E., and Miller, D.D.: Toxicity and elimination of trazodone after overdose. Clin. Pharm. *4*:97, 1985.

Kraft, T.B.: Psychosis following trazodone administration. Am. J. Psychiatry *140*:1383, 1983.

Rongioletti, F., and Rebora, A.: Drug eruption from trazodone. J. Am. Acad. Dermatol. *14*:274, 1986.

Class: Antipsychotic Agents

Generic Name: 1. Acetophenazine; 2. Butaperazine; 3. Carphenazine; 4. Chlorpromazine; 5. Diethazine; 6. Ethopropazine (Profenamine); 7. Fluphenazine; 8. Mesoridazine; 9. Methdilazine; 10. Methotrimeprazine (Levomepromazine); 11. Perazine; 12. Periciazine; 13. Perphenazine; 14. Piperacetazine; 15. Prochlorperazine; 16. Promazine; 17. Promethazine; 18. Propiomazine; 19. Thiethylperazine; 20. Thiopropazate; 21. Thioproperazine; 22. Thioridazine; 23. Trifluoperazine; 24. Triflupromazine; 25. Trimeprazine

Proprietary Name: 1. **Tindal**; 4. Amazin (S.Afr.), Chloractil (G.B.), Chlorazine (Switz.), Chlorpromanyl (Canad.), Clonazine (Ire.), Hibernal (Swed.), Hibernal-embonat (Swed.), Largactil (Austral., Canad., Fr., G.B., Ire., Ital., Neth., S. Afr., Span., Switz.), Protran (Austral.), Prozin (Ital.), **Thorazine**; 6. **Parsidol**, Parsitan (Canad.); 7. Anatensol (Ital., Neth.), Anatensol Decanoate (Neth.), Anatensol Hydrochloride (Austral.), Dapotum (Germ., Switz.), Dapotum D (Germ.), Dapotum D/D (Switz.), Fludecate (S. Afr.), Lyogen (Germ., Switz.), Lyogen Depot (Germ.), Modécate (Fr.), Modecate (Austral., Canad., G.B., Ire., S. Afr., Span.), Modecate Acutum (S. Afr.), Moditen (Fr., G.B., Ire., Neth., Switz.), Moditen Depot (Ital.), Moditen Enanthate (Canad.), Moditen HCL (Canad.), Moditen Retard (Fr.), Omca (Germ.), Pacinol (Swed.), **Permitil** (Canad.), **Prolixin, Prolixin Decanoate, Prolixin Enanthate**, Siqualone (Swed.), Siqualone decanoat (Swed.); 8. **Serentil** (Canad.); 9. Dilosyn (Austral.), **Tacaryl, Tacaryl Hydrochloride**; 10. Minozinan (Neth., Switz.), Neurocil (Germ.), Nozinan (Canad., Fr., G.B., Ire., Ital., Neth., Swed., Switz.), Sinogan (Span.); 11. Taxilan (Germ., Neth.); 12. Aolept (Germ.), Nemactil (Span.), Neulactil (Austral., G.B., Ire., S. Afr., Swed.), Neuleptil (Canad., Fr., Ital., Neth., Switz.); 13. Decentan (Germ., Span.), Decentan-Depot (Germ.), Fentazin (G.B., Ire.), **Trilafon** (Austral., Canad., Ital., Neth., S. Afr., Swed., Switz.), Trilafon Decanoaat (Neth.), Trilafon dekanoat (Swed.), Trilafon enantat (Swed.), Trilafon Enantato (Ital.), Trilafan (Fr.), Trilafan Retard (Fr.); 15. Anti-Naus (Austral.), Buccastem (G.B., Ire.), **Compazine** (Austral.), Mitil (S. Afr.), Prorazin (Canad.), Proziere (G.B.), Stemetil (Austral., Canad., G.B., Ire., Ital., Neth., S. Afr., Swed.), Témentil (Fr.), Vertigon (G.B., Ire.); 16. Prazine (Switz.), Protactyl (Germ.), **Sparine** (Austral., G.B., Ire., S. Afr.), Talofen (Ital.); 17. Allerfen (Ital.), Atosil (Germ.), Avomine (Austral., G.B., Ire.), Brunazine (S. Afr.), Crema Anitallergica Antipruriginosa (Ital.), Daralix (S. Afr.), Duplamin (Ital.), Eusedon (Germ.), Fargan (Ital.), Farganesse (Ital.), Fenazil (Ital.), Fenergan Topico (Span.), Frinova (Span.), Histantil (Canad.), Lergigan (Swed.), Phénergan (Fr., Switz.), **Phenergan** (Austral., Canad., G.B., Ire., Neth., S. Afr.), Phenhalal (G.B.), Progan (Austral.), Promahist (S. Afr.), **Promet 50**, Promkiddi (Germ.), Prothazine (Austral.), Sayomol (Span.), Sominex (G.B.); 18. Propavan (Swed.); 19. **Norzine**, Torécan (Fr., Switz.), **Torecan** (Austral., Canad., G.B., Germ., Ire., Ital., Neth., Span., Swed.); 20. Dartal (Canad.), Dartalan (Austral); 21. Majeptil (Canad., Fr., Span.); 22. Aldazine (Austral.), Mallorol (Swed.), Meleril (Span.), **Mellaril** (Canad.), **Mellaril-S**, Mellerette (Ital.), Melleretten (Germ., Neth.), Mellerettes (Switz.), Melleril (Austral., Fr., G.B., Germ., Ire., Ital., Neth., S. Afr., Switz.), Melzine (Ire.), Novoridazine (Canad.), Ridazine (S. Afr.), Thiozine (Ire.); 23. Calmazine (Austral.), Eskazine (Span.), Jatroneural (Germ.), Modalina (Ital.), Novoflurazine (Canad.), Solazine (Canad.), **Stelazine** (Austral., Canad., G.B., Ire., S. Afr.), Terfluzine (Fr., Neth.); 24. Psyquil (Germ., Switz.), Siquil (Neth.); 25. Nedeltran (Neth.), Panectyl (Canad.), **Temaril**, Theralen (Swed.), Théralène (Fr., Switz.), Theralene (Germ.), Vallergan (Austral., G.B., Ire., S. Afr.), Variargil (Span.)

Primary Use: These phenothiazines are used in the treatment of depressive, involutional, senile, or organic psychoses and various forms of schizophrenia. Some of the phenothiazines are also used as adjuncts to anesthesia, antiemetics, and in the treatment of tetanus.

Ocular Side Effects:
  A. Systemic Administration
     Not all of the ocular side effects listed have been reported for each phenothiazine.
     1. Decreased vision
     2. Decrease or paralysis of accommodation
     3. Night blindness
     4. Problems with color vision
        a. Color vision defect, red-green defect
        b. Objects have yellow or brown tinge
        c. Colored haloes around lights
     5. Cornea
        a. Pigmentary deposits
        b. Edema
        c. Punctate keratitis
     6. Pupils
        a. Mydriasis—may precipitate narrow-angle glaucoma
        b. Miosis—rare
        c. Decreased reaction to light
     7. Retina

      a. Pigmentary changes

      b. Edema

  8. Oculogyric crises

  9. Visual fields

      a. Scotomas—annular, central, or paracentral

      b. Constriction

10. Nuclear stellate cataracts

11. Visual hallucinations

12. Lacrimation

      a. Increased—rare

      b. Decreased

13. Horner's syndrome

14. Nystagmus

15. Jerky pursuit movements

16. Photophobia

17. Optic atrophy

18. Papilledema

19. Myopia

20. Toxic amblyopia

21. Eyelids or conjunctiva

      a. Allergic reactions

      b. Edema

      c. Hyperpigmentation

      d. Photosensitivity

      e. Angioneurotic edema

      f. Blepharospasm

      g. Lupoid syndrome

      h. Stevens-Johnson syndrome

      i. Exfoliative dermatitis

22. Myasthenic neuromuscular blocking effect

      a. Paralysis of extraocular muscles

      b. Ptosis

      c. Diplopia

23. Abnormal ERG or EOG

24. Subconjunctival or retinal hemorrhages secondary to drug-induced anemia

25. Ocular teratogenic effects

Clinical Significance: The phenothiazines as a class are among the more widely used drugs in the practice of medicine today. The most commonly prescribed drug in this group is chlorpromazine, which has been so thoroughly investigated that over 10,000 publications alone deal with its actions. Even so, these drugs are remarkably safe compared with previously prescribed antipsychotic agents. Their overall rate of side effects is estimated at only 3%. However, if patients are receiving phenothiazine therapy for a number of years, a 30% rate of ocular side effects has been reported. If therapy continues over 10 years, the rate of ocular side effects increases to nearly 100%. Side effects are dose and drug dependent, with the most significant side effects reported with chlorpromazine and thioridazine therapy, probably since they are most often prescribed. Critical ocular dosages are unknown since 800 mg in the United States and 600 mg in the United Kingdom are considered by the manufacturer as the maximum daily dosage for thioridazine. These drugs in high dosages can cause significant adverse effects within a few days, while the same reactions usually would take many years to develop in the normal dosage range. Each phenothiazine has the potential to cause ocular side effects, although it is not likely to cause all of those mentioned. The basic problem is that pinpointing specific toxic effects to a specific phenothiazine is extremely difficult because most patients have been receiving more than one type. The most common adverse ocular effect with this group of drugs is decreased vision, probably due to anticholinergic interference. Chlorpromazine, in chronic therapy, is the most common phenothiazine to cause pigmentary deposits in or on the eye, with multiple reports claiming that other phenothiazines can cause this as well. These deposits are first seen on the lens surface in the pupillary aperture, later near Descemet's membrane, and only in extreme cases in the corneal epithelium. Retinopathy, optic nerve disease, and blindness are exceedingly rare at the recommended dosage levels, and then they are almost only found in patients receiving chronic therapy. Retinal pigmentary changes are most frequently found with thioridazine. This reaction is dose-related and is seldom seen at recommended dosages. A phototoxic process has been postulated to be involved in both the increased ocular pigmentary deposits and the retinal degeneration. This group of drugs with piperidine side-chains, i.e., thioridazine, have a greater incidence of causing retinal problems than the phenothiazine derivatives with aliphatic side-chains, i.e., chlorpromazine, with relatively few retinal toxicities reported. The phenothiazines combine with ocular and dermal pigment and are only slowly released. This slow release has in part been given as the reason for the progression of adverse ocular reactions even after use of the drug is discontinued.

References:

Ball, W.A., and Caroff, S.N.: Retinopathy, tardive dyskinesia and low-dose thioridazine. Am. J. Psychiatry *143*:256, 1986.

Bejar, J.M.: Compazine-induced dyskinesia in a 14-month-old boy. Clin. Neuropharmacol. 7:171, 1984.

Cook, F.F., Davis, R.G., and Russo, L.S., Jr.: Internuclear ophthalmoplegia caused by phenothiazine intoxication. Arch. Neurol. *38*:465, 1981.

Crombie, A.L.: Drugs causing eye problems. Prescribers' J. *21*:222–227, 1981.

Deluise, V.P., and Flynn, J.T.: Asymmetric anterior segment changes induced by chlorpromazine. Ann. Ophthalmol. *13*:953, 1981.

Eichenbaum, J.W., and D'Amico, R.A.: Corneal injury by a Thorazine spansule. Ann. Ophthalmol. *13*:199, 1981.

Hamilton, J. DeV.: Thioridazine retinopathy within the upper dosage limit. Psychosomatics 26:823, 1985.

Kaeser, H.E.: Drug-induced myasthenic syndromes. Acta Neurol. Scand. 70(Suppl. 100):39, 1984.

Lam, R.W., and Remick, R.A.: Pigmentary retinopathy associated with low-dose thioridazine treatment. Can. Med. Assoc. J. 132:737, 1985.

Miller, F.A., and Rampling, D.: Adverse effects of combined propranolol and chlorpromazine therapy. Am. J. Psychiatry 139:1198, 1982.

Miyata, M., et al.: Changes in human electroretinography associated with thioridazine administration. Acta Ophthalmol. 181:175, 1980.

Ngen, C.C., Singh, P.: Long-term phenothiazine administration and the eye in 100 Malaysians. Br. J. Psychiatry 152:278–281, 1988.

Power, W.J., et al: Welding arc maculopathy and fluphenazine. Br. J. Ophthalmol. 75: 433–455, 1991.

Generic Name: 1. Chlorprothixene; 2. Thiothixene

Proprietary Name: 1. **Taractan** (Germ., Ital.), Tarasan (Canad.), Truxal (Germ., Neth., Swed., Switz.), Truxaletten (Germ., Switz.); 2. **Navane** (Austral., Canad., Neth., Swed.), Orbinamon (Germ.)

Primary Use: These thioxanthene derivatives are used in the management of schizophrenia. Chlorprothixene is also used in agitation neuroses and as an antiemetic.

Ocular Side Effects:
  A. Systemic Administration
      1. Decreased vision
      2. Decrease or paralysis of accommodation
      3. Oculogyric crises
      4. Pupils
         a. Mydriasis—may precipitate narrow-angle glaucoma
         b. Miosis
      5. Diplopia
      6. Cornea
         a. Fine particulate deposits
         b. Keratitis
      7. Lens
         a. Fine particulate deposits
         b. Stellate cataracts
      8. Retinal pigmentary changes
      9. Eyelids or conjunctiva
         a. Allergic reactions
         b. Photosensitivity
         c. Angioneurotic edema
         d. Urticaria

      e. Lupoid syndrome

      f. Exfoliative dermatitis

10. Subconjunctival or retinal hemorrhages secondary to drug-induced anemia

Clinical Significance: In short-term therapy, ocular side effects due to these thioxanthene derivatives are reversible and usually insignificant. In long-term therapy, however, cases of corneal or lens deposits (chlorprothixene) or lens pigmentation (thiothixene) have been reported. Retinal pigmentary changes are exceedingly rare.

References:

Drug Evaluations. 6th Ed., Chicago, American Medical Association, 1986, pp. 126–127.

Drugs for psychiatric disorders. Med. Lett. Drugs Ther. 25:45, 1983.

Drugs that cause photosensitivity. Med. Lett. Drugs Ther. 28:51, 1986.

McNevin, S., and MacKay, M.: Chlorprothixene-induced systemic lupus erythematosus. J. Clin. Psychopharmacol. 2:411, 1982.

———————

Generic Name: 1. Droperidol; 2. Haloperidol; 3. Trifluperidol

Proprietary Name: 1. Dehidrobenzperidol (Span.), Dehydrobenzperidol (Germ., Neth., Switz.), Dridol (Swed.), Droleptan (Austral., Fr., G.B., Ire.), Inapsin (S. Afr.), **Inapsine** (Canad.), Sintodian (Ital.); 2. Bioperidolo (Ital.), Cereen (S. Afr.), Dozic (G.B.), duraperidol (Germ.), Elaubat (Germ.), Fortunan (G.B.), **Haldol** (Canad., Fr., G.B., Germ., Ire., Ital., Neth., Swed., Switz.), Haldol decanoas (Switz.), Haldol Decanoas (Fr., Ital., Neth.), Haldol Decanoat (Germ.), **Haldol Decanoate** (G.B., Ire.), Haldol Depot (Swed.), Haldol LA (Canad.), **Halperon**, Novoperidol (Canad.), Peridol (Canad.), Serenace (Austral., G.B., Ire., S. Afr.), Serenase (Ital.), Sigaperidol (Germ., Switz.); 3. Psicoperidol (Ital.), Tripéridol (Fr.), Triperidol (G.B., Germ.)

Primary Use: These butyrophenone derivatives are used in the management of acute and chronic schizophrenia and manic-depressive, involutional, senile, organic, and toxic psychoses. Droperidol is also used as an adjunct to anesthesia and as an antiemetic.

Ocular Side Effects:

    A. Systemic Administration

        1. Decreased vision

        2. Oculogyric crises

        3. Decrease or paralysis of accommodation

        4. Pupils

    a. Mydriasis—may precipitate narrow-angle glaucoma

    b. Miosis—rare

5. Eyelids or conjunctiva

    a. Allergic reactions

    b. Photosensitivity

    c. Angioneurotic edema

    d. Blepharospasm

    e. Exfoliative dermatitis

6. Visual hallucinations

7. Subconjunctival or retinal hemorrhages secondary to drug-induced anemia

8. Decreased intraocular pressure

9. Capsular cataracts

10. Corneal decompensation

11. Myopia (haloperidol)

Clinical Significance: Ocular side effects due to these butyrophenone derivatives are often transient and reversible on withdrawal of the medication. There are a number of cases reported to the Registry of bilateral marked pupillary dilatation due to haloperidol. In the Japanese literature and similar case reports received by the Registry, these agents have been associated with the onset of capsular cataracts after long-term therapy. These appear as subepithelial changes near the equator. Histologically, they appear as large, round, balloon cells without proliferation of lens epithelium. A recent epidemiologic study by Isaac, et al. supports this. In some individuals, myopia associated with the use of haloperidol has occurred. This may be secondary to drug-induced hyponatremia. There is a report by Nishida, et al. that in rare individuals, who are often taking multiple tranquilizing agents, including haloperidol, the endothelium may be damaged and give a clinical picture of bilateral bullous keratopathy. Stopping the drugs allows for the corneas to return to normal. The decreased intraocular pressure due to these drugs is not of a sufficient amount to be of clinical value.

References:

Andrus, P.F.: Lithium and carbamazepine. J. Clin. Psychiatry 45:525, 1984.

Drugs that cause photosensitivity. Med. Lett. Drugs Ther. 28:51, 1986.

Honda, S.: Drug-induced cataract in mentally ill subjects. Jpn J. Clin. Ophthalmol. 28: 521, 1974.

Isaac, N.E., et al: Exposure to phenothiazine drugs and risk of cataract. Arch. Ophthalmol. 109:256–260, 1991.

Konikoff, F., et al.: Neuroleptic malignant syndrome induced by a single injection of haloperidol. Br. Med. J. 289:1228, 1984.

Laties, A.M.: Ocular toxicology of haloperidol. In Leopold, I.H., and Burns, R.P. (Eds.): Symposium on Ocular Therapy. New York, John Wiley & Sons, Vol. 9, 1976, pp. 87–95.

Mendelis, P.S.: Haldol (haloperidol) hyponatremia. ADR Highlights January 12, 1981.

Nishida, K., et al.: Endothelial decompensation in a schizophrenic patient receiving long-term treatment with tranquilizers. Cornea *11(5)*:475–478, 1992.

Patton, C.M., Jr.: Rapid induction of acute dyskinesia by droperidol. Anesthesiology *43*:126, 1975.

Selman, F.B., McClure, R.F., and Helwig, H.: Loxapine succinate: A double-blind comparison with haloperidol and placebo in schizophrenics. Curr. Therap. Res. *19*: 645–652, 1976.

Shapiro, A.K.: More on drug-induced blurred vision. Am. J. Psychiatry *134*:1449, 1977.

Generic Name: Lithium Carbonate

Proprietary Name: Camcolit (G.B., Neth., S.Afr.), Carbolith (Canad.), Duralith (Canad.), **Eskalith**, Hypnorex (Germ., Switz.), Lentolith (S.Afr.), leukominerase (Germ.), Liskonum (G.B.), **Lithane** (Canad.), Lithicarb (Austral.), Lithizine (Canad.), **Lithobid**, Manialit (Ital.), Phasal (G.B.), Plenur (Span.), Priadel (Austral., G.B., Neth., S.Afr.), Quilonorm retard (Switz.), Quilonum retard (Germ., S.Afr.), Téralithe (Fr.)

Primary Use: This lithium salt is used in the management of the manic phase of manic-depressive psychosis.

Ocular Side Effects:
A. Systemic Administration
   1. Decreased vision
   2. Nystagmus
     a. Horizontal
     b. Vertical
     c. Downbeat
   3. Scotomas
   4. Extraocular muscles
     a. Oculogyric crises
     b. Decreased spontaneous movements
     c. Lateral conjugate deviations
     d. Jerky pursuit movements
     e. Oscillopsia
   5. Eyelids or conjunctiva
     a. Conjunctivitis—nonspecific
     b. Edema
     c. Loss of eyelashes or eyebrows
   6. Nonspecific ocular irritation
     a. Lacrimation
     b. Photophobia
     c. Burning sensation
     d. Decreased lacrimation

7. Decreased accommodation
8. Visual hallucinations
9. Exophthalmos
10. Subconjunctival or retinal hemorrhages secondary to drug-induced anemia
11. Myasthenic neuromuscular blocking effect
12. Papilledema secondary to pseudotumor cerebri
13. Abnormal EOG or VEP
14. Decreased dark adaptation

Clinical Significance: Lithium salts are widely used and have proved effective in the treatment of bipolar-affected disorders. Lithium therapy is mainly prophylactic, with therapy lasting years to decades. Fraunfelder, Fraunfelder, and Jefferson is probably the definitive work on the effects of lithium on the human visual system. Lithium affects many areas of the visual system and clearly can cause nystagmus and other abnormalities of the extraocular muscles as a direct effect on the central nervous system. Secondary effects, such as exophthalmos, occur because of the direct effect of lithium on the thyroid or increased intracranial pressure with resultant papilledema. There is a direct cortical effect causing transient blindness. In general, ocular side effects of lithium are reversible upon withdrawal of the drug or lowering of the dosage. However, other side effects, such as downbeat nystagmus, can be permanent. Blurred vision is commonly experienced by patients taking lithium but is seldom significant enough to require the cessation of therapy. Usually with time, even while keeping the same dosage, blurred vision will disappear. Blurred vision, however, can be a signal of pending problems, such as pseudotumor cerebri. In most cases the patients who develop pseudotumor have been taking lithium for many years. Lithium can cause various forms of nystagmus, the most characteristic being downbeat. This can occur at therapeutic dosage ranges of lithium and may be the only adverse drug effect. While some patients have a full recovery after stopping or reducing the dosage of lithium, it can develop into the more severe form of downbeat nystagmus, which may be irreversible. If downbeat nystagmus occurs, one needs to re-evaluate the risk-benefit ratio of lithium therapy. Lithium can also cause other extraocular muscle abnormalities, especially in vertical or lateral far-gaze diplopia. Diplopia in these patients requires a workup for myasthenia gravis, especially if associated with ptosis. Ptosis can occur, however, without myasthenia gravis, although this is rare. Oculogyric crises have been reported primarily in patients also taking haloperidol. Thyroid-related eye disease in various forms secondary to hypo- or hyperthyroidism have been seen in patients receiving lithium therapy. While this is uncommon, exophthalmos has occurred secondary to lithium therapy. Lithium may decrease lacrimal secretion but initially can increase lacrimation. Occular irritation occurs secondary to the drug being secreted in the tears. Epiphora may then occur when the drug is first started, but it is rarely a reason for stopping the drug. Lithium probably aggravates sicca just for the above reasons. It has been reported that lithium has been deposited in the cornea and the conjunctiva, but the documentation for this has been poor. Ocular irritation in early cases may best be treated by the increased use of artificial tears. Lithium can cause a decrease in accommodation that may occur in up to 10% of patients. However, this primarily occurs in young patients and is rare in older patients. In general, this side effect is minimal and usually resolves after a few months even while taking the drug.

References:

Arden, G., Barada, A., and Kelsey, J.: New clinical test of retinal function based upon the standing potential of the eye. Br. J. Ophthalmol. 46:449–467, 1962.

Brenner, R., et al.: Measurement of lithium concentrations in human tears. Am. J. Psychiatry 139(5):678–679, 1982.

Corbett, J., et al.: Downbeating nystagmus and other ocular motor defects caused by lithium toxicity. Neurology 39:481–487, 1989.

Deleu, D., and Ebinger, G.: Lithium-induced internuclear ophthalmoplegia. Clin. Neuropharmacol. 12(3):224–226, 1989.

Dry, J., Aron-Rosa, A., and Pradalier, A.: Onset of exophthalmos during treatment with lithium carbonate. Biological hyperthyroidism. Therapie 29:701–708, 1974.

Emrich, H., et al.: Reduced dark-adaptation: An indication of lithium's neuronal action in humans. Am. J. Psychiatry 147(5):629–631, 1990.

Fenwick, P.B.C., and Robertson, R.: Changes in the visual evoked potential to pattern reversal with lithium medication. Electroencephalogr. Clin. Neurophysiol. 55:538, 1983.

Fraunfelder, F.T.: Lithium carbonate therapy and macular degeneration. JAMA 249: 2389, 1983.

Fraunfelder, F.T., Meyer, S.: Ocular toxicity of antineoplastic agents. Ophthalmology 90(1):1–3, 1983.

Fraunfelder, F.T., Fraunfelder, F.W., and Jefferson, J.W.: Monograph: The effects of lithium on the human visual system. J. Toxicol. Cut. & Ocular Toxicol., 11(2): 97–169, 1992.

Halmagyi, G., et al.: Downbeating nystagmus—a review of 62 cases. Arch. Neurol. 40:777–784, 1983.

Halmagyi, G., et al.: Lithium-induced downbeat nystagmus. Am. J. Ophthalmol. 107: 664–670, 1989.

Levine, S., and Puchalski, C.: Pseudotumor cerebri associated with lithium therapy in two patients. J. Clin. Psychiatry 51(6):251–253, 1990.

Levy, D.L., et al.: Pharmacologic evidence for specificity of pursuit dysfunction to schizophrenia. Lithium carbonate associated with abnormal pursuit. Arch. Gen. Psychiatry 42:335, 1985.

Pakes, G.: Eye irritation and lithium carbonate. Arch. Ophthalmol. 98:930, 1980.

Sandyk, R.: Oculogyric crisis induced by lithium carbonate. Eur. Neurol. 23:92, 1984.

Saul, R.F., Hamburger, H.A., Selhorst, J.B.: Pseudotumor cerebri secondary to lithium carbonate. JAMA 253(19):2869–2870, 1985.

Slonim, R., and McLarty, B.: Sixth cranial nerve palsy-unusual presenting symptom of lithium toxicity? Can. J. Psychiatry 30:443–444, 1985.

Thompson, C.H., and Baylis, P.H.: Asymptomatic Grave's disease during lithium therapy. Postgrad. Med. J. 62:295–296, 1986.
Tucker, W.: Visual disturbances with lithium therapy. Drug Ther. 5:61, 1975.
Ullrich, A., et al.: Lithium effects on ophthalmological-electrophysiological parameters in young healthy volunteers. Acta Psychiatr. Scand. 72:113–119, 1985

Generic Name: Loxapine

Proprietary Name: Desconex (Span.), Loxapac (Canad., Fr., G.B., Ital., Neth., Span.), **Loxitane, Loxitane C, Loxitane IM**

Primary Use: This dibenzoxazepine derivative represents a subclass of tricyclic antipsychotic agents used in the treatment of schizophrenia.

Ocular Side Effects:
    A. Systemic Administration
        1. Decreased vision
        2. Oculogyric crises
        3. Mydriasis—may precipitate narrow-angle glaucoma
        4. Decreased accommodation
        5. Eyelids or conjunctiva
            a. Edema
            b. Hyperpigmentation
            c. Photosensitivity
            d. Urticaria
        6. Ptosis
        7. Subconjunctival or retinal hemorrhages secondary to drug-induced anemia

Clinical Significance: Neuromuscular reactions, including oculogyric crises, are frequently reported, usually during the first few days of treatment with loxapine. These reactions occasionally require reduction or temporary withdrawal of the drug. The anticholinergic effects, blurred vision, mydriasis, and decreased accommodation, are more likely to occur with concomitant use of antiparkinsonian agents. The possibility of pigmentary retinopathy and lenticular pigmentation from loxapine cannot be excluded but seems quite rare or unlikely.

References:
McEvoy, G.K. (Ed.): American Hospital Formulary Service Drug Information 87. Bethesda, American Society of Hospital Pharmacists, 1987, pp. 1094–1096.
Moyano, C.Z.: A double-blind comparison of Loxitane, loxapine succinate and trifluoperazine hydrochloride in chronic schizophrenic patients. Dis. Nerv. Syst. 36:301, 1975.
Reynolds, J.E.F. (Ed.): Martindale: The Extra Pharmacopoeia. 28th Ed., London, Pharmaceutical Press, 1982, pp. 1544–1545.

Selman, F.B., McClure, R.F., and Helwig, H.: Loxapine succinate: A double-blind comparison with haloperidol and placebo in acute schizophrenics. Curr. Ther. Res. *19*:645, 1976.

Generic Name: Pimozide

Proprietary Name: Opiran (Fr.), **Orap** (Austral., Canad., Fr., G.B., Germ., Ire., Ital., Neth., S. Afr., Span., Swed., Switz.)

Primary Use: This diphenylbutylpiperidine derivative is used for suppression of motor and vocal tics of Tourette's syndrome.

Ocular Side Effects:
   A. Systemic Administration
      1. Decreased vision
      2. Decreased accommodation
      3. Visual hallucinations
      4. Oculogyric crises
      5. Eyelids
         a. Erythema
         b. Edema
      6. Decreased lacrimation

Clinical Significance: Approximately 10% to 15% of patients receiving the prescribed dosages of pimozide experience extra-pyramidal symptoms. Anticholinergic effects, such as blurred vision and difficulty with accommodation, are also common adverse ocular reactions, all of which are reversible.

References:
McEvoy, G.K. (Ed.): American Hospital Formulary Service Drug Information 87. Bethesda, American Society of Hospital Pharmacists, 1987, pp. 1098–1103.
Morris, P.A., MacKenzie, D.H., and Masheter, H.C.: A comparative double blind trial of pimozide and fluphenazine in chronic schizophrenia. Br. J. Psychiatry *117*:683, 1970.
Taub, R.N., and Baker, M.A.: Treatment of metastatic malignant melanoma with pimozide. Lancet *1*:605, 1979.

Class: Psychedelic Agents

Generic Name: 1. Dronabinol (Tetrahydrocannabinol, THC); 2. Hashish; 3. Marihuana

Proprietary Name: 1. **Marinol**

Street Name: 1. The one; 2. Bhang, Charas, Gram, Hash, Keif, Black Russian; 3. Ace, Acapulco gold, Baby, Belyando sprue, Bhang, Boo, Brown weed,

Bush, Cannabis, Charas, Dope, Gage, Ganja, Grass, Gungeon, Hay, Hemp, Herb, Home grown, Jay, Joint, Kick sticks, Lid, Locoweed, Mary Jane, Mexican green, MJ, Muggles, OJ (opium joint), Panama red, Pot, Rainy-day woman, Reefer, Roach, Rope, Stick, Tea, Twist, Weed, Wheat

Primary Use: These psychedelic agents are occasionally used as cerebral sedatives or narcotics commonly available on the illicit drug market. Dronabinol is also medically indicated for the treatment of the nausea and vomiting associated with chemotherapy.

Ocular Side Effects:
   A. Systemic Administration
      1. Visual hallucinations
      2. Problems with color vision
         a. Color vision defect
         b. Objects have yellow or violet tinge
         c. Colored flashing lights
         d. Heightened color perception
      3. Nystagmus
      4. Nonspecific ocular irritation
         a. Hyperemia
         b. Conjunctivitis
         c. Photophobia (variable)
         d. Burning sensation
      5. Decreased accommodation
      6. Decreased dark adaptation
      7. Diplopia
      8. Decreased vision
      9. Blepharospasm
      10. Impaired oculomotor coordination
      11. Decreased intraocular pressure
      12. Decreased lacrimation
      13. Pupils
         a. Miosis
         b. Anisocoria

Clinical Significance: Ocular side effects due to these drugs are transient and seldom of clinical importance. The current area of greatest clinical interest is with the cannabinols found in marihuana. These agents can decrease intraocular pressure, but this varies with the quality of marihuana, based on the quantity of the cannabinols contained in the plant. There is significant variation in an individual response to these agents as well as diminished desired response with time. Most patients taking this agent for glaucoma control cannot use it for prolonged periods due to side effects and lack of glaucoma control. Purified naturally occurring cannabinols have the problem that the central nervous system high cannot be separated from the ocular-pressure-lowering effect, so its value clinically is quite limited. Few patients are able to use marihuana to control their glaucoma and remain functional in the workplace. There is some evidence that marihuana decreases basal lacrimal secretion, decreases photosensitivity, increases dark adaptation, increases color-match limits, and increases Snellen visual acuity. Possibly within the first 5 to 15 minutes, some persons will get some pupillary constriction; however, most do not and, to date, there is no long-term pupillary effect noted. Conjunctival hyperemia is not uncommon and is more pronounced 15 minutes, rather than 90 minutes, after exposure. The sensory perception of one's external environment is altered while taking this agent. These drugs are occasionally used medically, primarily as an antinauseant in chemotherapy, but have no value in ophthalmology.

References:

Fried, P.A.: Marihuana use by pregnant women and effects on offspring: An update. Neurobehav. Toxicol. Teratol. *4*:451, 1982.

Green, K.: Marijuana and the eye-A review. J. Toxicol. Cut. Ocular Toxicol. *1*:3, 1982.

Green, K., and Roth, M.: Ocular effects of topical administration of Δ^9-tetrahydrocannabinol in man. Arch. Ophthalmol. *100*:265, 1982.

Jay, W.M., and Green, K.: Multiple-drop study of topically applied 1% Δ^9-tetrahydrocannabinol in human eyes. Arch. Ophthalmol. *101*:591, 1983.

Merritt, J.C., et al.: Topical Δ^9-tetrahydrocannabinol in hypertensive glaucomas. J. Pharm. Pharmacol. *33*:40, 1981.

Poster, D.S., et al.: Δ^9-Tetrahydrocannabinol in clinical oncology. JAMA *245*:2047, 1981.

Qazi, Q. H., et al.: Abnormal fetal development linked to intrauterine exposure to marijuana. Dev. Pharmacol. Ther. *8*:141, 1985.

Schwartz, R.H.: Marijuana: A crude drug with a spectrum of underappreciated toxicity. Pediatrics *73*:455, 1984.

Treffert, D.A., and Joranson, D.E.: Δ^9-Tetrahydrocannabinol and therapeutic research legislation for cancer patients. JAMA *249*:1469, 1983.

Weinberg, D., et al.: Intoxication from accidental marijuana ingestion. Pediatrics *71*: 848, 1983.

Generic Name: 1. LSD, Lysergide; 2. Mescaline; 3. Psilocybin

Proprietary Name: None

Street Name: 1. Acid, Barrels, Big D, Blotter acid, Blue acid, Brown dots, California sunshine, Crackers, Cubes, Cupcakes, Grape parfait, Green domes, Hawaiian sunshine, Lucy in the sky with diamonds, Micro dots, Purple barrels, Purple haze, Purple ozolone, Sunshine. The animal, The beast, The chief, The hawk, The ticket, Trips. Twenty-five, Yellow dimples, Windowpane; 2. Buttons, Cactus, Mesc, Peyote, The bad seed, Topi; 3. Magic mushroom, Shrooms

Primary Use: These experimental drugs are used in the treatment of chronic alcoholism, character neuroses, and sexual perversions.

Ocular Side Effects:
  A. Systemic Administration
    1. Pupils
       a. Mydriasis
       b. Anisocoria
       c. Decreased or absent reaction to light
    2. Visual hallucinations including micro- and macropsia
    3. Problems with color vision
       a. Color vision defect
       b. Heightened color perception
    4. Visual sensations
       a. Prolongation of after images
       b. Phosphene stimulation
       c. Colored flashing lights
    5. Decreased accommodation
    6. Decreased dark adaptation
    7. Decreased vision
    8. Abnormal ERG or VEP
    9. Ocular teratogenic effects
       a. Cataract
       b. Iris coloboma
       c. Microphthalmos
       d. Corneal opacities
       e. Persistent hyperplastic primary vitreous
       f. Retinal dysplasia
       g. Optic disc hypoplasia
       h. Optic nerve coloboma
       i. Anophthalmia

Clinical Significance: Ocular side effects due to these drugs are common, but seldom of significant importance, except when bizarre visual hallucinations aggravate an already disturbed sensorium. Some claim true visual hallucinations seldom occur with these drugs, but rather a complicated visual experience results from a perceptual disturbance. Perception changes include alterations in colors and shapes. Lysergide is 100 times more potent than psilocybin, which in turn is 4000 times more potent than mescaline. While these drugs are only occasionally used medically, they are easily obtained through illicit channels. While a significant number of cases of sun-gazing-induced macular damage have been reported in persons using lysergide, only one case of sustained or irreversible color discrimination impairment has been reported in a former lysergide user in a drug-free state.

References:

Abraham, H.D.: A chronic impairment of colour vision in users of LSD. Br. J. Psychiatry *140*:518, 1982.

Abraham, H.D.: Visual phenomenology of the LSD flashback. Arch. Gen. Psychiatry *40*:884, 1983.

Acute drug abuse reactions. Med. Lett. Drugs Ther. *27*:77, 1985.

Birch, J., et al.: Acquired color vision defects. *In* Pokorny, J., et al.: Congenital and Acquired Color Vision Defects. New York, Grune & Stratton, 1979, pp. 243–350.

Evans, H .L., and Garman, R. H.: Scotopic vision as an indicator of neurotoxicity. *In* Merigan, W.H., and Weiss, B. (Eds.): Neurotoxicity of the Visual System. New York, Raven Press, 1980, pp. 135–147.

Margolis, S., and Martin, L.: Anophthalmia in an infant of parents using LSD. Ann. Ophthalmol. *12*:1378, 1980.

Spaeth, G.L., Nelson, L.B., and Beaudoin, A.R.: Ocular teratology. *In* Jakobiec, F.A. (Ed.): Ocular Anatomy, Embryology and Teratology. Philadelphia, J.B. Lippincott, 1982, pp. 955–975.

Generic Name: Phencyclidine

Proprietary Name: None

Street Name: Angel Dust, Angel's Mist, Busy Bee, Crystal, DOA, Goon, Hog, Mist, Monkey Tranquilizer, PCP, Peace Pill, Rocket Fuel, Sheets, Super Weed, Tac, Tic

Primary Use: This nonbarbiturate anesthetic was removed from the market because of postoperative psychiatric disturbances; however, it is still commonly available on the illicit drug market.

Ocular Side Effects:

A. Systemic Administration
1. Extraocular muscles
   a. Nystagmus—horizontal, rotary, or vertical
   b. Diplopia
   c. Jerky pursuit movements
2. Pupils
   a. Miosis
   b. Decreased reaction to light
3. Decreased vision
4. Visual hallucinations
5. Ptosis
6. Oculogyric crises
7. Decreased corneal reflex
8. Increased intraocular pressure

Clinical Significance: Even with relatively low doses (5 mg), phencyclidine may give a characteristic type of nystagmus in which vertical, horizontal, and rotary eye movements occur in sudden bursts. In addition, this drug may produce hallucinations and visual defects, including distortion of body image, hallucinatory voices, and substitution of fairy-tale characters. Acute toxic reactions can last up to a week after a single dose, although the mental effects can linger for more than a month. These effects may keep recurring in sudden episodes, while the patient is apparently recovering. A state of sensory blockade or a blank stare in which the eyes remain conjugate and open but with little or no spontaneous movement is characteristic of phency-clidine coma.

References:

Acute drug abuse reactions. Med. Lett. Drugs Ther. 27:77, 1985.

Corales, R.L., Maull, K.I., and Becker, D.P.: Phencyclidine abuse mimicking head injury. JAMA 243:2323, 1980.

McCarron, M. M., et al.: Acute phencyclidine intoxication: Incidence of clinical find-ings in 1,000 cases. Ann. Emerg. Med. 10:237, 1981.

Pearlson, G.D.: Psychiatric and medical syndromes associated with phencyclidine (PCP) abuse. Johns Hopkins Med. J. 148:25, 1981.

Phencyclidine: The new American street drug. Br. Med. J. 281:1511, 1980.

Class: Sedatives and Hypnotics

Generic Name: Alcohol (Ethanol, Ethyl Alcohol)

Proprietary Name: AHD 2000 (Germ.)

Primary Use: This colorless liquid is used as a solvent, an antiseptic, a beverage, and as a nerve block in the management of certain types of intract-able pain.

Ocular Side Effects:

A. Systemic Administration—Acute Intoxication
1. Extraocular muscles
   a. Paralysis (coma)
   b. Diplopia
   c. Nystagmus—various types including downbeat nystagmus
   d. Esophoria or exophoria
   e. Convergent strabismus
   f. Decreased convergence
   g. Jerky pursuit movements
   h. Decreased spontaneous movements
2. Pupils
   a. Mydriasis
   b. Decreased or absent reaction to light

      c. Anisocoria
      d. Miosis (coma)
  3. Decreased vision
  4. Decreased accommodation
  5. Problems with color vision
      a. Color vision defect, blue-yellow or red-green defect
      b. Objects have blue tinge
  6. Decreased dark adaptation
  7. Decreased intraocular pressure
  8. Constriction of visual fields
  9. Decreased depth perception
10. Decreased optokinetic and peripheral gaze nystagmus
11. Visual hallucinations
12. Prolonged glare recovery
13. Ptosis (unilateral or bilateral)
14. Impaired oculomotor coordination
15. Toxic amblyopia
16. Abnormal ERG, VEP, or critical flicker fusion

B. Systemic Administration—Chronic Intoxication
  1. Extraocular muscles
      a. Paralysis
      b. Jerky pursuit movements
  2. Downbeat nystagmus
  3. Paralysis of accommodation
  4. Pupils
      a. Miosis
      b. Decreased or absent reaction to light
      c. Constrict or dilate poorly
  5. Decreased vision
  6. Scotomas—central
  7. Problems with color vision—color vision defect, red-green defect
  8. Oscillopsia
  9. Lacrimation
10. Decreased intraocular pressure
11. Visual hallucinations
12. Optic neuritis
13. Corneal deposits (arcus senilis)
14. Toxic amblyopia
15. Ocular teratogenic effects (fetal alcohol syndrome)
      a. Narrow palpebral fissure
      b. Hypertelorism
      c. Microphthalmos
      d. Epicanthus
      e. Ptosis

      f. Strabismus

      g. Retinal vascular tortuosity

      h. Pseudopapilledema (enlarged or pale discs)

      i. Myopia

      j. Duane's retraction syndrome

      k. Corneal endothelial abnormalities

      l. Microcornea

      m. Steep corneal curvature

      n. Shallow anterior chamber

      o. Corneal opacity

      p. Iris dysplasia

      q. Glaucoma

16. Subcapsular cataracts
17. May aggravate the following diseases
      a. Wernicke's encephalopathy
      b. Cerebellar degeneration
      c. Purtscher's retinopathy
      d. Diabetic retinopathy
18. May retard the following diseases
      a. Ocular arteriosclerosis
      b. Recurrent retrobulbar neuritis

C. Local Ophthalmic Use or Exposure—Retrobulbar Injection
1. Irritation
      a. Hyperemia
      b. Ocular pain
      c. Edema
2. Keratitis
3. Paralysis of extraocular muscles
4. Nystagmus
5. Ptosis
6. Corneal ulceration
7. Decreased vision
8. Depigmentation—eyelids

D. Inadvertent Ocular Exposure
1. Irritation
      a. Lacrimation
      b. Hyperemia
      c. Ocular pain
      d. Edema
      e. Burning sensation
2. Keratitis
3. Corneal necrosis or opacities

Clinical Significance: The large number of adverse ocular effects reported due to ethyl alcohol is in part due to the fact that this agent is second only to water in the volume humans consume. Transient amblyopia lasting up to 5 days is well documented in both acute and chronic alcoholism; however, permanent blindness directly caused by ethyl alcohol is debatable. So-called toxic alcohol amblyopia is probably secondary to a vitamin B deficiency, and if the alcoholic was taking vitamin supplements, it would probably not occur. It has, however, been increasingly recognized that ethyl alcohol and its metabolites may have direct neurotoxic effects on the nervous system. Intraocular pressure may be significantly lowered in the glaucomatous patient after 40 to 60 mL of ethyl alcohol; however, this effect lasts only for a few hours. Ethyl alcohol probably has some sensory effect on a person's ability to drive due to nystagmus, diplopia, and uncoordinated ocular movements. Saccadic eye movements in which the eyes are moved rapidly from one object of interest to another, are significantly slowed when the person is under the influence of this agent. There is now evidence that perceptual, cognitive, and ocular motor effects of alcohol and tetrahydrocannabinol are additive. The fetal alcohol syndrome is a well-defined entity seen in off-springs whose mothers had high alcohol consumption during pregnancy. Recently, Duane's retraction syndrome, corneal decreased density polymegathism, and hexagonality have been added to the ocular portion of the fetal alcohol syndrome. The popularity of retrobulbar injections of alcohol is probably not as great today as it was in the past because of numerous untoward, often permanent, ocular and periocular effects.

References:

Alvarez, S.L., Jacobs, N.A., and Murray, I.J.: Visual changes mediated by beer in retrobulbar neuritis—An investigative case report. Br. J. Ophthalmol. 70:141, 1986.

Carones, F., Brancato, R., and Venturi, E.: Corneal endothelial anomalies in the fetal alcohol syndrome. Arch. Ophthalmol. 110:1128–1131, 1992.

Erwin, C.W., and Linnoila, M.: Effect of ethyl alcohol on visual evoked potentials. Alcoholism: Clin. Exp. Res. 5:49, 1981.

Eshagian, J.: Human posterior subcapsular cataracts. Trans. Ophthalmol. Soc. U.K. 102:364, 1982.

Ewing, J.A., and Rouse, B.A.: Corneal arcus as a sign of possible alcoholism. Alcoholism: Clin. Exp. Res. 4:104, 1980.

Giarelli, L., et al.: Decreased ocular (retinal and choroidal) arteriosclerosis in alcoholism. Ann. Ophthalmol. 12:815, 1980.

Holzman, A.E., Chrousos, G.A., and Kozma, C.: Duane's retraction syndrome in the fetal alcohol syndrome. Am. J. Ophthalmol. 110(5):565–566, 1990.

Kobatake, K., et al.: Impairment of smooth pursuit eye movement in chronic alcoholics. Eur. Neurol. 22:392, 1983.

Melgaard, B.: The neurotoxicity of ethanol. Acta Neurol. Scand. 67:131, 1983.

Miller, M., Israel, J., and Cuttone, J.: Fetal alcohol syndrome. J. Pediatr. Ophthalmol. 18:6, 1981.

Rubin, L.S.: Pupillometric studies of alcoholism. Int. J. Neurosci. 11:301, 1980.

Young, R.J., et al.: Alcohol: Another risk factor for diabetic retinopathy? Br. Med. J. 288:1035, 1984.

Zasorin, N.L.,and Baloh, R.W.: Downbeat nystagmus with alcoholic cerebellar degeneration. Arch. Neurol. *41*:1301, 1984.

Generic Name: 1. Amobarbital; 2. Aprobarbital; 3. Barbital; 4. Butabarbital; 5. Butalbital; 6. Butethal; 7. Cyclobarbital; 8. Hexobarbital; 9. Mephobarbital (Methylphenobarbital); 10. Metharbital; 11. Methohexital; 12. Pentobarbital; 13. Phenobarbital; 14. Primidone; 15. Secobarbital; 16. Talbutal; 17. Thiamylal; 18. Thiopental

Proprietary Name: 1. **Amytal** (Canad., G.B.), **Amytal Sodium** (Austral., Canad.), Neur-Amyl (Austral.), Sodium Amytal (G.B., Ire.); 2. **Alurate**; 4. **Butisol Sodium** (Canad.); 6. Soneryl (Austral., G.B., Ire., S. Afr.); 7. Somnupan C (Germ.); 9. **Mebaral** (Canad.), Prominal (Austral., Span., G.B.); 11. Brevimytal Natrium (Germ.), **Brevital Sodium**, Briétal Sodique (Fr.), Brietal (Neth., Swed.), Brietal Sodium (Austral., Canad., G.B., S. Afr.); 12. Barbopent (Austral.), Carbrital (Austral.), Medinox Mono (Germ.), Nembutal (Austral.), **Nembutal Sodium** (Canad.), Neodorm (Germ.), Nova (Canad.), Repocal (Germ.), Sopental (S. Afr.); 13. Aparoxal (Fr.), Comizial (Ital.), Fenemal (Swed.), Gardénal (Fr.), Gardenal (S. Afr., Span.), Gardenal Sodium (G.B.), Gardenale (Ital.), Lethyl (S. Afr.), Luminal (Germ., Span., Switz.), Luminale (Ital.), Luminaletas (Span.), Luminalette (Ital.), Luminaletten (Germ.), Nervolitan S (Germ.), Phenaemal (Germ.), Phenaemaletten (Germ.), **Solfoton**; 14. Liskantin (Germ.), Mylepsin (Swed.), Mylepsinum (Germ.), **Mysoline** (Austral., Canad., Ire., Fr., G.B., Ital., Neth., S. Afr., Span., Switz.), Resimatil (Germ.), Sertan (Canad.); 15. Imménoctal (Fr.), **Seconal Sodium** (Canad., G.B., Ire., S. Afr.); 17. **Surital**; 18. Farmotal (Ital.), Intraval Sodium (Austral., G.B., S. Afr.), Nesdonal (Neth.), **Pentothal**, Pentothal Natrium (Swed.), Pentothal Sodico (Span.), Pentothal Sodium (Austral., Canad., Ital.), Sandothal (S. Afr.), Tiobarbital Miro (Span.), Trapanal (Germ.)

Street Name: 1-18. Barbs, Bluebirds, Blues, Tooies, Yellow jackets

Primary Use: These barbituric acid derivatives vary primarily in duration and intensity of action and are used as central nervous system depressants, hypnotics, sedatives, and anticonvulsants.

Ocular Side Effects:
    A. Systemic Administration
        1. Eyelids
            a. Ptosis
            b. Blepharoclonus
        2. Pupils
            a. Mydriasis
            b. Miosis (coma)

  c. Decreased reaction to light

  d. Hippus

 3. Extraocular muscles

  a. Diplopia

  b. Decreased convergence

  c. Paresis or paralysis

  d. Jerky pursuit movements

  e. Random ocular movements

  f. Vertical gaze palsy

 4. Oscillopsia

 5. Nystagmus

  a. Downbeat, gaze-evoked, horizontal, jerk, or vertical

  b. Depressed or abolished optokinetic, latent, positional, voluntary, or congenital nystagmus

 6. Decreased vision

 7. Visual fields

  a. Scotomas

  b. Constriction

 8. Problems with color vision

  a. Color vision defect

  b. Objects have yellow or green tinge

 9. Visual hallucinations

10. Eyelids or conjunctiva

  a. Allergic reactions

  b. Conjunctivitis—nonspecific

  c. Edema

  d. Photosensitivity

  e. Angioneurotic edema

  f. Urticaria

  g. Lupoid syndrome

  h. Erythema multiforme

  i. Stevens-Johnson syndrome

  j. Exfoliative dermatitis

  k. Lyell's syndrome

  l. Symblepharon

  m. Conjunctival bullae

11. Decreased accommodation (primidone)

12. Keratoconjunctivitis sicca (primidone)

13. Decreased intraocular pressure

14. Toxic amblyopia

15. Retinal vasoconstriction

16. Optic nerve disorders

  a. Retrobulbar or optic neuritis

  b. Papilledema

  c. Optic atrophy

17. Abnormal ERG, VEP, or critical flicker fusion
18. Subconjunctival or retinal hemorrhages secondary to drug-induced anemia
19. Ocular teratogenic effects (primidone)
    a. Optic atrophy
    b. Ptosis
    c. Hypertelorism
    d. Epicanthus
    e. Strabismus
20. Cortical blindness (thiopental)

Clinical Significance: Numerous adverse ocular side effects have been attributed to barbiturate usage, yet nearly all significant ocular side effects are found in habitual users or in barbiturate poisoning. Few toxic ocular reactions are found due to barbiturate usage at therapeutic dosages or in short-term therapy. The most common ocular abnormalities are disturbances of ocular movement, such as decreased convergence, paresis of extraocular muscles, or nystagmus. The pupillary response to barbiturate intake is quite variable, but usually miosis occurs except in the most toxic states when mydriasis is the most frequent side effect. Transient or permanent visual loss is primarily found in patients who are in barbiturate coma. Barbital and phenobarbital have the most frequently reported ocular side effects; however, all barbiturates may produce adverse ocular effects. Chronic barbiturate users have a ''tattle tale'' ptosis and blepharoclonus. Normally, a tap on the glabella area of the head produces a few eyelid blinks, but in the barbiturate addict the response will be a rapid fluttering of the eyelids. Bilateral blindness or decreased vision, primarily after recovery from barbiturate-induced coma with or without retinal or disc findings, usually has returned to normal vision. The above findings may occur with acute poisoning as well. Optic neuropathy with complete recovery in a 12-year-old boy from chronic phenobarbital medication is a unique case (Homma, Wakakura, and Ishikawa). The barbiturates do not appear to have teratogenic effects, except possibly primidone.

References:

Alpert, J. N.: Downbeat nystagmus due to anticonvulsant toxicity. Ann. Neurol. *4*:471, 1978.

Amarenco, P., Royer, I., and Guillevin, L.: Ophthalmoplegia externa in barbiturate poisoning. Presse Med. *13*:2453, 1984.

Clarke, R.S.J., Fee, J.H., and Dundee, J.W.: Hypersensitivity reactions to intravenous anaesthetics. In Watkins, J., and Ward, A. (Eds.): Adverse Response to Intravenous Drugs. New York, Grune & Stratton, 1978, pp. 41–47.

Crosby, S.S., et al.: Management of Stevens-Johnson syndrome. Clin. Pharm. *5*:682, 1986.

Homma, K., Wakakura, M., and Ishikawa, S.: A case of phenobarbital-induced optic neuropathy. Neuro-Ophthalmol. *9(6)*:357–359, 1989.

Murphy, D.F.: Anesthesia and intraocular pressure. Anesth. Analg. *64*:520, 1985.

Nakame, Y., et al.: Multi-institutional study on the teratogenicity and fetal toxicity of antiepileptic drugs: A report of a collaborative study group in Japan. Epilepsia *21*: 663, 1980.

Raitta, C., et al.: Changes in the electroretinogram and visual evoked potentials during general anesthesia. Graefes Arch. Clin. Exp. Ophthalmol. *211*:139, 1979.

Tedeschi, G., et al.: Specific oculomotor deficits after amylobarbitone. Psychopharmacology *79*:187, 1983.

Tseng, S.C.G., et al.: Topical retinoid treatment for various dry-eye disorders. Ophthalmology *92*:717, 1985.

Wallar, P.H., Genstler, D.E., and George, C.C.: Multiple systemic and periocular malformations associated with the fetal hydantoin syndrome. Ann. Ophthalmol. *10*: 1568, 1978.

Generic Name: Bromide

Proprietary Name: None

Primary Use: This nonbarbiturate sedative-hypnotic is primarily effective as an anticonvulsant in recalcitrant epilepsy.

Ocular Side Effects:
    A. Systemic Administration
1. Decreased vision
2. Pupils
   a. Mydriasis
   b. Miosis
   c. Decreased or absent reaction to light
   d. Anisocoria
3. Problems with color vision—color vision defect
4. Visual hallucinations—mainly Lilliputian
5. Eyelids or conjunctiva
   a. Allergic reactions
   b. Erythema
   c. Blepharoconjunctivitis
   d. Stevens-Johnson syndrome
6. Decreased accommodation
7. Decreased convergence
8. Diplopia
9. Nystagmus
10. Extraocular muscles
    a. Decreased spontaneous movements
    b. Jerky pursuit movements
11. Photophobia
12. Decreased corneal reflex
13. Apparent movement of stationary objects

14. Visual fields
   a. Scotomas
   b. Constriction

Clinical Significance: The medical use of bromides has been drastically reduced by newer agents since the therapeutic blood level of bromide is so close to its toxic level. Nearly all ocular side effects are reversible after use of the drug is discontinued; however, in acute toxic states, both central and peripheral visual loss may be permanent. It is currently banned in the United States.

References:

Barbour, R.F., Pilkington, F., and Sargant, W.: Bromide intoxication. Br. Med. J. 2: 957, 1936.

Bucy, P.C., Weaver, T.A., and Camp, E. H.: Bromide intoxication of unusual severity and chronicity resulting from self medication with bromoseltzer. JAMA *117*:1256, 1941.

Kunze, U.: Chronic bromide intoxication with a severe neurological deficit. J. Neurol. *213*:149, 1976.

Levin, M.: Eye disturbances in bromide intoxication. Am. J. Ophthalmol. *50*:478, 1960.

Perkins, H.A.: Bromide intoxication: Analysis of cases from a general hospital. Arch. Intern. Med. *85*:783, 1950.

Roy, A.: Bromide intoxication. Br. J. Psychiatry *127*:415, 1975.

Walsh, F.B., and Hoyt, W.F.: Clinical Neuro-Ophthalmology. 3rd Ed., Baltimore, Williams & Wilkins, Vol. III, 1969, pp. 2541, 2618, 2641.

Generic Name: 1. Bromisovalum (Bromisoval*); 2. Carbromal

Proprietary Name: 1. *Available in multi-ingredient preparations only; 2. Mirfudorm

Primary Use: These brominated monoureides are effective in the management of mild insomnia.

Ocular Side Effects:

A. Systemic Administration
   1. Decreased vision
   2. Nystagmus—horizontal or vertical
   3. Pupils
      a. Mydriasis
      b. Miosis
      c. Decreased reaction to light
      d. Anisocoria
   4. Visual fields
      a. Scotomas—central
      b. Constriction

5. Retrobulbar or optic neuritis
6. Eyelids or conjunctiva—Stevens-Johnson syndrome
7. Diplopia
8. Decreased convergence (bromisovalum)
9. Ptosis (carbromal)
10. Retinal edema (carbromal)
11. Optic atrophy

Clinical Significance: Adverse ocular side effects due to these agents are rare except in overdose situations. Except for signs or symptoms related to optic nerve disease, the effects are reversible. Both drugs can elevate serum bromide levels, and this in part may account for some adverse ocular side effects. It is said that nystagmus and diplopia are seen more frequently with bromide poisoning than with these brominated monoureides. One case of acute reversible cataracts has been reported with carbromal use.

References:

Berndt, K., and Piper, H.F.: Eye changes from intoxication with bromcarbamide containing sleeping medications. Klin. Monatsbl. Augenheilkd. *174*:123, 1979.

Copas, D.E., Kay, W.W., and Longman, V.H.: Carbromal intoxication. Lancet *1*:703, 1959.

Crawford, R.: Toxic cataract. Br. Med. J. 2:1231, 1959.

Harenko, A.: Irreversible cerebello-bulbar syndrome as the sequela of bromisovalum poisoning. Ann. Med. Interne. Fenn. *56*:29, 1967.

Harenko, A.: Neurologic findings in chronic bromisovalum poisoning. Ann. Med. Interne. Fenn. *56*:181, 1967.

Heuer, H.: Eye involvement in bromine intoxication. Klin. Monatsbl. Augenheilkd. *172*:400, 1978.

Koch, H.R., and Hockwin, O.: Iatrogenic cataracts. Ther. Ggw. *114*:1450, 1975.

Manthey, K. F.: Eye changes after chronic abuse of bromide-containing sleeping medication. Klin. Monatsbl. Augenheilkd. *172*:400, 1978.

Generic Name: Chloral Hydrate

Proprietary Name: Chloraldurat (Germ., Neth., Switz.), Chloralix (Austral.), Dormel (Austral.), Elix-Nocte (Austral.), Médianox (Switz.), **Noctec** (Austral., Canad., G.B.), Welldorm (G.B., Ire.)

Primary Use: This nonbarbiturate sedative-hypnotic is effective in the treatment of insomnia.

Ocular Side Effects:

A. Systemic Administration
1. Decreased vision
2. Pupils
   a. Mydriasis—toxic states
   b. Miosis

   3. Visual hallucinations—mainly Lilliputian
   4. Ptosis
   5. Decreased convergence
   6. Eyelids or conjunctiva
     a. Allergic reactions
     b. Hyperemia
     c. Edema
   7. Lacrimation
   8. Nonspecific ocular irritation
   9. Nystagmus
  10. Extraocular muscles
     a. Paralysis
     b. Jerky pursuit movements—toxic states

Clinical Significance: While the more serious ocular side effects due to chloral hydrate occur at excessive dosage levels, decreased convergence, miosis, and occasionally ptosis are seen even at recommended therapeutic dosages. Lilliputian hallucinations (in which objects appear smaller than their actual size) are said to be almost characteristic for chloral hydrate-induced delirium. Mydriasis only occurs in severely toxic states.

References:

Goldstein, J.H.: Effects of drugs on cornea, conjunctiva, and lids. Int. Ophthalmol. Clin. *11(2)*: 13, 1971.

Hermans, G.: Les psychotropes. Bull. Soc. Belge Ophtalmol. *160*:15, 1972.

Lane, R.J.M., and Routledge, P.A.: Drug-induced neurological disorders. Drugs *26*: 124, 1983.

Levy D.L., Lipton, R.B., and Holzman, P.S.: Smooth pursuit eye movements: Effects of alcohol and chloral hydrate. J. Psychiatr. Res. *16*:1, 1981.

Lubeck, M.J.: Effects of drugs on ocular muscles. Int. Ophthalmol. Clin. *11(2)*:35, 1971.

Mowry, J.B., and Wilson, G.A.: Effect of exchange transfusion in chloral hydrate overdose. Vet. Human Toxicol. *25*(Suppl. 1):15, 1983.

Walsh, F.B., and Hoyt, W.F.: Clinical Neuro-Ophthalmology. 3rd Ed., Baltimore, Williams & Wilkins, Vol. III, 1969, p. 2619.

Generic Name: Ethchlorvynol

Proprietary Name: Placidyl (Canad.)

Primary Use: This nonbarbiturate sedative-hypnotic is effective in the treatment of simple insomnia. It is also used as a daytime sedative.

Ocular Side Effects:
  A. Systemic Administration
    1. Decreased vision

2. Diplopia
3. Nystagmus—horizontal or gaze
4. Visual hallucinations
5. Problems with color vision
    a. Color vision defect
    b. Objects have yellow tinge
6. Visual fields
    a. Scotomas—central or centrocecal
    b. Constriction
7. Decreased accommodation
8. Toxic amblyopia
9. Anisocoria
10. Optic neuritis

Clinical Significance: Nearly all ocular side effects due to ethchlorvynol are reversible after discontinuation of the drug. In rare cases, visual defects may be permanent after prolonged therapy. Upon withdrawal of the drug, visual hallucinations are common in patients who have been receiving high doses. Although horizontal coarse nystagmus is usually seen in patients who have ingested large amounts of ethchlorvynol, positional central "vestibular" nystagmus has also been reported.

References:

Brust, J.C.M.: Drug abuse and nervous system toxins. *In* Rosenberg, R.N. (Ed.): Neurology: Science and Practice of Clinical Medicine. New York, Grune & Stratton, Vol. 5, 1980, pp. 540–569.

Fogle, J.A., and Spyker, D.A.: Management of chemical and drug injury to the eye. *In* Haddad, L.M., and Winchester, J.F. (Eds.): Clinical Management of Poisoning and Drug Overdose. Philadelphia, W.B. Saunders, 1983, pp. 140–154.

Heston, L.L., and Hastings, D.: Psychosis with withdrawal from ethchlorvynol. Am. J. Psychiatry *137*:249, 1980.

––––––––––––

Generic Name: 1. Glutethimide; 2. Methyprylon

Proprietary Name: 2. Noludar (Canad.)

Primary Use: These piperidinedione derivatives are effective in the treatment of simple insomnia or as mild daytime sedatives.

Ocular Side Effects:
    A. Systemic Administration
        1. Decreased vision
        2. Pupils
            a. Mydriasis

   b. Miosis (methyprylon)
   c. Decreased or absent reaction to light—toxic states
3. Nystagmus—horizontal or vertical
4. Diplopia
5. Decreased accommodation
6. Visual hallucinations
7. Eyelids or conjunctiva
   a. Allergic reactions
   b. Urticaria
   c. Purpura
   d. Exfoliative dermatitis
8. Subconjunctival or retinal hemorrhages secondary to drug-induced anemia
9. Decreased corneal reflex
10. Papilledema

Clinical Significance: At the recommended dosage, few ocular side effects due to these agents are seen; however, in overdose situations ocular side effects, especially with glutethimide, are common. Papilledema and dilated fixed pupils have only been found in near terminal patients.

References:
Critchley, E.M.R.: Drug-induced diseases. Drug-induced neurological disease. Br. Med. J. *1*:862, 1979.

Diagnosis and management of reactions to drug abuse. Med. Lett. Drugs Ther. *27*:77, 1985.

McEvoy, G.K. (Ed.): American Hospital Formulary Service Drug Information 87. Bethesda, American Society of Hospital Pharmacists, 1987, pp. 1161–1162, 1169–1170.

Generic Name: Methaqualone

Proprietary Name: Normi-Nox (Germ.), Pallidan (Span.), Somnomed (Span.)

Street Name: 714s, Ludes, Sopor Quaaludes

Primary Use: This nonbarbiturate sedative-hypnotic is effective in the treatment of simple insomnia or as a daytime sedative.

Ocular Side Effects:
   A. Systemic Administration
      1. Nystagmus
      2. Lacrimation
      3. Pupils

      a. Mydriasis—toxic states

      b. Decreased reaction to light—toxic states

      c. Anisocoria

  4. Eyelids or conjunctiva

      a. Urticaria

      b. Purpura

      c. Erythema multiforme

  5. Diplopia

  6. Decreased vision

  7. Problems with color vision—objects have yellow tinge

  8. Visual hallucinations

  9. Subconjunctival or retinal hemorrhages

Clinical Significance: All ocular side effects due to methaqualone appear to be transient and reversible. Methaqualone has come to be widely abused, and the abuser may employ doses of 75 mg to 2 g per day. Pupillary abnormalities and papilledema are seen primarily in acute toxic states.

References:

Brust, J.C.M.: Drug abuse and nervous system toxins. *In* Rosenberg, R.N. (Ed.): Neurology: Science and Practice of Clinical Medicine. New York, Grune & Stratton, Vol. 5, 1980, pp. 540–569.

Davidson, S.I.: Reports of ocular adverse reactions. Trans. Ophthalmol. Soc. U.K. *93*: 495, 1973.

Drugs for psychiatric disorders. Med. Lett. Drugs Ther. *25*:52, 1983.

Parish, L.C., et al.: Erythema multiforme due to methaqualone. Acta Derm. Venereol. *61*:88, 1981.

Trese, M.: Retinal hemorrhage caused by overdose of methaqualone (Quaalude). Am. J. Ophthalmol. *91*:201, 1981.

III Analgesics, Narcotic Antagonists, and Agents Used to Treat Arthritis

Class: Agents Used to Treat Gout

Generic Name: Allopurinol

Proprietary Name: Allo-300-Tablinen (Germ., Switz.), allo-basan (Switz.), Allo-efeka (Germ.), Allop.-Gry (Germ.), Alloprin (Canad.), Allopur (Switz.), Allo-Puren (Germ.), Allopurin (Span.), Alloremed (Austral.), Allpargin (Germ.), Allural (Span.), Allurit (Ital.), Aloral (G.B.), Apulonga (Germ.), Apurin (Neth.), Bleminol (Germ.), Caplenal (G.B., Ire.), Capurate (Austral.), Cellidrin (Germ.), Cellidrine (Switz.), Cosuric (G.B.), Dabroson (Germ.), dura AL (Germ.), Embarin (Germ.), Epidropal (Germ.), Foligan (Germ., Switz.), Hamarin (G.B.), **Lopurin**, Lo-Uric (S. Afr.), Lysuron (Switz.), Méphanol (Switz.), Novopurol (Canad.), Progout (Austral.), Puricos (S. Afr.), Purinol (Canad., Ire.), Redurate (S. Afr.), Remid (Germ.), Rimapurinol (G.B.), Sigapurol (Switz.), Suspendol (Germ.), Tipuric (Ire.), Uredimin (Switz.), Uribenz (Germ.), Uricemil (Ital.), Uriconorme (Switz.), Uripurinol (Germ.), Urosin (Germ.), Urozyl-SR (S. Afr.), urtias (Germ.), Xanthomax (G.B.), Xanturic (Fr.), **Zyloprim** (Austral., Canad., S. Afr.), Zyloric (Fr., G.B., Germ., Ire., Ital., Neth., Span., Swed., Switz.)

Primary Use: This potent xanthine oxidase inhibitor is primarily used in the treatment of chronic hyperuricemia.

Ocular Side Effects:
A. Systemic Administration
1. Decreased vision
2. Cataracts
3. Eyelids or conjunctiva
   a. Allergic reactions
   b. Erythema
   c. Conjunctivitis—nonspecific
   d. Edema

      e. Photosensitivity
      f. Ulceration
      g. Urticaria
      h. Purpura
      i. Lupoid syndrome
      j. Erythema multiforme
      k. Stevens-Johnson syndrome
      l. Exfoliative dermatitis
      m. Lyell's syndrome
      n. Loss of eyelashes or eyebrows
   4. Subconjunctival or retinal hemorrhages secondary to drug-induced anemia

Clinical Significance: The only ocular side effects of major clinical importance are the probable lens changes associated with prolonged use of this agent. Research by Lerman, Megaw, and Gardner implicates the role of ultraviolet radiation as a cofactor of this process. Data support the finding that cataracts do not develop at any different rate than in the normal population when this drug is used in environments of limited sunlight. Leske, Chylack, and Wu implicate the gout medications as second only to steroids as a major risk factor in cataractogenesis. The lens changes seen with allopurinol are anterior and posterior capsule changes with anterior subcapsular vacuoles. With time, wedge-shaped anterior and posterior cortical haze occurs. This may progress to dense posterior subcapsular opacities. Clinically and histologically, there is no characteristic identifying feature of these lens changes. We recommend to patients taking this agent who are exposed to high levels of sunlight or occupational ultraviolet light exposure that they may benefit from U.V. blocking lenses. While there are a few cases of macular changes reported in the literature and a number in the Registry, there is to date no clear-cut association between allopurinol and macular changes. Allopurinol is, however, a photosensitizing agent, and if one concurs with sunlight playing a role in macular degeneration, then protective lenses may be indicated, especially in the pseudophakic patient.

References:

Dan, M., et al.: Allopurinol-induced toxic epidermal necrolysis. Int. J. Dermatol. *23*: 142, 1984.

Fraunfelder, F.T., and Lerman, S.: Allopurinol and cataracts. Am. J. Ophthalmol. *99*: 215, 1985.

Fraunfelder, F.T., et al.: Cataracts associated with allopurinol therapy. Am. J. Ophthalmol. *94*:137, 1982.

Jick, H., and Brandt, D.E.: Allopurinol and cataracts. Am. J. Ophthalmol. *98*:355, 1984.

Laval, J.: Allopurinol and macular lesions. Arch. Ophthalmol. *80*:415, 1968.

Leske, M.C., Chylack, L.T., and Wu, S.: The lens opacities case-control study. Risk factors for cataract. Arch. Ophthalmol. *109*:244–251, 1991.

Lerman, S., Megaw, J.M., and Gardner, K.: Allopurinol therapy and human cataractogenesis. Am. J. Ophthalmol. *94*:141, 1982.
Pennell, D.J., et al.: Fatal Stevens-Johnson syndrome in a patient on captopril and
allopurinol. Lancet *1*:463, 1984.
Pinnas, G.: Possible association between macular lesions and allopurinol. Arch. Ophthalmol. *79*:786, 1968.

Generic Name: Colchicine

Proprietary Name: Colgout (Austral.)

Primary Use: This alkaloid is used in the prophylaxis and treatment of acute
gout.

Ocular Side Effects:
    A. Systemic Administration
        1. Cornea
            a. Delayed wound healing
            b. Dellen or erosion
            c. Keratitis
        2. Subconjunctival or retinal hemorrhages secondary to drug-
induced anemia
        3. Papilledema—toxic states
    B. Inadvertent Ocular Exposure
        1. Decreased vision
        2. Conjunctival hyperemia
        3. Corneal clouding

Clinical Significance: Colchicine rarely causes adverse ocular side effects
and when it does, they are usually insignificant and transitory. This antimi-
totic agent arrests cell division in metaphase, and it is well documented that
corneal epithelial replication can be so arrested. With the recent interest in
the limbal approach to rectus muscle surgery, there may be an increase in
limbal edema and perilimbal epithelial disturbances. There are reports that
some patients taking colchicine have had difficulty in healing of dellen, or
have experienced peripheral corneal erosions. Significant ocular side effects
have occurred in toxic states and include paresis of extraocular muscles,
keratitis, hypopyon, papilledema, and cataracts. The lens changes may have
been due to severe dehydration. Although optic atrophy secondary to systemic colchicine has been reported in animals, there have been no similar
reports in humans.

References:
Biedner, B.Z., et al.: Colchicine suppression of corneal healing after strabismus surgery.
Br. J. Ophthalmol. *61*:496, 1977.

Estable, J.J.: The ocular effect of several irritant drugs applied directly to the conjunc-
tiva. Am. J. Ophthalmol. *31*:837, 1948.
Heaney, D., et al.: Massive colchicine overdose: A report on the toxicity. Am. J. Med.
Sci. *271*:233, 1976.
Naidus, R.M., Rodvien, R., and Mielke, C.H., Jr.: Colchicine toxicity. A multisystem
disease. Arch. Intern. Med. *137*:394, 1977.
Stapczynski, J.S., et al.: Colchicine overdose: Report of two cases and review of the
literature. Ann. Emerg. Med. *10*:364, 1981.

Class: Antirheumatic Agents

Generic Name: 1. Auranofin; 2. Aurothioglucose; 3. Gold ^{198}Au; 4. Gold
Sodium Thiomalate (Sodium Aurothiomalate); 5. Gold Sodium Thiosulfate
(Sodium Aurothiosulfate)

Proprietary Name: 1. Crisinor (Span.), Crisofin (Ital.), **Ridaura** (Austral.,
Canad., G.B., Germ., Ire., Ital., Neth., S. Afr. Span., Swed., Switz.), Ri-
dauran (Fr.); 2. Aureotan (Germ.), Auromyose (Neth.), Gold-50 (Austral.),
Solganal (Canad.); 4. Miocrin (Span.), **Myochrysine** (Canad.), Myocrisin
(Austral., G.B., Ire., S. Afr., Swed.), Tauredon (Germ., Switz.)

Primary Use: These heavy metals are used in the treatment of active rheumatoid arthritis and nondisseminated lupus erythematosus. Radioactive gold
(^{198}Au) is also employed for its radiation effects in treating neoplastic
growths.

Ocular Side Effects:
    A. Systemic Administration
        1. Red, violet, purple, or brown gold deposits
           a. Eyelids
           b. Conjunctiva
           c. Superficial and deep cornea
           d. Surface of lens
        2. Eyelids or conjunctiva
           a. Allergic reactions
           b. Hyperemia—including ciliary body
           c. Erythema
           d. Blepharoconjunctivitis
           e. Edema
           f. Photosensitivity
           g. Symblepharon
           h. Angioneurotic edema
           i. Urticaria
           j. Purpura
           k. Lupoid syndrome

          l. Erythema multiforme
         m. Stevens-Johnson syndrome
         n. Exfoliative dermatitis
         o. Lyell's syndrome
      3. Photophobia
      4. Cornea
         a. Keratitis
         b. Ulceration
         c. Stromal melting
      5. Iritis
      6. Myasthenic neuromuscular blocking effect
         a. Paralysis of extraocular muscles
         b. Ptosis
         c. Diplopia
      7. May activate the following diseases
         a. Herpes infections
         b. Guillain-Barre syndrome
      8. Nystagmus
      9. Subconjunctival or retinal hemorrhages secondary to drug-induced anemia
    B. Inadvertent Ocular Exposure
      1. Irritation
      2. Corneal clouding
      3. Iritis

Clinical Significance: Although gold deposition in the conjunctiva and superficial cornea is not uncommon, deposition of gold in the lens or deep cornea is uncommon, except in chronic high dosage. Corneal deposition occurs within the epithelium or deep to the epithelium, possibly in the region of the basal lamina. It is usually diffuse, but in some patients the visual axis is spared and the perilimbal corneal area is more involved. Gold deposition in the cornea may only be in the Hudson-Stähli line region, or it may take a vortex distribution as in Fabry's disease; the gold deposits tend to be increased in areas of corneal scarring. Deep stromal involvement is unusual and possibly only associated with large dosages. These deposits will be located in the posterior half of the cornea and are denser inferiorly; the superior cornea and perilimbal areas are usually spared. Lens deposits of gold are much less frequent than corneal deposits and of little to no clinical importance. They are totally reversible after stopping gold therapy. Visual acuity is unaffected, and deposition of gold in the cornea or lens is not an indication for cessation of therapy unless inflammatory complications occur. In general, 1 g of this drug is needed before corneal changes are seen. In total dosages of 1.5 g, from 40% to 80% of patients will have gold deposition in the cornea. While lens deposits have previously been considered rare, 55% of patients taking daily dosages over 1 g for 3 or more years have been reported to develop lens deposits. Corneal deposits may be seen as early as 1 month after starting therapy; once therapy is ceased, clearing is usually complete within 3 to 12 months. Corneal ulceration is a rarely encountered manifestation of gold therapy and is theorized to be an allergic reaction to gold. Ptosis, diplopia, and nystagmus due to gold therapy are rare. It has been suggested that gold deposits in the cornea and anterior chamber are secondary to metal from the aqueous fluid.

References:

Dick, D., and Raman, D.: The Guillain-Barre syndrome following gold therapy. Scand. J. Rheumatol. *11*:119, 1982.

Evanchick, C.C., and Harrington, T.M.: Transient monocular visual loss after aurothioglucose. J. Rheumatol. *12*:619, 1985.

Fam, A.G., Paton, T.W., and Cowan, D.H.: Herpes zoster during gold therapy. Ann. Intern. Med. *94*:712, 1981.

Kincaid, M.C., et al.: Ocular chrysiasis. Arch. Ophthalmol. *100*:1791, 1982.

McCormick, S.A., et al.: Ocular chrysiasis. Ophthalmology *92*:1432, 1985.

Moore, A.P., et al.: Penicillamine-induced myasthenia reactivated by gold. Br. Med. J. *288*:192, 1984.

Segawa, K.: Electron microscopy of the trabecular meshwork in open-angle glaucoma associated with gold therapy. Glaucoma *3*:257, 1981.

Weidle, E.G.: Lenticular chrysiasis in oral chrysotherapy. Am. J. Ophthalmol. *103*: 240, 1987.

Generic Name: Fenoprofen

Proprietary Name: Fenopron (G.B., S. Afr.), Fepron (Ital., Neth.), **Nalfon** (Canad.), Nalgésic (Fr.), Progesic (G.B., Ire.)

Primary Use: This nonsteroidal anti-inflammatory agent is used in the management of rheumatoid arthritis.

Ocular Side Effects:
A. Systemic Administration
   1. Decreased vision
   2. Diplopia
   3. Optic neuritis
   4. Visual fields
      a. Scotomas—centrocecal or paracentral
      b. Enlarged blind spot
      c. Constriction
   5. Eyelids or conjunctiva
      a. Erythema
      b. Conjunctivitis—nonspecific
      c. Angioneurotic edema
      d. Urticaria

    e. Erythema multiforme
    f. Stevens-Johnson syndrome
    g. Exfoliative dermatitis
  6. Subconjunctival or retinal hemorrhages secondary to drug-
     induced anemia

Clinical Significance: Ocular side effects are seldom of clinical significance
with fenoprofen. The most common adverse events are transient blurred
vision and diplopia. Many of the adverse events associated with other nonsteroidal anti-inflammatories have been reported to the Registry with fenoprofen; however, the numbers are small. Again, as with others in this group
of drugs, there appears to be a rare idiosyncratic optic nerve response that
may be associated with the use of this drug. There have been five cases
reported to the Registry of a unilateral or bilateral marked decrease in visual
acuity ranging from 20/80 to 20/200 after 6 months of therapy. Visual fields
may show various types of scotomas. If the medication is stopped, the visual
acuity usually returns to normal in 1 to 3 months. It has, however, taken
over 8 months for color vision to return. If this drug is not discontinued,
the possibility of permanent visual loss may result. It is not possible to state
a positive cause-and-effect relationship between optic neuritis and this drug.
It is prudent, however, to stop the medication if optic neuritis occurs. There
are no reports in the literature of this agent causing pseudotumor cerebri.

References:

Bigby, M., and Stern, R.: Cutaneous reactions to nonsteroidal anti-inflammatory drugs.
    A review. J. Am. Acad. Dermatol. *12*:866, 1985.
Fraunfelder, F.T., Samples, J.R., and Fraunfelder, F.W.: Possible optic nerve side ef-
    fects associated with nonsteroidal anti-inflammatory drugs. J. Toxicol. Cut. & Ocu-
    lar Toxicol. *13(4)*:311–316, 1994.
McEvoy, G.K. (Ed.): American Hospital Formulary Service Drug Information 87.
    Bethesda, American Society for Hospital Pharmacists, 1987, pp. 914–917.
Reynolds, J.E.F. (Ed.): Martindale: The Extra Pharmacopoeia. 29th Ed., London, Phar-
    maceutical Press, 1982, pp. 253–254.
Treusch, P.J., et al.: Agranulocytosis associated with fenoprofen. JAMA *241*:2700,
    1979.

Generic Name: Flurbiprofen

Proprietary Name: *Systemic*: **Ansaid** (Canad.), Cebutid (Fr.), Froben
(Canad., G.B., Germ., Ire., Ital., Neth., S. Afr., Span., Switz.), Ocufen
(Canad., G.B., Ire., S. Afr.), Ocuflur (Germ., Switz.) *Ophthalmic*: Ocufen
(Canad., G.B., Ire., S. Afr.)

Primary Use: *Systemic*: This nonsteroidal anti-inflammatory agent is used
in the treatment of rheumatoid arthritis. *Ophthalmic*: Flurbiprofen is used
for the inhibition of intraoperative miosis.

Ocular Side Effects:
A. Systemic Administration
    1. Decreased vision
    2. Eyelids or conjunctiva
       a. Erythema
       b. Conjunctivitis—nonspecific
       c. Urticaria
    3. Diplopia
    4. Subconjunctival or retinal hemorrhages secondary to drug-induced anemia
B. Local Ophthalmic Use or Exposure
    1. Irritation
       a. Hyperemia
       b. Burning sensation
    2. Cornea
       a. Punctate keratitis
       b. Delayed wound healing
    3. May aggravate herpes infections
    4. Increased ocular or periocular bleeding

Clinical Significance: Ocular side effects secondary to systemic administration are infrequent. While side effects reported with other nonsteroidal anti-inflammatory agents must be looked for, to date no cases of optic neuritis or pseudotumor cerebri have been reported to the Registry. Generally, short-term therapy with ophthalmic flurbiprofen has been well tolerated; the most frequent adverse reactions have been mild transient stinging and burning upon instillation. Flurbiprofen has been shown to inhibit corneal scleral wound healing, decrease leukocytes in tears, and increase complications of herpetic keratitis. Flurbiprofen is one of the more potent nonsteroidal anti-inflammatory drugs that can interfere with thrombocyte aggregation. This may cause intraoperative bleeding as a rare event. This is more common if the patient is already taking oral agents, i.e., other nonsteroidal anti-inflammatory drugs, aspirin, etc., or if topical ocular flurbiprofen is used excessively.

References:

Bergamini, M.V.W.: Pharmacology of flurbiprofen, a nonsteroidal anti-inflammatory drug. Int. Ophthalmol. Rep. 6:2, 1981.

Feinstein, N.C.: Toxicity of flurbiprofen sodium. Arch. Ophthalmol. 106:311, 1988.

Flurbiprofen—an ophthalmic NSAID. Med. Lett. Drugs Ther. 29:58, 1987.

Gimbel, H.V.: The effect of treatment with topical nonsteroidal anti-inflammatory drugs with and without intraoperative epinephrine on the maintenance of mydriasis during cataract surgery. Ophthalmology 96(5):585–588, 1989.

Miller, D., et al.: Topical flurbiprofen or prednisolone. Effect on corneal wound healing in rabbits. Arch. Ophthalmol. 99:681, 1981.

Samples, J.R.: Sodium flurbiprofen for surgically induced miosis and the control of inflammation. J. Toxicol. Cut. & Ocular Toxicol. *8(2)*:163–166, 1989.

Trousdale, M.D., Dunkel, E.C., and Nesburn, A.B.: Effect of flurbiprofen on herpes simplex keratitis in rabbits. Invest. Ophthalmol. Vis. Sci. *19*:267, 1980.

Generic Name: Ibuprofen

Proprietary Name: Abbifen (S. Afr.), Aciril (Ital.), Actifen (Span.), Actiprofen (Canad.), **Advil** (Canad., Fr.), Aktren (Germ.), Aldospray Analgesico (Span.), Algiasdin (Span.), Algifor (Switz.), Algisan (Span.), Algofen (Ital.), Altior (Span.), Amersol (Canad.), Anadin Ibuprofen (G.B.), Analgyl (Fr.), Anco (Germ.), Antalgil (Ital.), Antalgit (Switz.), Antiflam (S. Afr.), Apsifen (G.B.), Arfen (Ital.), Arthrofen (G.B.), Artrene (Ital.), Benflogin (Ital.), Betagesic (S. Afr.), Betaprofen (S. Afr.), Brufen (Austral., Fr., G.B., Germ., Ire., Ital., Neth., S. Afr., Swed., Switz.), Brufort (Ital.), Bufedon (Neth.), Bufigen (Ire.), Cesra (Germ.), Contraneural (Germ.), Cunil (Ire.), Cuprofen (G.B.), Cusialgil (Span.), Dignoflex (Germ.), Dimidon (Germ.), Dismenol N (Germ.), Dolgit (Fr., Germ., Switz.), Dolocyl (Span., Switz.), Dolo-Dolgit (Germ.), Dolo-Neos (Germ.), DoLo-Puren (Germ.), Dorival (Span.), dura-Ibu (Germ.), duralbuprofen (Germ.), Dysdolen (Germ.), Ebufac (G.B.), Ecoprofen (Switz.), Ediluna (Span.), Esprenit (Germ.), Evasprin (Span.), exneural (Germ.), Fénalgic (Fr.), Femafen (G.B.), Femapirin (Neth.), Femidol (Span.), Fenbid (G.B.), Flubenil (Ital.), Focus (Ital.), Ibenon (Span.), Ibol (Germ.), Ibosure (Neth.), Ibrufhalal (G.B.), ibu-Attritin (Germ.), Ibu-Cream (Austral.), Ibufac (G.B.), Ibufen-L (Switz.), Ibufug (Germ.), Ibugel (G.B.), Ibuhexal (Germ.), Ibular (G.B.), Ibuleve (G.B.), Ibumetin (Neth., Swed.), Ibuphlogont (Germ.), **Ibuprohm, Ibu-Tab**, Ibutad (Germ.), Ibutop (Germ.), Ibu-vivimed (Germ.), Imbun (Germ.), Inabrin (Ital.), Incefal (Span.), Inflam (Austral.), Inoven (G.B.), Inza (S. Afr.), Ipren (Swed.), Iproben (Switz.), Irfen (Switz.), Isdol (Span.), Isisfen (G.B.), Junifen (G.B.), Kos (Ital.), Lacondan (Span.), Leonal (Span.), Librofem (G.B.), Lidifen (G.B.), Lisi-Budol (Span.), **Medipren** (Canad.), Melfen (Ire.), **Midol 200 Advanced Pain Formula,** Migrafen (G.B.), Mobilat (Germ.), Moment (Ital.), **Motrin** (Canad., G.B.), Narfen (Span.), Neobrufen (Span.), Nerofen (Neth.), Novaprin (G.B.), Novogent (Germ.), Novoprofen (Canad.), **Nuprin**, Nurofen (Austral., Fr., G.B., Ire., Ital., Span., Swed., Switz.), Optalidon (Germ.), Optifen (Switz.), Opturem (Germ.), Pacifene (G.B.), Parsal (Germ.), **Pedia-Profen**, Phor Pain (G.B.), Posidolor (Span.), Proflex (G.B.), Prontalgin (Ital.), Rafen (Austral.), Relcofen (G.B.), Rimafen (G.B.), Rofen (S. Afr.), **Rufen, Saleto**, Sedaspray (Span.), Solufen (S. Afr.), Spedifen (Switz.), stadasan (Germ.), Tabalon (Germ.), Trauma-Dolgit (Germ.), Urem (Germ.))

Primary Use: This antipyretic analgesic is used in the treatment of rheumatoid arthritis and osteoarthritis.

Ocular Side Effects:
A. Systemic Administration
  1. Decreased vision
  2. Diplopia
  3. Problems with color vision
    a. Color vision defect, red-green defect
    b. Colors appear faded
  4. Abnormal visual sensations
    a. Moving mosaic of colored lights
    b. Shooting streaks
  5. Optic or retrobulbar neuritis
  6. Myopia
  7. Papilledema secondary to pseudotumor cerebri
  8. Abnormal ERG or VEP
  9. Visual fields
    a. Scotomas—centrocecal or paracentral
    b. Constriction
    c. Hemianopsia
    d. Enlarged blind spot
  10. Toxic amblyopia
  11. Keratoconjunctivitis sicca
  12. Photophobia
  13. Visual hallucinations
  14. Eyelids or conjunctiva
    a. Erythema
    b. Conjunctivitis—nonspecific
    c. Edema
    d. Photosensitivity
    e. Angioneurotic edema
    f. Urticaria
    g. Purpura
    h. Lupoid syndrome
    i. Erythema multiforme
    j. Stevens-Johnson syndrome
    k. Lyell's syndrome
  15. Nystagmus—toxic states
  16. Subconjunctival or retinal hemorrhages secondary to drug-induced anemia

Clinical Significance: Ibuprofen is one of the largest selling antiarthritic agents in the world. The adverse ocular event most commonly associated with this drug is transient blurred vision. In those patients who have experienced a drug rechallenge, refractive error changes, diplopia, photophobia, dry eyes, and decrease in color vision appear to be well documented. There may be a rare idiosyncratic optic nerve response associated with the use of this drug. The typical sequence is that after a few months of therapy, a unilateral or bilateral marked decrease in visual acuity occurs, with vision receding to the 20/80 to 20/200 range. Visual fields may show various types of scotomas. If the medication is stopped, visual acuity usually returns to normal in 1 to 3 months, but it may take up to 8 months for color vision to return to normal. If ibuprofen is not discontinued, permanent visual loss may result. For a drug so commonly used, often in combination with other agents, it is not possible to specifically implicate this agent. However, many of the cases are outside the usual multiple sclerosis age group and occur shortly after starting this medication. Therefore, patients taking this drug should be told to stop this medication if a sudden decrease in vision occurs. Ibuprofen, as well as with other nonsteroidal anti-inflammatories, can cause pseudotumor cerebri. This is more common if used in combination with other antiarthritic agents that can also induce this side effect. If there is an unexplained decrease in vision that occurs while taking ibuprofen, tests to rule out optic nerve abnormalities are important.

References:

Asherov, J., et al.: Diplopia following ibuprofen administration. JAMA *248*:649, 1982.

Birch, J., et al.: Acquired color vision defects. In Pokorny, J., et al. (Eds.): Congenital and Acquired Color Vision Defects. New York, Grune & Stratton, 1979, pp. 243–350.

Court, H., Streete, P., and Volans, G.N.: Acute poisoning with ibuprofen. Human Toxicol. *2*:381, 1983.

Dukes, M.N.G. (Ed.): Meyler's Side Effects of Drugs. Amsterdam, Excerpta Medica, Vol. X, 1984, pp. 162–163.

Fraunfelder, F.T.: Interim report: National Registry of Possible Drug-Induced Ocular Side Effects. Ophthalmology *87*:87, 1980.

Fraunfelder, F.T., Samples, J.R., and Fraunfelder, F.W.: Possible optic nerve side effects associated with nonsteroidal anti-inflammatory drugs. J. Toxicol. Cut. & Ocular Toxicol. *13(4)*:311–316, 1994.

Hamburger, H.A., Beckman, H., and Thompson, R.: Visual evoked potentials and ibuprofen (Motrin) toxicity. Ann. Ophthalmol. *16*:328, 1984.

Melluish, J.W., et al.: Ibuprofen and visual function. Arch. Ophthalmol. *93*:781, 1975.

Palmer, C.A.L.: Toxic amblyopia from ibuprofen. Br. Med. J. *3*:765, 1972.

Quinn, J.P., et al.: Eosinophilic meningitis and ibuprofen therapy. Neurology *34*:108, 1984.

Tullio, C.J.: Ibuprofen-induced visual disturbance. Am. J. Hosp. Pharm. *38*:1362, 1981.

Generic Name: 1. Indomethacin (Indometacin); 2. Sulindac

Proprietary Name: 1. Ainscrid (Fr.), Aliviosin (Span.), Amuno (Germ.), Arthrexin (Austral., S. Afr.), Articulen (S. Afr.), Artracin (G.B.), Artrinovo (Span.), Betacin (S. Afr.), Bonidon (Switz.), Boutycin (Ital.), Butidil (Span.), Chibro-Amuno (Germ.), Chrono-Indocid (Fr.), Cidalgon (Ital.), Cidomel (Ire.), Confortid (Germ., Swed., Switz.), Dolazol (Neth.), Dometin

(Neth.), durametacin (Germ.), Elmetacin (Germ., S. Afr., Switz.), Flamecid (S. Afr.), Flexin Continus (G.B., Ire.), Flogoter (Span.), Imbrilon (G.B., Ire.), Imet (Ital.), Inacid (Span.), Inacid Dap (Span.), Indo Framan (Span.), Indocaf (Span.), Indocid (Austral., Canad., Fr., G.B., Neth., S. Afr., Switz.), Indocid PDA (Canad., G.B., Neth.), **Indocin**, Indocollyre (Fr.), Indocontin (Germ.), Indoftol (Span.), Indolar SR (G.B.), Indolgina (Span.), Indomax (G.B.), Indomed (S. Afr.), Indomee (Swed.), Indomet-ratiopharm (Germ.), Indomisal (Germ.), Indomod (G.B.), Indo-Phlogont (Germ.), Indophtal (Switz.), Indoptic (Switz.), Indoptol (Neth.), Indorektal (Germ.), Indo-Spray (Austral.), Indo-Tablinen (Germ.), Indoxen (Ital.), Mederreumol (Span.), Metacen (Ital.), Methabid (S. Afr.), Mobilan (G.B.), Neo-Decabutin (Span.), Novomethacin (Canad.), Peralgon (Ital.), Restameth-SR (S. Afr.), Reumo (Span.), Reusin (Span.), Rheumacin (Austral., G.B.), Rimacid (G.B.), Slo-Indo (G.B.) Vonum (Germ.); 2. Apo-Sulin (Canad.), Arthrocine (Fr.), Citi-reuma (Ital.), **Clinoril** (Austral., Canad., G.B., Ital., Neth., S. Afr., Swed., Switz.), Clisundac (Ital.), Lyndak (Ital.), Novosundac (Canad.), Reumyl (Ital.), Sudac (Ital.), Sulartrene (Ital.), Sulen (Ital.), Sulic (Ital.), Sulindal (Span.), Sulinol (Ital.), Sulreuma (Ital.)

Primary Use: *Systemic:* These nonsteroidal anti-inflammatory drugs are methylated indole derivates used as antipyretic, analgesic, or anti-inflammatory agents in the treatment of rheumatoid arthritis, rheumatoid spondylitis, and degenerative joint disease. *Ophthalmic:* Indometacin has been advocated for the treatment of cystoid macular edema or preoperatively to enhance mydriasis at cataract surgery. It has also been advocated in the management of symptoms due to corneal scars, edema, or erosions.

Ocular Side Effects:
  A. Systemic Administration
    1. Decreased vision
    2. Diplopia
    3. Eyelids or conjunctiva
      a. Erythema
      b. Blepharoconjunctivitis
      c. Edema
      d. Photosensitivity
      e. Angioneurotic edema
      f. Urticaria
      g. Lupoid syndrome
      h. Erythema multiforme
      i. Stevens-Johnson syndrome
      j. Lyell's syndrome
      k. Exfoliative dermatitis
    4. Subconjunctival or retinal hemorrhages
    5. Cornea

        a. Keratitis
        b. Deposits (indomethacin)
        c. Erosions (indomethacin)
    6. Keratoconjunctivitis sicca
    7. Optic neuritis—retrobulbar neuritis
    8. Visual hallucinations
    9. Problems with color vision—color vision defect, blue-yellow defect (indomethacin)
  10. Abnormal ERG or EOG—(indomethacin)
  11. Papilledema secondary to pseudotumor cerebri
  12. Paralysis of extraocular muscles
  13. Retina or macula
        a. Edema
        b. Degeneration
        c. Retinal thinning
        d. Pigment mottling
  14. Visual fields
        a. Scotoma
        b. Constriction
        c. Enlarged blind spot
B. Local Ophthalmic Use or Exposure—Topical Ocular
    1. Irritation
    2. Superficial punctate keratitis
    3. Eyelids
        a. Edema
        b. Erythema
    4. Burning sensation
    5. Decreases miosis during intraocular surgery (weak)

Clinical Significance: Systemic adverse drug effects from indomethacin can occur in up to 35% to 50% of patients receiving normal dosage levels after taking the drug for many months. Sulindac has many fewer side effects. As with all nonsteroidal anti-inflammatories, decreased vision can occur in rare cases, and one needs to rule out a secondary optic neuritis or papilledema from pseudotumor cerebri as the cause. These are extremely rare events but well documented. If diplopia occurs, it is usually always transitory. Subconjunctival and retinal hemorrhages are secondary to a direct toxic effect of the drug on the hemopoietic system and are usually a sign of anemia. Reversible corneal deposits have occurred with both of these drugs, as have recurrent corneal erosions. While there are a number of reports of corneal melts and perforations in the Registry, a cause-and-effect relationship has not been clearly established. There has been significant discussion regarding the relationship of these drugs with macular or retinal disease; however, these data are not clear-cut. There are a number of reports implicating this drug as retinal toxic, especially in high dosages given over a prolonged period. The cases include color vision, EOG, and ERG abnormalities. These drugs are photosensitizers, and the potential of macular phototoxicity exists as with all photosensitizers, especially in the aphake. Still, there is debate as to a true cause-and-effect relationship. At worst, these are extremely rare findings. Other than retinal findings, all side effects seem to be reversible with time once the drug is discontinued. Topical ocular indomethacin is not available commercially, and ''home'' mixtures have been associated with ocular burning and irritation, including superficial punctate keratitis. These all seem to be reversible and cause no significant adverse effect. There has been a case, however, of acute asthma from topical ocular indomethacin.

References:

Birch, J., et al.: Acquired color vision defects. *In* Pokorny, J., et al.: Congenital and Acquired Color Vision Defects. New York, Grune & Stratton, 1979, pp. 243–350.

Carr, R.E., Siegel, I.M.: Retinal function in patients treated with indomethacin. Am. J. Ophthalmol. *75*:302–306, 1973.

Fraunfelder, F.T., Samples, J.R., and Fraunfelder, F.W.: Possible optic nerve side effects associated with nonsteroidal anti-inflammatory drugs. J. Toxicol. Cut. & Ocular Toxicol. *13(4)*:311–316, 1994.

Gimbel, H.W.: The effect of treatment with topical nonsteroidal anti-inflammatory drugs with and without intraoperative epinephrine on the maintenance of mydriasis during cataract surgery. Ophthalmology *96(5)*:585–588, 1989.

Graham, C.M., and Blach, R.K.: Indomethacin retinopathy: case report and review. Brit. J. Ophthalmol. *72*:434–438, 1988.

Henkes, H.E., van Lith G.H.M., and Canta, L.R.: Indomethacin retinopathy. Am. J. Ophthalmol. *73*:846–856, 1972.

Katz, I.M.: Indomethacin. Ophthalmology *88*:455, 1981.

Katzman, B., et al.: Pseudotumor cerebri: An observation and review. Ann. Ophthalmol. *13*:887, 1981.

Rich, L.F.: Toxic drug effects on the cornea. J. Toxicol. Cut. & Ocular Toxicol. *1*: 267, 1982–1983.

Sheehan G.J., and Kutzner M.R.: Acute Asthma Attack Due to Ophthalmic Indocin. Ann. Intl. Med., *111*:337–338, 1989.

Yoshizumi, M.O., Schwartz, S., and Peterson M.: Ocular toxicity of topical indomethacin eye drops. J. Toxicology *10(3)*:201–206, 1991.

Generic Name: Ketoprofen

Proprietary Name: Alrheumat (G.B., Ire.), Alrheumun (Germ.), Apo-Keto (Canad.), Arcental (Span.), Artrosilene (Ital.), Bi-Profénid (Fr.), Dexal (Ital.), europan (Germ.), Extraplus (Span.), Fastum (Ital., Span.), Flexen (Ital.), Iso-K (Ital.), Kefenid (Ital.), Ketalgin (Ital.), Ketartrium (Ital.), Keto (Ital.), Ketofen (Ital.), Ketosolan (Span.), Meprofen (Ital.), **Orudis** (Austral., Canad., G.B., Germ., Ire., Ital., Neth., S. Afr., Span., Swed.), Oruvail (G.B., Ire., S. Afr.), Oscorel (Neth.), Profénid (Fr.), Profenid (Switz.), Reumoquin

(Span.), Reuprofen (Ital.), Rhodis (Canad.), Salient (Ital.), Sinketol (Ital.), Tafirol (Span.)

Primary Use: This nonsteroidal anti-inflammatory drug with antipyretic and analgesic properties is used in the treatment of rheumatoid arthritis, osteo-arthritis, ankylosing spondylitis, and gout.

Ocular Side Effects:
  A. Systemic Administration
    1. Decreased vision
    2. Eyelids or conjunctiva
      a. Erythema
      b. Conjunctivitis—nonspecific
      c. Edema
      d. Discoloration
      e. Photosensitivity
      f. Urticaria
      g. Purpura
      h. Exfoliative dermatitis
      i. Eczema
    3. Nonspecific ocular irritation
      a. Hyperemia
      b. Ocular pain
    4. Paralysis of extraocular muscles
    5. May aggravate the following diseases
      a. Myasthenia gravis
      b. Herpes infections
    6. Visual hallucinations
    7. Subconjunctival or retinal hemorrhages secondary to systemic anemia

Clinical Significance: As with other propionic acid nonsteroidal anti-inflam-matory drugs, the full gamut of possible adverse ocular events associated with this group of drugs should be looked for. However, in general, this agent has few ocular side effects. There is only one case each of pseudo-tumor cerebri or possible optic neuritis reported to the Registry, so a causa-tive relationship is highly unlikely. Ketoprofen, however, has been associ-ated with precipitating cholinergic crises. It has also been associated with aggravating herpes simplex systemically and ocularly. We are not convinced that this agent causes keratoconjunctivitis sicca; however, since the drug is secreted in the tears it would have the potential to aggravate patients with borderline sicca or those with pre-existing sicca. Since this agent is a photo-sensitizing agent, selective use of UV blocking lenses might be considered in selected cases that may be affected by phototoxicity, i.e., cornea, lens, or retina.

References:

Alomar, A.: Ketoprofen photodermatitis. Contact Dermatitis *12*:112, 1985.

Dukes, M.N.G. (Ed.): Meyler's Side Effects of Drugs. Amsterdam, Excerpta Medica, Vol. X, 1984, p. 163.

Fraunfelder, F.T., Samples, J.R., and Fraunfelder, F.W.: Possible optic nerve side effects associated with nonsteroidal anti-inflammatory drugs. J. Toxicol. Cut. & Ocular Toxicol. *13(4)*:311–316, 1994.

Larizza, D., et al.: Ketoprofen causing pseudotumor cerebri in Bartter's syndrome. N. Engl. J. Med. *300*:796, 1979.

McDowell, I.F.W., and McConnell, J.B.: Cholinergic crisis in myasthenia gravis precipitated by ketoprofen. Br. Med. J. *291*:1094, 1985.

Umez-Eronini, E.M.: Conjunctivitis due to ketoprofen. Lancet 2:737, 1978.

Generic Name: Naproxen

Proprietary Name: Aliviomas (Span.), Alpoxen (Swed.), **Anaprox** (Canad.), Antalgin (Span.), Apo-Napro-Na (Canad.), Apranax (Fr., Germ., Switz.), Arthrosin (G.B.), Arthroxen (G.B.), Artroxen (Ital.), Axer (Ital.), Denaxpren (Span.), Dysmenalgit (Germ.), Femex (Neth.), Floginax (Ital.), Flogogin (Ital.), Floxalin (Ital.), Genoxen (Ire.), Gibinap (Ital.), Gibixen (Ital.), Laraflex (G.B.), Laser (Ital.), Leniartril (Ital.), Lundiran (Span.), Nafasol (S. Afr.), Napmel (Ire.), Naprex (Ire.), Naprium (Ital.), Naprius (Ital.), Naprogesic (Austral.), Naprokes (Span.), Naprorex (Ital.), **Naprosyn** (Austral., Canad., G.B., Ital., S. Afr., Span., Swed., Switz.), Naprosyne (Fr., Neth.), Naproval (Span.), Naxen (Austral., Canad., S. Afr.), Novonaprox (Canad.), Novonaprox Sodium (Canad.), Nycopren (G.B.), Pranoxen Continus (G.B.), Prexan (Ital.), Primeral (Ital.), Pronaxen (Swed.), Prosaid (G.B.), Proxen (Germ., Span., Switz.), Rheuflex (G.B.), Rimoxyn (G.B.), Rofanten (Span.), Sobronil (Span.), Synflex (Canad., G.B., Ital., S. Afr.), Valrox (G.B.), Xenar (Ital.)

Primary Use: This antipyretic analgesic is used in the treatment of rheumatoid arthritis, osteoarthritis, and ankylosing spondylitis.

Ocular Side Effects:

A. Systemic Administration
  1. Decreased vision
  2. Decreased accommodation
  3. Problems with color vision
      a. Color vision defect
      b. Objects have green or red tinge
  4. Optic or retrobulbar neuritis
  5. Papilledema secondary to pseudotumor cerebri
  6. Photophobia
  7. Corneal opacities—verticillate pattern

    8. Visual field defects
       a. Scotomas—centrocecal or paracentral
       b. Constriction
       c. Hemianopsia
       d. Enlarged blind spot
    9. Keratoconjunctivitis sicca
  10. Paresis of extraocular muscles
  11. Eyelids or conjunctiva
       a. Allergic reactions
       b. Erythema
       c. Conjunctivitis—nonspecific
       d. Edema
       e. Photosensitivity
       f. Angioneurotic edema
       g. Urticaria
       h. Purpura
       i. Erythema multiforme
       j. Stevens-Johnson syndrome
       k. Exfoliative dermatitis
       l. Lyell's syndrome
  12. Subconjunctival or retinal hemorrhages secondary to drug-induced anemia

Clinical Significance: With the increased use of this nonsteroidal anti-inflammatory agent, more adverse ocular effects have been reported. Although some patients complain of decreased vision, this is seldom a significant finding and occurs in less than 5% of patients. It is possible, but not probable, that in rare instances this agent can cause optic or retrobulbar neuritis. This, however, is not proven, although this group of drugs can cause numerous CNS side effects. Typically, these patients are taking the drug about a year before the optic neuritis, often unilateral, presents. The drug should be discontinued. Pseudotumor cerebri is well documented to occur with naproxen. Both of these findings are probably idiosyncratic responses. Whether or not this agent causes anterior or posterior cataracts is unknown; there are 20 such reports in the Registry, but there is no proof to date of a cause-and-effect relationship. Whorl-like corneal opacities have been associated with the use of naproxen, and the Registry has also received several reports of corneal ulcerations. This agent is one of the more potent photosensitizing nonsteroidal anti-inflammatory agents. Theoretically, this could enhance retinal disease, especially in the pseudophake who has macular disease or necrotizing vasculitis. There is data to support that naproxen has been associated with systemic vascular disorders.

References:
Diffey, B.L., Daymond, T.J., and Fairgreaves, H.: Phototoxic reactions to piroxicam, naproxen and tiaprofenic acid. Br. J. Rheumatol. 22:239,1983.

Fraunfelder, F.T.: Interim report: National Registry of Possible Drug-Induced Ocular Side Effects. Ophthalmology 86:126, 1979.

Fraunfelder, F.T., Samples, J.R., and Fraunfelder, F.W.: Possible optic nerve side effects associated with nonsteroidal anti-inflammatory drugs. J. Toxicol. Cut. & Ocular Toxicol. 13(4):311–316, 1994.

Harry, D.J., and Hicks, H.: Naproxen hypersensitivity. Hosp. Form. 18:648, 1983.

McEvoy, G.K. (Ed.): American Hospital Formulary Service Drug Information 87. Bethesda, American Society of Hospital Pharmacists, 1987, pp. 942–946.

Mordes, J.P., Johnson, M.W., and Soter, N.A.: Possible naproxen-associated vasculitis. Arch. Intern. Med. 140:985, 1980.

Shelley, W.B., et al.: Naproxen photosensitization demonstrated by challenge. Cutis 38:169, 1986.

Svihovec, J.: Anti-inflammatory analgesics and drugs used in gout. In Dukes, M.N.G. (Ed.): Meyler's Side Effects of Drugs. Amsterdam, Excerpta Medica, Vol. IX, 1980, p. 152.

Szmyd, L., Jr., and Perry, H.D.: Keratopathy associated with the use of naproxen. Am. J. Ophthalmol. 99:598, 1985.

Generic Name: 1. Oxyphenbutazone; 2. Phenylbutazone

Proprietary Name: 1. Californit (Germ.), Otone (S. Afr.), Oxybutazone (Canad.), Phlogont (Germ.), Tanderil (G.B., Germ., Ire., Switz.); 2. Butacote (G.B., Ire.), Butadion (Switz.), Butadiona (Span.), Butazina (Ital.), Butazolidin (Austral., Canad., Germ., Ire., Neth., Swed.), Butazolidina (Ital., Span.), Butazolidine (Fr., Switz.), Butazone (G.B.), Butrex (S. Afr.), Carudol (Fr., Ital., Span., Switz.), Exrheudon N (Germ.), Inflazone (S. Afr.), Intrabutazone (Canad.), Kadol (Ital.), Novobutazone (Canad.), Ticinil (Ital.)

Primary Use: These pyrazolone derivatives are effective in the management of acute gout, ankylosing spondylitis, osteoarthritis, and musculoskeletal disorders.

Ocular Side Effects:
    A. Systemic Administration
        1. Decreased vision
        2. Eyelids or conjunctiva
            a. Allergic reactions
            b. Hyperemia
            c. Conjunctivitis—nonspecific
            d. Edema
            e. Photosensitivity
            f. Urticaria
            g. Lupoid syndrome
            h. Erythema multiforme
            i. Stevens-Johnson syndrome
            j. Exfoliative dermatitis

        k. Lyell's syndrome
        l. Pemphigoid lesion with symblepharon (phenylbutazone)
   3. Subconjunctival or retinal hemorrhages
   4. Paralysis of extraocular muscles
   5. Diplopia
   6. Problems with color vision—color vision defect, red-green
      defect
   7. Cornea
        a. Peripheral stromal vascularization
        b. Opacities
        c. Keratitis
        d. Scarring
        e. Ulceration
   8. Photophobia
   9. Optic or retrobulbar neuritis
 10. Visual fields
        a. Scotoma
        b. Altitudinal defects
 11. Visual hallucinations

Clinical Significance: Ocular side effects due to these drugs are not uncommon and can be severe. At least 10% to 15% of patients taking these agents must discontinue their use due to systemic toxic reactions. This is due, in part, to the high dosages necessary in some patients to control their disease. Unlike most drugs, these act so that the older the patient, the more likely an untoward side effect occurs. Side effects are so common in patients older than the age of 60 that the manufacturers recommend treatment only at weekly intervals. The most common ocular side effect is decreased vision. It has been suggested that this is due to increased lens hydration. Phenylbutazone-induced hypermetropia up to 3 to 4 diopters has been reported to the Registry. Eyelid or conjunctival changes followed by retinal hemorrhages, not necessarily associated with a drug-induced anemia, are the next most frequent adverse ocular reactions. This group of drugs can elicit an allergic reaction that induces a lupus syndrome with its associated ocular side effects; some of the reported conjunctival or corneal adverse reactions may be due to lupoid effects rather than a direct drug effect. These drugs are photosensitizers, and the potential for eyelid and anterior and posterior segment phototoxicity does exist. Optic and retrobulbar neuritis have been associated with these agents. The mean onset occurs after 3 or more years of use. No pseudotumor cerebri has been reported with these agents as has been the case with other nonsteroidal anti-inflammatory agents.

References:
Bigby, M., and Stern, R.: Cutaneous reactions to nonsteroidal anti-inflammatory drugs. A review. J. Am. Acad. Dermatol. *12*:866, 1985.

Class: Antirheumatic Agents

color vision defects. *In* Pokorny, J., et al. (Eds.): Congenital
Birch, J., et al.: Acq¹ Vision Defects. New York, Grune & Stratton, 1979, pp.
and Acquired
243–350.   ions on drug-induced toxic epidermal necrolysis in Singapore. J.
Chan, H.L.: Qlatol. *10*:973, 1984.
    Am. A   hotosensitivity. Med. Lett. Drugs Ther. *28*:51, 1986.
Drugs th Ed.): Meyler's Side Effects of Drugs. Amsterdam, Excerpta Medica,
       r, pp. 153–156.
Duke, T, Samples, J.R., and Fraunfelder, F.W.: Possible optic nerve side effects
    1 with nonsteroidal anti-inflammatory drugs. J. Toxicol. Cut. & Ocular
    F *13(4)*:311–316, 1994.
    .: Toxic drug effects on the cornea. J. Toxicol. Cut. & Ocular Toxicol. *1*:
    1982–1983.
    ), V., and Pisani, M.: Induced pemphigus. Arch. Dermatol. Res. *274*:123, 1982.

---

neric Name: Piroxicam

Proprietary Name: Antiflog (Ital.), Artroxicam (Ital.), Brexin (Ital.), Bruxicam (Ital.), Cicladol (Ital.), Cicladol L (Ital.), Dexicam (Ital.), Doblexan (Span.), Felden (Germ., Swed., Switz.), Feldène (Fr.), **Feldene** (Austral., Canad., G.B., Ital., Neth., S. Afr., Span.), Flogobene (Ital.), Improntal (Span.), Lampoflex (Ital.), Larapam (G.B.), Nirox (Ital.), Novopirocam (Canad.), Piroftal (Ital.), Pirozip (G.B.), Polipirox (Ital.), Reucam (Ital.), Reudene (Ital.), Reumagil (Ital.), Riacen (Ital.), Roxene (Ital.), Roxenil (Ital.), Roxicam (S. Afr.), Roxiden (Ital.), Roxim (Ital.), Sasulen (Span.), Vitaxicam (Span.), Zacam (Ital.), Zunden (Ital.)

Primary Use: This nonsteroidal anti-inflammatory drug is used in the treatment of osteoarthritis and rheumatoid arthritis.

Ocular Side Effects:

A. Systemic Administration
1. Decreased vision
2. Eyelids or conjunctiva
   a. Erythema
   b. Conjunctivitis—nonspecific
   c. Photosensitivity
   d. Angioneurotic edema
   e. Urticaria
   f. Purpura
   g. Erythema multiforme
   h. Stevens-Johnson syndrome
   i. Exfoliative dermatitis
   j. Lyell's syndrome
   k. Pemphigoid lesion

    l. Eczema
    m. Loss of eyelashes or eyebrows
3. Nonspecific ocular irritation
    a. Lacrimation
    b. Hyperemia
    c. Edema
    d. Burning sensation
4. Visual hallucinations
5. Decreased accommodation
6. Diplopia
7. Optic neuritis

Clinical Significance: Worldwide, piroxicam is one of the most widely prescribed nonsteroidal anti-inflammatory drugs and appears to have no serious ocular side effects except a questionable optic neuritis. This possible drug-related event is described by Fraunfelder, Samples, and Fraunfelder. This is one of the few nonsteroidal anti-inflammatory agents with which pseudotumor cerebri has not been reported. Other ocular side effects are infrequent and usually transient. This agent is a strong photosensitizing agent, and sunglasses may be indicated in selected cases.

References:

Duro, J.C., et al.: Piroxicam-induced erythema multiforme. J. Rheumatol. *11*:554, 1984.

Fraunfelder, F.T., Samples, J.R., and Fraunfelder, F.W.: Possible optic nerve side effects associated with nonsteroidal anti-inflammatory drugs. J. Toxicol. Cut. & Ocular Toxicol. *13(4)*:311–316, 1994.

Halasz, C.L.G.: Photosensitivity to the nonsteroidal anti-inflammatory drug piroxicam. Cutis *39*:37, 1987.

Roujeau, J.C., et al.: Sjögren-like syndrome after drug-induced toxic epidermal necrolysis. Lancet *1*:609, 1985.

Rolando, M., et al.: Piroxicam eyedrops for the control of inflammation after argon laser trabeculoplasty. Glaucoma *7*:195, 1985.

Stern, R.S., and Bigby, M.: An expanded profile of cutaneous reactions to nonsteroidal anti-inflammatory drugs. Reports to a specialty-based system for spontaneous reporting of adverse reactions to drugs. *JAMA 252*:1433, 1984.

Vale, J.A., and Meredith, T.J.: Acute poisoning due to nonsteroidal anti-inflammatory drugs. Clinical features and management. Med. Toxicol. *1*:21, 1986.

Class: Mild Analgesics

Generic Name: 1. Acetaminophen; 2. Acetanilide; 3. Phenacetin

Proprietary Name: 1. Abenol (Canad.), Acétalgine (Switz.), Acertol (Span.), Acetamol (Ital.), Actron (Fr., G.B., Span.), Aféradol (Fr.), Akindol (Fr., Span.), **Alba-Temp 300**, Alginina (Span.), **Alka-Seltzer Advanced Formula**, Alvedon (G.B., Swed.), **Anacin-3** (Canad.), Anadin Paracetamol

(G.B.), Anaflon (Germ.), Analter (Span.), Anti-Algos (Germ.), Antidol (Span.), Apiretal (Span.), Arcanagesic (S. Afr.), Aspac (Span.), Asplin (Span.), Aspro Paraclear (G.B.), Asprol (Austral.), Atasol (Canad.), Bebesan N (Switz.), Ben-u-ron (Germ., Switz.), Brunomol (S. Afr.), Calmanticold (Span.), Calpol (G.B., Ire., Ital., S. Afr.), Captin (Germ.), Ceetamol (Austral.), Cetamol (Ire.), Claradol (Fr.), Compu-Pain (S. Afr.), Cupanol (G.B., Span.), Dafalgan (Fr., Switz.), Desfebre (Span.), Dignocetamol (Germ.), Disprol (G.B.), Dolarist (Germ.), Dolgesic (Span.), Doliprane (Fr.), Dolofugin (Germ.), Doloreduct (Germ.), Dolorfug (Germ.), Dolorol (S. Afr.), Dolostop (Span.), Dolprone (Switz.), **Dorcol Children's Fever & Pain Reducer**, Dorocoff (Germ.), Drazin (Span.), Duorol (Span.), duracetamol (Germ.), Dymadon (Austral.), Efferalgan (Fr., Ital., Span.), Elkamol (G.B.), Enelfa (Germ.), Ennagesic (S. Afr.), Exdol (Canad.), Exdol Strong (Canad.), **Extra-strength Datril**, Fanalgic (G.B.), Febrectal Simple (Span.), Fennings Children's Powders (G.B.), Fensum (Germ.), Fevamol-P (S. Afr.), **Fevernol**, Finimal kindertabletten (Neth.), Finiweh (Germ.), Freka-cetamol (Germ.), Gelocatil (Span.), Gynospasmine Sarein (Fr.), Hedex (G.B., Neth., Span.), Junior Disprol (Austral.), Kiddycalm (Austral.), Kinderfinimal (Neth.), Lemsip (G.B., Swed.), Lonarid mono (Germ.), Malgis (Fr.), Maxadol-P (S. Afr.), Melabon Infantil (Span.), Miradol (G.B.), Mogil (Germ.), Mono Praecimed (Germ.), Mono-Trimedil (Germ.), Napamol (S. Afr.), Nina (Switz.), Nofedol (Span.), Octadon N (Germ.), Ortensan (Switz.), Painamol (S. Afr.), Paldesic (G.B.), Panacete (Austral.), Panado (S. Afr.), **Panadol** (Austral., Canad., Fr., G.B., Ire., Ital., Neth., Span., Switz.), Panaleve (G.B.), Panamax (Austral.), Panodil (Swed.), Panrectal (Span.), Paracets (G.B.), Paraclear (G.B.), Paralgin (Austral.), Paralief (Ire.), Paralyoc (Fr.), Paramin (G.B.), Parasin (Austral.), Parasol (Ire.), Paraspen (Austral.), Parmol (Austral.), Pediapirin (Span.), **Phenaphen**, Pirinasol (Span.), Prolief (S. Afr.), Prontina (Span.), Puernol (Ital.), Pyragesic (S. Afr.), Pyromed S (Germ.), Reliv (Swed.), Robigesic (Canad.), Rounox (Canad.), Salzone (G.B.), Sanipirina (Ital.), Setamol (S. Afr.), Sinaspril Paracetamol (Neth.), Sinpro junior (Germ.), Sinpro-N (Germ.), **Snaplets-FR**, Sudafed Co (Span.), Suotex (Ire.), Tachipirina (Ital.), Temol (S. Afr.), Temperal (Span.), **Tempra** (Austral., Canad., Span.), Termalgin (Span.), Treupel P (Germ.), Treuphadol (Switz.), **Tylenol** (Austral., Canad., Fr., Ire., Span , Switz.), **Uni-Ace**, Verlapyrin N (Germ.), Winpain (S. Afr.), Zatinol (Span.), Zolben (Span., Switz.)

Primary Use: These para-aminophenol derivatives are used in the control of fever and mild pain.

Ocular Side Effects:
    A. Systemic Administration
        1. Decreased vision
        2. Eyelids or conjunctiva
           a. Allergic reactions

   b. Erythema
   c. Conjunctivitis—nonspecific
   d. Edema
   e. Angioneurotic edema
   f. Urticaria
   g. Erythema multiforme
   h. Stevens-Johnson syndrome
   i. Lyell's syndrome
   j. Pemphigoid lesion (phenacetin)
   k. Icterus
  3. Problems with color vision—objects have yellow tinge (acetaminophen, phenacetin)—toxic states
  4. Visual hallucinations
  5. Green or chocolate discoloration of subconjunctival or retinal blood vessels
  6. Pupils
   a. Mydriasis—toxic states
   b. Decreased reaction to light—toxic states
  7. Subconjunctival or retinal hemorrhages secondary to drug-induced anemia

Clinical Significance: Ocular side effects due to these analgesics are quite rare; however, some adverse ocular reactions have occurred at quite low doses, implying a drug idiosyncrasy or a peculiar sensitivity. The most frequent toxic responses have been reported due to acetanilid, followed by phenacetin, and the fewest are due to acetaminophen. In chronic therapy, all of these drugs can produce sulfhemoglobinemia, which accounts for the greenish or chocolate color change in the subconjunctival or retinal blood vessels. Optic tract demyelination has been reported in an elderly man who was addicted for years to a mixture of phenacetin and aminopyrine. No definitive association can be made.

References:

Gerard, A., et al.: Drug-induced Lyell's syndrome. Nine cases. Therapie *37*:475, 1982.

Johnson, D.A.W.: Drug-induced psychiatric disorders. Drugs *22*:57, 1981.

Kashihara, M., et al.: Bullous pemphigoid-like lesions induced by phenacetin. Report of a case and an immunopathologic study. Arch. Dermatol. *120*:1196, 1984.

Kneezel, L.D., and Kitchens, C.S.: Phenacetin-induced sulfhemoglobinemia: Report of a case and review of the literature. Johns Hopkins Med. J. *139*:175, 1976.

Krenzelok, E.P., Best, L., and Manoguerra, A.S.: Acetaminophen toxicity. Am. J. Hosp. Pharm. *34*:391, 1977.

Neetans, A., et al.: Possible iatrogenic action of phenacetin at the levels of the visual pathway. Bull. Soc. Belge Ophtalmol. *178*:65, 1977.

Malek-Ahmadi, P., and Ramsey, M.: Acute psychosis associated with codeine and acetaminophen: A case report. Neurobehav. Toxicol. Teratol. *7*:193, 1985.

Generic Name: Antipyrine (Phenazone)

Proprietary Name: Aurone (S. Afr.), Eu-Med mono (Germ.), Oto-Phen (S. Afr.), Spondylon N (Germ.), Tropex (Ire.)

Primary Use: This pyrazolone derivative is used as a mild analgesic and antipyretic.

Ocular Side Effects:
  A. Systemic Administration
    1. Eyelids or conjunctiva
      a. Allergic reactions
      b. Conjunctivitis—nonspecific
      c. Edema
      d. Discoloration
      e. Urticaria
      f. Erythema multiforme
      g. Stevens-Johnson syndrome
      h. Lyell's syndrome
    2. Decreased vision
    3. Keratitis
    4. Toxic amblyopia (overdose)
    5. Subconjunctival or retinal hemorrhages secondary to drug-induced anemia

Clinical Significance: Adverse ocular reactions due to antipyrine are not uncommon, with allergic reactions being the most frequent. Fixed eruptions (those occurring at the same site on re-exposure) have also been reported. Conjunctivitis and keratitis are rare; however, fine superficial gray punctate keratitis with peripheral fine stromal infiltrates have been reported (Lewin and Guillery; Sattler). A transitory decrease in vision or even blindness may occur and last for a few minutes or a number of days. Optic atrophy has been reported in two instances, but a cause-and-effect relationship has not been proven.

References:
Adams, R.M., and Farber, E.M.: Treatment dermatitis. 2. Dermatitis medicamentosa. Postgrad. Med. *45*:125, 1969.
Goldstein, J.H.: Effects of drugs on cornea, conjunctiva, and lids. Int. Ophthalmol. Clin. *11(2)*:13, 1971.
Hotz, F.C.: A case of antipyrin amaurosis induced by 130 grains taken in 48 hours. Arch. Ophthalmol. *35*:160, 1906.
Landwehr, A.J., and van Ketel, W.G.: Delayed-type allergy to phenazone in a patient with erythema multiforme. Contact Dermatitis *8*:283, 1982.
Lewin, L., Guillery, H.: Die Wirkungen von Arzneimitteln und Giften auf das Auge, 2nd ed. Berlin, August Hirschwald, 1913.

Lucas, D.R., and Newhouse, J.P.: Action of metabolic poisons on the isolated retina. Br. J. Ophthalmol. *43*:147–158, 1959.

Sattler, C.H.: Augenveranderungen bei Intoxikationen. *In* Kurzes Handbuch der Ophthalmologie. Berlin, Springer, 1932, vol 7, pp. 229–290.

Generic Name: 1. Aspirin (Acetylsalicylic Acid); 2. Sodium Salicylate

Proprietary Name: 1. AAS (Span.), Acesal (Ital.), Acetard (Swed.), Acetylin (Germ.), Actispirine (Fr.), Adiro (Span.), Albyl (Swed.), Angettes (G.B.), Apernyl (Germ.), Arthrisin (Canad.), **Arthritis Strength Bufferin**, Artria (Canad.), **A.S.A.**, Asadrine (Canad.), Asaferm (Swed.), Asalite (Swed.), Aspalox (Germ.), Aspinfantil (Span.), Aspirina (Ital.), Aspirinetta (Ital.), Aspro (Austral., G.B., Germ., Ital., Neth., Span., Switz.), ASS (Germ.), Astrix (Austral.), Bamycor (Swed.), Bamyl (Swed.), Bonakiddi (Germ.), **Bufferin** (Ital.), Calmantina (Span.), Caprin (G.B.), Cardiprin (Austral.), Cartia (Austral.), Cemirit (Ital.), Claraigne (Fr.), Codalgina Retard (Span.), Colfarit (Germ., Switz.), Contradol (Germ.), Contrheuma (Germ.), Dispril (Swed.), Disprin (Austral., G.B., S. Afr.), Doléan pH 8 (Switz.), Doleron (Swed.), Domupirina (Ital.), Dreimal (Ital.), Dulcipirina (Span.), **Easprin**, **Ecotrin** (Austral., Canad.), Endydol (Ital.), Entérosarine (Switz.), Entrophen (Canad.), **Extra Strength Tri-Buffered Bufferin**, Gepan (Germ.), Helver Sal (Span.), Kilios (Ital.), Kynosina (Ital.), Magnecyl (Swed.), Melabon (Germ.), monobeltin 350 (Germ.), Novasen (Canad.), Nu-Seals (G.B., Ire.), Okal Infantil (Span.), Orravina (Span.), Platet (G.B.), Protectin-OPT (Germ.), Rectosalyl (Ital.), Resprin (Ire.), Reumyl (Swed.), Rhonal (Fr., Neth., Span., Switz.), Sal (Canad.), Salicilina (Span.), Sanocapt (Germ.), Santasal (Germ.), Saspryl (Span.), Sinaspril (Neth.), Solprin (Austral.), SRA (Austral.), Supasa (Canad.), Superaspidin (Span.), Temagin ASS (Germ.), Togal ASS (Switz.), Trombyl (Swed.), Winsprin (Austral.), **ZORprin**; 2. Fennings Mixture (G.B.), Jackson's Febrifuge (G.B.), Rhumax (Austral.), S-60 (Canad.)

Primary Use: These salicylates are used as antipyretics, analgesics, and in the management of gout, acute rheumatic fever, rheumatoid arthritis, subacute thyroiditis, and renal calculi.

Ocular Side Effects:
    A. Systemic Administration
        1. Eyelids or conjunctiva
            a. Allergic reactions
            b. Conjunctivitis—nonspecific
            c. Edema
            d. Angioneurotic edema
            e. Urticaria
            f. Purpura

       g. Erythema multiforme
       h. Stevens-Johnson syndrome
       i. Lyell's syndrome
       j. Pemphigoid lesion
   2. Decreased vision
   3. Problems with color vision
       a. Color vision defect, red-green defect
       b. Objects have yellow tinge
   4. Paralysis of extraocular muscles
   5. Diplopia
   6. Visual hallucinations
   7. Myopia—transient
   8. Decreased intraocular pressure
   9. Nystagmus
 10. Pupils
       a. Mydriasis
       b. Decreased or absent reaction to light
 11. Visual fields
       a. Scotomas
       b. Constriction
       c. Hemianopsia
 12. Scintillating scotomas
 13. Papilledema
 14. Retinal edema
 15. Subconjunctival or retinal hemorrhages—increased rebleeds
 16. Toxic amblyopia
 17. Keratitis
 18. Drug found in tears
 19. Hyphema (traumatic)—increased rebleeds
 20. Optic atrophy—toxic
  B. Inadvertent Ocular Exposure
   1. Conjunctival edema or scarring
   2. Keratitis with or without ulceration

Clinical Significance: While ocular side effects due to salicylates are quite rare, significant adverse effects may occur at therapeutic dosage levels. This is probably due to a drug idiosyncrasy or hypersensitivity. Adverse drug-induced ocular reactions are primarily due to acid-base imbalances, metabolic disturbances, toxic encephalopathy, hemorrhagic phenomena, or hypersensitivity reactions. Sodium salicylate appears to have more toxic ocular reactions than aspirin; however, aspirin has a much higher percentage of hypersensitivity reactions. Toxic responses are more frequent and more severe in infants and children. Neuro-ophthalmologic defects have been primarily seen with sodium salicylate and are much less frequent with aspirin. A transitory blindness that lasts for hours, days, or even weeks may occur. Optic atrophy with permanent blindness has, however, also been reported. In a retrospective study of traumatic hyphemas, the incidence of rebleeding was significantly increased with aspirin administration. Salicylates have been found to be excreted in tears in a dose-dependent relationship proportional to the plasma concentration, and corneal grafts from donors receiving high doses of salicylates may have the potentiality of subjecting corneal endothelial cells to cytotoxic concentrations of the drug. Recent data suggest that therapeutic doses of aspirin do not cause fetal damage in humans. Topical ocular aspirin powder has been used for self-mutilation and has caused various degrees of conjunctival and corneal damage. In patients taking high doses of aspirin for rheumatoid or osteoarthritis, acetazolamide may increase the nonionized salicylates in the blood stream. The nonionized salicylates penetrate the central nervous system more easily than the ionized form. Therefore, some carbonic anhydrase inhibitors may increase the risk of salicylate intoxication with its resultant adverse drug effects. These agents do not appear to have a protective effect in preventing cataracts. Chew, et al. have shown that aspirin (650 mg/d), which diabetics require for treatment of cardiovascular disease or other medical indications, does not significantly affect the severity or duration of vitreous/preretinal hemorrhages.

References:

Basu, P.K., et al.: Should corneas from donors receiving a high dose of salicylate be used as grafts: An animal experimentation. Exp. Eye Res. *39*:393, 1984.

Benawra, R., Mangurten, H.H., and Duffell, D.R.: Cyclopia and other anomalies following maternal ingestion of salicylates. J. Pediatr. *96*:1069, 1980.

Birch, J., et al.: Acquired color vision defects. *In* Pokorny, J., et al. (Eds.): Congenital and Acquired Color Vision Defects. New York, Grune & Stratton, 1979, pp. 243–350.

Black, R.A., and Bensinger, R.E.: Bilateral subconjunctival hemorrhage after acetylsalicylic acid overdose. Ann. Ophthalmol. *14*:1024, 1982.

Cheng, H.: Aspirin and cataract (Editorial). Br. J. Ophthalmol. *76*:257–258, 1992.

Early Treatment Diabetic Retinopathy Study Research Group. Effects of aspirin treatment on diabetic retinopathy. Ophthalmology *98*:757-765, 1991.

Chew, E.Y., et al.: Effects of aspirin on vitreous/preretinal hemorrhage in patients with diabetes mellitus. Arch. Ophthalmol. *113*:52–55, 1995.

Ganley, J. P., et al.: Aspirin and recurrent hyphema after blunt ocular trauma. Am. J. Ophthalmol. *96*:797, 1983.

Makela, A. L., Lang, H., and Korpela, P.: Toxic encephalopathy with hyperammonaemia during high-dose salicylate therapy. Acta Neurol. Scand. *61*:146, 1980.

Paris, G.L., and Waltuch, G.F.: Salicylate-induced bleeding problem in ophthalmic plastic surgery. Ophthalmic Surg. *13*:627, 1982.

Ruocco, V., and Pisani, M.: Induced pemphigus. Arch. Dermatol. Res. *274*:123, 1982.

Spaeth, G.L., Nelson, L.B., and Beaudoin, A.R.: Ocular teratology. *In* Jakobiec, F.A. (Ed.): Ocular Anatomy, Embryology and Teratology. Philadelphia, J.B. Lippincott, 1982, pp. 955–975.

Valentic, J.P., Leopold, I.H., and Dea, F.J.: Excretion of salicylic acid into tears following oral administration of aspirin. Ophthalmology 87:815, 1980.

Generic Name: 1. Codeine; 2. Propoxyphene

Proprietary Name: 1. Actacode (Austral.), Bronchoforton Kodeinsaft (Germ.), Codate (Austral.), Codeisan (Span.), Codelix (Austral.), codicept (Germ.), Codicompren (Germ.), Cod in (Austral.), Contrapect (Germ.), contrapect Infant N (Germ.), Evacode (G.B.), Galcodine (G.B.), Paveral (Canad.), Rami Kinderhoestsiroop (Neth.), Solcodein (Span.), Tricodein (Germ., Switz.); 2. 642 (Canad.), Artalvic (Fr.), **Darvon** (Span.), **Darvon-N** (Canad.), Deprancol (Span.), Depronal (Neth.), Depronal retard (Switz.), Develin (Germ.), Dexofen (Swed.), Dolo-Neurotrat (Germ.), Dolotard (Swed.), Doloxene (Austral., G.B., Ire., S. Afr., Swed.), Liberen (Ital.), Novopropoxyn (Canad.)

Primary Use: These mild analgesics are used for the relief of mild to moderate pain. Codeine is also used as an antitussive agent.

Ocular Side Effects:
    A. Systemic Administration
        1. Pupils
            a. Miosis—acute and toxic states
            b. Pinpoint pupils—initial and coma
            c. Mydriasis—withdrawal or extreme hypoxia
        2. Decreased vision
        3. Myopia (codeine)
        4. Eyelids or conjunctiva
            a. Angioneurotic edema (codeine)
            b. Urticaria (codeine)
            c. Erythema multiforme (codeine)
            d. Exfoliative dermatitis (codeine)
        5. Visual hallucinations
        6. Keratoconjunctivitis sicca (propoxyphene)
        7. Lacrimation—withdrawal states
        8. Optic atrophy—toxic states (propoxyphene)

Clinical Significance: Codeine and propoxyphene seldom cause significant ocular side effects. While codeine may produce miosis, propoxyphene does so only in overdose situations. Visual disturbances are usually insignificant. Codeine has been reported to cause transient myopia that is idiosyncratic, acute, and transient. Darvocet-N, a compound containing propoxyphene and acetaminophen, has been reported to reduce tear secretion, which resulted in soft contact lens dehydration and corneal epithelial abrasion. In addition, bilateral optic atrophy has been possibly associated with an overdose of

Darvon, a compound containing propoxyphene, aspirin, and caffeine; however, other contributing factors in this patient may have been acidosis, hypokalemia, or hypoxia.

References:

Bergmanson, J.P.G., and Rios, R.: Adverse reaction to painkiller in Hydrogel lens wearer. Am. Optom. Assoc. J. *52*:257, 1981.

Golden, N.L., King, K.C., and Sokol, R. J.: Propoxyphene and acetaminophen. Possible effects on the fetus. Clin. Pediatr. *21*:752, 1982.

Leslie, P. J., Dyson, E.H., and Proudfoot, A.T.: Opiate toxicity after self poisoning with aspirin and codeine. Br. Med. J. *292*:96, 1986.

Ostler, H.B., Conant, M.A., and Groundwater, J.: Lyell's disease, the Stevens-Johnson syndrome, and exfoliative dermatitis. Trans. Am. Ophthalmol. Otolaryngol. *74*:1254, 1970.

Ponte, C.D.: A suspected case of codeine-induced erythema multiforme. Drug Intell. Clin. Pharm. *17*:128, 1983.

Wall, R., Linford, S.M.J., and Akhter, M.I.: Addiction to Distalgesic (dextropropoxyphene). Br. Med. J. *280*:1213, 1980.

Weiss, I.S.: Optic atrophy after propoxyphene overdose. Report of a case. Ann. Ophthalmol. *14*:586, 1982.

Generic Name: Mefenamic Acid

Proprietary Name: Coslan (Span.), Dysman (G.B.), Ecopan (Switz.), Lysalgo (Ital.), Mefac (Ire.), Mefalgic (S. Afr.), Méfénacide (Switz.), Mefic (Austral.), Parkemed (Germ.), Pinalgesic (Ire.), Ponalar (Germ.), Ponalgic (Ire.), Ponstan (Austral., Canad., G.B., Ire., S. Afr., Switz.), **Ponstel**, Ponstyl (Fr.)

Primary Use: This anthranilic acid derivative is used for the relief of mild to moderate pain.

Ocular Side Effects:
  A. Systemic Administration
      1. Decreased vision
      2. Problems with color vision—nonspecific
      3. Nonspecific ocular irritation
      4. Eyelids or conjunctiva
          a. Erythema
          b. Conjunctivitis
          c. Edema
          d. Stevens-Johnson syndrome
          e. Urticaria
          f. Pemphigoid lesion
      5. Subconjunctival or retinal hemorrhages secondary to drug-induced anemia

Clinical Significance: Ocular side effects due to mefenamic acid are rare, transitory, and seldom require discontinuation of the use of the drug.

References:
Chan, J.C.N., Lai, F.M., and Critchley J.: A case of Stevens-Johnson Syndrome, cholestatic hepatitis and haemolytic anaemia associated with use of mefenamic acid. Drug Safety *6(3)*:230–234, 1991.
Shepherd, A.N., et al.: Mefenamic acid-induced bullous pemphigoid. Post-grad. Med. J. *62*:67, 1986.
Shipton, E.A., and Muller, F.O.: Severe mefenamic acid poisoning. A case report. S. Afr. Med. J. *67*:823, 1985.

Class: Narcotic Antagonists

Generic Name: 1. Levallorphan; 2. Nalorphine; 3. Naloxone; 4. Naltrexone

Proprietary Name: 2. Lethidrone (Austral.); 3. **Narcan** (Austral., Canad., Fr., G.B., Ital., S. Afr., Switz.), Narcanti (Germ., Swed.); 4. Antaxone (Ital.), Celupan (Span.), Nalorex (Fr., G.B., Ital.), **Trexan**

Primary Use: These narcotic antagonists are used primarily in the management of narcotic-induced respiratory depression.

Ocular Side Effects:
   A. Systemic Administration
      1. Pupils
         a. Mydriasis—may precipitate narrow-angle glaucoma—if a prior narcotic has been given
         b. Miosis
      2. Decreased vision
      3. Visual hallucinations
      4. Pseudoptosis
      5. Lacrimation—withdrawal states
      6. Eyelids or conjunctiva
         a. Allergic reactions
         b. Erythema
         c. Photosensitivity (naltrexone)
         d. Urticaria
         e. Erythema multiforme (naloxone)
         f. Exfoliative dermatitis (naltrexone)
      7. Nonspecific ocular irritation (naltrexone)
         a. Photophobia
         b. Ocular pain
         c. Edema
         d. Burning sensation

B. Local Ophthalmic Use or Exposure (Nalorphine, Naloxone)
   1. Pupils
      a. Mydriasis—may precipitate narrow-angle glaucoma—if a prior narcotic has been given
      b. Miosis

Clinical Significance: Although ocular side effects due to these narcotic antagonists are common, they have little clinical significance other than as a screening test to discover narcotic users. These narcotic antagonists produce either a miosis or no effect on the pupils when administered to nonaddicts; however, in addicts they cause mydriasis. Vivid visual hallucinations are seen both as an adverse ocular reaction and as a withdrawal symptom. Naloxone has only been reported to cause pupillary changes and erythema multiforme.

References:

Bellini, C., et al.: Naloxone anisocoria: A non-invasive inexpensive test for opiate addiction. Int. J. Clin. Pharm. Res. *11*:55, 1982.
Drago, F., et al.: Ocular instillation of naloxone increases intraocular pressure in morphine-addicted patients: A possible test for detecting misuse of morphine. Experimentia *41*:266, 1985.
Fanciullacci, M., et al.: The naloxone conjunctival test in morphine addiction. Eur. J. Pharmacol. *61*:319, 1980.
Jasinski, D.R., Martin, W.R., and Haertzen, C.: The human pharmacology and abuse potential of N-Allylnoroxymorphone. (Naloxone). J. Pharmacol. Exp. Ther. *157*: 420, 1967.
Martin, W.R.: Opioid antagonists. Pharmacol. Rev. *19*:463, 1967.
Nomof, N., Elliott, H.W., and Parker, K.D.: The local effect of morphine, nalorphine, and codeine on the diameter of the pupil of the eye. Clin. Pharmacol. Ther. *9*:358, 1968.

Class: Strong Analgesics

Generic Name: Diacetylmorphine (Diamorphine, Heroin)

Proprietary Name: None

Street Name: Boy, Brother, Brown sugar, Caballo, Ca-ca, Crap, H, Harry, Horse, Junk, Poison, Scag, Schmeck, Shit, Smack, Stuff, Tecata

Primary Use: This potent narcotic analgesic is administered preoperatively and postoperatively and in the terminal stage of cancer for the relief of severe pain.

Ocular Side Effects:
   A. Systemic Administration
      1. Pupils

    a. Miosis
    b. Pinpoint pupils—toxic states
    c. Absence of reaction to light
    d. Mydriasis—withdrawal states
    e. Anisocoria—withdrawal states
2. Decreased accommodation
3. Nonspecific ocular irritation
    a. Lacrimation
    b. Photophobia
4. Eyelids or conjunctiva
    a. Hyperemia
    b. Erythema
    c. Edema
    d. Urticaria
    e. Decreased blink rate
5. Decreased intraocular pressure
6. Horner's syndrome
    a. Ptosis
    b. Increased sensitivity to sympathetic agents
7. Intranuclear ophthalmoplegia (toxic)

Clinical Significance: This potent narcotic seldom causes significant ocular side effects. However, heroin addiction has been associated with bacterial and fungal endophthalmitis, probably due to the method of administration and impurities on an embolus basis. If undiagnosed and incompletely treated, these indirect drug-related entities can result in permanent loss of vision. Horner's syndrome has been reported in chronic addicts. Withdrawal of diacetylmorphine in the addict may cause excessive tearing, irregular pupils, and decreased accommodation.

References:

Alinlari, A., and Hashem, B.: Effect of opium addiction on intraocular pressure. Glaucoma 7:69, 1985.

Caradoc-Davies, T.H.: Opiate toxicity in elderly patients. Br. Med. J. 283:905, 1981.

Cosgriff, T.M.: Anisocoria in heroin withdrawal. Arch. Neurol. 29:200, 1973.

Crandall, D.C., and Leopold, I.H.: The influence of systemic drugs on tear constituents. Ophthalmology 86:115, 1979.

Dally, S., Thomas, G., and Mellinger, M.: Loss of hair, blindness and skin rash in heroin addicts. Vet. Human Toxicol. 24(Suppl.):62, 1982.

Gomez Manzano, C., et al.: Internuclear ophthalmopathy associated with opiate overdose. Medicina Clinica 94:637, 1990.

Hawkins, K.A., Bruckstein, A.H., and Guthrie, T.C.: Percutaneous heroin injection causing heroin syndrome. JAMA 237:1963, 1977.

Hogeweg, M., and De Jong, P.T.V.M.: Candida endophthalmitis in heroin addicts. Doc. Ophthalmol. 55:63, 1983.

Rathod, N.H., De Alarcón, R., and Thomson, I.G.: Signs of heroin usage detected by drug users and their parents. Lancet 2:1411, 1967.

Salmon, J.F., Partridge, B.M., and Spalton, D.J.: Candida endophthalmitis in a heroin addict: A case report. Br. J. Ophthalmol. 67:306, 1983.

Siepser, S.B., Magargal, L.E., and Augsburger, J.J.: Acute bilateral retinal microembolization in a heroin addict. Ann. Ophthalmol. 13:699, 1981.

Tarr, K.H.: Candida endophthalmitis and drug abuse. Aust. J. Ophthalmol. 8:303, 1980.

Vastine, D.W., et al.: Endogenous *Candida* endophthalmitis associated with heroin use. Arch. Ophthalmol. 94:1805, 1976.

Generic Name: 1. Hydromorphone (Dihydromorphinone); 2. Oxymorphone

Proprietary Name: 1. **Dilaudid** (Canad., Germ., Ire.); 2. **Numorphan** (Canad.)

Primary Use: These hydrogenated ketones of morphine are used for the relief of moderate to severe pain.

Ocular Side Effects:
    A. Systemic Administration
        1. Decreased vision
        2. Decreased accommodation
        3. Pupils
            a. Miosis
            b. Pinpoint pupils—toxic states
            c. Mydriasis—hypoxic states
        4. Eyelids or conjunctiva
            a. Allergic reactions
            b. Urticaria

Clinical Significance: Adverse ocular effects due to these drugs, although not uncommon, are rarely significant. All ocular side effects are reversible and transitory. Difficulty in focusing is probably the most frequent complaint.

References:
Acute drug abuse reactions. Med. Lett. Drugs Ther. 27:77, 1985.

Drug Evaluations. 6th Ed., Chicago, American Medical Association, 1986, p. 59.

Gilman, A.G., Goodman, L.S., and Gilman, A. (Eds.): The Pharmacological Basis of Therapeutics. 6th Ed., New York, Macmillan, 1980, pp. 495–511.

Reynolds, J.E.F. (Ed.): Martindale: The Extra Pharmacopoeia. 28th Ed., London, Pharmaceutical Press, 1982, pp. 1014, 1023.

Generic Name: Meperidine (Pethidine)

Proprietary Name: Centralgine (Switz.), Demerol (Canad.), **Demerol Hydrochloride**, Dolantin (Germ.), Dolantina (Span.), Dolantine (Switz.), Dolosal (Fr.)

Primary Use: This phenylpiperidine narcotic analgesic is used for the relief of pain, as a preoperative medication, and to supplement surgical anesthesia.

Ocular Side Effects:
  A. Systemic Administration
      1. Pupils
          a. Mydriasis (overdose)
          b. Miosis
          c. Decreased reaction to light
      2. Decreased intraocular pressure
      3. Decreased vision
      4. Eyelids or conjunctiva
          a. Allergic reactions
          b. Erythema
          c. Urticaria
      5. Visual hallucinations
      6. Nystagmus
  B. Inadvertent Ocular Exposure
      1. Blepharitis
      2. Conjunctivitis—nonspecific

Clinical Significance: None of the ocular side effects due to meperidine are of major importance, and all are transitory. Miosis is uncommon at therapeutic dosages and seldom significant. Mydriasis and decreased pupillary light reflexes are only seen in acute toxicity or in long-term addicts. Decrease in intraocular pressure is minimal. Ocular side effects, such as blepharitis or conjunctivitis, have been seen secondary to meperidine dust.

References:

Acute drug abuse reactions. Med. Lett. Drugs Ther. 27:77, 1985.

Bron, A.J.: Vortex patterns of the corneal epithelium. Trans. Ophthalmol. Soc. U.K. 93:455, 1973.

Goetting, M.G., and Thirman, M.J.: Neurotoxicity of meperidine. Ann. Emerg. Med. 14:1007, 1985.

Hovland, K.H.: Effects of drugs on aqueous humor dynamics. Int. Ophthalmol. Clin. 11(2):99, 1971.

Johnson, D.A.W.: Drug-induced psychiatric disorders. Drugs 22:57, 1981.

Lubeck, M.J.: Effects of drugs on ocular muscles. Int. Ophthalmol. Clin. 11(2):35, 1971.

Waisbren, B.A., and Smith, M.B.: Hypersensitivity to meperidine. JAMA 239:1395, 1978.

Generic Name: Methadone

Proprietary Name: Dolophine Hydrochloride, Eptadone (Ital.), Metasedin (Span.), Physeptone (Austral., G.B., Ire., S. Afr.), Symoron (Neth.)

Street Name: Dolly

Primary Use: This synthetic analgesic is useful in the treatment of chronic painful conditions and in the detoxification treatment of patients dependent on heroin or other morphine-like agents.

Ocular Side Effects:
   A. Systemic Administration
      1. Decreased vision
      2. Pupils
         a. Miosis—toxic states
         b. Pinpoint pupils—toxic states
         c. Mydriasis—withdrawal states
      3. Eyelids—urticaria
      4. Decreased spontaneous eye movements
      5. Talc retinopathy
      6. Teratogenic—increased incidences of strabismus

Clinical Significance: Methadone seldom causes significant ocular side effects. Although miosis is uncommon but may occur at therapeutic dosages, it may be so severe in toxic states as to give "pinpoint" pupils. Talc emboli, appearing as small white glistening dots in the macular area, have been reported in addicts who intravenously inject oral methadone that contains talc as a filler. A case of cortical blindness, apparently secondary to anoxia, has been reported in a child who experienced severe respiratory depression. Nelson, et al. reported increased incidences of strabismus in infants of methadone-dependent mothers.

References:

Aronow, R., Paul, S.D., and Wooley, P.V.: Childhood poisoning, an unfortunate consequence of methadone availability. J. Am. Med. Assoc. *219*:321–324, 1972.

Murphy, S.B., Jackson, W.B., and Pare, J.A.P.: Talc retinopathy. Can. J. Ophthalmol. *13*:152, 1978.

Nelson, L.B., et al: Occurrence of strabismus in infants born to drug-dependent women. Am. J. Dis. Child. *141*:175–178, 1987.

Rothenberg, S., et al.: Methadone depression of visual signal detection performance. Pharmacol. Biochem. Behav. *11*:521, 1979.

Rothenberg, S., et al.: Specific oculomotor deficit after acute methadone. I. Saccidic eye movements. Psychopharmacology *67*:221, 1980.

Rothenberg, S., et al.: Specific oculomotor deficit after acute methadone. II. Smooth pursuit eye movements. Psychopharmacology *67*:229, 1980.

Generic Name: 1. Morphine; 2. Opium

Proprietary Name: 1. **Astramorph PF**, Dolcontin (Swed.), **Duramorph**, Epimorph (Canad.), Morfina Miro (Span.), Morfina Serra (Span.), Morphitec (Canad.), M.O.S. (Canad.), Moscontin (Fr.), **MS Contin** (Canad., Ital., Neth.), **MSIR**, MST (Germ.), MST Continus (G.B., Ire., S. Afr., Span., Switz.), Oramorph (G.B.), **RMS, Roxanol**, Sevredol (G.B.), SRM-Rhotard (G.B.), Statex (Canad.)

Street Name: 1. M, Morf, White Stuff

Primary Use: These opioids are used for the relief of severe pain. Morphine is the alkaloid that gives opium its analgesic action.

Ocular Side Effects:
  A. Systemic Administration
      1. Pupils
          a. Miosis
          b. Pinpoint pupils—toxic states
          c. Mydriasis—withdrawal or extreme toxic states
          d. Irregularity—withdrawal states
      2. Decreased vision
      3. Decreased accommodation
      4. Decreased convergence
      5. Decreased intraocular pressure
      6. Myopia
      7. Lacrimation
          a. Increased—withdrawal states
          b. Decreased
      8. Accommodative spasm
      9. Diplopia
      10. Eyelids or conjunctiva
          a. Allergic reactions
          b. Conjunctivitis—nonspecific
          c. Urticaria
      11. Ptosis (opium)
      12. Keratoconjunctivitis
  B. Local Ophthalmic Use or Exposure—Morphine
      1. Miosis
      2. Decreased intraocular pressure
  C. Epidural Exposure
      1. Vertical nystagmus

Clinical Significance: These narcotics seldom cause significant ocular side effects, and all proven drug-induced toxic effects are transitory. Miosis is the most frequent ocular side effect and is seen routinely even at usual dosage levels. Ocular side effects reported in long-term addicts may show color vision or visual field changes that are probably due to vitamin deficiency rather than to the drug itself. Withdrawal of morphine or opium in the addict may cause excessive tearing, irregular pupils, decreased accommodation, and diplopia. Epidural opioids have been reported to cause vertical nystagmus (Fish and Rosen).

References:

Aminlari, A., and Hashem, B.: Effect of opium addiction on intraocular pressure. Glaucoma 7:69, 1965.

Andersen, P.T.: Alopecia areata after epidural morphine. Anesth. Analg. 63:1142, 1984.

Crandall, D.C., and Leopold, I.H.: The influence of systemic drugs on tear constituents. Ophthalmology 86:115, 1979.

Fish, D.J., and Rosen, S.M.: Epidural opioids as a cause of vertical nystagmus. Anesthesiology 73:785–786, 1990.

Murphy, D.F.: Anesthesia and intraocular pressure. Anesth. Analg. 64:520, 1985.

Shelly, M.P., and Park, G.R.: Morphine toxicity with dilated pupils. Br. Med. J. 289: 1071, 1984.

Generic Name: Pentazocine

Proprietary Name: Fortal (Fr.), Fortalgesic (Swed., Switz.), Fortral (Austral., G.B., Germ., Ire., Neth.), Liticon (Ital.), Ospronim (S. Afr.), Pentafen (Ital.), Pentalgina (Ital.), Sosegon (Span.), Sosenol (S. Afr.), **Talwin** (Canad., Ital.), Talwin-TAB (Ital.)

Primary Use: This benzomorphan narcotic analgesic is used for the relief of pain, as a preoperative medication, and to supplement surgical anesthesia.

Ocular Side Effects:

A. Systemic Administration
 1. Miosis
 2. Decreased vision
 3. Visual hallucinations
 4. Nystagmus
 5. Diplopia
 6. Lacrimation—abrupt withdrawal states
 7. Decreased accommodation
 8. Eyelids or conjunctiva
   a. Erythema
   b. Conjunctivitis-nonspecific
   c. Edema
   d. Urticaria
 9. Decreased spontaneous eye movements

Clinical Significance: Ocular side effects due to pentazocine are usually insignificant and reversible. Miosis is the most frequent and is seen routinely even at suggested dosage levels. Although visual complaints are seldom of major consequence, diplopia may be incapacitating. Vivid visual hallucinations, some of which are threatening, have been reported with this drug; once pentazocine is discontinued, the hallucinations cease. All other ocular side effects are rare.

References:

Belleville, J.P., Dorey, F., and Belville, J.W.: Effects of nefopam on visual tracking. Clin. Pharmacol. Ther. *26*:457, 1979.

Davidson, S.I.: Reports of ocular adverse reactions. Trans. Ophthalmol. Soc. U.K. *93*: 495–510, 1973.

Gould, W.M.: Central nervous disturbance with pentazocine. Br. Med. J. *1*:313–314, 1972.

Jones, K.D.: A novel side-effect of pentazocine. Br. J. Clin. Pract. *29*:218, 1975.

Martin, W.R.: Opioid antagonists. Pharmacol. Rev. *19*:463, 1967.

IV   Agents Used in Anesthesia

Class: Adjuncts to Anesthesia

Generic Name: Hyaluronidase

Proprietary Name: Hyalase (Austral., Canad., G.B., S. Afr.), Jalovis (Ital.), Jaluran (Ital.), Kinetin (Germ.), **Wydase** (Canad.)

Primary Use: This enzyme is added to local anesthetic solutions to enhance the effect of infiltrative anesthesia. It has also been used in paraphimosis, lepromatous nerve reactions, and the management of carpal tunnel syndrome.

Ocular Side Effects:
A. Subconjunctival or Retrobulbar Injection
    1. Eyelids or conjunctiva
        a. Allergic reactions
        b. Conjunctivitis—follicular
    2. Irritation
    3. Myopia
    4. Astigmatism
    5. Decreases the length of action of local anesthetics
    6. Increases the frequency of local anesthetic reactions
    7. Cystoid macular edema
    8. Allergic reaction simulated expulsive choroidal hemorrhage

Clinical Significance: Adverse ocular reactions due to periocular injection of hyaluronidase are either quite rare or masked by the postoperative surgical reactions. Subconjunctival injection of this drug causes myopia and astigmatism secondary to changes in the corneal curvature. This is a transitory phenomenon with recovery occurring within a few weeks. Irritative or allergic reactions are stated to be due to impurities in the preparation since pure hyaluronidase is believed to be nontoxic. Minning reported allergic reactions secondary to retrobulbar hyaluronidase. This occurred as an acute process simulating an expulsive choroidal or retrobulbar hemorrhage. Massive retrobulbar, peribulbar, and intraorbital swelling may occur. Hyaluronidase decreases the duration of action of local anesthetic drugs by allowing them to diffuse out of the tissue more rapidly. Side effects of the local anesthetic are probably more frequent when it is used with hyaluronidase, since its absorption rate is increased. A prospective double blind study that suggests that cystoid macular edema is possibly caused by the use of hyaluronidase is of marked clinical importance. To date, these data are not completely accepted. If the patient is taking heparin or if there is associated bleeding in the area of injection, the effect of hyaluronidase may be decreased since both human serum and heparin inhibit this agent.

References:

Barton, D.: Side reactions to drugs in anesthesia. Int. Ophthalmol. Clin. *11(2)*:185, 1971.

Minning, C.A.: Hyaluronidase allergy simulating expulsive choroidal hemorrhage. Case reports. Arch. Ophthal. *112*:585, 1994.

Roper, D.L., and Nisbet, R.M.: Effect of hyaluronidase on the incidence of cystoid macular edema. Ann. Ophthalmol. *10*:1673, 1978.

Salkie, M.L.: Inhibition of Wydase by human serum. Can. Med. Assoc. J. *121*:845, 1979.

Taylor, I.S., and Pollowitz, J.A.: Little known phenomenon. Ophthalmology *91*:1003, 1984.

Treister, G., Romano, A., and Stein, R.: The effect of subconjunctivally injected hyaluronidase on corneal refraction. Arch. Ophthalmol. *81*:645, 1969.

Generic Name: 1. Methscopolamine; 2. Scopolamine (Hyoscine)

Proprietary Name: *Systemic*: 2. Boro-Scopol (Germ.), Buscapina (Span.), Buscopan (Austral., Canad., Fr., G.B., Germ., Ital., Neth., S. Afr., Swed., Switz.), Holopon (Germ.), Hyospasmol (S. Afr.), Joy-Rides (G.B.), Kwells (Austral., G.B.), **Pamine** (Austral.), Scop (Austral.), Scopex (S. Afr.), Scopoderm (Swed.), Scopoderm TTS (Fr., G.B., Germ., Neth., S. Afr., Switz.), Scopolamina Lux (Ital.), Scopos (Fr.), Skopyl (Germ.), Transcop (Ital.), Transderm-V (Canad.), Vorigeno (Span.) *Ophthalmic*: 2. **Isopto Hyoscine** *Topical*: 2. **Transderm Scop**

Primary Use: *Systemic*: These quaternary ammonium derivatives are used as preanesthetic medications to decrease bronchial secretions, as sedatives and antispasmodics, and in the prophylaxis of motion sickness. *Ophthalmic*: Scopolamine, a topical parasympatholytic mydriatic and cycloplegic agent, is used in refractions, accommodative spasm, and the management of uveitis. *Topical*: Scopolamine is used in the prevention of nausea and vomiting associated with motion sickness.

Ocular Side Effects:
   A. Systemic Administration
      1. Mydriasis—may precipitate narrow-angle glaucoma
      2. Decrease or paralysis of accommodation
      3. Decreased vision
      4. Decreased lacrimation
      5. Visual hallucinations
      6. Decreased tear lysozymes
   B. Local Ophthalmic Use or Exposure
      1. Decreased vision
      2. Mydriasis—may precipitate narrow-angle glaucoma
      3. Decrease or paralysis of accommodation
      4. Eyelids or conjunctiva
         a. Allergic reactions
         b. Conjunctivitis—follicular
         c. Eczema
      5. Irritation
         a. Hyperemia
         b. Photophobia
         c. Edema
      6. Increased intraocular pressure
      7. Decreased lacrimation
      8. Visual hallucinations
   C. Systemic Absorption from Topical Application to the Skin
      1. Pupils
         a. Mydriasis—may precipitate narrow-angle glaucoma
         b. Anisocoria
         c. Absent reaction to light—toxic states
      2. Decrease or paralysis of accommodation
      3. Decreased vision
      4. Decreased lacrimation
      5. Visual hallucinations
      6. Nystagmus

Systemic Side Effects:
   A. Local Ophthalmic Use or Exposure
      1. Psychosis
      2. Agitation
      3. Confusion
      4. Hallucinations
      5. Hostility
      6. Amnesia
      7. Ataxia
      8. Vomiting
      9. Urinary incontinence

10. Somnolence
11. Fever
12. Vasodilation

Clinical Significance: Although ocular side effects from systemic administration of these drugs are common, they are reversible and seldom serious. Occasionally, patients taking scopolamine have aggravated keratoconjunctivitis sicca problems due to decreased tear production. This is the only autonomic drug that has been reported to cause decreased tear lysozymes. Mydriasis and paralysis of accommodation are intended ocular effects resulting from topical ophthalmic application of scopolamine but may occur from oral administration. This drug may elevate the intraocular pressure in open-angle glaucoma and can precipitate narrow-angle glaucoma. Allergic reactions are not uncommon after topical ocular application. Transient impairment of ocular accommodation, including blurred vision and mydriasis, have also been reported following the application of transdermal scopolamine patches. Several case reports of unilateral dilated pupils with associated blurred vision and narrow-angle glaucoma have been published, and inadvertent finger-to-eye contamination has been suspected as the cause. Systemic side effects from topical ophthalmic use of scopolamine have been reported infrequently and are similar to those seen secondary to topical ophthalmic atropine. Toxic psychosis, however, especially in the elderly or visually impaired, has been reported in the literature and to the Registry.

References:

Fraunfelder, F.T.: Transdermal scopolamine precipitating narrow-angle glaucoma. N. Engl. J. Med. *307*:1079, 1982.

Gleiter, C.H., et al.: Transdermal scopolamine and basal acid secretion. N. Engl. J. Med. *311*:1378, 1984.

Goldfrank, L., et al.: Anticholinergic poisoning. J. Toxicol. Clin. Toxicol. *19*:17, 1982.

Kortabarria, R.P., Duran J.A., and Chaco, J.R.: Toxic psychosis following cycloplegic eyedrops. DICP, Ann. Pharmacotherapy *24*:708–709. 1990.

Namborg-Petersen, B., Nielsen, M.M., and Thordal, C.: Toxic effect of scopolamine eye drops in children. Acta Ophthalmol. *62*:485, 1984.

Namill, M.B., Suelflow, J.A., and Smith, J.A.: Transdermal scopolamine delivery system (Transderm-V) and acute angle-closure glaucoma. Ann. Ophthalmol. *15*:1011, 1983.

McBride, W.G., Vardy, P.H., and French, J.: Effects of scopolamine hydrobromide on the development of the chick and rabbit embryo. Aust. J. Biol. Sci. *35*:173, 1982.

MacEwan, G.W., et al.: Psychosis due to transdermally administered scopolamine. Can. Med. Assoc. J. *133*:431, 1985.

Price, B.H.: Anisocoria from scopolamine patches. JAMA *253*:1561, 1985.

Rengstorff, R.H., and Doughty, C.B.: Mydriatic and cycloplegic drugs: A review of ocular and systemic complications. Am. J. Optom. Physiol. Optics *59*:162, 1982.

Seenhauser, F. H., and Schwarz, H.P.: Toxic psychosis from transdermal scopolamine in a child. Lancet *2*:1033, 1986.

Generic Name: 1. Metocurine Iodide; 2. Tubocurarine

Proprietary Name: 1. **Metubine Iodide** (Canad.); 2. Jexin (G.B.), Tubarine (Austral., Canad., G.B., Ital.)

Primary Use: These neuromuscular blocking agents are used as adjuncts to anesthesia, primarily as skeletal muscle relaxants.

Ocular Side Effects:
A. Systemic Administration
1. Decreased convergence
2. Diplopia
3. Nystagmus
4. Paresis or paralysis of extraocular muscles
5. Ptosis
6. Decreased intraocular pressure—minimal
7. Eyelids
a. Erythema
b. Urticaria

Clinical Significance: The extraocular muscles, especially the abductors, are selectively affected as the first signs of toxicity due to these curare agents. These drugs, unlike succinylcholine, do not cause a transitory elevation of intraocular pressure, so they are safe to use if the globe is perforated.

References:
Cunningham, A.J., et al.: The effect of intravenous diazepam on rise of intraocular pressure following succinylcholine. Can. Anaesth. Soc. J. 28:591, 1981.
Duncalf, D.: Anesthesia and intraocular pressure. Trans. Am. Acad. Ophthalmol. Otolaryngol. 79:562, 1975.
Lim, M., and Churchill-Davidson, H.C.: Adverse effects of neuromuscular blocking drugs. In Thornton, J.A. (Ed.): Adverse Reactions to Anaesthetic Drugs. New York, Elsevier, 1981, pp. 65–136.
Stevens, J.K., et al.: Paralysis of the awake human: visual perceptions. Vision Res. 16:93–98, 1976.

Generic Name: Succinylcholine (Suxamethonium)

Proprietary Name: Anectine (Austral., Canad., G.B., Span.), Celocurin-klorid (Swed.), Curalest (Neth.), Lysthenon (Germ., Switz.), Midarine (Ital., Switz.), Mioflex (Span.), Myotenlis (Ital.), Quelicin Chloride (Canad.), Scoline (Austral., G.B., S. Afr.), Succinolin (Switz.), Succinyl (Germ., Neth., Switz.)

Primary Use: This neuromuscular blocking agent is used as an adjunct to general anesthesia to obtain relaxation of skeletal muscles.

Ocular Side Effects:
  A. Systemic Administration
      1. Extraocular muscles
         a. Eyelid retraction
         b. Enophthalmos
         c. Globe rotates inferiorly
         d. Paralysis
         e. Adduction of abducted eyes
         f. Alters forced duction tests
      2. Intraocular pressure
         a. Increased—initial
         b. Decreased
         c. Narrow-angle glaucoma
      3. Ptosis
      4. Diplopia
      5. Eyelids or conjunctiva
         a. Allergic reactions
         b. Erythema
         c. Edema
         d. Urticaria

Clinical Significance: All ocular side effects of succinylcholine are transitory. The importance of the possible side effect of this drug affecting the "open" eye is an ongoing debate among ophthalmologists and anesthesiologists. Some feel a transient contraction of extraocular muscles may cause 5 to 15 mm Hg of intraocular pressure elevations within 1 minute after succinylcholine is given, lasting from 1 to 4 minutes. While this short-term elevation of intraocular pressure has little or no effect in the normal or glaucomatous eye, some feel it has the potential to cause expulsion of the intraocular contents in a surgically opened or perforated globe. Moreno, et al. state that they are unaware of a documented case of vitreous loss directly attributed to succinylcholine use. McGoldrick considers the drug safe in human "open" eyes with the benefits far outweighing the "unproven" risks. There are at least 20 publications taking both sides of this argument. To be on the safe side, one may want to consider not using this agent with an "open" eye. However, if this requires your anesthesiologist to use an agent that he or she is not familiar with, the risk may well be much greater not to use it. Eldor, et al. report two cases of this agent inducing acute glaucoma. Extraocular muscle contraction induced by succinylcholine may cause lid retraction or an enophthalmos, which may cause the surgeon to misjudge the amount of resection needed in ptosis procedures. Eyelid retraction may be due to a direct action on Muller's muscle. Both eyelid retraction and enophthalmos seldom last for over 5 minutes after drug administration. Succinylcholine may cause abnormal forced duction tests, however, up to 20 minutes after the drug is administered. In anesthetized patients, succinylcholine may cause abduction-deviated eyes to return to a normal position. Prolonged respiratory paralysis may follow administration of succinylcholine during general anesthesia in patients with recent exposure to topical ocular echothiophate or anticholinesterase insecticides or in those with cholinesterase deficiency.

References:

Eldor, J., Admoni, M.: Acute glaucoma following nonophthalmic surgery. Isr. J. Med. Sci. *25*:293–294, 1989.

Cook, J.H.: The effect of suxamethonium on intraocular pressure. Anaesthesia *36*:359, 1981.

France, N.K., et al.; Succinylcholine alteration of the forced duction test. Ophthalmology *87*:1282, 1980.

Goldstein, J.H., Gupta, M.K., and Shah, M.D.: Comparison of intramuscular and intravenous succinylcholine on intraocular pressure. Ann. Ophthalmol. *13*:173, 1981.

Indu, B., et al.: Nifedipine attenuates the intraocular pressure response to intubation following succinylcholine. Can. J. Anesthesiol. *36*:269–272, 1989.

Kelly, R.E., et al.: Succinylcholine increases intraocular pressure in the human eye with the extraocular muscles detached. Anesthesiology *79*:948, 1993.

Letter-to-the-Editor. Succinylcholine in open eyes. Ophthalmology *98(11)*:1607–1609, 1991.

Lim, M., and Churchill-Davidson, N.C.: Adverse effects of neuromuscular blocking drugs. *In* Thorton, J.A. (Ed.): Adverse Reactions to Anaesthetic Drugs. New York, Elsevier, 1981, pp. 65–136.

McGoldrick, K.E.: The open globe: is an alternative to succinylcholine necessary? J. Clin. Anesthesia. *5(1)*:1–4, 1993.

Metz, H.S., and Venkatesh, B.: Succinylcholine and intraocular pressure. J. Pediatr. Ophthalmol. Strabismus *18*:12, 1981.

Meyers, E.F., Singer, P., and Otto, A.: A controlled study of the effect of succinylcholine self-taming on intraocular pressure. Anesthesiology *53*:72, 1980.

Mindel, J.S., et al.: Succinylcholine-induced return of the eyes to the basic deviation. Ophthalmology *87*:1288, 1980.

Moreno, et al.: Effect of succinylcholine on the intraocular contents of open globes. Ophthalmology *98*:636–638, 1991.

Nelson, L.B., Wagner, R.S., and Harley, R.D.: Prolonged apnea caused by inherited cholinesterase deficiency after strabismus surgery. Am. J. Ophthalmol. *96*:392, 1983.

Class: General Anesthetics

Generic Name: Chloroform (Anesthetic Chloroform)

Proprietary Name: As chloroform and available in multi-ingredient preparations.

Primary Use: This potent inhalation anesthetic, analgesic, and muscle relaxant is used in obstetrical anesthesia. It is also used as a solvent.

Ocular Side Effects:
A. Systemic Administration
    1. Pupils—dependent on plane of anesthesia
        a. Mydriasis—reactive to light (initial)
        b. Miosis—reactive to light (deep level of anesthesia)
        c. Mydriasis—nonreactive to light (coma)
    2. Strabismus—convergent or divergent
    3. Nystagmus
    4. Decreased intraocular pressure
    5. Decreased vision
B. Inadvertent Ocular Exposure
    1. Irritation
        a. Lacrimation
        b. Hyperemia
        c. Ocular pain
        d. Edema
        e. Burning sensation
    2. Keratitis
    3. Corneal opacities
    4. Corneal ulceration

Clinical Significance: Ocular side effects due to chloroform are common, transitory, and seldom of clinical significance other than as an aid in judging the level of anesthesia. During early levels of anesthesia induction, the eyes are convergent; however, with deeper levels they become divergent. Nystagmus most often occurs during the recovery phase of anesthesia. Blindness has been reported secondary to central anoxic episodes.

References:

Duncalf, D.: Anesthesia and intraocular pressure. Bull. N Y Acad. Med. *51*:374, 1975.
Gilman, A.G., et al. (Eds.): The Pharmacological Basis of Therapeutics. 8th Ed., Elmsford, N.Y., Pergamon Press, 1990, p. 1623.
Hovland, K.R.: Effects of drugs on aqueous humor dynamics. Int. Ophthalmol. Clin. *11(2)*:99, 1971.
Smith, M.B.: Handbook of Ocular Toxicology. Acton, Publishing Sciences Group, 1976, p. 355.
Tripathi, R.C., and Tripathi, B.J.: The eye. *In* Riddell, R.H. (Ed.): Pathology of Drug-Induced and Toxic Diseases. New York, Churchill Livingstone, 1982, pp. 377–450.

Generic Name: Ether (Anesthetic Ether)

Proprietary Name: O.G. (Odontalgico Gazzoni) (Ital.)

Primary Use: This potent inhalation anesthetic, analgesic, and muscle relaxant is used during induction of general anesthesia.

Ocular Side Effects:
  A. Systemic Administration
      1. Pupils—dependent on plane of anesthesia
          a. Mydriasis—reactive to light (initial)
          b. Miosis—reactive to light (deep level of anesthesia)
          c. Mydriasis—nonreactive to light (coma)
      2. Extraocular muscles—dependent on plane of anesthesia
          a. Slow oscillations (initial)
          b. Eccentric placement of globes (initial)
          c. Concentric placement of globes (coma)
      3. Nonspecific ocular irritation
      4. Conjunctival hyperemia
      5. Lacrimal secretion—dependent on plane of anesthesia
          a. Increased (initial)
          b. Decreased (coma)
          c. Abolished (coma)
      6. Decreased intraocular pressure
      7. Decreased vision
  B. Inadvertent Ocular Exposure
      1. Irritation
          a. Hyperemia
          b. Edema
      2. Punctate keratitis
      3. Corneal opacities

Clinical Significance: Adverse ocular reactions due to ether are common, reversible, and seldom of clinical importance other than in the determination of the plane of anesthesia. Ether decreases intraocular pressure probably on the basis of increasing the facility of outflow. Ether vapor is an irritant to all mucous membranes, including the conjunctiva. Regardless of this irritant effect, ether vapor has, in addition, a vasodilator property. Permanent corneal opacities have been reported due to direct contact of liquid ether with the cornea. Blindness after induction of general anesthesia is probably due to asphyxic cerebral cortical damage.

References:

Gilman, A.G., et al. (Eds.): The Pharmacological Basis of Therapeutics. 8th Ed., Elmsford, N.Y., Pergamon Press, 1990, pp. 269–270.

Murphy, D.F.: Anesthesia and intraocular pressure. Anesth. Analg. *64*:520, 1985.

Reynolds, J.E.F (Ed.): Martindale: The Extra Pharmacopoeia. 30th Ed., London, Pharmaceutical Press, 1993, p. 913.

Smith, M.B.: Handbook of Ocular Toxicology. Acton, Publishing Sciences Group, 1976, pp. 356–357.

Tripathi, R.C., and Tripathi, B.C.: The eye. In Riddell, R.H. (Ed.): Pathology of Drug-Induced and Toxic Diseases. New York, Churchill Livingstone, 1982, pp. 377–450.

Generic Name: Ketamine

Proprietary Name: Kétalar (Fr.), **Ketalar** (Austral., Canad., G.B., Ital., Neth., S. Afr., Swed., Switz.), Ketanest (Germ.), Ketolar (Span.)

Primary Use: This intravenous nonbarbiturate anesthetic is used for short-term diagnostic or surgical procedures. It may also be used as an adjunct to anesthesia.

Ocular Side Effects:
    A. Systemic Administration
        1. Decreased vision
        2. Diplopia
        3. Horizontal nystagmus
        4. Postsurgical visually induced "emergence reactions"
        5. Extraocular muscles
          a. Abnormal conjugate deviations
          b. Random ocular movements
        6. Lacrimation
        7. Visual hallucinations
        8. Increased intraocular pressure—minimal (deep level of anesthesia)

Clinical Significance: All ocular side effects due to ketamine are transient and reversible. After ketamine anesthesia, diplopia may persist up to 30 minutes during the recovery phase and may be particularly bothersome to some patients. "Emergence reactions" occur in 12% of patients and may consist of various psychological manifestations varying from pleasant dream-like states to irrational behavior. The incidence of these reactions is increased by visual stimulation as the effect of the drug is wearing off. Three cases of transient blindness following ketamine anesthesia have also been reported. The blindness lasts about half an hour with complete restoration of sight and no apparent sequelae. This is thought to be a toxic cerebral-induced phenomenon. The effect of ketamine on intraocular pressure is somewhat confusing, with various authors obtaining different results. Probably, if intraocular pressure is taken before this drug increases muscle tone (just prior to anesthesia), there is an 8- to 10-minute period when intraocular pressure is not elevated. Ketamine is also being used by lay people for its psychedelic effect, and abusers may develop visual hallucinations, coarse horizontal nystagmus, abnormal conjugate eye deviations, and diplopia.

References:
Ausinsch B., et al.: Ketamine and intraocular pressure in children. Anesth. Analg. *55*: 773, 1976.

Crandall, D.C., and Leopold, I.H.: The influence of systemic drugs on tear constituents. Ophthalmology 86:115, 1979.
Drugs that cause psychiatric symptoms. Med. Lett. Drugs Ther. 28:81, 1986.
Fine, J., Weissman, J., and Finestone, S.C.: Side effects after ketamine anesthesia: Transient blindness. Anesth. Analg. 53:72, 1974.
MacLennan, F.M.: Ketamine tolerance and hallucinations in children. Anaesthesia 37: 1214, 1982.
Meyers, E.F., and Charles, P.; Prolonged adverse reactions to ketamine in children. Anesthesiology 49:39, 1979.
Shaw, I.H., and Moffett, S.P.: Ketamine and video nasties. Anaesthesia 45:422, 1990.
Whitwam, J.G.: Adverse reactions to intravenous agents: Side effects. In Thorton, J.A. (Ed.): Adverse Reactions to Anaesthetic Drugs. New York, Elsevier, 1981, pp. 47–57.

Generic Name: Methoxyflurane

Proprietary Name: Penthrane (Austral., Germ.)

Primary Use: This methyl ether is used as an inhalation anesthetic with good analgesic and muscle relaxant properties.

Ocular Side Effects:
    A. Systemic Administration
        1. Decreased intraocular pressure
        2. "Flecked retinal syndrome"
        3. Myasthenic neuromuscular blocking effect
            a. Paralysis of extraocular muscles
            b. Ptosis

Clinical Significance: Ocular side effects due to methoxyflurane are rare, but a unique adverse ocular reaction has been reported. If this drug is used for an extended period, especially in a patient with renal insufficiency, irreversible renal failure may occur. Oxalosis occurs for unknown reasons, with calcium oxalate crystal deposits throughout the body. These deposits have a predilection for the retinal pigment epithelium and around retinal arteries and arterioles. They may be found in any ocular tissue, but mainly in vascularized tissue. Seldom does this interfere with vision. The deposition of these crystals in the retina gives the clinical picture of an apparent "flecked retinal syndrome." This drug can also aggravate or unmask myasthenia gravis.

References:
Albert, D.M., et al.: Flecked retina secondary to oxalate crystals from methoxyflurane anesthesia: Clinical and experimental studies. Trans. Am. Acad. Ophthalmol. Otolaryngol. 79:817, 1975.

Argov, Z., and Mastaglia, F.L.: Disorders of neuromuscular transmission caused by drugs. N. Engl. J. Med. *301*:409, 1979.

Bullock, J.D., and Albert, D.M.: Flecked retina. Arch. Ophthalmol. *93*:26, 1975.

Kaeser, H.E.: Drug-induced myasthenic syndromes. Acta Neurol. Scand. *70*(Suppl. 100):39, 1984.

Reynolds, J.E.F. (Ed.): Martindale: The Extra Pharmacopoeia. 28th Ed., London, Pharmaceutical Press, 1982, pp. 754–755.

Schettini, A, Owre, E.S., and Fink, A.I.: Effect of methoxyflurane anesthesia on intraocular pressure. Can. Anaesth. Soc. J. *15*:172, 1968.

Tammisto, O., Hamalainen, L., and Tarkkanen, L.: Halothane and methoxyflurane in ophthalmic anesthesia. Acta. Anaesth. Scand. 9:173–177, 1965.

Generic Name: Nitrous Oxide

Proprietary Name: Stickoxydul (Germ.)

Primary Use: This inhalation anesthetic and analgesic is used in dentistry, in the second stage of labor in pregnancy, and during induction of general anesthesia.

Ocular Side Effects:
   A. Systemic Administration
       1. Pupils—dependent on plane of anesthesia
           a. Mydriasis—reactive to light (initial)
           b. Miosis—reactive to light (deep level of anesthesia)
           c. Mydriasis—nonreactive to light (coma)
       2. Intraocular pressure
           a. Increased
           b. Decreased
       3. Decreased vision
       4. Decreased lacrimation
       5. Abnormal ERG or VEP

Clinical Significance: Pupillary changes due to nitrous oxide are common; however, other than aiding in determination of the anesthetic plane, they are seldom of importance. Nitrous oxide, as well as other anesthetics, produces the transitory effect of decreased basal tear production during general anesthesia. Although decreased vision or blindness after induction of general anesthesia is quite rare, this phenomenon is more frequent with nitrous oxide than with most other general anesthetics. Visual loss is probably secondary to asphyxic cerebral cortical damage. Because nitrous oxide increases the rate of absorption of intraocular air by 25%, most ophthalmologists who use nitrous oxide will have the anesthesiologist administer another general anesthetic 20 to 25 minutes before air must be injected.

References:

Boucher, M.C., and Meyers, E.: Effects of nitrous oxide anesthesia on intraocular air volume. Can. J. Ophthalmol. *18*:246, 1983.

Crandall, D.C., and Leopold, I.H.: The influence of systemic drugs on tear constituents. Ophthalmology *86*:115, 1979.

Fenwick P.B.C., et al.: Changes in the pattern reversal visual evoked potential as a function of inspired nitrous oxide concentration. Electroencephalogr. Clin. Neurophysiol. *57*:178, 1984.

Lane, G.A., et al.: Anesthetics as teratogens: Nitrous oxide is fetotoxic, xenon is not. Science *210*:899, 1980.

Ratta, C., et al.: Changes in the electroretinogram and visual evoked potentials during general anaesthesia. Graefes Arch. Clin. Exp. Ophthalmol. *211*:139, 1979.

Sebel, P.S., Flynn, P.J., and Ingram, D.A.: Effect of nitrous oxide on visual, auditory and somatosensory evoked potentials. Br. J. Anaesth. *56*:1403, 1984.

Generic Name: Propofol

Proprietary Name: Diprivan (Austral., Fr., G.B., Ital., Neth., S. Afr., Swed.), Disoprivan (Germ., Switz.)

Primary Use: An intravenous sedative-hypnotic used in the induction and maintenance of anesthesia or sedation.

Ocular Side Effects:
    A. Intravenous Administration
        1. Blurred vision
        2. Extraocular muscles
            a. Diplopia
            b. Palsy
            c. Paresis
        3. Inability to open eyes
        4. Eyelids
            a. Rash
            b. Edema
        5. Exposure keratitis

Clinical Significance: Propofol is an intravenous medication that can cause transitory visual complications. To date, none of the reported events in the literature or in the Registry have been permanent. One of the most unusual side effects is that after patients have recovered from anesthesia, i.e., respond to verbal commands and have a return of muscular power, they are unable to open their eyes either spontaneously or in response to a command from 3 to 20 minutes. This may include the transitory loss of all ocular or periocular muscle movements, including the lids and rectus muscles. Blurred vision can occur, but it is usually inconsequential, and associated keratitis results from exposure due to lack of eyelid control and restriction of Bell's phenomena. While nystagmus has been reported to the Registry, it is difficult to prove a cause-and-effect relationship.

References:
Kumar, C.M., and McNeela, B.J.: Ocular manifestation of propofol allergy. Anaesthesia *44*:266, 1989.
Marsch, S.C.U., Schaefer, H.G.: Problems with eye opening after propofol anesthesia. Anesth. and Analg. *70*:127–128, 1990.

Generic Name: Trichloroethylene

Proprietary Name: Trilene (G.B.)

Primary Use: This potent inhalation anesthetic is used primarily for short-term diagnostic or surgical procedures and in obstetrics. It may also be used as an adjunct to anesthesia.

Ocular Side Effects:
 A. Systemic Administration
  1. Extraocular muscles
   a. Paresis or paralysis
   b. Diplopia
   c. Pain on ocular movements
   d. Limitation of ocular movements
  2. Ptosis
  3. Decreased vision
  4. Visual fields
   a. Scotomas—central or paracentral
   b. Constriction
   c. Enlarged blind spot
  5. Photophobia
  6. Paralysis of accommodation
  7. Eyelids or conjunctiva
   a. Conjunctivitis—nonspecific
   b. Exfoliative dermatitis
  8. Pupils
   a. Decreased or absent reaction to light
   b. Anisocoria
  9. Problems with color vision—color vision defect
  10. Horizontal nystagmus
  11. Decreased lacrimation
  12. Retrobulbar or optic neuritis
  13. Optic atrophy
  14. Toxic amblyopia
  15. Decreased intraocular pressure

16. Peripapillary hemorrhages
17. Decreased corneal reflex
18. Retinal edema
19. Retinal vasoconstriction
20. Visual hallucinations
21. Corneal ulceration
B. Inadvertent Ocular Exposure
  1. Irritation
    a. Lacrimation
    b. Hyperemia
    c. Edema
    d. Burning sensation
  2. Punctate keratitis
  3. Corneal opacities

Clinical Significance: Ocular side effects due to trichloroethylene are uncommon since the discovery that most of the adverse reactions were due to toxic decomposition products of the drug. With adjustments in anesthetic equipment and technique, such as using this drug for only short procedures, adverse ocular reactions are seldom seen. The most severe toxic response occurs in the central nervous system, and the cranial nerves are the most susceptible. Trichloroethylene may cause toxic ocular side effects, however, from industrial exposure. A comprehensive review of this agent industrially and clinically is given in the 4th edition of Grant and Schuman's "Toxicology of the Eye."

References:

Annau, Z.: The neurobehavioral toxicity of trichloroethylene. Neurobehav. Toxicol. Teratol. *3*:417, 1981.

Conde-Salazar, L., et al.: Subcorneal pustular eruption and erythema from occupational exposure to trichloroethylene. Contact Dermatitis *9*:235, 1983.

Hovland, K.R.: Effects of drugs on aqueous humor dynamics. Int. Ophthalmol. Clin. *11(2)*:99, 1971.

Grant, W.M., and Schuman, J.S.: Toxicology of the Eye. In Charles C. Thomas (Ed.), 4th Ed., Springfield, IL, 1993, pp. 1448–1455.

Lachapelle, P., and Molotchnikoff, S.: The effect of acute trichloroethylene exposure on electroretinogram components. *In* Proceedings of the second meeting of the International Neurotoxicology Association. E. Rodriguez-Farre (Ed.), Neurotoxicol. Teratol. *12(6)*:1990, pp. 633–636.

Murphy, D.F.: Anesthesia and intraocular pressure. Anesth. Analg. *64*:520, 1985.

Vernon, R.J., and Ferguson, R.K.: Effects of trichloroethylene on visual motor performance. Arch. Environ. Health *18*:894, 1969.

Class: Local Anesthetics

Generic Name: 1. Bupivacaine; 2. Chloroprocaine; 3. Etidocaine; 4. Lidocaine; 5. Mepivacaine; 6. Prilocaine; 7. Procaine; 8. Propoxycaine

Proprietary Name: 1. Carbostesin (Germ.), Carbostésine (Switz.), Carbostésine hyperbare (Switz.), Macaine (S. Afr.), Marcain (Austral., G.B., Swed.), Marcain Spinal Heavy (Austral.), Marcaina (Ital.), Marcaïne (Fr.), Marcaïne Rachianesthésie (Fr.), Marcaine (Canad., Neth.), **Marcaine Hydrochloride**, **Marcaine Spinal**, Regibloc (S. Afr.), **Sensorcaine, Sensorcaine Spinal**; 2. Nesacaïne (Switz.), **Nesacaine** (Canad.); 3. **Duranest** (Austral., Swed.); 4. Aeroderm (Span.), **Anestacon**, Anestecidan Simple (Span.), **Banadyne-3**, Bonjela (G.B.), Cidancaina Simple (Span.), Corafusin (Germ.), Dentiform (Neth.), Dentinox (Neth.), Heweneural (Germ.), Laryng-O-Jet (G.B.), Lidesthesin (Germ.), Lidojek (Germ.), Lignostab (G.B.), Luan (Ital.), Mouth Gel (G.B.), neo-Novutox (Germ.), Odontalg (Ital.), Ortodermina (Ital.), Otalgan (Neth.), Peterkaine (S. Afr.), Pharmacaine (S. Afr.), Rapidocaïne (Switz.), Remicaine (S. Afr.), Remicard (S. Afr.), sagittaproct (Germ.), Solarcaine (Switz.), Xylesine (Switz.), Xylocain (Germ., Swed.), Xylocain f.d. Kardiologie (Germ.), Xylocain Schwer (Germ.), Xylocain tung (Swed.), Xylocaina (Ital., Span.), Xylocaïne (Fr., Switz.), **Xylocaine** (Austral., Canad., G.B., Ire., Neth., S. Afr.), Xylocaine Accordion (G.B.), Xylocaine Heavy (Austral., S. Afr.), Xylocard (Austral., Canad., Fr., G.B., Ire., Neth., Swed.), Xyloneural (Germ., Switz.), Xylonor (Ital.), Xylotox (G.B., S. Afr.), Xylotox 2% Plain SE (S. Afr.); 5. Carbocain (Swed.), Carbocaina (Ital.), Carbocaine (Austral., Canad., S. Afr.), **Carbocaine Hydrochloride**, Isocaine 3% (Canad.), Meaverin (Germ.), Meaverin 3% Woelm (Germ.), Meaverin 4% hyperbar (Germ.), Mepicaton (Switz.), Mepivastesin (Germ.), **Polocaine** (Canad.), Scandicaïne (Switz.), Scandicain (Germ.), Scandicaïne (Switz.), Scandicaine (Neth.), Scandinibsa (Span.); 6. Citanest (G.B., Neth., Swed.), Citanest 15 (Austral.), Citanest Plain (Austral., Canad.), Xylonest (Germ., Switz.); 7. Géro (Fr.), Lenident (Ital.), **Novocain** (Canad., Germ.), Pasconeural-Injektopas (Germ.), Syntocaïne (Switz.), Venocaina Miro (Span.); 8. **Ravocaine**

Primary Use: These amides or esters of para-aminobenzoic acid are used in infiltrative, epidural block, and peripheral or sympathetic nerve block anesthesia or analgesia.

Ocular Side Effects:
  A. Nonocular Administration
   1. Decreased vision
   2. Horner's syndrome (transitory—lumbar extradural blockade)
     a. Miosis
     b. Ptosis
   3. Extraocular muscles
     a. Paresis or paralysis
     b. Diplopia
     c. Nystagmus

      d. Jerky pursuit movements—toxic states
      e. Abnormal doll's head movements—toxic states
    4. Eyelids or conjunctiva
      a. Allergic reactions
      b. Hyperemia
      c. Blepharoconjunctivitis
      d. Edema
      e. Urticaria
      f. Exfoliative dermatitis
      g. Blepharoclonus
    5. Pupils
      a. Mydriasis—toxic states
      b. Anisocoria—toxic states
    6. Problems with color vision—color vision defect (lidocaine)
    7. Visual hallucinations (lidocaine)
B. Systemic Administration—Injection (Spinal)
    1. Decreased vision
    2. Miosis
    3. Paralysis of extraocular muscles
    4. Diplopia
    5. Blepharoclonus
    6. Photosensitivity (dibucaine)
    7. Macular edema
C. Local Ophthalmic Use or Exposure—Retrobulbar Injection
   (Bupivacaine, Etidocaine, Lidocaine, Mepivacaine, Procaine)
    1. Decreased vision
    2. Paresis or paralysis of extraocular muscles
    3. Decreased intraocular pressure
    4. Hyperpigmentation of eyelids (lidocaine with sodium
      bicarbonate)
D. Inadvertent Intraocular Injection
    1. Vision loss
    2. Corneal edema
    3. Endothelial cell loss
    4. Elevated intraocular pressure (transitory)
    5. Uveitis
    6. Hypotony
    7. Decreased pupillary function
    8. Pigment dispersion syndrome
    9. Cataracts
    10. Chronic Descemet's membrane wrinkling
E. Inadvertent Posterior Segment Injection (All Transitory)
    1. Vision loss
    2. Elevated intraocular pressure

        3. Pupillary dilatation
        4. Corneal edema
    F. Inadvertent Ocular Exposure (Lidocaine)
        1. Pupils
            a. Mydriasis
            b. Absence of reaction to light
        2. Decreased vision
        3. Visual field defects
        4. Abnormal ERG

Systemic Side Effects:
    A. Local Ophthalmic Use or Exposure—Retrobulbar Injection
        1. Convulsion
        2. Apnea
        3. Cardiac arrest

Clinical Significance: Spinal injections of local anesthetics rarely cause ocular side effects; however, when they do, the event may be within a few hours or delayed many days. The most common ocular adverse event is an extraocular nerve palsy or paralysis. This may start with or without a headache followed by a weakness of the 6th nerve, although 3 and 4 may be involved. This may occur as soon as 2 hours after the spinal or up to 3 weeks later. Recovery usually occurs in 3 days to 3 weeks but may require up to 18 months. Acute bilateral central scotomas, possibly due to hypotension and macular ischemia, have been reported. Inadvertent intraocular injection of a local anesthetic into the anterior chamber is a rare but potential devastating event. While little is published, there are a number of reports in the Registry. To differentiate between the effects of the force of the fluid coming out through a small-gauge needle (fire hose effect) and that from the drug itself is not always clear-cut. It is apparent that initially there is a marked rise in intraocular pressure, but within a few hours to days a uveitis with resultant decrease in pressure and hypotony may occur. Endothelial cell loss from both a fire hose shearing effect and/or the toxicity of the drug plus uveitis may cause corneal edema. Many cases have come to corneal transplant since endothelial loss appears permanent. The lens may or may not become cataractous. Pigment dispersion is common, and much of this may be mechanical due to the fire hose effect. Pupillary function is often decreased and even absent, in part due to acute secondary glaucoma, synechiae, or direct toxic drug effect. The spectrum of injury is broad; however, if the posterior segment is not involved and chronic glaucoma avoided, the prognosis may be good with a corneal graft. Unlike the anterior segment, the outcome of inadvertent local anesthetic injected in the posterior segment is more dependent on the direct effect of the needle penetration. Although a double perforation often has a better prognosis than a single perforation, an injection through the pars plana may be devoid of significant effects other than the acute rise in intraocular pressure. The immediate effect of the injection is a marked increase in intraocular pressure, with or without pupillary dilation, corneal edema, and loss of vision. All of the above are transitory since there appear to be no significant long-term toxic effects of the local anesthetic on the retina or optic nerve. The chief concern is control of the acute rise in pressure that may be severe enough to cause central retinal venous or arterial occlusion. Next are the problems from retinal perforation, vitreous adhesion, or retinal detachment. Lemagne, et al. reported a case of Purtscher-like retinopathy with a retrobulbar injection of a local anesthetic in a 41 year old. The exudates and hemorrhages disappeared; however, a localized paracentral scotoma and afferent pupil defect were permanent. Numerous systemic reactions from topical ocular applications of local anesthetics have been reported. Many of these occur in part from the fear of the impending procedure or possibly an oculocardiac reflex. Side effects include syncope, convulsions, and anaphylactic shock.

References:

Antoszyk, A.N., and Buckley, E.G.: Contralateral decreased visual acuity and extraocular palsies following retrobulbar anesthesia. Ophthalmology *93*:462, 1986.

Beltranena, H.P., et al.: Complications of retrobulbar Marcaine injection. J. Clin. Neurol. Ophthalmol. *2*:159, 1982.

Breslin, C.W., Hershenfeld, S., and Motolko, M.: Effect of retrobulbar anesthesia on ocular tension. Can. J. Ophthalmol. *18*:223, 1983.

Brookshire, G.L., Gleitsmann, K.Y., and Schenk, E.C.: Life-threatening complication of retrobulbar block. A hypothesis. Ophthalmology *93*:1476, 1986.

Carroll, R.P.: Blindness following lacrimal nerve block. Ophthalmic Surg. *13*:812, 1982.

Duker, J.S., et al.: Inadvertent globe perforation during retrobulbar and peribulbar anesthesia. Patient characteristics, surgical management, and visual outcome. Ophthalmology *98(4)*:519–526, 1991.

Esswein, M.B., and Von Noorden, G.K.: Paresis of a vertical rectus muscle after cataract extraction. Am. J. Ophthalmol. *116*:424–430, 1993.

Gild, W.M., et al.: Eye injuries associated with anesthesia. A closed claims analysis. Anesthesiology *76*:204–208, 1992.

Gupta, M.K., Goldstein, J.H., and Shah, M.: Epidural anesthesia and VI nerve palsy. Ann. Ophthalmol. *12*:571, 1980.

Haddad, R.: Fibrinous iritis due to oxybuprocaine. Br. J. Ophthalmol. *73*:76–77, 1989.

Lemagne, J.M., et al.: Purtscher-like retinopathy after retrobulbar anesthesia. Ophthalmology *97(7)*:859–861, 1990.

Lincoff, H., et al.: Intraocular injection of lidocaine. Ophthalmology *92*:1587, 1985.

Sullivan, K.L., et al.: Retrobulbar anesthesia and retinal vascular obstruction. Ophthalmology *90*:373, 1983.

Wittpenn, J.R., et al.: Respiratory arrest following retrobulbar anesthesia. Ophthalmology *93*:867, 1986.

Class: Therapeutic Gases

Generic Name: Carbon Dioxide

Proprietary Name: None

Primary Use: This odorless, colorless gas is used as a respiratory stimulant to increase cerebral blood flow and in the maintenance of acid-base balance.

Ocular Side Effects:
A. Systemic Administration
   1. Decreased vision
   2. Decreased convergence
   3. Paralysis of accommodation
   4. Decreased dark adaptation
   5. Photophobia
   6. Visual fields
      a. Constriction
      b. Enlarged blind spot
   7. Problems with color vision
      a. Color vision defect
      b. Objects have yellow tinge
   8. Retinal vascular engorgement
   9. Pupils
      a. Mydriasis
      b. Absence of reaction to light
   10. Visual hallucinations
   11. Diplopia
   12. Abnormal conjugate deviations
   13. Papilledema
   14. Increased intraocular pressure
   15. Ptosis
   16. Decreased corneal reflex
   17. Proptosis

Clinical Significance: Although ocular side effects due to carbon dioxide are lengthy, they are rare; nearly all significant findings are in toxic states. Transient elevation of intraocular pressure has been reported in the inhalation of 10% carbon dioxide.

References:
Duke-Elder, S.: Systems of Ophthalmology. St. Louis, C.V. Mosby, Vol. XIV, Part 2, 1972, pp. 1350–1351.
Freedman, A., and Sevel, D.: The cerebro-ocular effects of carbon dioxide poisoning. Arch. Ophthalmol. 76:59, 1966.

Lincoff, A., et al: Selection of xenon gas for rapidly disappearing retinal tamponade. Arch. Ophthalmol. *100*:996–997, 1982.

Peczon, J.D., Grant, W.M., and Lambert, B.: Systemic vasodilators, intraocular pressure and chamber depth in glaucoma. Am. J. Ophthalmol. *72*:74–78, 1971.

Sevel, D., and Freedman, A.: Cerebro-retinal degeneration due to carbon dioxide poisoning. Br. J. Ophthalmol. *51*:475, 1967.

Sieker, H.O., and Hickam, J.B.: Carbon dioxide intoxication: The clinical syndrome, its etiology and management, with particular reference to the use of mechanical respirators. Medicine *35*:389, 1956.

Walsh, F.B., and Hoyt, W.F.: Clinical Neuro-Ophthalmology. 3rd Ed., Baltimore, Williams & Wilkins, Vol. III, 1969, pp. 2601–2602.

Wolbarsht, M.L., et al.: Speculation on carbon dioxide and retrolental fibroplasia. Pediatrics *71*:859, 1983.

Generic Name: Oxygen

Proprietary Name: None

Primary Use: This colorless, odorless, tasteless gas is used in inhalation anesthesia and in hypoxia.

Ocular Side Effects:
   A. Systemic Administration
      1. Retinal vascular changes
         a. Constriction
         b. Spasms
         c. Hemorrhages
      2. Decreased vision
      3. Visual fields
         a. Constriction
      4. Retrolental fibroplasia—in newborns or young infants
      5. Heightened color perception
      6. Retinal detachment
      7. Abnormal ERG
      8. Decreased dark adaptation
      9. Myopia
      10. Cataracts—nuclear

Clinical Significance: The toxic ocular effects due to oxygen are most prominent in premature infants, but some may be found in any age group under hyperbaric conditions at increased, elevated atmospheric pressures. Ocular side effects secondary to the usual use of oxygen therapy are otherwise rare. While the ocular changes due to retrolental fibroplasia are irreversible, most other side effects are transient after use of oxygen is discontinued. Permanent bilateral blindness probably due to 80% oxygen during general anesthesia has been reported. It has been suggested that in some susceptible people, severe retinal vasoconstriction or even direct retinal toxicity may occur from oxygen therapy. Bilateral retinal hemorrhages with permanent partial visual loss were reported secondary to sudden increase in CSF pressure after an excessive volume of oxygen was used to increase a myelogram contrast. A slow increase in myopia following prolonged hyperbaric oxygen has been seen in premature infants and adults. In addition, oxidative damage to the lens proteins has been postulated as a cause of nuclear cataracts in patients exposed to hyperbaric oxygen treatments.

References:

Anderson, B., Jr., and Farmer, J.C., Jr.: Hyperoxic myopia. Trans. Am. Ophthalmol. Soc. *76*:116, 1978.

Ashton, N.: Oxygen and the retinal vessels. Trans. Ophthalmol. Soc. U.K. *100*:359, 1980.

Campbell, P.B., et al.: Incidence of retinopathy of prematurity in a tertiary newborn intensive care unit. Arch. Ophthalmol. *101*:1686, 1983.

Fisher, A.B.: Oxygen therapy. Side effects and toxicity. Am. Rev. Respir. Dis. *122*: 61, 1980.

Gallin-Cohen, P.F., Podos, S.M., and Yablonski, M.E.: Oxygen lowers intraocular pressure. Invest. Ophthalmol. Vis. Sci. *19*:43, 1980.

Handelman, I.L., et al.: Retinal toxicity of therapeutic agents. J. Toxicol. Cut. Ocular Toxicol. 2:131, 1983.

Kalina, R.E., and Karr, D.J.: Retrolental fibroplasia. Ophthalmology *89*:91, 1982.

Lyne, A.J.: Ocular effects of hyperbaric oxygen. Trans. Ophthalmol. Soc. U.K. *98*:66, 1978.

Miller, E.F.: Effect of breathing 100% oxygen upon visual field and visual acuity. J. Aviation Med. *29*:598–602, 1958.

Nissenkorn, I., et al.: Myopia in premature babies with and without retinopathy of prematurity. Br. J. Ophthalmol. *67*:170, 1983.

Oberman, J., Cohn, H., and Grand, M.G.: Retinal complications of gas myelography. Arch. Ophthalmol. *97*:1905, 1979.

Palmquist, B.M., Philipson, B., and Barr, P.O.: Nuclear cataract and myopia during hyperbaric oxygen therapy. Br. J. Ophthalmol. *68*:113, 1984.

V Gastrointestinal Agents

Class: Agents Used to Treat Acid Peptic Disorders

Generic Name: Cimetidine

Proprietary Name: Aciloc (Swed.), Acinil (Swed.), Biomag (Ital.), Brumetidina (Ital.), Cimal (Swed.), Cimeldine (Ire.), Cinulcus (Span.), Citimid (Ital.), Dina (Ital.), Duogastril (Span.), Duractin (Austral.), Dyspamet (G.B., Ire.), Edalene (Fr.), Eureceptor (Ital.), Fremet (Span.), Galenamet (G.B.), Gastro H2 (Span.), Gastromet (Ital.), Lenamet (S. Afr.), Mansal (Span.), Novocimetine (Canad.), Peptimax (G.B.), Peptol (Canad.), Phimetin (G.B.), Stomet (Ital.), Tagagel (Germ.), Tagamet (Austral., Canad., Fr., G.B., Germ., Ire., Ital., Neth., S. Afr., Span., Swed., Switz.), Tametin (Ital.), Temic (Ital.), Ulcedin (Ital.), Ulcodina (Ital.), Ulcofalk (Ital.), Ulcomedina (Ital.), Ulis (Ital.), Valmagen (Ital.)

Primary Use: This histamine H2 receptor antagonist is used in the treatment of confirmed duodenal ulcers.

Ocular Side Effects:
    A. Systemic Administration
        1. Decreased vision
        2. Visual hallucinations
        3. Photophobia
        4. Eyelids or conjunctiva
            a. Hyperemia
            b. Erythema
            c. Conjunctivitis—nonspecific
            d. Urticaria
            e. Purpura
            f. Stevens-Johnson syndrome
            g. Exfoliative dermatitis
        5. Decreased accommodation

6. Pupils
   a. Mydriasis—may precipitate narrow-angle glaucoma—toxic states
   b. Decreased reaction to light-toxic states
7. Subconjunctival or retinal hemorrhages secondary to drug-induced anemia

Clinical Significance: Adverse ocular effects secondary to cimetidine are uncommon, considering this drug is in the top ten prescription products. While the Registry has hundreds of possible adverse ocular reactions with this agent, there are few patterns, and most just background "noise." Still, transient myopia, yellow or pink tinge to objects, and sicca-like symptoms are possibly related. Visual hallucinations have occurred, particularly with high doses, in elderly patients with renal impairment. All adverse ocular reactions are transient and disappear with withdrawal of drug therapy. Although one recent report found no change in intraocular pressure secondary to cimetidine therapy in normal and medically controlled glaucoma patients, there have been reports of angle-closure glaucoma and exacerbation of glaucoma following administration of cimetidine.

References:
Adler, L.E., Sadja, L., and Wilets, G.: Cimetidine toxicity manifested as paranoia and hallucinations. Am. J. Psychiatry *137*:1112, 1980.
Agarwal, S.K.: Cimetidine and visual hallucinations. *JAMA 240*:214, 1978.
Ahmed, A.H., et al.: Stevens-Johnson syndrome during treatment with cimetidine. Lancet 2:433, 1978.
Cimetidine—reversible visual disturbance of myopia. Lakartidinger *78*:2752, 1981.
Dobrilla, G., et al.: Exacerbation of glaucoma associated with both cimetidine and ranitidine. Lancet *1*:1078, 1982.
Feldman, F., and Cohen, M.M.: Effect of histamine-2 receptor blockade by cimetidine on intraocular pressure in humans. Am. J. Ophthalmol. *93*:351, 1982.
Hoskyns, B.L.: Cimetidine withdrawal. Lancet *1*:254, 1977.
Nelson, P.G.: Cimetidine and mental confusion. Lancet 2:928, 1977.
Papp, K.A., and Curtis, R.M.: Cimetidine-induced psychosis in a 14-year-old girl. Can. Med. Assoc. J. *131*:1081, 1984.
Veitch, G.B.A., et al.: Prospective monitoring of adverse reactions to cimetidine: The role of the pharmacist. Br. J. Pharm. Pract. *6*:196, 1984.

Generic Name: Ranitidine

Proprietary Name: Azantac (Fr.), Coralen (Span.), Mauran (Ital.), Nodol (Ital.), Novoranidine (Canad.), Quantor (Span.), Ran H2 (Span.), Raniben (Ital.), Ranibloc (Ital.), Ranidil (Ital.), Ranidin (Span.), Ranilonga (Span.), Raniplex (Fr.), Ranix (Span.), Ranuber (Span.), Sostril (Germ.), Tanidina (Span.), Terposen (Span.), Toriol (Span.), Trigger (Ital.), Ulcex (Ital.), Ulkobrin (Ital.), **Zantac** (Austral., Canad., G.B., Ire., Ital., Neth., S. Afr., Span., Swed.), Zantic (Germ., Switz.)

Primary Use: This histamine H2 receptor antagonist is used in pathologic hypersecretory conditions or intractable duodenal ulcers.

Ocular Side Effects:
  A. Systemic Administration
    1. Decreased vision
    2. Eyelids or conjunctiva
       a. Erythema
       b. Conjunctivitis—nonspecific
       c. Angioneurotic edema
       d. Urticaria
    3. Visual hallucinations
    4. Problems with color vision—color vision defect
    5. Subconjunctival or retinal hemorrhages secondary to drug-induced anemia

Clinical Significance: Ocular side effects due to ranitidine are uncommon and predominantly occur in children or severely ill elderly patients. Ocular pain, blurred vision and increased intraocular pressure recurred in one patient with chronic glaucoma when 150 mg of ranitidine were given; these same symptoms had occurred 1 year earlier with cimetidine.

References:
De Giacomo, C., Maggiore, G., and Scotta, M.S.: Ranitidine and loss of colour vision in a child. Lancet 2:47, 1984.
Dobrilla, G., et al.: Exacerbation of glaucoma associated with both cimetidine and ranitidine. Lancet 2:1078, 1982.
Ranitidine (Zantac). Med. Lett. Drugs Ther. 24:111, 1982.
Sonnenblick, M., and Yinnon, A.: Mental confusion as a side effect of ranitidine. Am. J. Psychiatry 143:257, 1986.

Class: Antacids

Generic Name: 1. Acid Bismuth Sodium Tartrate; 2. Bismuth Oxychloride; 3. Bismuth Sodium Tartrate; 4. Bismuth Sodium Thioglycollate; 5. Bismuth Sodium Triglycollamate; 6. Bismuth Subcarbonate; 7. Bismuth Subsalicylate

Proprietary Name: 7. In Pepto-Bismol (G.B.)

Primary Use: Bismuth salts are primarily used as antacids and in the treatment of syphilis and yaws.

Ocular Side Effects:
  A. Systemic Administration
    1. Eyelids or conjunctiva
      a. Blue discoloration
      b. Exfoliative dermatitis
      c. Lyell's syndrome
    2. Subconjunctival hemorrhages
    3. Corneal deposits
    4. Visual hallucinations—toxic states

Clinical Significance: Adverse ocular reactions to bismuth preparations are extremely rare and seldom of clinical significance except in toxic states. Bismuth-containing corneal deposits have been documented. Only one case of decreased vision has been reported after an overdose of bismuth.

References:

Cohen, E.L.: Conjunctival haemorrhage after bismuth injection. Lancet *1*:627, 1945.
Fischer, F.P.: Bismuthiase secondaire de la cornee. Ann. Oculist (Paris) *183*:615, 1950.
Goas, J.Y., et al.: Encephalopathie myoclinique par le sous-nitrate de Bismuth. Une observation recente. Nouv. Presse Med. *10*:3855, 1981.
Granstein, R.D., and Sober, A.J.: Drug- and heavy metal-induced hyperpigmentation. J. Am. Acad. Dermatol. *5*:1, 1981.
Supino-Viterbo, V., et al.: Toxic encephalopathy due to ingestion of bismuth salts: Clinical and EEG studies of 45 patients. J. Neurol. Neurosurg. Psychiatry *40*:748, 1977.
Zurcher, K., and Krebs, A.: Cutaneous Side Effects of Systemic Drugs. Basel, S. Karger, 1980, p. 302.

Class: Antiemetics

Generic Name: 1. Chlorcyclizine; 2. Cyclizine; 3. Meclizine (Meclozine)

Proprietary Name: 1. Di-Paralene (Swed.); 2. Happy-Trip (Neth.), Marezine, Marzine (Canad., Fr., Ital., Neth., Switz.), Marziné (Swed.), Motozina (Ital.), Triazine (S.Afr.), Valoid (G.B., Ire., S. Afr.); 3. Ancolan (Austral.), Antivert (Canad.), Bonamine (Canad., Germ.), Bonine, Calmonal (Germ.), Chiclida (Span.), Dramine (Span.), D-Vert 30, Neo-Istafene (Ital.), Peremesin (Germ.), Prmsine (Switz.), Postafen (Germ., Swed.), Sea-legs (G.B.), Suprimal (Neth.)

Primary Use: These piperazine antihistaminic derivatives are effective in the management of nausea and vomiting.

Ocular Side Effects:
  A. Systemic Administration
    1. Decreased vision

   2. Pupils (toxic—cyclizine)
      a. Mydriasis—may precipitate narrow-angle glaucoma
      b. Decreased reaction to light
   3. Decreased tolerance to contact lenses
   4. Diplopia
   5. Visual hallucinations
   6. May aggravate keratoconjunctivitis sicca

Clinical Significance: Ocular side effects due to these drugs are rare, reversible, and usually of little clinical significance. Pupillary changes and visual hallucinations primarily occur in overdose situations. A few reports of ocular teratogenic abnormalities have been reported with cyclizine and meclizine therapy; however, these findings may be coincidental. The FDA makes no mention of ocular teratogenic properties in their extensive review of this drug.

References:

Algan, B., and Afarchal, H.: Concerning two observations of drug-induced teratogenesis: tapetoretinal degeneration produced in a brother and sister by cyclizine hydrochloride. Excerpta Med. Int. Cong. Series *154*:63, 1967. (French)

Brand, J.J., Colquhoun, W.P., and Perry, W.L.M.: Side-effects of l-hyoscine and cyclizine studied by objective tests. Aerospace Med. *39*:999–1002, 1969.

Gott, P.H.: Cyclizine toxicity. Intentional drug abuse of a proprietary antihistamine. N. Engl. J. Med. *279*:596, 1968.

McBride, W.: Cyclizine and congenital abnormalities. Br. Med. J. *1*:1157, 1963.

Shapiro, S., et al.: Meclizine in pregnancy in relation to congenital malformations. Br. Med. J. *1*:483, 1978.

Generic Name: Metoclopramide

Proprietary Name: Abbemetic (S. Afr.), Ananda (Ital.), Anausin (Fr.), Antimet (Ire.), Apo-Metoclop (Canad.), Betaclopramide (S. Afr.), Citroplus (Ital.), Clopamon (S. Afr.), Clopan (Ital.), Contromet (S. Afr.), Cronauzan (Ital.), duraclamid (Germ.), Emex (Canad.), Enterosil (Ital.), Gastrobid Continus (G.B., Ire.), Gastroflux (G.B.), Gastromax (G.B.), Gastronerton (Germ.), Gastrosil (Germ., Switz.), Gastro-Tablinen (Germ.), Gastrotem (Germ.), Gastro-Timelets (Germ., Switz.), Gastrotranquil (Germ.), Gastrotrop (Germ.), Maxeran (Canad.), Maxolon (Austral., G.B., Ire., S. Afr.), MCP-ratiopharm (Germ.), Metamide (Austral.), Metoclamid (Germ.), Metocobil (Ital.), Metocyl (Ire.), Metramid (G.B.), Mygdalon (G.B.), Nadir (Ital.), Octamide, Opram (Ire.), Parmid (G.B.), Paspertin (Germ., Switz.), Plasil (Ital.), Pramin (Austral.), Primpran (Fr., Switz.), Primperan (G.B., Ire., Neth., S. Afr., Span., Swed.), Prokinyl (Mon.), Prostal (S. Afr.), Randum (Ital.), Regastrol (Ital.), Reginerton (Germ.), Reglan (Canad.), Setin (S. Afr.)

Primary Use: This orthopramide is used as adjunctive therapy in roentgen-ray examination of the stomach and duodenum and for the prevention and treatment of irradiation sickness.

Ocular Side Effects:
  A. Systemic Administration
      1. Extraocular muscles
          a. Oculogyric crises
          b. Diplopia
          c. Paralysis
          d. Nystagmus
          e. Strabismus
      2. Decreased vision
      3. Eyelids or conjunctiva
          a. Edema
          b. Angioneurotic edema
          c. Urticaria
      4. Problems with color vision—color vision defect
      5. Mydriasis—may precipitate narrow-angle glaucoma
      6. Photophobia

Clinical Significance: Ocular side effects secondary to metoclopramide are rare; however, the drug can produce acute dystonic reactions, particularly in children. This includes transitory oculogyric crises, inability to close the eyes, nystagmus, and various extraocular muscle abnormalities. These dystonic reactions usually occur within 36 hours of starting treatment and subside within 24 hours after stopping the drug.

References:
Berkman, N., Frossard, C., and Moury, F.: Oculogyric crises and metoclopramide. Bull. Soc. Ophtalmol. Fr. *81*:153, 1981.

Bui, N.B., Marit, G., and Hoerni, B.: High-dose metoclopramide in cancer chemotherapy-induced nausea and vomiting. Cancer Treat. Rep. *66*:2107, 1982.

Hyser, C.L., and Drake, M.E., Jr.: Myoclonus induced by metoclopramide therapy. Arch. Intern. Med. *143*:2201, 1983.

Kofoed, P.E., and Kamper, J.: Extrapyramidal reactions caused by antiemetics during cancer chemotherapy. J. Pediatr. *105*:852, 1984.

Laroche, J., and Laroche, C.: Etude de l'action d'un 4e groupe de medicaments sur la discrimination des couleurs et recapitulation des resultats acquis. Ann. Pharm. Fr. *38*:323, 1980.

Terrin, B.N., McWilliams, N.B., and Maurer, H.M.: Side effects of metoclopramide as an antiemetic in childhood cancer chemotherapy. J. Pediatr. *104*:138, 1984.

Class: Antilipidemic Agents

Generic Name: Clofibrate

Proprietary Name: Arterioflexin (Austral.), atherolipin (Germ.), Atromidin (Ital., Swed.), Atromid-S (Austral., Canad., G.B., Ire., S. Afr.), Claripex

(Canad.), Clofi (Neth.), Clofibral (Fr.), Clofinit (Ital.), Clofirem (Fr.), Geromid (Ital.), Lipavil (Ital.), Lipavlon (Fr.), Neo Atromid (Span.), Novofibrate (Canad.), Regelan (Switz.), Regelan N (Germ.), Sepik (Ital.), Skleromexe (Germ.)

Primary Use: This aryloxyisobutyric acid derivative is effective in the treatment of hypercholesterolemia and/or hypertriglyceridemia.

Ocular Side Effects:
A. Systemic Administration
   1. Decreased vision
   2. Eyelids or conjunctiva
      a. Erythema
      b. Conjunctivitis—nonspecific
      c. Edema
      d. Urticaria
      e. Purpura
      f. Lupoid syndrome
      g. Blepharoclonus
      h. Loss of eyelashes or eyebrows
   3. Subconjunctival or retinal hemorrhages secondary to drug-induced anemia
   4. Myopia
   5. Decreased intraocular pressure

Clinical Significance: Ocular side effects due to clofibrate are quite rare and seldom of major clinical significance. All reactions seem to clear on cessation of the drug. There are two reports that suggest this agent, by decreasing blood viscosity, has made glaucoma more easily managed. This, however, has not been proven. Regression of xanthomas and diabetic retinopathy has been claimed as well. The drug can make hair more brittle, and alopecia has occurred. One case in the Registry seems to suggest a $+2.50$ refractive change, lasting for 6 weeks after cessation of the drug.

References:
Arif, M.A., and Vahrman, J.: Skin eruption due to clofibrate. Lancet 2:1202, 1975.
Clements, D.B., Elsby, J.M., and Smith, W.D.: Retinal vein occlusion. A comparative study of factors affecting the prognosis, including a therapeutic trial of Atromid S in this condition. Br. J. Ophthalmol. 52:111, 1968.
Cullen, J.F.: Clofibrate in glaucoma. Lancet 2:892. 1967.
Orban, T.: Clofibrate in glaucoma. Lancet 1:47, 1968.

Class: Antispasmodics

Generic Name: 1. Ambutonium; 2. Anisotropine (Octatropine); 3. Clidinium; 4. Dicyclomine (Dicycloverine); 5. Diphemanil; 6. Glycopyrrolate; 7. Hexocyclium; 8. Isopropamide; 9. Mepenzolate; 10. Methantheline; 11. Methixene; 12. Methylatropine Nitrate (Atropine Methonitrate); 13. Oxyphencyclimine; 14. Oxyphenonium; 15. Pipenzolate (Pipenzolone); 16. Piperidolate; 17. Poldine; 18. Propantheline; 19. Tridihexethyl

Proprietary Name: 2. **Valpin 50**, Vapin (Span.); 3. **Quarzan**; 4. **Bentyl** (Ital.), Bentylol (Canad., Span.), Formulex (Canad.), Lomine (Canad.), Medicyclomine (S. Afr.), Merbentyl (Austral., G.B., S. Afr.), Protylol (Canad.), Spasmoban (Canad.); 5. Prantal (Austral., Fr., Ital.); 6. **Robinul** (Austral., Canad., G.B., Germ., Neth., S. Afr., Swed., Switz.); 8. **Darbid** (Canad.), Dipramid (Ital.), Priamide (Neth.), Tyrimide (Austral.); 9. **Cantil** (Austral., Fr., G.B., Swed.); 10. Vagantin (Germ.); 11. Trmaril (Switz.), Tremaril (Ital., Neth., Span.), Tremarit (Germ.), Tremonil (G.B., Ire.), Tremoquil (Swed.); 13. Daricol (Swed.), **Daricon** (Neth.), Vagogastrin (Ital.); 14. Antrnyl (Switz.), Antrenyl (Neth.), Spastrex (S. Afr.); 15. Piper (Ital.), Piptal (Austral., Fr., G.B., Ital.); 17. Nacton (G.B., Ire.); 18. Corrigast (Germ.), Ercorax Roll-on (Switz.), Ercotina (Swed.), Pantheline (Austral.), **Probamide**, Probanthine (Fr.), **Pro-Banthine** (Austral., Canad., G.B., Ire., Neth., S. Afr., Span., Swed., Switz.), Propanthel (Canad.); 19. **Pathilon**

Primary Use: *Systemic*: These anticholinergic agents are effective in the management of gastrointestinal tract spasticity and peptic ulcers. *Ophthalmic*: These topical anticholinergic mydriatic and cycloplegic agents are used in refractions and fundus examinations.

Ocular Side Effects:
   A. Systemic Administration
      1. Decreased vision
      2. Mydriasis—may precipitate narrow-angle glaucoma
      3. Paralysis of accommodation
      4. Photophobia
      5. Diplopia
      6. Problems with color vision
         a. Color vision defect (piperidolate)
         b. Colored flashing lights (propantheline)
      7. Flashing lights (piperidolate)
      8. Eyelids or conjunctiva
         a. Allergic reactions
         b. Exfoliative dermatitis
   B. Local Ophthalmic Use or Exposure
      1. Mydriasis—may precipitate narrow-angle glaucoma
      2. Photophobia
      3. Paralysis of accommodation
      4. Eyelids or conjunctiva (oxyphenonium)

      a. Allergic reactions
      b. Conjunctivitis—nonspecific
   5. Increased intraocular pressure (oxyphenonium)
 C. Inadvertent Ocular Exposure
   1. Pupils (propantheline)
      a. Mydriasis
      b. Absence of reaction to light

Clinical Significance: Ocular side effects due to these anticholinergic agents vary depending on the drug; however, adverse ocular reactions are seldom significant and are reversible. None of the preceding drugs have little more than 10% to 15% of the anticholinergic activity of atropine. The most frequent ocular side effects are decreased vision, mydriasis, decreased accommodation, and photophobia. While these effects are common, only rarely are they severe enough to modify the use of the drug. The weak anticholinergic effect of these agents seldom aggravates open-angle glaucoma; however, it has the potential to precipitate narrow-angle glaucoma attacks. Nissen and Nielsen reported two cases of unilateral pupillary dilatation in patients who inadvertently got antiperspirants containing propantheline on their fingers and transferred it to their eyes.

References:

Brown, D.W., and Guilbert, G.D.: Acute glaucoma in patient with peptic ulcer. Am. J. Ophthalmol. *36*:1735–1736, 1953.

Cholst, M., Goodstein, S., and Bernes, C.: Glaucoma in medical practice, danger of use of systemic antispasmodic drugs in patients predisposed to or having glaucoma. JAMA *166*:1276–1280, 1958.

Grant, W.M.: Toxicology of the eye, 1st Ed. Springfield, Thomas, p. 160, 1962.

Henry, D.A., and Langman, M.J.S.: Adverse effects of anti-ulcer drugs. Drugs *21*:444, 1981.

Hufford, A.R.: Bentyl hydrochloride: Successful administration of a parasympatholytic antispasmodic in glaucoma patients. Am. J. Dig. Dis. *19*:257–258, 1952.

McHardy, G., and Brown, D.C.: Clinical appraisal of gastrointestinal antispasmodics. South Med. J. *45*:1139–1144, 1952.

Mody, M.V., and Keeney, A.H.: Propantheline (Pro-Banthine) bromide in relation to normal and glaucomatous eyes: Effects on intraocular tension and pupillary size. JAMA *159*:113–114, 1955.

Nissen, S.N., and Nielsen, P.G.: Unilateral mydriasis after use of propantheline bromide in an antiperspirant. Lancet 2:1134, 1977.

Schwartz, N., and Apt, L.: Mydriatic effect of anticholinergic drugs used during reversal of nondepolarizing muscle relaxants. Am. J. Ophthalmol. *88*:609, 1979.

Generic Name: 1. Atropine; 2. Belladonna; 3. Homatropine

Proprietary Name: *Systemic*: 1. Atropinol (Germ.); 2. Atrobel (Austral.), Belladonna Extract, Leaf, or Tincture, Belladonnysat Brger (Germ.), Bel-

lafolin (Germ.), Bellafolina (Ital., Span.), Tremoforat (Germ.); 3. Novatrop-
ina (Ital., Span.) *Ophthalmic*: 1. **Atropine-1, Atropine Care, Atropine
Sulfate Ophthalmic Ointment, Atropine Sulfate Solution, Atropine Sulfate S.O.P.**, Atropisol, Atropt (Austral.), Isopto Atropine, Liotropina (Ital.),
Skiatropine (Switz.), Spersatropine (S. Afr.), Vitatropine (Fr.); 3. **AK-Hom-
atropine**, Homat (Austral.), Homatro (Span.), **Homatropine HBr Solution**,
Isopto Homatropine *Topical*: 1. **Ocean-A/S**

Primary Use: *Systemic:* These anticholinergic agents are used in the management of gastrointestinal tract spasticity and peptic ulcers, and to decrease
secretions of the respiratory tract. Atropine is also used in the treatment of
hyperactive carotid sinus reflex and Parkinson's disease. Homatropine is
also used in the treatment of dysmenorrhea. *Ophthalmic:* These topical
anticholinergic mydriatic and cycloplegic agents are used in refractions,
semiocclusive therapy, accommodative spasms, and uveitis.

Ocular Side Effects:
A. Systemic Administration
   1. Decreased vision
   2. Pupils
      a. Mydriasis—may precipitate narrow-angle glaucoma
      b. Absence of reaction to light—toxic states
   3. Decrease or paralysis of accommodation
   4. Photophobia
   5. Micropsia
   6. Decreased lacrimation
   7. Visual hallucinations
   8. Problems with color vision
      a. Color vision defect
      b. Objects have red tinge
   9. Eyelids or conjunctiva—Stevens-Johnson syndrome
      (belladonna)
B. Local Ophthalmic Use or Exposure—Topical Application
   1. Decreased vision
   2. Decrease or paralysis of accommodation
   3. Mydriasis—may precipitate narrow-angle glaucoma
   4. Irritation
      a. Hyperemia
      b. Photophobia
      c. Ocular pain
      d. Edema
   5. Increased intraocular pressure
   6. Eyelids or conjunctiva
      a. Allergic reactions
      b. Blepharoconjunctivitis—follicular and papillary

      7. Micropsia
      8. Decreased lacrimation
      9. Visual hallucinations
   C. Local Ophthalmic Use or Exposure—Subconjunctival Injection
      1. Brawny scleritis

Systemic Side Effects:
   A. Local Ophthalmic Use or Exposure—Topical Application
      1. Agitation
      2. Confusion
      3. Psychosis
      4. Delirium
      5. Hallucinations
      6. Ataxia
      7. Hostility
      8. Fever
      9. Dry mouth
    10. Vasodilation
    11. Dysarthria
    12. Tachycardia (atropine)
    13. Convulsion (atropine)

Clinical Significance: Atropine and homatropine have essentially the same ocular side effects whether they are administered systemically, via aerosols, or by topical ocular application. Systemic administration causes fewer and less severe ocular side effects, since significantly smaller amounts of the drug reaches the eye. However, transient loss of vision following an intravenous injection of atropine has been reported. Topical ocular atropine and homatropine may elevate the intraocular pressure in eyes with open-angle glaucoma. Probably the most common side effect that requires the discontinuation of these agents is contact dermatitis. Conjunctival papillary hypertrophy usually suggests a hypersensitivity reaction, while a follicular response suggests a toxic or irritative reaction to these agents. Atropine, but not homatropine, is said to produce a greater and faster pupillary response in patients with Down's syndrome. Permanent fixed, dilated pupils may result from chronic atropinization, or a large dose of atropine, such as that needed for resuscitation. Although chronic atropinization of post-keratopathy for keratoconus has recently been reported to not produce irreversible mydriasis (Geyer, Rothkoff, and Lazar), cases of this adverse event have been reported to the Registry. Unilateral atropinization during visual immaturity may cause amblyopia. In the primate, topical ocular atropine appears to decrease or slow echothiophate-induced lens changes. Systemic reactions may occur after ocular instillation of these anticholinergic drugs, particularly in children or elderly patients. Symptoms of systemic toxicity include dryness of the mouth and skin, flushing, fever, rash, thirst, tachycardia, irritability, hyperactivity, ataxia, confusion, somnolence, hallucinations, and delirium. These reactions have been observed most frequently after the use of atropine. Rarely, convulsions, coma, and death have occurred after ocular instillation of atropine in infants and children, especially when the solution form was used. The possibility of atropine overdose can be distinguished by applying topical ocular 1.0% pilocarpine.

References:

Boothe, R.G., Kiorpes, L., and Hendrickson, A.: Anisometropic amblyopia in Macaca nemestrina monkeys produced by atropinization of one eye during development. Invest. Ophthalmol. Vis. Sci. *22*:228, 1982.

Geyer, O., Rothkoff, L., and Lazar, M.: Atropine in keratoplasty for keratoconus. Cornea *10(5)*:372–373, 1991.

Gooding, J.M., and Holcomb, M.C.: Transient blindness following intravenous administration of atropine. Anesth. Analg. *56*:872, 1977.

Kaufman, P.L., Axelsson, U., and Barany, E.H.: Atropine inhibition of echothiophate cataractogenesis in monkeys. Arch. Ophthalmol. *95*:1262, 1977.

Merli, G.J., et al.: Cardiac dysrhythmias associated with ophthalmic atropine. Arch. Intern. Med. *146*:45, 1986.

O'Brien, D., Haake, M.W., and Braid, B.: Atropine sensitivity and serotonin in mongolism. J. Dis. Child. *100*:873–874, 1960.

Sanitato, J.J., and Burke, M.J.: Atropine toxicity in identical twins. Ann. Ophthalmol. *15*:380, 1983.

Smith, E.L., III, et al.: Permanent alterations in muscarinic receptors and pupil size produced by chronic atropinization in kittens. Invest. Ophthalmol. Vis. Sci. *25*:239, 1984.

Verma, N.P.: Drugs as a cause of fixed, dilated pupils after resuscitation. JAMA *255*: 3251, 1986.

von Noorden, G.K.: Amblyopia caused by unilateral atropinization. Ophthalmology *88*:131, 1981.

Wark, N.J., Overton, J.H., and Marian, P.: The safety of atropine premedication in children with Downs syndrome. Anaesthesia *38*:871, 1983.

Wilson, F.M., II: Adverse external ocular effects of topical ophthalmic medications. Surv. Ophthalmol. *24*:57, 1979.

Class: Gastrointestinal and Urinary Tract Stimulants

Generic Name: Bethanechol

Proprietary Name: Duvoid (Canad.), Myo Hermes (Span.), Myocholine (Germ., Switz.), **Myotonachol**, Myotonine (G.B.), **Urecholine** (Austral., Canad., S. Afr.), Urecholine Chloruro (Ital.), Urocarb (Austral.)

Primary Use: This quaternary ammonium parasympathomimetic agent is effective in the management of postoperative abdominal distention and nonobstructive urinary retention.

Ocular Side Effects:
  A. Systemic Administration
    1. Nonspecific ocular irritation
      a. Lacrimation
      b. Hyperemia
      c. Burning sensation
    2. Decreased accommodation
    3. Miosis

Clinical Significance: Adverse ocular reactions due to bethanechol are unusual, but they may continue after use of the drug is discontinued. Some advocate use of this agent in the treatment of Riley Day syndrome and ocular pemphigoid because of the possible increase in lacrimal secretion.

References:

Crandall, D.C., and Leopold, I.H.: The influence of systemic drugs on tear constituents. Ophthalmology *86*:115, 1979.
McEvoy, G.K. (Ed.): American Hospital Formulary Service Drug Information 87. Bethesda, American Society of Hospital Pharmacists, 1987, pp. 521–523.
Perritt, R.A.: Eye complications resulting from systemic medications. Ill. Med. J. *117*: 423, 1960.

Generic Name: Carbachol

Proprietary Name: *Systemic*: Doryl (Germ., Switz.), Miostat (Canad., Neth., Switz.) Ophthalmic: Carbamann (Germ.), **Isopto Carbachol**, Isopto Karbakolin (Swed.), Miostat, Spersacarbachol (Switz.)

Primary Use: *Systemic*: This quaternary ammonium parasympathomimetic agent is effective in the management of postoperative intestinal atony and urinary retention. *Ophthalmic*: This topical or intraocular agent is used in open-angle glaucoma.

Ocular Side Effects:
  A. Systemic Administration
    1. Decreased accommodation
  B. Local Ophthalmic Use or Exposure—Topical Application
    1. Miosis
    2. Decreased vision
    3. Decreased intraocular pressure
    4. Accommodative spasm
    5. Eyelids or conjunctiva
      a. Allergic reactions
      b. Hyperemia

      c. Conjunctivitis—follicular
      d. Pemphigoid lesion with symblepharon
  6. Irritation
      a. Lacrimation
      b. Ocular pain
  7. Blepharoclonus
  8. Myopia
  9. Retinal detachment
  10. Problems with color vision—objects have yellow tinge
C. Local Ophthalmic Use or Exposure—Intracameral Injection
  1. Miosis
  2. Corneal edema
  3. Decreased vision

Systemic Side Effects:
A. Local Ophthalmic Use or Exposure—Topical Application
  1. Dizziness
  2. Vomiting
  3. Diarrhea
  4. Stomach pain
  5. Intestinal cramps
  6. Bradycardia
  7. Arrhythmia
  8. Hypotension
  9. Syncope

Clinical Significance: Probably the most frequent ocular side effect due to carbachol is a decrease in vision secondary to miosis or accommodative spasms. In the younger age groups, transient drug-induced myopia may also occur. Follicular conjunctivitis is common after long-term therapy, but this in general has minimal clinical significance. Miotics can induce retinal detachments but probably only in eyes with a pre-existing retinal pathologic condition. If there are abrasions of the conjunctiva or corneal epithelium, care must be taken to not apply topical ocular carbachol since the incidences of systemic side effects are increased dramatically. Otherwise, systemic reactions to carbachol are rare, usually occurring after excessive use of the medication. In addition, this topical ocular medication used in glaucoma therapy may be one of the more toxic agents on the corneal epithelium. N-demethylated carbachol in a 6% or 9% solution has demonstrated ocular hypotensive actions in patients with open-angle glaucoma.

References:
Beasley, H., and Fraunfelder, F.T.: Retinal detachments and topical ocular miotics. Ophthalmology 86:95, 1979.
Beasley, H., et al.: Carbachol in cataract surgery. Arch. Ophthalmol. 80:39, 1968.

Crandall, D.C., and Leopold, I.H.: The influence of systemic drugs on tear constituents. Ophthalmology *86*:115, 1979.

Fraunfelder, F.T.: Corneal edema after use of carbachol. Arch. Ophthalmol. *97*:975, 1979.

Hesse, R.J., et al.: The effect of carbachol combined with intraoperative viscoelastic substances on postoperative IOP response. Ophthalmic Surg. *19*:224, 1988.

Hung, P.T., Hsieh, J.W., and Chiou, G.C.Y.: Ocular hypotensive effects of N-demethylated carbachol on open-angle glaucoma. Arch. Ophthalmol. *100*:262, 1982.

Krejci, L., and Harrison, R.: Antiglaucoma drug effects on corneal epithelium. A comparative study in tissue culture. Arch. Ophthalmol. *84*:766, 1970.

Mönig, H., et al.: Kreislaufkollaps durch carbachol-haltige augentropfen. Dtsch. Med. Wochenschr. *114(47)*:1860, 1989.

Olson, R.J., et al.: Commonly used intraocular medications and the corneal endothelium. Arch. Ophthalmol. *98*:2224–2226, 1980.

Pape, L.G., and Forbes, M.: Retinal detachment and miotic therapy. Am. J. Ophthalmol. *85*:558, 1978.

Vaughn, E.D., Hull, D.S., and Green, K.: Effect of intraocular miotics on corneal endothelium. Arch. Ophthalmol. *96*:1897, 1978.

VI   Cardiac, Vascular, and Renal Agents

Class: Agents Used to Treat Migraine

Generic Name: 1. Ergonovine (Ergometrine); 2. Ergotamine; 3. Methylergonovine; 4. Methysergide

Proprietary Name: 1. Ergometron (S. Afr.), **Ergotrate Maleate** (Austral., Canad., S. Afr.); 2. Ergate (S. Afr.), ergo sanol SL (Germ.), Ergo-Kranit mono (Germ.), Ergomar (Canad.), **Ergostat**, Ergotan (Ital.), Gynergeen (Neth.), Gynergen (Canad., Germ., Ital.), Gynergeno (Span.), Lingraine (Austral., G.B., Ire.), **Medihaler-Ergotamine** (Austral., Canad., G.B.); 3. Méthergin (Fr., Switz.), Methergin (Germ., Ital., Neth., Span., Swed.), **Methergine**; 4. Déséril (Switz.), Deseril (Austral., G.B., Germ., Ire., Neth., S. Afr., Span.), Désernil-Sandoz (Fr.), Deserril (Ital.), **Sansert** (Canad., Swed.)

Primary Use: These ergot alkaloids and derivatives are effective in the management of migraine or other vascular types of headaches and as oxytocic agents.

Ocular Side Effects:
   A. Systemic Administration
   1. Decreased vision
   2. Retinal vascular disorders
      a. Spasms
      b. Constriction
      c. Stasis
      d. Thrombosis
      e. Occlusion
   3. Miosis (ergotamine)
   4. Decreased intraocular pressure—minimal
   5. Visual fields
      a. Scotomas
      b. Hemianopsia

6. Decreased accommodation (methysergide)
7. Problems with color vision
   a. Color vision defect, red-green defect
   b. Objects have red tinge
8. Eyelids or conjunctiva
   a. Allergic reactions
   b. Erythema
   c. Edema
   d. Lupoid syndrome
9. Visual hallucinations (methysergide)
10. Decreased dark adaptation

Clinical Significance: Ocular side effects due to these ergot alkaloids are rare; however, patients taking standard therapeutic dosages may develop significant adverse ocular effects. This is probably due to an unusual susceptibility, sensitivity, or a pre-existing disease that is exacerbated by the ergot preparations. Increased ocular vascular complications have been seen in patients with a pre-existing occlusive peripheral vascular disease. Crews reported on a healthy 19-year-old in whom a standard therapeutic injection of ergotamine apparently precipitated a central retinal artery occlusion. Gupta and Strobos reported a bilateral ischemic optic neuritis that may have been due to ergotamine. Merhoff and Porter reported a case with possible drug-induced central scotoma, retinal vasospasms, and retinal pallor. Heider, Berninger, and Brunk reported the case of a long-term ergot user who developed reversible decreased vision with decreased sensitivity in the central 30° in his visual field. A case observed by Creze, et al., possibly due to methylergonovine-induced cerebral vasospasm, may have caused transitory cortical blindness. There are sporadic reports of cataracts in the literature, but these are rare and it is difficult to prove a cause-and-effect relationship.

References:

Birch, J., et al.: Acquired color vision defects. *In* Pokorny, J., et al. (Eds.): Congenital and Acquired Color Vision Defects. New York, Grune & Stratton, 1979, pp. 243–350.

Crews, S.J.: Toxic effects on the eye and visual apparatus resulting from the systemic absorption of recently introduced chemical agents. Trans. Ophthalmol. Soc. UK *82*: 387–406, 1963.

Creze, B., et al.: Transitory cortical blindness after delivery using Methergin. Rev. Fr. Gynecol. Obstet. *71*:353, 1976.

Gupta, D.R., and Strobos, R.J.: Bilateral papillitis associated with Cafergot therapy. Neurology *22*:793, 1972.

Heider, W., Berninger, T., and Brunk, G.: Electroophthalmological and clinical findings in a case of chronic abuse of ergotamine. Fortschr. Ophthalmol. *83*:539–541, 1986.

Merhoff, G.C., and Porter, J.M.: Ergot intoxication. Ann. Surg. *180*:773, 1974.

Mindel, J.S., Rubenstein, A.E., and Franklin, B.: Ocular ergotamine tartrate toxicity during treatment of Vacor-induced orthostatic hypotension. Am. J. Ophthalmol. *92*: 492, 1981.

Wollensak, J., and Grajewski, O.: Bilateral vascular papillitis following ergotamine medication. Klin. Monatsbl. Augenheilkd. *173*:731, 1978.

Class: Antianginal Agents

Generic Name: Amiodarone

Proprietary Name: Amiodar (Ital.), Corbionax (Fr.), Cordarex (Germ.), **Cordarone** (Canad., Fr., Ital., Neth., Swed., Switz.), Cordarone X (Austral., G.B., S. Afr.), Ortacrone (Span.), Rythmarone (Fr.), Trangorex (Span.)

Primary Use: This benzofuran derivative is effective in the treatment of life-threatening recurrent ventricular arrhythmia.

Ocular Side Effects:
A. Systemic Administration
    1. Cornea
        a. Yellow-brown deposits
        b. Epithelial breakdown
        c. Decreased sensation
        d. Endothelial deposits
    2. Decreased vision
    3. Problems with color vision
        a. Color vision defect
        b. Colored haloes around lights (blue-green)
    4. Eyelids or conjunctiva
        a. Yellow-brown deposits
        b. Blepharoconjunctivitis
        c. Discoloration (blue-gray)
        d. Photosensitivity
        e. Urticaria
        f. Stevens-Johnson syndrome
        g. Lyell's syndrome
        h. Chalazia
        i. Loss of eyelashes or eyebrows
    5. Keratoconjunctivitis sicca
    6. Photophobia
    7. Cataracts
    8. Papilledema secondary to pseudotumor cerebri
    9. Optic neuropathy
        a. Edema
        b. Hemorrhage
    10. Thyroid eye disease

11. Nystagmus
12. Visual field defects
    a. Baring of the blind spot
    b. Arcuate scotomas
    c. Central scotomas
    d. Enlarged blind spot
    e. Generalized constriction
13. Retinal depigmentation
14. Opsoclonus

Clinical Significance: Corneal microdeposits due to amiodarone probably occur in nearly all patients who are using the drug long term. The corneal epithelial whorl-like drug-related deposition is indistinguishable from that due to chloroquine. Although these deposits are dose- and time-related, it is not possible to accurately predict the degree of keratopathy either from daily or cumulative dosage. In some patients, the keratopathy appears to reach a steady state with no progression even with continued drug use. The usual pattern for corneal deposition initially is a horizontal, irregular, branching line near the junction of the mid and outer one-third of the cornea (stage 1). In stage 2, this increases so that 6 to 10 branches increase in length and curve superiorly. Any increase in the number of branches constitutes stage 3. Stage 4 is the whorl pattern with clumping deposits. The deposits may be seen as early as 2 weeks after starting the drug and probably occur in most patients by 4 months. In general, visible keratopathy develops in most patients within 6 weeks after initiation of amiodarone therapy and reaches its peak within 3 to 6 months. Patients taking 100 to 200 mg/day have only minimal or even no corneal deposits. At dosages of 400 mg or more, however, almost all patients will show corneal deposits. Possibly, if the drug is withheld for 1 week every 1 to 2 months, this side effect will not occur. Once the drug is stopped, most deposits totally regress in 3-7 months. However, in rare instances it may take up to 2 years. Visual changes are unusual and most often consist of complaints of hazy vision or colored haloes around lights. Occasionally, a patient may complain that bright lights, especially headlights at night, will cause a significant glare problem. Sicca has been reported, but since the drug is secreted in tears this may, in some instances, aggravate borderline sicca cases. A possible autoimmune reaction with dry mouth, dry eyes, peripheral neuropathy, and pneumonitis has been reported secondary to this drug. Slate-gray periocular skin pigmentation or blue skin discoloration has been seen secondary to photosensitivity reactions. Corneal ulcerations that appear during treatment with amiodarone have been reported to heal without complications other than microcyst formation. An acute rise in intracranial pressure associated with papilledema and visual field defects has been reported secondary to amiodarone, but this has not been reconfirmed. Optic neuropathy secondary to amiodarone is well documented with at least seven publications in the literature. This entity can occur at dosages from 200 to 1200 mg/day, and has been reported to occur as early as 1 month and as late as 72 months after starting therapy. The characteristics are generally milder than those with anterior ischemic optic neuropathy. Many patients are even unaware of any visual abnormality which follows the nonarteritic pattern of ischemic optic neuropathy. Amiodarone is prescribed for intractable ventricular tachycardia, and this ocular side effect is only a relative risk and not necessarily a reason for modifying drug therapy. However, depending on the degree of ocular involvement or the availability of other forms of therapy, decreasing or discontinuing this drug may be indicated since either method has been associated with visual recovery. The cause of this neuropathy may be due to the drug-induced lipidosis with intracytoplasmic lamellar inclusions seen in all ocular tissue. Flach and Dolan first described subtle anterior subcapsular lens opacities in all patients who were taking this agent for many years. These changes occur primarily in the pupillary area and are yellow-white, loosely packed deposits, which do not interfere with vision. The authors point out that the location of the deposits suggests a photosensitizing effect on the lens from the drug. There is no documented evidence that this drug causes human retinal damage, although the intracytoplasmic granulations have been found in the retinal pigment epithelium and choroid as well as the ciliary body, iris, cornea, conjunctiva, and lens. This drug is a photosensitizing agent and in selected cases for lens and retinal reasons, sunglasses that block to 400 nm may be considered.

References:

Dickerson, E.J., and Wolman, R.L.: Sicca syndrome associated with amiodarone therapy. Br. Med. J. *293*:510, 1986.

Feiner, L.A., et al.: Optic neuropathy and amiodarone therapy. Mayo Clin. Proc. *62*: 702, 1987.

Fikkers, B.G., et al.: Pseudotumor cerebri with amiodarone. J. Neurol. Neurosurg. Psychiatry *49*:606, 1986.

Flach, A.J., et al.: Amiodarone-induced lens opacities. Arch. Ophthalmol. *101*:1554, 1983.

Flach, A.J., and Dolan, B.J.: Amiodarone-induced lens opacities: An 8-year follow-up study. Arch. Ophthalmol. *108*:1668–1669, 1990.

Fraunfelder, F.T., and Meyer, S.M.: Amiodarone keratopathy. Trans. Ophthalmol. Soc. NZ *36*:33, 1984.

Garrett, S.N., Kearney, J.J., and Schiffman, J.S.: Amiodarone optic neuropathy. J. Clin. Neuro-op. *8*:105–110, 1988.

Ghosh, M., and McCulloch, C.: Amiodarone-induced ultrastructural changes in human eyes. Can. J. Ophthalmol. *19*:178, 1984.

Gittinger, J.W., and Asdourian, G.K.: Papillopathy caused by amiodarone. Arch. Ophthalmol. *105*:349, 1987.

Kaplan, L.J., and Cappaert, W.E.: Amiodarone keratopathy. Correlation to dosage and duration. Arch. Ophthalmol. *100*:601, 1982.

Klingele, T.G., Alves, L.E., and Rose, E.P.: Amiodarone keratopathy. Ann. Ophthalmol. *16*:1172, 1984.

Lopez, A.C., et al.: Acute intracranial hypertension during amiodarone infusion. Crit. Care Med. *13*:688, 1985.

Orlando, R.G., Dangel, M.E., and Schaal, S.F.: Clinical experience and grading of amiodarone keratopathy. Ophthalmology *91*:1184, 1984.

Palakurthy, P.R., et al: Amiodarone induced encephalopathy and diabetes insipidus. J. Kentucky Med. Assoc. *85*:373–374, 1987.

Palakurthy, P.R., Iyer, V., and Meckler, R.J.: Unusual neurotoxicity associated with amiodarone therapy. Arch. Intern. Med. *147*:881–884, 1987.

Reifler, D.M., et al.: Multiple chalazia and rosacea in a patient treated with amiodarone. Am. J. Ophthalmol. *103*:594, 1987.

Roberts, J.E., et al.: Exposure to bright light and the concurrent use of photosensitizing drugs. N. Engl. J. Med. *326*(22):1500, 1992.

Weiss, S. R., Lim, H.W., and Curtis, G.: Amiodarone. J. Am. Acad. Dermatol. *11*: 898–900, 1984.

Wilson, J.S., and Podrid, P.J.: Side effects from amiodarone. Am. Heart J. *121*:158–171, 1991

Generic Name: Amyl Nitrite

Proprietary Name: None

Primary Use: This short-acting nitrite antianginal agent is effective in the treatment of acute attacks of angina pectoris.

Ocular Side Effects:
    A. Inhalation Administration
        1. Mydriasis
        2. Decreased vision
        3. Problems with color vision
          a. Objects have yellow tinge
          b. Colored haloes around objects—mainly blue or yellow
        4. Decreased intraocular pressure—transient
        5. Color hallucinations
        6. Eyelids or conjunctiva—allergic reactions
        7. Retinal vasodilatation

Clinical Significance: Ocular side effects due to amyl nitrite are transient and reversible. Adverse ocular reactions are common and seldom of clinical significance. There is no evidence that this drug has precipitated narrow-angle glaucoma. Amyl nitrite ordinarily causes a fall in intraocular pressure for only 10 to 20 minutes. Prior reports of elevation of intraocular pressure with this drug are being questioned.

References:
Cristini, G., and Pagliarani, N.: Amyl nitrite test in primary glaucoma. Br. J. Ophthalmol. *37*:741, 1953.

Cristini, G., and Pagliarani, N.: Slitlamp study of the aqueous veins in simple glaucoma during the amyl nitrite test. Br. J. Ophthalmol. *39*:685, 1955.

Grant, W.M.: Physiological and pharmacological influences upon intraocular pressure. Pharmacol. Rev. *7*:143, 1955.

Robertson, D., and Stevens, R.M.: Nitrates and glaucoma. JAMA *237*:117, 1977.

Variations and patterns of IOP. Ann. Ophthalmol. *8*:1027–1028, 1976 (Glaucoma Report by the Editors).

Generic Name: 1. Diltiazem; 2. Nifedipine; 3. Verapamil

Proprietary Name: 1. Adizem (G.B.), Altiazem (Ital.), Angiozem (G.B.), Angizem (Ital.), Apo-Diltiaz (Canad.), Britiazim (G.B.), **Cardizem** (Austral., Canad., Swed.), Coridil (Switz.), **Dilacor XR**, Diladel (Ital.), Dilem (Ital.), Diltam (Ire.), Dilzem (Germ., Ire., Switz.), Dilzene (Ital.), Dinisor (Span.), Entrydil (Swed.), Herbesser (Jap.), Tilazem (S. Afr.), Tildiem (Fr., G.B., Ire., Ital., Neth.), Zilden (Ital.); 2. **Adalat** (Austral., Canad., G.B., Germ., Ire., Ital., Neth., S. Afr., Span., Swed., Switz.), Adalate (Fr.), Angiopine (G.B.), Anifed (Ital.), Anpine (Austral.), Antamex (Switz.), Apo-Nifed (Canad.), Aprical (Germ.), Calcilat (G.B.), Cardifen (S. Afr.), Citilat (Ital.), Coracten (G.B.), Coral (Ital.), Cordicant (Germ.), Cordilan (Span.), Corotrend (Germ., Switz.), Dignokonstant (Germ.), Dilcor (Span.), duranifin (Germ.), Ecodipine (Switz.), nifé-basan (Switz.), Nifecor (Germ.), Nifed (Ire.), Nifedicor (Ital.), Nifedin (Ital.), Nifedipat (Germ.), Nifehexal (Germ.), Nifelat (Germ.), Nifensar XL (G.B.), Nife-Puren (Germ.), Nife-Wolff (Germ.), Nifical (Germ.), Nifidine (S. Afr.), Novonifedin (Canad.), Pidilat (Germ.), Pinifed (Ire.), **Procardia**, Systepin (Ire.), Vasad (G.B.), Vasofed (Ire.); 3. Anpec (Austral.), Apo-Verap (Canad.), Azupamil (Germ.), Berkatens (G.B., Ire.), **Calan**, Cardiagutt (Germ.), cardibeltin (Germ.), Coraver (Swed.), Cordilox (Austral., G.B.), Dignover (Germ.), durasoptin (Germ.), Flamon (Switz.), Geangin (G.B., Neth.), Half Securon (G.B.), **Isoptin** (Canad., Germ., Ire., Ital., Neth., S. Afr., Swed., Switz.), Isoptine (Fr.), Manidon (Span.), Novoveramil (Canad.), Praecicor (Germ.), Quasar (Ital.), Securon (G.B.), Univer (G.B.), Vasomil (S. Afr.), Véracim (Switz.), Veradil (Austral.), Veradurat (Germ.), Verahexal (Germ.), Veraloc (Swed.), Veramex (Germ.), Veranorm (Germ.), **Verelan** (Ire.), Veroptinstada (Germ.), Verpamil (S. Afr.)

Primary Use: These calcium channel blockers are used in the treatment of vasospastic angina and chronic stable angina.

Ocular Side Effects:
   A. Systemic Administration
      1. Decreased vision
      2. Periorbital edema (nifedipine)
      3. Eyelids or conjunctiva

   a. Erythema
   b. Conjunctivitis—nonspecific
   c. Photosensitivity
   d. Angioneurotic edema
   e. Urticaria
   f. Purpura
   g. Erythema multiforme
   h. Exfoliative dermatitis (diltiazem)
   i. Lyell's syndrome (diltiazem)
   j. Loss of eyelashes or eyebrows
  4. Visual hallucinations
  5. Nonspecific ocular irritation
   a. Lacrimation
   b. Photophobia (nifedipine)
   c. Ocular pain (nifedipine)
   d. Edema
  6. Nystagmus—rotary (nifedipine, verapamil)
  7. Retinal vascular disorders (diltiazem, nifedipine)
   a. Thrombosis
   b. Hemorrhages
  8. Subconjunctival or retinal hemorrhages secondary to drug-induced anemia
   a. Increased intraocular pressure (transient)
   b. Local ophthalmic use or exposure

Clinical Significance: Ocular side effects secondary to calcium channel blockers consist primarily of blurred vision and ocular irritation with periorbital edema. Nifedipine has more ocular side effects than the other agents. Transient blindness at peak plasma levels has been observed in several patients. Apart from the ischemic responses affecting the myocardial circulation, such symptoms may also arise from the cerebral and the retinal circulation. Although toxic doses of calcium channel blockers have been noted to cause cataracts in animals, a well-documented study found no evidence of changes in lens transparency in patients receiving long-term treatment with high doses of verapamil. Intraocular pressure does not appear to be affected by calcium channel blockers, except there are questionable data that glaucoma patients may be more difficult to control while taking these agents. Nifedipine attenuates the intraocular pressure response to intubation following succinylcholine. Verapamil eyedrops have been shown to produce a slight transient rise in intraocular pressure. There is increasing suggestion that topical ocular beta blockers given to patients who are taking calcium channel blockers may, in exceedingly rare cases, cause an arrhythmia. The theory to explain this occurrence is that each agent acts in a different way to decrease the heart rate, so the effects may be additive, causing an arrhythmia.

References:

Anastassiades, C.J.: Nifedipine and beta-blocker drugs. Br. Med. J. *281*:1251–1252, 1980.

Beatty, J.F., et al.: Elevation of intraocular pressure by calcium channel blockers. Arch. Ophthalmol. *102*:1072, 1984.

Gill, J.S., et al.: Rupture of a cerebral aneurysm associated with nifedipine treatment. Postgrad. Med. J. *62*:1029, 1986. Grunwald, J.E., and Furubayashi, C.: Effect of topical timolol maleate on the ophthalmic artery blood pressure. Inv. Ophthalmol. Vis. Sci. *30*:1095–1100, 1989.

Hockwin, O., et al.: Evaluation of the ocular safety of verapamil. Scheimpflug photography with densitometric image analysis of lens transparency in patients with hypertrophic cardiomyopathy subjected to long-term therapy with high doses of verapamil. Ophthalmic Res. *16*:264, 1984.

Indu, B., et al.: Nifedipine attenuates the intraocular pressure response to intubation following succinylcholine. Can. J. Anaesth. *36*:269–272, 1989.

Kelly, S.P., and Walley, T.J.: Eye pain with nifedipine. Br. Med. J. *296*:1401, 1988.

Opie, L.H., and White, D.A.: Adverse interaction between nifedipine and B-blockade. Br. Med. J. *281*:1462, 1980.

Pitlik, S., et al.: Transient retinal ischaemia induced by nifedipine. Br. Med. J. *287*: 1845, 1983.

Silverstone, P.H.: Periorbital oedema caused by nifedipine. Br. Med. J. *288*:1654, 1984.

Sinclair, N.I., and Benzie, J.L.: Timolol eyedrops and verapamil-A dangerous combination. Med. J. Aust. *1*:549, 1983.

Staffurth, J.S., and Emery, P.: Adverse interaction between nifedipine and beta-blockade. Br. Med. J. *282*:225, 1981.

Tordjman, K., Rosenthal, T., and Bursztyn, M.: Nifedipine-induced periorbital edema. Am. J. Cardiol. *55*:1445, 1985

Generic Name: 1. Erythrityl Tetranitrate; 2. Isosorbide Dinitrate; 3. Mannitol Hexanitrate; 4. Pentaerythritol Tetranitrate; 5. Trolnitrate

Proprietary Name: 1. **Cardilate** (Canad., Ital.), Cardiwell (Fr.); 2. Acordin (Switz.), Cardopax (Swed.), Carvasin (Ital.), Cedocard (Canad., G.B., Neth.), Coradur (Canad.), Coronex (Canad.), Corovliss (Germ.), Dignonitrat (Germ.), Dilanid (S. Afr.), **Dilatrate-SR**, Disorlon (Fr.), duranitrat (Germ.), EureCor (Germ.), Imtack (G.B.), Isdin (Germ.), Iso (Span.), Iso Mack (Germ., S. Afr., Switz.), **Iso-Bid**, Isocard-Spray (Fr.), isoforce (Germ.), isoket (G.B., Germ., Switz.), Iso-Puren [Germ.), **Isordil** (Austral. Canad., G.B., Ire., Neth. S. Afr., Span.), Isostenase (Germ.), Isotrate (Austral.), Langoran (Fr.), Maycor (Germ., Span.), Nitrosorbide (Ital.), Nitrosorbon (Germ.), Nitro-Spray (Austral.), Nitro-Tablinen (Germ.), Novosorbide (Canad.), Prodicard (Neth.), Rifloc (Germ.), Risordan (Fr.), Soni-Slo (G.B.), Sorbangil (Swed.), Sorbichew (G.B.), Sorbid (G.B.), Sorbidilat (Germ., Switz.), **Sorbitrate** (Fr., G.B.), TD Spray Iso Mack (Germ.), Vascardin (G.B., Ire.), Vermicet (Germ.); 4. Dilcoran (Germ.), **Duotrate**, Mycardol (G.B., Ire.), Niscodil (Ital.), Nitrodex (Switz.), Nitrodex Chronules (Fr.), Péritrate (Fr.), **Peritrate** (Austral., Canad., Ital., S. Afr., Span.)

Primary Use: These long-acting vasodilators are used in the treatment of chronic angina pectoris.

Ocular Side Effects:
A. Systemic Administration
    1. Decreased vision—transitory
    2. Intraocular pressure—decreased
    3. Myopia—transitory (isosorbide dinitrate)
    4. Eyelids—exfoliative dermatitis

Clinical Significance: Ocular side effects due to the nitrate vasodilators are uncommon, transitory, and reversible. The primary adverse ocular reaction is transitory blurred vision. Use of these vasodilators is probably not contraindicated in glaucomatous patients; however, there have been rare reports to the contrary. Clinically, no adverse glaucomatous effects of any practical importance have been reported to date. Mueller and Meienberg reported a single case of unilateral headache with ipsilateral ptosis and miosis in a patient receiving isosorbide dinitrate therapy. Dangel, Weber, and Leier reported on a woman who, after each ingestion of isosorbide dinitrate, developed blurred vision within one-half hour; this blurred vision lasted for 1-2 hours secondary to myopia. This was associated with decreased amplitude of accommodation, a reduction of the AC/A ratio, and a decrease in the anterior chamber depth. The authors believed this was due to a drug-induced ciliary spasm. In addition, transient cerebral ischemia may be precipitated when long-acting nitrates are used in patients with concurrent cerebrovascular disease.

References:

Dangel, M.E., Weber, P.A., and Leier, C.B.: Transient myopia following isosorbide dinitrate. Ann. Ophthalmol. *15*:1156, 1983.

Leydhecker, H.C.W.: Glaukom und gefässerweiternde Medikamente. Dtsch. Med. Wochenschr. *104*:1330, 1979.

McEvoy, G.K. (Ed.): American Hospital Formulary Service Drug Information 87. Bethesda, American Society of Hospital Pharmacists, 1987, pp. 868–869, 872–873.

Mueller, R.A., and Meienberg, O.: Hemicrania with oculosympathetic paresis from isosorbide dinitrate. N. Engl. J. Med. *308*:458, 1983.

Purvin, V., and Dunn, D.: Nitrate-induced transient ischemic attacks. South. Med. J. *74*:1130, 1981.

Robertson, D., and Stevens, R.M.: Nitrates and glaucoma. JAMA *237*:117, 1977.

Wizemann, A.J.S., and Wizemann, V.: Organic nitrate therapy in glaucoma. Am. J. Ophthalmol. *90*:106, 1980

Generic Name: 1. Flecainide; 2. Mexiletine; 3. Tocainide

Proprietary Name: 1. Almarytm (Ital.), Apocard (Span.), Corflene (Span.), Flécaïne (Fr.), **Tambocor** (Austral., Canad., G.B., Germ., Neth., Swed.,

Switz.); 2. **Mexitil** (Austral., Canad., Fr., G.B., Germ., Ital., Neth., S. Afr., Span., Swed., Switz.); 3. **Tonocard** (Canad., G.B., Ire., Neth., Swed.), Xylotocan (Germ.)

Primary Use: These primary amine analogs of lidocaine are used in the treatment of resistant ventricular arrhythmia.

Ocular Side Effects:
   A. Systemic Administration
      1. Decreased vision
      2. Decreased accommodation
      3. Nystagmus
      4. Visual hallucinations
      5. Diplopia
      6. Corneal deposits (flecainide)
      7. Eyelids or conjunctiva
         a. Erythema
         b. Angioneurotic edema
         c. Urticaria (flecainide)
         d. Lupoid syndrome
         e. Exfoliative dermatitis (flecainide)
         f. Loss of eyelashes or eyebrows
      8. Nonspecific ocular irritation (flecainide)
         a. Photophobia
         b. Ocular pain
      9. Subconjunctival or retinal hemorrhages secondary to drug-induced anemia

Clinical Significance: The most frequent adverse effects of these drugs involve the CNS. These drugs, especially flecainide, may transitorily interfere with accommodation. Infrequently, blurred vision and nystagmus may occur; these ocular side effects are transient and usually respond to dose reduction. Moller, Thygesen, and Kruit recently reported two patients taking flecainide who developed superficial gray whorl corneal deposits. High-pressure liquid chromatography suggests flecainide and peptide corneal deposition. Stopping the drug resulted in corneal clearing over a 3-month period. Painful eye movements accompanied by lateral rectus spasm have been reported in one patient.

References:

Cetnarowski, A.B., and Rihn, T.L.: Adverse reactions to tocainide and mexiletine. Cardiovasc. Rev. Reports 6:1335, 1985.
Clarke, C.W.F., and el-Mahdi, E.O.: Confusion and paranoia associated with oral tocainide. Postgrad. Med. J. 61:79, 1985.

Gentzkow, G.D., and Sullivan, J.Y.: Extracardiac adverse effects of flecainide. Am. J. Cardiol. *53*:101B–105B, 1984.

Keefe, D.L.D., Kates, R.E., and Harrison, D.C.: New antiarrhythmic drugs: Their place in therapy. Drugs 22:363, 1981.

Møller, H.U., Thygesen, and Kruit, P.J.: Corneal deposits associated with flecainide. Br. Med. J. *302*:506–507, 1991.

Ramhamadany, E., et al.: Dysarthria and visual hallucinations due to flecainide toxicity. Postgrad. Med. J. *62*:61, 1986.

Skander, M., and Issacs, P.E.T.: Flecainide, ocular myopathy, and antinuclear factor. Br. Med. J. *291*:450, 1985.

Vincent, F.M., and Vincent, T.: Tocainide encephalopathy. Neurology *35*:1804, 1985.

Generic Name: Nitroglycerin

Proprietary Name: Adesitrin (Ital.), Anginine (Austral.), Angiospray (Ital.), Angiplex (Swed.), Angised (Ire., S. Afr.), Angitrine (Fr.), Angonit (Neth.), Aquo-Trinitrosan (Germ.), Colenitral (Span.), Corangin Nitro (Germ.), Corditrine (Fr.), Coro-Nitro (G.B., Germ.), deponit (Germ.), **Deponit** (G.B., Ital., Neth., Switz.), Diafusor (Fr., Span.), Gilustenon (Germ.), Glytrin (G.B.), Lénitral (Fr.), Maycor (Germ.), Millisrol (Jap.), **Minitran,** Natirose (Fr.), Natispray (Fr., Ital., Switz.), Neos Nitro N (Germ.), Niong retard (Switz.), Nitradisc (Austral., Germ., S. Afr., Span.), Nitriderm TTS (Fr.), Nitro Dur (Span.), Nitro Mack (Germ., Switz.), Nitro Pohl (Germ., Neth.), Nitro Rorer (Germ.), Nitrobaat (Neth.), **Nitro-Bid** (Austral., Canad.), **Nitrocine** (G.B.), Nitrocontin Continus (G.B., Ire.), Nitrocor (Ital.), Nitroderm TTS (Germ., Ital., S. Afr., Span., Switz.), **Nitrodisc, Nitro-Dur** (G.B., Ital., Switz.), **Nitrogard**, Nitrogard-SR (Canad.), Nitro-Gesanit (Germ.), Nitroglin (Germ.), Nitroglyn (Swed.), Nitroject (Canad.), Nitrokapseln-ratiopharm (Germ.), **Nitrol** (Canad.), Nitrolate (Austral.), **Nitrolingual** (Canad., G.B., Germ., Neth., S. Afr., Swed., Switz.), Nitromex (Swed.), Nitromint (Switz.), Nitronal (G.B., Germ., S. Afr., Switz.), **Nitrong** (Canad., Ital., Neth., S. Afr., Swed.), nitroperlinit (Germ.), Nitro-Pflaster-ratiopharm (Germ.), Nitrorectal (Germ.), Nitro-Retard (Ital.), **Nitrospan, Nitrostat** (Canad., Neth.), Nitrotard (Span.), Nitrozell (Germ., Neth.), **NTS**, Percutol (G.B., Ire.), perlinganit (Germ., Swed., Switz.), Probucard (Neth.), Solinitrina (Span.), Suscard (G.B., Ital., Swed.), Sustac (G.B.), **Transdermal-NTG, Transderm-Nitro** (Canad.), Transiderm-Nitro (Austral., G.B., Ire., Neth., Swed.), **Tridil** (Austral., Canad., G.B., S. Afr.), Trinitran (Fr.), Trinitrina (Ital.), Trinitrine (Switz.), Trinitrosan (Germ.), Venitrin Flebo (Ital.), Vernies (Span.)

Primary Use: This short-acting trinitrate vasodilator is effective in the treatment of acute attacks of angina pectoris.

Ocular Side Effects:
  A. Systemic Administration
    1. Decreased vision

   2. Intraocular pressure—decreased
   3. Retinal vasodilatation
   4. Problems with color vision—colored haloes around lights, mainly yellow or blue
   5. Subconjunctival or retinal hemorrhages secondary to drug-induced anemia
   6. Eyelids—exfoliative dermatitis
   7. Papilledema secondary to pseudotumor cerebri

Clinical Significance: Ocular side effects due to nitroglycerin are uncommon, transient, and reversible. No clinically important evidence of significant ocular pressure elevation due to nitroglycerin usage exists in patients with open- or narrow-angle glaucoma. Theoretically, however, the drug does have the potential to precipitate narrow-angle glaucoma. Transitory and reversible blindness due to ingestion of nitroglycerin has been seen, and in one instance, optic atrophy was reported. Long-acting nitrates can cause sustained cerebral vasodilatation that increases cerebral blood flow and possibly shunts blood away from narrowed vessels, thus producing transient cerebral ischemia.

References:

Leydhecker, W.: Glaukom und gefässerweiternde Medikamente. Dtsch. Med. Wochenschr. *104*:1330, 1979.

Ohar, J.M., et al.: Intravenous nitroglycerin-induced intracranial hypertension. Crit. Care Med. *13*:867, 1985.

Purvin, V., and Dunn, D.: Nitrate-induced transient ischemic attacks. South. Med. J. *74*:1130, 1981.

Robertson, D., and Stevens, R.M.: Nitrates and glaucoma. JAMA *237*:117, 1977.

Shorey, J., Bhardwaj, N., and Loscalzo, J.: Acute Wernicke's encephalopathy after intravenous infusion of high-dose nitroglycerin. Ann. Intern. Med. *101*:500, 1984.

Sveska, K.: Nitrates may not be contraindicated in patients with glaucoma. Drug Intell. Clin. Pharm. *19*:361, 1985.

Wizemann, A.J.S., and Wizemann, V.: Organic nitrate therapy in glaucoma. Am. J. Ophthalmol. *90*:106,1980.

Generic Name: Perhexiline

Proprietary Name: Pexid (Austral., Fr., Germ.)

Primary Use: This antianginal agent reduces the severity of anginal attacks in patients with coronary artery disease.

Ocular Side Effects:
   A. Systemic Administration
      1. Decreased vision
      2. Nystagmus

3. Papilledema secondary to pseudotumor cerebri
4. Problems with color vision—color vision defect
5. Enlarged blind spot
6. Retinal vascular disorders
   a. Thrombosis
   b. Hemorrhages
   c. Engorgement

Clinical Significance: Neurologic complications are common among the adverse effects of perhexiline, and several cases of bilateral papilledema have been reported. Normally, the papilledema improved within 6 weeks of discontinuing the drug; but permanent changes may ensue if the drug-induced increased intracranial pressure remains unrecognized. Nystagmus may occur secondary to equilibrium disorders induced by this agent. A case of keratitis sicca and lipidosis in a verticullata pattern has been reported.

References:

Atkinson, A.B., McAreavey, D., and Trope, G.: Papilloedema and hepatic dysfunction apparently induced by perhexiline maleate (Pexid). Br. Heart J. *43*:490, 1980.

Caruzzo, C., et al.: Toxic polyneuritis and toxic hepatitis related to long-term perhexiline maleate therapy. Am. Heart J. *100*:270, 1980.

Detilleux, J.M., and Rausin, G.: Papilledema and perhexiline maleate. Bull. Soc. Belge Ophtalmol. *180*:27, 1978.

Gibson, J.M., et al.: Severe ocular side effects of perhexiline maleate. Br. J. Ophthalmol. *68*:553, 1984.

Laroche, J., and Laroche, C.: Nouvelles recherches sur la modification de la vision des couleurs sous l'action des medicaments a dose therapeutique. Ann. Pharm. Fr. *35*:173, 1977.

McQueen, E.G.: New Zealand committee on adverse drug reactions: Fifteenth annual report 1980. NZ Med. J. *93*:194, 1981.

Mandelcorn, M., Murphy, J., and Colman, J.: Papilledema without peripheral neuropathy in a patient taking perhexiline maleate. Can. J. Ophthalmol. *17*:173, 1982.

Poisson, M., et al.: Thrombose post-arteriographique des veines ophtalmiques dans 2 cas de neuropathie peripherique au maleate de perhexiline avec signes neurologiques centraux. Nouv. Presse Med. *6*:3550, 1977.

Stephens, W.P., et al.: Raised intracranial pressure due to perhexiline maleate. Br. Med. J. *1*:21, 1978.

Turut, P., et al.: Ophthalmologic complications of Pexid. Bull. Soc. Ophtalmol. Fr. *77*:1003, 1977.

Class: Antiarrhythmic Agents

Generic Name: Disopyramide

Proprietary Name: Dicorynan (Span.), Dirythmin SA (G.B., Ire.), Dirytmin (Neth., Swed.), Diso-Duriles (Germ.), Durbis (Swed.), Isomide (G.B.),

Isomide CR (G.B.), **Norpace** (Austral., Canad., Germ., S. Afr., Switz.), Ritmodan (Ital.), Ritmodan Retard (Ital.), Ritmoforine (Neth.), Rythmodan (Austral., Canad., Fr., G.B., Ire., Neth., S. Afr.), Rythmodul (Germ.)

Primary Use: This anticholinergic agent is indicated for suppression and prevention of recurrence of cardiac arrhythmias.

Ocular Side Effects:
A. Systemic Administration
1. Decreased vision
2. Eyelids or conjunctiva
   a. Erythema
   b. Conjunctivitis—nonspecific
   c. Photosensitivity
3. Mydriasis—may precipitate narrow-angle glaucoma
4. Decreased accommodation
5. Decreased lacrimation
6. Visual hallucinations
7. Photophobia

Clinical Significance: The anticholinergic effects of disopyramide can cause blurred vision and fluctuation of visual acuity. The drug can cause mydriasis and has precipitated narrow-angle glaucoma. There are cases in the literature and the Registry of narrow-angle glaucoma occurring shortly after or up to 3 weeks after the patient started taking the medication. A few cases of diplopia and paralysis of extraocular muscles have also been reported to the Registry; some of these patients were also taking digitalis drugs as well and some had pre-existent myasthenia gravis that could have been aggravated.

References:
Ahmad, S.: Disopyramide: Pulmonary complications and glaucoma. Mayo Clin. Proc. 65:1030–1031, 1990.

Frucht, J., Freimann, I., and Merin, S.: Ocular side effects of disopyramide. Br. J. Ophthalmol. 68:890, 1984.

Keefe, D.L.D., Kates, R.E., and Harrison, D.C.: New antiarrhythmic drugs: Their place in therapy. Drugs 22:363, 1981.

McEvoy, G.K. (Ed.): American Hospital Formulary Service Drug Information 87. Bethesda, American Society of Hospital Pharmacists, 1987, pp. 729–732.

Schwartz, J.B., Keefe, D., and Harrison, D.C.: Adverse effects of antiarrhythmic drugs. Drugs 21:23, 1981.

Trope, G.E., and Hind, V.M.D.: Closed-angle glaucoma in patient on disopyramide. Lancet 1:329, 1978.

Wayne, K., Manolas, E., and Sloman, G.: Fatal overdose with disopyramide. Med. J. Aust. 1:231, 1980.

Generic Name: Methacholine
Proprietary Name: Provocholine

Primary Use: *Systemic*: This quaternary ammonium parasympathomimetic agent is primarily used in the management of paroxysmal tachycardia, Raynaud's syndrome, and scleroderma. *Ophthalmic*: This topical agent is used in the management of narrow-angle glaucoma and in the diagnosis of Adie's pupil.

Ocular Side Effects:
  A. Systemic Administration
      1. Decreased accommodation
      2. Lacrimation
  B. Local Ophthalmic Use or Exposure
      1. Pupils
          a. No effect—normal pupil
          b. Miosis—Adie's pupil
      2. Decreased intraocular pressure
      3. Eyelids or conjunctiva
          a. Allergic reactions
          b. Hyperemia
      4. Myopia
      5. Bloody tears
      6. Blepharoclonus
      7. Lacrimation

Systemic Side Effects:
  A. Local Ophthalmic Use or Exposure—Retrobulbar Injection
      1. Nausea
      2. Vomiting
      3. Heart block
      4. Incontinence
      5. Cardiac arrest

Clinical Significance: Topical ocular application of methacholine causes a number of ocular side effects; however, all are reversible and of minimal clinical importance. While miosis normally occurs with topical ocular 10% methacholine solutions, no effect is seen with 2.5% solutions, except in patients with Adie's pupil or familial dysautonomia.

References:
Crandall, D.C., and Leopold, I.H.: The influence of systemic drugs on tear constituents. Ophthalmology *86*:115, 1979.
Ellis, P.P.: Ocular Therapeutics and Pharmacology. 6th Ed., St. Louis, C.V. Mosby, 1981, p. 57.

Gilman, A.G., Goodman, L.S., and Gilman, A. (Eds.): The Pharmacological Basis of Therapeutics. 6th Ed., New York, Macmillan, 1980, pp. 91–96.

Havener, W.H.: Ocular Pharmacology. 5th Ed., St. Louis, C.V. Mosby, 1983, pp. 316–317.

Leopold, I.H.: The use and side effects of cholinergic agents in the management of intraocular pressure. *In* Drance, S.M., and Neufeld, A.H. (Eds.): Glaucoma: Applied Pharmacology in Medical Treatment. New York, Grune & Stratton, 1984, pp. 357–393.

Reynolds, J.E.F. (Ed.): Martindale: The Extra Pharmacopoeia. 29th Ed., London, Pharmaceutical Press, 1982, p. 1042.

Spaeth, G. L.: The effect of autonomic agents on the pupil and the intraocular pressure of eyes treated with dexamethasone. Br. J. Ophthalmol. *64*:426, 1980.

Generic Name: Oxprenolol

Proprietary Name: Apsolox (G.B.), Corbeton (Austral.), Lo-Tone (S. Afr.), Ornel (S. Afr.), Oxyprenix (G.B.), Slow-Pren (G.B.), Slow-Trasicor (Canad., G.B., Ire., S. Afr., Switz.), Trasicor (Austral., Canad., Fr., G.B., Germ., Ire., Ital., Neth., S. Afr., Span., Swed., Switz.)

Primary Use: This beta-adrenergic blocking agent is effective in the management of cardiac arrhythmias, angina pectoris, and hypertension.

Ocular Side Effects:
    A. Systemic Administration
        1. Decreased vision
        2. Eyelids or conjunctiva
            a. Allergic reactions
            b. Hyperemia
            c. Erythema
            d. Conjunctivitis—nonspecific
            e. Edema
            f. Hyperpigmentation
            g. Purpura
        3. Visual hallucinations
        4. Decreased lacrimation
        5. Nonspecific ocular irritation
            a. Photophobia
            b. Ocular pain
            c. Burning sensation
        6. Diplopia
        7. Myasthenic neuromuscular blocking effect
    B. Local Ophthalmic Use or Exposure
        1. Decreased intraocular pressure
        2. Miosis
        3. Punctate keratitis

Clinical Significance: This beta blocker only rarely causes ocular side effects, and these are usually transitory and insignificant. There was a suspicion initially that oxprenolol has the potential to cause an oculomucocutaneous syndrome similar to that seen with practolol. However, for as long as this drug has been on the market, there have been no such reported cases. There are cases of sudden onset keratoconjunctivitis sicca with marked conjunctival hyperemia after starting this medication. Transient diplopia has also been reported.

References:

Almog, Y., et al.: The effect on oral treatment with beta-blockers on the tear secretion. Metab. Pediatr. Syst. Ophthalmol. 6:343, 1982.

Bucci, M.G.: Topical administration of oxprenolol (beta blocking agent) in the therapy of the glaucoma. Preliminary note. Boll. Oculist. 54:235,1975.

Cocco, G., et al.: A review of the side effects of B-adrenoceptor blocking drugs on the skin, mucosae and connective tissue. Curr. Therap. Res. 31:362, 1982.

Holt, P.J.A., and Waddington, E.: Oculocutaneous reaction to oxprenolol. Br. Med. J. 2:539, 1975.

Kaeser, H.E.: Drug-induced myasthenic syndromes. Acta Neurol. Scand. 70(Suppl. 100):39, 1984.

Knapp, M.S., and Galloway, N.R.: Ocular reactions to beta-blockers. Br. Med. J. 2: 557, 1975.

Lewis, B.S., Setzen, M., and Kokoris, N.: Ocular reaction to oxprenolol. A case report. S. Afr. Med. J. 50:482, 1976.

Lyall, J.R.W.: Ocular reactions to beta-blockers. Br. Med. J. 2:747, 1975.

Petounis, A.D., and Akritopoulos, P.: Influence of topical and systemic beta-blockers on tear production. Int. Ophthalmol. 13:75–80, 1989.

Singer, L., and Knobel, B.: Influence of systemic administration beta-blockers on tear secretion. Ann. Ophthalmol. 16:728–729, 1984.

Steinert, J., and Pugh, C.R.: Two patients with schizophrenic-like psychosis after treatment with beta-adrenergic blockers. Br. Med. J. 1:790, 1979.

Weber, J.C.P.: Beta-adrenoreceptor antagonists and diplopia. Lancet 2:826, 1982.

Generic Name: Practolol

Proprietary Name: None

Primary Use: This beta-adrenergic blocking agent is effective in the management of angina pectoris, certain arrhythmias, and hypertension. It is also used as an adjunct to anesthesia and as a bronchodilator.

Ocular Side Effects:

A. Systemic Administration
1. Oculomucocutaneous syndrome—keratoconjunctivitis sicca
2. Nonspecific ocular irritation
   a. Lacrimation

    b. Photophobia
    c. Ocular pain
    d. Burning sensation
  3. Decreased lacrimation
  4. Decreased vision
  5. Conjunctiva
    a. Hyperemia
    b. Conjunctivitis—nonspecific
    c. Prominence of papillary tufts
    d. Areas of increased or decreased vascularity
    e. Scarring
    f. Keratinization
    g. Shrinkage—with obliteration of fornix
    h. Edema
    i. Pemphigoid lesion
  6. Cornea
    a. Dense yellow or white stromal opacities
    b. Loss of stroma
    c. Perforation
    d. Ulceration
  7. Eyelids
    a. Edema
    b. Erythema
    c. "Cafe au lait" pigmentation
    d. Lupoid syndrome
    e. Urticaria
    f. Exfoliative dermatitis
    g. Eczema
  8. Decreased tear lysozymes
  9. Myasthenic neuromuscular blocking effect
    a. Ptosis
    b. Diplopia
  10. Visual hallucinations
  11. Decreased intraocular pressure
B. Local Ophthalmic Use or Exposure
  1. Decreased intraocular pressure

Clinical Significance: Although this drug is used rarely and with major restrictions, it is included here, in part for significant historical reasons. Ocular side effects due to practolol occur in approximately 0.2% of patients. The severity of the practolol-induced ocular changes is directly proportional to the length of time the patient has been taking the drug. If at the first signs of ocular involvement the drug is discontinued, all the ocular changes are reversible. However, if it remains unrecognized, this may lead to severe irreversible ocular changes, including blindness. The most frequent adverse ocular reaction includes various degrees of keratoconjunctivitis sicca. This may progress to severe keratinization, scarring, and loss of conjunctival fornices. Sudden onset of corneal opacities with loss of stromal thickness leading to perforation has been seen. Adverse ocular reactions due to practolol may be unique since a serum intercellular antibody has been found in several patients. This antibody has also been found in the epithelium of eyes with practolol-induced disease. Possibly, this syndrome is due to an antibody that is a metabolite of practolol. While many of the signs and symptoms improve on withdrawal of the drug, reduction of tear secretion persists in most patients. The drug has been withdrawn from the market for general use but is still available in an injectable form for hospital use. To date, no clear-cut oculomucocutaneous syndrome has been seen with any other beta-blocking drug.

References:

Amos, H.E., Brigden, W.D., and McKerron, R.A.: Untoward effects associated with practolol: Demonstration of antibody binding to epithelial tissue. Br. Med. J. *1*:598, 1975.

Amos, H.E., Lake, B.G., and Artis, J.: Possible role of antibody specific for a practolol metabolite in the pathogenesis of oculomucocutaneous syndrome. Br. Med. J. *1*: 402, 1978.

Felix R.H., Ive, F.A., and Dahl, M.G.C.: Cutaneous and ocular reactions to practolol. Br. Med. J. *4*:321, 1974.

Hughes, R.O., and Zacharias, F.J.: Myasthenic syndrome during treatment with practolol. Br. Med. J. *1*:460, 1976.

Karlin, K.M., Zimmerman, T. J., and Nardin, G.: Beta blockers in ophthalmology. J. Toxicol. Cut. Ocular Toxicol. *1*:155, 1982.

Rahi, A.H.S., et al.: Pathology of practolol-induced ocular toxicity. Br. J. Ophthalmol. *60*:312, 1976.

Van Joost, T.H., Crone, R.A., and Overdijk, A.D.: Ocular cicatricial pemphigoid associated with practolol therapy. Br. J. Dermatol. *94*:447, 1976.

Wright, P., and Fraunfelder, F.T.: Practolol-induced oculomucocutaneous syndrome. *In* Leopold, I.H., and Burns, R.P. (Eds.): Symposium on Ocular Therapy. New York, John Wiley & Sons, Vol. IX, 1976, pp. 97–110.

Wright, P.: Untoward effects associated with practolol administration: Oculomucocutaneous syndrome. Br. Med. J. *1*:595, 1975

Generic Name: Propranolol

Proprietary Name: Angilol (G.B.), Antarol (Ire.), Apsolol (G.B.), Bedranol S.R. (G.B.), Beprane (Fr.), Berkolol (G.B., Ire.), Beta Prograne (G.B.), Beta-dur CR (G.B.), Beta-Tablinen (Germ.), Beta-Timelets (Germ.), Cardinol (Austral., G.B.), Cardispare (S. Afr.), Detensol (Canad.), Dociton (Germ.), Duranol (Ire.), Efektolol (Germ.), Elbrol (Germ.), Half-Betadur CR (G.B.), Half-Inderal (G.B., Ire.), **Inderal** (Austral., Canad., G.B., Ire., Ital., Neth., S. Afr., Swed., Switz.), Indobloc (Germ.), Intermigran (Germ.), Novopranol

(Canad.), Prodorol (S. Afr.), Propabloc (Germ.), Propal (Swed.), Propanix (G.B.), Prophylux (Germ.), Propranur (Germ.), Propra-ratiopharm (Germ.), Pur-Bloka (S. Afr.), Sloprolol (G.B.), Sumial (Span.), Tiperal (Ire.)

Primary Use: This beta-adrenergic blocking agent is effective in the management of angina pectoris, certain arrhythmias, hypertrophic subaortic stenosis, pheochromocytoma, and certain hypertensive states.

Ocular Side Effects:
  A. Systemic Administration
   1. Diplopia
   2. Decreased vision
   3. Eyelids or conjunctiva
       a. Allergic reactions
       b. Erythema
       c. Conjunctivitis—nonspecific
       d. Urticaria
       e. Purpura
       f. Lupoid syndrome
       g. Erythema multiforme
       h. Stevens-Johnson syndrome
       i. Exfoliative dermatitis
       j. Pemphigoid lesion
   4. Decreased intraocular pressure
   5. Visual hallucinations
   6. Decreased lacrimation
   7. Nonspecific ocular irritation
       a. Lacrimation
       b. Photophobia
       c. Ocular pain
   8. Decreased accommodation
   9. Exophthalmos—withdrawal states
   10. Myasthenic neuromuscular blocking effect
       a. Paralysis of extraocular muscles
       b. Ptosis
  B. Local Ophthalmic Use or Exposure
   1. Decreased corneal reflex
   2. Irritation
       a. Hyperemia
       b. Ocular pain
       c. Burning sensation
   3. Decreased intraocular pressure
   4. Miosis
   5. Local anesthetic effect

Clinical Significance: Adverse ocular side effects due to propranolol are usually insignificant and transient. As with all beta-adrenergic blocking agents, one needs to be aware of the possibility of sicca-like syndrome. There now seem to be enough cases in the literature and in the Registry to implicate this drug in causing a keratoconjunctivitis sicca-like syndrome. If, however, this does occur, it is a rare event. In the Registry's experience, one of the most bothersome side effects is transient diplopia. This may resolve even if the drug is continued. One possible case suggested that this agent had caused an inflammatory lymphoid process of the iris and ciliary body, which resolved without treatment when propranolol was discontinued. Topical ocular use has little clinical application, although it has been advocated for thyrotoxic lid retraction and glaucoma therapy. While propranolol is structurally similar to practolol, to date there has been no oculocutaneous syndrome associated with this agent.

References:
Almog, Y., et al.: The effect of oral treatment with beta-blockers on the tear secretion. Metab. Pediatr. Syst. Ophthalmol. 6:343, 1982.

Dollery, C.T., et al.: Eye symptoms in patients taking propranolol and other hypotensive agents. Br. J. Clin. Pharmacol. 4:295, 1977.

Draeger, J., and Winter, R.: Corneal sensitivity and intraocular pressure. In Krieglstein, G.K., and Leydhecker, W. (Eds.): Glaucoma Update II. New York, Springer-Verlag, 1983, pp. 63–67.

Felminger, R.: Visual hallucinations and illusions with propranolol. Br. Med. J. 1: 1182, 1978.

Gilbert, G.J.: An occurrence of complicated migraine during propranolol therapy. Headache 22:81, 1982.

Malm, L.: Propranolol as cause of watery nasal secretion. Lancet 1:1006, 1981.

Ohrstrom, A.: Oral beta-blockers in glaucoma. Glaucoma 5:102, 1983.

Ohrstrom, A., and Pandolfi, M.: Regulation of intraocular pressure and pupil size by β-blockers and epinephrine. Arch. Ophthalmol. 98:2182, 1980.

Pecori-Giraldi, J., et al.: Topical propranolol in glaucoma therapy and investigations on the mechanism of action. Glaucoma 6:31, 1984.

Ruocco, V., and Pisani, M.: Induced pemphigus. Arch. Dermatol. Res. 274:123, 1982.

Singer, L., Knobel, B., and Romem, M.: Influence of systemic administered beta-blockers on tear secretion. Ann. Ophthalmol. 16:728–729, 1984.

Weber, J.C.P.: Beta-adrenoreceptor anatagonists and diplopia. Lancet 2:826–827, 1982.

Yeomans, S.M., et al.: Ocular inflammatory pseudotumor associated with propranolol therapy. Ophthalmology 90:1422, 1983.

Generic Name: Quinidine

Proprietary Name: Biquin Durules (Canad.), **Cardioquin** (Canad., Neth.), Cardioquine (Fr., Span.), Chinteina (Ital.), **Duraquin**, Galactoquin (Germ.), Kiditard (G.B., Neth.), Kinidin (Austral., Ire., Swed.), Kinidin Duriles (Switz.), Kinidin Durules (G.B.), Kinidine (Neth.), Naticardina (Ital.), Neochinidin (Ital.), Optochinidin retard (Germ.), **Quinaglute** (Canad., Ital., S.

Afr.), **Quinalan**, Quinate (Canad.), Quinicardina (Span.), **Quinidex** (Austral., Canad.), Quinidoxin (Austral.), Quinidurule (Fr.), **Quinora**, Ritmocor (Ital.), Solfachinid (Ital.)

Primary Use: This isomer of quinine is effective in the treatment and prevention of atrial, nodal, and ventricular arrhythmias.

Ocular Side Effects:
A. Systemic Administration
1. Decreased vision, blurred vision
2. Problems with color vision—color vision defect, red-green defect
3. Mydriasis
4. Visual fields
   a. Scotomas
   b. Constriction
5. Photophobia
6. Diplopia
7. Night blindness
8. Eyelids or conjunctiva
   a. Allergic reactions
   b. Hyperpigmentation
   c. Photosensitivity
   d. Angioneurotic edema
   e. Urticaria
   f. Lupoid syndrome
   g. Exfoliative dermatitis
9. Corneal deposits
10. Keratoconjunctivitis sicca
11. Visual hallucinations
12. Subconjunctival or retinal hemorrhages secondary to drug-induced anemia
13. Optic neuritis
14. Myasthenic neuromuscular blocking effect
15. Anterior uveitis, granulomatous uveitis
16. Toxic amblyopia

Clinical Significance: Ocular side effects due to quinidine are rare, and most are transitory and reversible with discontinued use of the drug. Adverse ocular reactions are primarily dose-dependent and are cumulative. A presumably allergic reaction, including keratic precipitates, flare and cells, and Koeppe nodules, has been described secondary to quinidine.

References:
Birch, J., et al.: Acquired color vision defects. *In* Pokorny, J., et al. (Eds.): Congenital and Acquired Color Vision Defects. New York, Grune & Stratton, 1979, pp. 243–350.

Drugs that cause psychiatric symptoms. Med. Lett. Drugs Ther. 28:81, 1986.

Fisher, C.M.: Visual disturbances associated with quinidine and quinine. Neurology 31:1569, 1981.

Hustead, J.D.: Granulomatous Uveitis and Quinidine Hypersensitivity. Am. J. Ophthalmol. 112(4):461–462, 1991.

Kaeser, H.E.: Drug-induced myasthenic syndromes. Acta Neurol. Scand. 70(Suppl. 100):39, 1984.

Mahler, R., Sissons, W., and Watters, K.: Pigmentation induced by quinidine therapy. Arch. Dermatol. 122:1062, 1986.

Naschitz, J.E., and Yeshurun, D.: Quinidine-induced sicca syndrome. J. Toxicol. Clin. Toxicol. 20:367, 1983.

Spitzberg, D.H.: Acute anterior uveitis secondary to quinidine sensitivity. Arch. Ophthalmol. 97:1993, 1979.

Zaidman, G.W.: Quinidine keratopathy. Am. J. Ophthalmol. 97:247, 1984.

Class: Antihypertensive Agents

Generic Name: 1. Acebutolol; 2. Atenolol; 3. Labetolol; 4. Metoprolol; 5. Nadolol; 6. Pindolol

Proprietary Name: 1. Acecor (Ital.), Alol (Ital.), Monitan (Canad.), Neptal (Germ.), Prent (Germ., Ital, Neth., Switz.), **Sectral** (Canad., Fr., G.B., Ire., Ital., Neth., S. Afr., Span., Switz.); 2. Alinor (Swed.), Amolin (Ire.), Antipressan (G.B., Ire.), Atecor (Ire.), Atehexal (Germ.), Atendol (Germ.), Aténil (Switz.), Atenix (G.B.), Atenol (Ital.), Atenomel (Ire.), Aterol (S. Afr.), Blocotenol (Germ.), Blokium (Span.), Cardaxen (Switz.), Cuxanorm (Germ.), Dignobeta (Germ.), duratenol (Germ.), Juvental (Germ.), Neatenol (Span.), Noten (Austral.), Seles Beta (Ital.), Selinol (Swed.), Taraskon (Germ.), Ten-Bloka (S. Afr.), teno-basan (Germ.), **Tenormin** (Austral., Canad., G.B., Germ., Ire., Ital., Neth., S. Afr., Span., Swed., Switz.), Ténormine (Fr.), Tonoprotect (Germ.), Totamol (G.B.), Trantalol (Ire.), Uniloc (Swed.), Vasaten (G.B.); 3. Abetol (Ital.), Alfabetal (Ital.), Amipress (Ital.), Ipolab (Ital.), Labrocol (G.B.), Lolum (Ital.), Mitalolo (Ital.), **Normodyne**, Presolol (Austral.), Pressalolo (Ital.), **Trandate** (Austral., Canad., Fr., G.B., Germ., Ire., Ital., Neth., S. Afr., Span., Swed., Switz.); 4. Arbralene (G.B.), Beloc (Germ.), Beprolo (Ital.), Betaloc (Austral., Canad., G.B., Ire.), Loprésor (Switz.), Lopresor (Austral., Canad., G.B., Germ., Ire., Ital, Neth., S. Afr., Span.), Loprésor OROS (Switz.), Lopresor Oros (S. Afr.), **Lopressor** (Fr.), Mepranix (G.B.), Metohexal (Germ.), Metoproferm (Swed.), Metoros (G.B.), Novometoprol (Canad.), Prelis (Germ.), Selokeen (Neth.), Seloken (Fr., Ital., Span., Swed.); 5. Apo-Nadol (Canad.), **Corgard** (Canad., Fr., G.B., Ire., Ital., S. Afr., Span., Switz.), Solgol (Germ., Span.); 6. Apo-Pindol (Canad.), Barbloc (Austral.), Betapindol (Switz.), durapindol (Germ.), Glauco-Stullin (Germ.), Hexapindol (Swed.), Pectobloc (Germ.), Pinbetol (Germ.), Pindoptan (Germ.), Viskeen (Neth.), Viskén (Swed.), **Visken**

(Austral., Canad., Fr., G.B., Germ., Ire., Ital., S. Afr., Span.), Viskène (Switz.)

Primary Use: *Systemic*: These adrenergic blockers are used in the management of mild to severe hypertension, myocardial infarction, and chronic stable angina pectoris. *Ophthalmic*: These adrenergic blockers are used in the treatment of elevated intraocular pressure.

Ocular Side Effects:
A. Systemic Administration
    1. Decreased vision
    2. Visual hallucinations
    3. Decreased intraocular pressure
    4. Eyelids or conjunctiva
       a. Hyperemia (metoprolol)
       b. Erythema
       c. Blepharoconjunctivitis (metoprolol)
       d. Urticaria (labetalol, metoprolol)
       e. Purpura (metoprolol)
       f. Lupoid syndrome (acebutolol, labetalol)
       g. Eczema (metoprolol)
       h. Exacerbation psoriasis
    5. Nonspecific ocular irritation (labetalol, metoprolol)
       a. Photophobia
       b. Ocular pain
    6. Myasthenic neuromuscular blocking effect
       a. Paresis of extraocular muscles
       b. Ptosis
       c. Diplopia
    7. Decreased lacrimation
    8. Subconjunctival or retinal hemorrhages secondary to drug-induced anemia
B. Local Ophthalmic Use or Exposure
    1. Decreased intraocular pressure
    2. Irritation
       a. Lacrimation
       b. Burning sensation
    3. Keratitis
    4. Decreased corneal reflex
    5. Keratoconjunctivitis sicca

Systemic Side Effects:
A. Local Ophthalmic Use or Exposure
    1. Bradycardia
    2. Hypotension

Clinical Significance: Visual disturbances and vivid visual hallucinations are the most common ocular side effects seen with these drugs. Hallucinations appear with an increase in drug dosage and tend to disappear with reduction of drug dosage or withdrawal of the drug. Beta blockers may worsen myasthenia gravis, and occasional patients experience diplopia while taking these medications. Patients who exhibit an extraocular paresis may need to be evaluated for myasthenia. Not all the listed possible ocular side effects have been reported with each agent; however, in general, these drugs may decrease tear secretion, possibly enhance migraine ocular scotoma, and decrease ocular pressure. Topically, sicca symptoms, decreased tear film break-up times, corneal anesthesia, and ocular irritation may be observed. Systemic side effects from these topical ophthalmic beta blockers appear to be minimal; measurements of plasma concentrations of these ocularly applied drugs were below those levels known to induce minimal systemic beta-blockade. Regardless, one must be aware that some of these agents have been blamed for systemic beta blocker side effects after topical ocular application.

References:
Almog, Y., et al.: The effect of oral treatment with beta-blockers on the tear secretion. Metab. Pediatr. Syst. Ophthalmol. *6*:343–345, 1982.

Teicher, A., Rosenthall, T., and Kissin, E.: Labetalol-induced toxic myopathy. Br. Med. J. *282(6)*:1824–1825, 1981.

Cervantes, R., Hernandez, H.H., and Frati, A.: Pulmonary and heart rate changes associated with nonselective beta-blocker glaucoma therapy. J. Toxicol. Cut. Ocul. Toxicol. *5*:185–193, 1986.

Cocco, G., et al.: A review of the effects of p-adrenoceptor blocking drugs on the skin, mucosae and connective tissue. Curr. Ther. Res. *31*:362,1982.

Kaul, S., et al.: Nadolol and papilledema. Ann. Intern. Med. *97*:454, 1982.

Kumar, K.L., and Cooney, T.G.: Visual symptoms after atenolol therapy for migraine. Ann. Intern. Med. *112(1)*:712–713, 1990.

Nielsen, P.C., et al.: Metaprolol eyedrops 3%, a short-term comparison with pilocarpine and a five-month follow-up study. Acta Ophthalmol. *60*:347, 1982.

Scott, D.: Another beta-blocker causing eye symptoms? Br. Med. J. *2*:1221, 1977.

Weber, J.C.P.: Beta-adrenoreceptor antagonists and diplopia. Lancet *2*:826, 1982.

Generic Name: 1. Alkavervir; 2. Cryptenamine; 3. Protoveratrines A and B; 4. Veratrum Viride Alkaloids

Proprietary Name: None

Primary Use: These veratrum alkaloids are used in the management of mild to moderate hypertension and various forms of renal dysfunction.

Ocular Side Effects:
    A. Systemic Administration
        1. Decreased vision

    2. Mydriasis—may precipitate narrow-angle glaucoma
    3. Extraocular myotonia

Clinical Significance: Few ocular side effects have been reported for these drugs. All adverse ocular effects are reversible and rarely of clinical significance. However, in some glaucoma patients a decrease in blood pressure may cause progression of optic nerve damage.

References:
Beasley, J., and Robinson, K.: Intolerance to "verloid." Br. Med. J. *1*:316, 1954.
Brown, J.Q.: Antihypertensive drugs and danger to vision. JAMA *237*:118, 1977.
Bullock, J .D.: Antihypertensive drugs and danger to vision. JAMA *237*:2186, 1977.
Heilmann, K.: Glaukom und Hypertonie. MMW *116*:1821, 1974.
Kolb, E.J., and Korein, J.: Neuromuscular toxicity of veratrum alkaloids. Neurology *11*:159, 1961

Generic Name: 1. Alseroxylon; 2. Deserpidine; 3. Rauwolfia Serpentina; 4. Rescinnamine; 5. Reserpine; 6. Syrosingopine

Proprietary Name: 3. **Raudixin** (Austral.), Rivadescin (Germ.); 4. **Moderil**; 5. **Sandril**, Serpasil (Canad., Ital.), Serpasol (Span.); 6. Neoreserpan (Ital.)

Primary Use: These rauwolfia alkaloids are used in the management of hypertension and agitated psychotic states.

Ocular Side Effects:
    A. Systemic Administration
        1. Conjunctival hyperemia
        2. Horner's syndrome
            a. Miosis
            b. Ptosis
            c. Increased sensitivity to topical ocular epinephrine preparations
        3. Nonspecific ocular irritation
            a. Lacrimation
            b. Hyperemia
        4. Extraocular muscles
            a. Oculogyric crises
            b. Decreased spontaneous movements
            c. Abnormal conjugate deviations
            d. Jerky pursuit movements
        5. Decreased vision
        6. Retinal hemorrhages
        7. Decreased intraocular pressure
        8. Mydriasis—may precipitate narrow-angle glaucoma

9. Problems with color vision
   a. Color vision defect
   b. Objects have yellow tinge
10. Eyelids or conjunctiva—lupoid syndrome

Clinical Significance: Most of the preceding ocular side effects have been primarily due to reserpine instead of the other rauwolfia alkaloids. Ocular conjunctival hyperemia is not uncommon with reserpine but of no basic importance. Ocular side effects are otherwise rare, and nearly all are reversible.

References:

Alarcón-Segovia, D.: Drug-induced antinuclear antibodies and lupus syndromes. Drugs *12*:69, 1976.

Crandall, D.C., and Leopold, I.H.: The influence of systemic drugs on tear constituents. Ophthalmology *86*:115, 1979.

Freedman, D.X., and Benton, A.J.: Persisting effects of reserpine in man. N. Engl. J. Med. *264*:529, 1961.

Raymond, L.F.: Ocular pathology in reserpine sensitivity: Report of two cases. J. Med. Soc. N.J. *60*:417, 1963.

Spaeth, G.L., Nelson, L.B., and Beaudoin, A.R.: Ocular teratology. *In* Jakobiec, F.A. (Ed.): Ocular Anatomy, Embryology and Teratology. Philadelphia, J.B. Lippincott, 1982, pp. 955–975.

Generic Name: 1. Captopril; 2. Enalapril

Proprietary Name: 1. Acepress (Ital.), Acepril (G.B.), Alopresin (Span.), **Capoten** (Austral., Canad., G.B., Ire., Ital., Neth., S. Afr., Span., Swed.), Captolane (Fr.), Cesplon (Span.), cor tensobon (Germ.), Dilabar (Span.), Garranil (Span.), Lopirin (Germ., Switz.), Lopril (Fr.), Tensobon (Germ., Switz.), Tensoprel (Span.); 2. Acetensil (Span.), Amprace (Austral.), Baripril (Span.), Bitensil (Span.), Clipto (Span.), Controlvas (Span.), Converten (Ital.), Crinoren (Span.), Dabonal (Span.), Ditensor (Span.), Enapren (Ital.), Hipoartel (Span.), Innovace (G.B.), Nacor (Span.), Naprilene (Ital., Span.), Neotensin (Span.), Pres (Germ.), Pressitan (Span.), Presyndral (Span.), Renitec (Austral., Fr., Neth., S. Afr., Span., Swed.), Reniten (Switz.), **Vasotec** (Canad.), Xanef (Germ.)

Primary Use: These angiotensin converting enzyme inhibitors are used in the management of hypertension.

Ocular Side Effects:

A. Systemic Administration
   1. Decreased vision
   2. Eyelids or conjunctiva

    a. Erythema
    b. Blepharoconjunctivitis
    c. Edema
    d. Brown discoloration
    e. Photosensitivity
    f. Angioneurotic edema
    g. Urticaria
    h. Lupoid syndrome
    i. Erythema multiforme
    j. Stevens-Johnson syndrome
    k. Exfoliative dermatitis
    l. Pemphigoid lesion
    m. Eczema
3. Subconjunctival or retinal hemorrhages secondary to drug-induced anemia
4. Visual hallucinations

Clinical Significance: Ocular side effects due to these drugs are rare and seldom of clinical significance. All adverse ocular reactions are reversible with discontinued drug use. Enalapril has been well documented to cause angioneurotic edema. This may only occur around the eyes or may involve a well-demarcated erythema with nonpitting edema of subcutaneous tissue mainly of the head and neck. This usually occurs within 1 to 3 weeks after starting the drug but has occurred as late as 3 years. Necrotizing blepharitis was the first clinical sign of drug-induced agranulocytosis secondary to captopril in one patient.

References:
Ahmad, S.: Enalapril and reversible alopecia. Arch. Intern. Med. *151*:404, 1991.

Gianos, M.E., et al.: Enalapril induced angioedema. Am. J. Emerg. Med. *8*:124–126, 1990.

Gillman, M.A., and Sandyk, R.: Reversal of captopril-induced psychosis with naloxone. Am. J. Psychiatry *142*:270, 1985.

Gonnering, R.S., and Hirsch, S.R.: Delayed drug-induced periorbital angioedema. Am. J. Ophthalmol. *110(5)*:566–568, 1990.

Goodfield, M.J., and Millard, L.G.: Severe cutaneous reactions to captopril. Br. Med. J. *290*:1111, 1985.

Kubo, S.H., and Cody, R.J.: Enalapril, a rash, and captopril. Ann. Intern. Med. *100*: 616, 1984.

Pennell, D.J., et al.: Fatal Stevens-Johnson syndrome in a patient on captopril and allopurinal. Lancet *1*:463, 1984.

Suarez, M., et al.: Angioneurotic edema, agranulocytosis and fatal septicemia following captopril therapy. Am. J. Med. *81*:336, 1986.

Wizemann, A.: Nekrotisierende Blepharitis nach Captopril-induzierter Agranulozytose. Klin. Monatsbl. Augenheilkd. *182*:82, 1983

Generic Name: Clonidine

Proprietary Name: *Systemic*: **Catapres** (Austral., Canad., G.B., S. Afr.), Catapresan (Germ., Ital., Neth., Span., Swed., Switz.), Catapressan (Fr.), **Catapres-TTS**, Clonistada (Germ.), Dixarit (Austral., Canad., G.B., Germ., Neth., S. Afr.), Ipotensium (Ital.), Isoglaucon (Germ.), Ital., Span.), Tenso-Timelets (Germ.) *Ophthalmic*: Isoglaucon (Germ., Ital., Span.), **Iopidine**

Primary Use: *Systemic*: This alpha-adrenergic agonist is used in the management of hypertension. *Ophthalmic*: Topical ocular clonidine has been used investigationally to reduce intraocular pressure.

Ocular Side Effects:
    A. Systemic Administration
        1. Decreased vision
        2. Decreased intraocular pressure
        3. Eyelids or conjunctiva
            a. Angioneurotic edema
            b. Urticaria
        4. Nonspecific ocular irritation—burning sensation
        5. Visual hallucinations
        6. Pupils
            a. Miosis—toxic states
            b. Mydriasis—toxic states
            c. Absence of reaction to light—toxic states
        7. Decreased lacrimation
        8. Abnormal EOG
    B. Local Ophthalmic Use or Exposure
        1. Decreased intraocular pressure
        2. Eyelids or conjunctiva
            a. Angioneurotic edema
            b. Urticaria
        3. Miosis

Systemic Side Effects:
    A. Local Ophthalmic Use or Exposure
        1. Hypotension

Clinical Significance: Ocular side effects associated with clonidine have been inconsequential and ceased after discontinuation of the drug. While there is a question whether glaucoma patients exposed to systemic clonidine experience progression of visual field defects resulting from decreased systolic and diastolic blood pressure, there are no data to support this. Systemic clonidine has a minimal effect on pupillary changes, except in toxic dosages.

Although miosis is the most commonly reported ocular symptom in clonidine overdose, mydriasis may occasionally be a clinical feature. Clonidine-induced visual hallucinations may resolve with continued drug usage. Since systemic clonidine has been reported to cause vulval pemphigoid, one should be alert; but to date, there are no data as to drug-related ocular cicatricial pemphigoid. Topical ocular clonidine has been found to reduce intraocular pressure up to 30% while reducing blood pressure 10%. The eyedrops are well tolerated and produce miosis in the treated and contralateral eye. Local ophthalmic use of clonidine reduces ophthalmic arterial and episcleral venous pressure when concentrations greater than 0.125% are administered.

References:

Banner, W., Jr., Lund, M.E., and Clawson, L.: Failure of naloxone to reverse clonidine toxic effect. Am. J. Dis. Child. *137*:1170, 1983.

Gaasterland, D.E.: Efficacy in glaucoma treatment—The potential of marijuana. Ann. Ophthalmol. *12*:448, 1980.

Hodapp, E., et al.: The effect of topical clonidine on intraocular pressure. Arch. Ophthalmol. *99*:1208, 1981.

Kaskel, D., Becker, H., and Rudolf, H.: Early effects of clonidine, epinephrine, and pilocarpine on the intraocular pressure and the episcleral venous pressure in normal volunteers. Graefes Arch. Clin. Exp. Ophthalmol. *213*:251, 1980.

Krieglstein, G.K.: The uses and side effects of adrenergic drugs in the management of intraocular pressure. *In* Drance, S.M., and Neufeld, A.H. (Eds.): Glaucoma: Applied Pharmacology in Medical Treatment. New York, Grune & Stratton, 1984, pp. 255–276.

Krieglstein, G.K., Langham, M.E., and Leydhecker, W.: The peripheral and central neural actions of clonidine in normal and glaucomatous eyes. Invest. Ophthalmol. Vis. Sci. *17*:149, 1978.

Lee, D.A., Topper, J.E., and Brubaker, R.F.: Effect of clonidine on aqueous humor flow in normal human eyes. Exp Eye Res. *38*:239, 1984.

Mathew, P.M., Addy, D.P., and Wright, N.: Clonidine overdose in children. Clin. Toxicol. *18*:169, 1981.

Petursson, G., Cole, R., and Hanna, C.: Treatment of glaucoma using minidrops of clonidine. Arch. Ophthalmol. *102*:1180, 1984.

Turacli, M.E.: The clonidine side effect in the human eye. Ann. Ophthalmol. *6*:699, 1974.

Van Joost, T.H., Faber, W.R., and Manuel, H.R.: Drug-induced anogenital pemphigoid. Br. J. Dermatol. *102*:715, 1980

Generic Name: Diazoxide

Proprietary Name: Eudemine (G.B., Ire.) **Hyperstat** (Austral., Canad., Fr., Ital., Neth., S. Afr., Span., Swed., Switz.), Hypertonalum (Germ.), Proglicem (Fr., Germ., Ital., Neth., Switz.), **Proglycem** (Canad.)

Primary Use: This nondiuretic benzothiadiazine derivative is used in the emergency treatment of malignant hypertension.

Ocular Side Effects:
A. Systemic Administration
1. Lacrimation
2. Eyelids or conjunctiva
   a. Allergic reactions
   b. Erythema
3. Decreased vision
4. Oculogyric crises
5. Hypertrichosis
6. Ring scotomas
7. Diplopia
8. Subconjunctival or retinal hemorrhages secondary to drug-induced anemia

Clinical Significance: Ocular side effects due to diazoxide are uncommon except for increased lacrimation, which occurs in up to 20% of patients taking this agent. In some instances, the lacrimation continued long after the diazoxide was discontinued. The cause of this unusual phenomenon is unknown. Cove, et al. reported blindness occurring secondary to a rapid decrease of malignant hypertension, as is seen with other potent antihypertensive agents.

References:
Cove, D.H., et al.: Blindness after treatment for malignant hypertension. Br. Med. J. 2:245–246, 1979.
Crandall, D.C., and Leopold, I.H.: The influence of systemic drugs on tear constituents. Ophthalmology 86:115, 1979.
Drug Evaluations. 6th Ed., Chicago, American Medical Association, 1986, pp. 533–534.
Fenton, D.A.: Hypertrichosis. Semin. Dermatol. 4:58, 1985.
McEvoy, G.K. (Ed.): American Hospital Formulary Service Drug Information 87. Bethesda, American Society of Hospital Pharmacists, 1987, pp. 809–812.
Neary, D., Thurston, H., and Pohl, J.E.F.: Development of extrapyramidal symptoms in hypertensive patients treated with diazoxide. Br. Med. J. 3:474, 1973.
Reynolds, J.E.F. (Ed.): Martindale: The Extra Pharmacopoeia. 28th Ed., London, Pharmaceutical Press, 1982, pp. 142–144.
Thomasen, A., et al.: Clinical observations on an antihypertensive chlorothiazide analogue devoid of a diuretic activity. Can. Med. Assoc. J. 87:1306, 1962

Generic Name: Furosemide. *See under Class: Diuretics.*

Generic Name: Guanethidine

Proprietary Name: *Systemic*: Isméline (Fr., Switz.), **Ismelin** (Canad., G.B., Ire., Neth., S. Afr.) *Ophthalmic*: Isméline (Fr.), Ismelin (G.B., Ire., Switz.), Visutensil (Ital.)

Primary Use: *Systemic*: This adrenergic blocker is effective in the treatment of moderate to severe hypertension. *Ophthalmic*: This topical adrenergic blocker is used in the management of open-angle glaucoma and lid retraction due to thyroid disorders.

Ocular Side Effects:
- A. Systemic Administration
    1. Decreased vision
    2. Nonspecific ocular irritation
        a. Hyperemia
        b. Photophobia
        c. Edema
    3. Horner's syndrome
        a. Miosis
        b. Ptosis
    4. Diplopia
    5. Decreased intraocular pressure
    6. Accommodative spasm
    7. Flashing lights
    8. Subconjunctival or retinal hemorrhages secondary to drug-induced anemia
- B. Local Ophthalmic Use or Exposure
    1. Irritation
        a. Hyperemia
        b. Photophobia
        c. Ocular pain
        d. Edema
        e. Burning sensation
    2. Horner's syndrome
        a. Miosis
        b. Ptosis
        c. Enophthalmos
    3. Decreased intraocular pressure
    4. Mydriasis
    5. Punctate keratitis
    6. Eyelids
        a. Contact dermatitis

Clinical Significance: Topical ocular application or systemic administration of guanethidine frequently causes ocular side effects. These adverse ocular reactions are reversible and transitory with discontinued use of the drug. Topical ocular administration of guanethidine produces a decreased intraocular pressure that is poorly maintained. Conjunctival epidermalization can be associated with guanethidine eyedrops, as with all chronic ocular medications.

References:
Cant, J.S., and Lewis, D.R.H.: Unwanted pharmacological effects of local guanethidine in the treatment of dysthyroid upper lid retraction. Br. J. Ophthalmol. *53*:239–245, 1969.

Davidson, S.I.: Reports of ocular adverse reactions. Trans. Ophthalmol. Soc. U.K. *93*: 495, 1973.

Gloster, J.: Guanethidine and glaucoma. Trans. Ophthalmol. Soc. U.K. *94*:573, 1974.

Hoyng, Ph.F.J., and Dake, C.L.: The aqueous humor dynamics and biphasic response to intraocular pressure induced by guanethidine and adrenaline in the glaucomatous eye. Graefes Arch. Clin. Exp. Ophthalmol. *214*:263, 1980.

Jones, D.E.P., Norton, D.A., and Davies, D.J.G.: Control of glaucoma by reduced dosage guanethidine-adrenaline formulation. Br. J. Ophthalmol. *63*:813, 1979.

Krieglstein, G.K.: The uses and side effects of adrenergic drugs in the management of intraocular pressure. *In* Drance, S.M., and Neufeld, A.H. (Eds.): Glaucoma: Applied Pharmacology in Medical Treatment. New York, Grune & Stratton, 1984, pp. 255–276.

McEvoy, G.K. (Ed.): American Hospital Formulary Service Drug Information 87. Bethesda, American Society of Hospital Pharmacists, 1987, pp. 826–828.

Wright, P.: Squamous metaplasia or epidermalization of the conjunctiva as an adverse reaction to topical medication. Trans. Ophthalmol. Soc. U.K. *99*:244, 1979

Generic Name: Hexamethonium

Proprietary Name: None

Primary Use: This ganglionic blocking agent is used primarily in emergency hypertensive crises.

Ocular Side Effects:
  A. Systemic Administration
    1. Decreased vision
    2. Mydriasis—may precipitate narrow-angle glaucoma
    3. Paralysis of accommodation
    4. Macular edema
    5. Decreased lacrimation
    6. Decreased intraocular pressure
    7. Visual fields
      a. Constriction
      b. Hemianopsia
    8. Conjunctival edema
    9. Problems with color vision—color vision defect, red-green defect
    10. Retinal vasodilatation
    11. Optic atrophy
    12. Toxic amblyopia

Clinical Significance: Hexamethonium frequently causes adverse ocular reactions, but the drug itself is rarely used except in severe end-stage hypertension or in a hypertensive crisis. While decreased vision, mydriasis, and paralysis of accommodation are common and reversible, most other ocular side effects are infrequent. Many of the drug-induced ocular side effects can be explained by rapid changes in blood pressure. Articles by Bruce as well as by Goldsmith and Hewer have described major visual losses, including constricted visual fields and bilateral optic atrophy. These may well be drug related, possibly on a vascular or hypotensive basis; however, these events are extremely rare.

References:

Barnett, A.J.: Ocular effects of methonium compounds. Br. J. Ophthalmol. *36*:593, 1952.

Birch, J., et al.: Acquired color vision defects. *In* Pokorny, J., et al. (Eds.): Congenital and Acquired Color Vision Defects. New York, Grune & Stratton, 1979, pp. 243–350.

Bruce, G.M.: Permanent bilateral blindness following use of hexamethonium chloride. Arch. Ophthalmol. *54*:422, 1955.

Cameron, A.J., and Burn, R.A.: Hexamethonium and glaucoma. Br. J. Ophthalmol. *36*:482, 1952.

Goldsmith, A.J., and Hewer, A.J.: Unilateral amaurosis with partial recovery after using hexamethonium iodide. Br. Med. J. 2:759, 1952.

Walsh, F.B., and Hoyt, W.F.: Clinical Neuro-Ophthalmology. 3rd Ed., Baltimore, Williams & Wilkins, Vol. III, 1969, pp. 2667–2668.

Generic Name: Hydralazine

Proprietary Name: Alphapress (Austral.), Apresolin (Ital.,Swed.), **Apresoline** (Austral., Canad., G.B., Ire., Neth.), Hydrapres (Span.), Hyperex (S. Afr.), Hyperphen (S. Afr.), Ipolina (Ital.), Novohylazin (Canad.), Rolazine (S. Afr.), Slow-Aprésoline (Switz.), Supres (Austral.)

Primary Use: This phthalazine derivative is effective in the management of essential or malignant hypertension, hypertensive complications of pregnancy, and hypertension associated with acute glomerulonephritis.

Ocular Side Effects:
    A. Systemic Administration
        1. Decreased vision
        2. Nonspecific ocular irritation
            a. Lacrimation
            b. Photophobia
            c. Ocular pain
        3. Eyelids or conjunctiva

  a. Allergic reactions
  b. Erythema
  c. Conjunctivitis—nonspecific
  d. Edema
  e. Urticaria
  f. Lupoid syndrome
 4. Periorbital edema
 5. Colored flashing lights
 6. Subconjunctival or retinal hemorrhages secondary to drug-induced anemia

Clinical Significance: All ocular side effects due to hydralazine are reversible, transient, and seldom of clinical significance. A syndrome resembling systemic lupus erythematosus associated with hydralazine therapy is generally considered a benign condition that resolves without permanent sequelae. Several patients with hydralazine-induced lupus syndrome with ocular manifestations, including retinal vasculitis, episcleritis, and exophthalmos, have been described.

References:

Crandall, D.C., and Leopold, I.H.: The influence of systemic drugs on tear constituents. Ophthalmology *86*:115, 1979.

Doherty, M., Maddison, P.J., and Grey, R.H.B.: Hydralazine-induced lupus syndrome with eye disease. Br. Med. J. *290*:675, 1985.

Johansson, M., and Manhem, P.: SLE-syndrome with exophthalmus after treatment with hydralazin. Lakartidningen *72*:153, 1975.

Mansilla-Tinoco, R., et al.: Hydralazine, antinuclear antibodies, and the lupus syndrome. Br. Med. J. *284*:936, 1982.

Peacock, A., and Weatherall, D.: Hydralazine-induced necrotising vasculitis. Br. Med. J. *282*:1121, 1981.

Reynolds, J.E.F. (Ed.): Martindale: The Extra Pharmacopoeia. 28th Ed., London, Pharmaceutical Press, 1982, pp. 148–150.

Walsh, F.B., and Hoyt, W.F.: Clinical Neuro-Ophthalmology. 3rd Ed., Baltimore, Williams & Wilkins, Vol. III, 1969, p. 2668.

Generic Name: 1. Mecamylamine; 2. Pentolinium; 3. Tetraethylammonium; 4. Trimethaphan (Trimetaphan)

Proprietary Name: 1. **Inversine**; 3. Available in multi-ingredient preparations; 4. **Arfonad** (Canad., G.B., Ire., Ital., Span.)

Primary Use: These ganglionic blocking agents are used in the management of moderate to severe hypertension and to produce controlled hypotension for the reduction of surgical hemorrhage.

Ocular Side Effects:
  A. Systemic Administration
    1. Decreased vision
    2. Mydriasis—may precipitate narrow-angle glaucoma
    3. Paralysis of accommodation
    4. Conjunctival edema
    5. Decreased intraocular pressure
    6. Myasthenic neuromuscular blocking effect
       (tetraethylammonium, trimethaphan)
       a. Ptosis
    7. Colored flashing lights (mecamylamine)
    8. Eyelids—urticaria (trimethaphan)

Clinical Significance: Although ocular side effects due to the ganglionic blocking agents are common, they are transitory, reversible, and seldom of major significance. Since these drugs can cause profound hypotensive episodes, visual complaints probably occur on a cerebral basis. Mydriasis and cycloplegic effects are probably due to the parasympatholytic effect of these drugs. Side effects tend to become less pronounced as administration of the drug is continued.

References:

Argov, Z., and Mastaglia, F.L.: Disorders of neuromuscular transmission caused by drugs. N. Engl. J. Med. *301*:409, 1979.

Dias, P.L.R., Andrew, D.S., and Romanes, G.J.: Effect on the intraocular pressure of hypotensive anaesthesia with intravenous trimetaphan. Br. J. Ophthalmol. *66*:721, 1982.

Drucker, A.P., Sadove, M.S., and Unna, K.: Ocular manifestations of intravenous tetraethylammonium chloride in man. Am. J. Ophthalmol. *33*:1564, 1950.

Kaeser, H.E.: Drug-induced myasthenic syndromes. Acta Neurol. Scand. *70*(Suppl. 100):39, 1984.

McEvoy, G.K. (Ed.): American Hospital Formulary Service Drug Information 87. Bethesda, American Society of Hospital Pharmacists, 1987, pp. 839–840, 863–865.

Walsh, F.B., and Hoyt, W.F.: Clinical Neuro-Ophthalmology. 3rd Ed., Baltimore, Williams & Wilkins, Vol. 111, 1969, p. 2668.

Generic Name: Methyldopa

Proprietary Name: Aldomet (Austral., Canad., Fr., G.B., Ital., Neth., S. Afr., Span., Swed., Switz.), Arcanadopa (S. Afr.), Dopagen (Ire.), Dopamet (Canad., G.B., Ire., Swed., Switz.), Elanpres (Ire.), Elanpress (Ital.), Equibar (Fr.), Hydopa (Austral.), Hy-Po-Tone (S. Afr.), Medomet (G.B.), Medopren (Ital.), Meldopa (Ire.), Metalpha (G.B.), Normopress (S. Afr.), Novomedopa (Canad.), Nu-Medopa (Canac.), Presinol (Germ., Ital.), Sembrina (Germ., Neth.), Sinepress (S. Afr.)

Primary Use: This adrenergic blocker is effective in the management of acute or severe hypertension.

Ocular Side Effects:
A. Systemic Administration
1. Decreased vision
2. Decreased intraocular pressure—minimal
3. Eyelids or conjunctiva
   a. Allergic reactions
   b. Hyperemia
   c. Conjunctivitis—nonspecific
   d. Edema
   e. Urticaria
   f. Lupoid syndrome
   g. Eczema
4. Subconjunctival or retinal hemorrhages secondary to drug-induced anemia
5. Paralysis of extraocular muscles
6. Keratoconjunctivitis sicca
7. Visual hallucinations
8. Photophobia

Clinical Significance: Adverse ocular side effects due to methyldopa are rare and insignificant. Lowering of intraocular pressure due to this drug has been documented; however, this decrease is only minimal. There have been a number of reports associating this drug with the onset of keratoconjunctivitis sicca. Although a cause-and-effect relationship is difficult to prove, some cases of keratoconjunctivitis sicca improved upon discontinuation of the drug.

References:
Alarcón-Segovia, D.: Drug-induced antinuclear antibodies and lupus syndromes. Drugs *12*:69, 1976.

Chan, W.: Less common side effects of methyldopa. Med. J. Aust. *2*:14, 1977.

Cove, D.H., et al.: Blindness after treatment for malignant hypertension. Br. Med. J. *2*:245, 1979.

Davidson, S.I.: Reports of ocular adverse reactions. Trans. Ophthalmol. Soc. U.K. *93*: 495, 1973.

Drug Evaluations. 6th Ed., Chicago, American Medical Association, 1986, pp. 517–518.

Endo, M., Hirai, K., and Ohara, M.: Paranoid-hallucinatory state induced in a depressive patient by methyldopa: A case report. Psychoneuroendocrinology *3*:211, 1978.

McEvoy, G.K. (Ed.): American Hospital Formulary Service Drug Information 87. Bethesda, American Society of Hospital Pharmacists, 1987, pp. 840–844.

Okun, R., et al.: Long-term effectiveness of methyldopa in hypertension. Calif. Med. *104*:46, 1966.

Peczon, J.D.: Effect of methyldopa on intraocular pressure in human eyes. Am. J. Ophthalmol. *60*:82, 1965.

Suda, K., et al.: On the hypotensive effect of Aldomet. J. Clin. Ophthalmol. *18*:191, 1964.

Tassinari, J.: Methyldopa-related convergence insufficiency. J. Am. Optom. Assoc. *60*: 311–314, 1989

Generic Name: Minoxidil

Proprietary Name: Alopexil (Fr.), Alostil (Fr.),Crecisan (Span.), Kapodin (Span.), **Loniten** (Austral., Canad., G.B., Ire., Ital., S. Afr., Span., Switz.), Lonnoten (Neth.), Lonolox (Germ.), Lonoten (Fr.), **Minodyl**, Minotricon (Ital.), Minoximen (Ital.), Neocapil (Switz.), Néoxidil (Fr.), Normoxidil (Ital.), Pierminox (Ital.), Pilovital (Span.), Piloxil (Fr.), Prexidil (Ital.), Regaine (Fr., G.B., Ire., Ital., Neth., S. Afr., Span., Swed., Switz.), Riteban (Span.), **Rogaine** (Canad.), Tricoxidil (Ital.)

Primary Use: This vasodilator is used in the treatment of severe hypertension resistant to other drugs and to treat alopecia.

Ocular Side Effects:
  A. Systemic Administration
    1. Eyelids or conjunctiva
      a. Hyperemia
      b. Erythema
      c. Conjunctivitis—nonspecific
      d. Hyperpigmentation
      e. Stevens-Johnson syndrome
      f. Discoloration of eyelashes or eyebrows
      g. Hypertrichosis
    2. Decreased vision
    3. Optic neuritis
  B. Topical Application
    1. Keratitis
    2. Decreased vision
    3. Dry skin
    4. Amaurosis

Clinical Significance: Minoxidil can cause an increase in the growth of fine hair that is darker and longer in 80% of the patients taking this drug. This usually occurred in 3 to 6 weeks after exposure, and often occurred first between the eyebrows and between the eyebrows and the forehead hairline. This side effect regresses and disappears 1 to 6 months after stopping the drug. There are more than 60 reports in the Registry of a nonspecific conjunctivitis with or without ocular pain associated with the oral use of this agent. Gombos reports a case of bilateral optic neuritis associated with minoxidil usage. The topical minoxidil in solution to treat alopecia can cause significant ocular irritation with inadvertent ocular exposure. These effects are transitory.

References:

Degreef H., et al.: Allergic contact dermatitis to minoxidil. Contact Dermatitis *13*:194, 1985.

DiSantis, D.J., and Flanagan, J.: Minoxidil-induced Stevens-Johnson syndrome. Arch. Intern. Med. *141*:1515, 1981.

Gombos, G.M.: Bilateral optic neuritis following minoxidil administration. Ann. Ophthalmol. *15*:259, 1983.

Mitchell, H.C., and Pettinger, W.A.: Long-term treatment of refractory hypertensive patients with minoxidil. JAMA *239*:2131, 1978.

Traub, Y.M., et al.: Treatment of severe hypertension with minoxidil. Isr. J. Med. Sci. *11*:991, 1975.

Weinberg, R.S., Haynes, J.H., and Ferry, A.P.: Toxic keratitis following topical minoxidil use for baldness. *In* Cavanagh, H.D.: The Cornea: Transactions of the world congress on cornea III. New York, Raven Press, 1988, p. 141–145.

Generic Name: Pargyline

Proprietary Name: None

Primary Use: This nonhydrazine monoamine oxidase inhibitor is used in the treatment of moderate to severe hypertension.

Ocular Side Effects:

    A. Systemic Administration
        1. Pupils—toxic states
          a. Mydriasis
          b. Decreased reaction to light
        2. Decreased accommodation
        3. Visual hallucinations
        4. Hyperactive eye movements—toxic states
        5. Problems with color vision—color vision defect, red-green defect

Clinical Significance: Significant ocular side effects due to pargyline are rare, and those reported are primarily in overdose situations. Optic nerve damage has not been found as a side effect of this drug, although it has been seen with other monoamine oxidase inhibitors. A well-documented study has reported a significant decrease in intraocular pressure in patients with chronic simple or absolute glaucoma following application of topical ocular pargyline.

References:

Grant, W. M.: Toxicology of the Eye. 3rd Ed., Springfield, Charles C Thomas, 1986, p. 701.

Lipkin, D., and Kushnick, T.: Pargyline hydrochloride poisoning in a child. JAMA *201*:135, 1967.

Mehra, K.S., Roy, P.N., and Singh, K.: Pargyline drops in glaucoma. Arch. Ophthalmol. *92*:453, 1974.

Sutnick, A.I., et al.: Psychotic reactions during therapy with pargyline. JAMA *188*: 610, 1964.

Walsh, F.B., and Hoyt, W.F.: Clinical Neuro-Ophthalmology. 3rd Ed., Baltimore, Williams & Wilkins, Vol. III, 1969, p. 2628.

Generic Name: Prazosin

Proprietary Name: Alphavase (G.B.), duramipress (Germ.), Eurex (Germ.), Hypovase (G.B.), Minipres (Span.), **Minipress** (Austral., Canad., Fr., Germ., Ital., Neth., S. Afr., Switz.), Peripress (Swed.), Pratsiol (S. Afr.)

Primary Use: This quinazoline derivative is used in the treatment of hypertension.

Ocular Side Effects:
A. Systemic Administration
   1. Decreased vision
   2. Eyelids or conjunctiva
      a. Erythema
      b. Conjunctivitis—nonspecific
      c. Edema
      d. Urticaria
   3. Visual hallucinations
   4. May aggravate keratoconjunctivitis sicca

Clinical Significance: Ocular side effects seen secondary to prazosin are uncommon and usually of little clinical significance. Schachat reported two cases of retrobulbar optic neuritis possibly related to prazosin therapy. The Registry has received several cases of aggravated dry eyes following the administration of this agent. While there have been numerous reports of lens and retinal pigmentary mottling to the Registry, the data are soft and not conclusive.

References:

Chin, D.K.F., Ho, A.K.C., and Tse, C.Y.: Neuropsychiatric complications related to use of prazosin in patients with renal failure. Br. Med. J. *293*:1347, 1986.

McEvoy, G.K. (Ed.): American Hospital Formulary Service Drug Information 87. Bethesda, American Society of Hospital Pharmacists, 1987, pp. 854–857.

Rosendorff, C.: Prazosin: Severe side effects are dose-dependent. Br. Med. J. *2*:508, 1976.

Ruzicka, T., and Ring, J.: Hypersensitivity to prazosin. Lancet *1*:473, 1984.

Schachat, A.: Retrobular optic neuropathy associated with prazosin therapy. Ophthalmol. *88*(Suppl. 9):97, 1981.

Generic Name: Timolol. See under *Class: Agents Used to Treat Glaucoma.*

Class: Digitalis Glycosides

Generic Name: 1. Acetyldigitoxin; 2. Deslanoside; 3. Digitoxin; 4. Digoxin; 5. Gitalin; 6. Lanatoside C; 7. Ouabain

Proprietary Name: 1. Acylanide (Fr.); 2. Cedilanid (Canad., Span.), **Cedilanid-D**, Cédilanide (Fr.), Desaci (Ital.); 3. Coramedan (Germ.), Digicor (Germ.), Digimed (Germ.), Digimerck (Germ.), Digipural (Germ.), Digitaline (Neth., Span., Switz.), Digitrin (Swed.), Ditaven (Germ.), mono-glycocard (Germ.), Tardigal (Germ.); 4. Cardioreg (Ital.), Coragoxine (Fr.), Digacin (Germ.), Digomal (Ital.), Eudigox (Ital.), Lanacard (Germ.), Lanacordin (Span.), Lanacrist (Swed.), Lanicor (Germ., Ital., Neth.), **Lanoxicaps** (Neth.), **Lanoxin** (Austral., Canad., G.B., Ire., Ital., Neth., S. Afr., Swed., Switz.), Lenoxin (Germ.), Novodigal (Germ.), Purgoxin (S. Afr.); 6. Cedilanid (Germ., Ire., Ital., S. Afr., Span.), Celadigal (Germ.), Celanate (Switz.); 7. Purostrophan (Germ.), Strodival (Germ.)

Primary Use: Digitalis glycosides are effective in the control of congestive heart failure and certain arrhythmias.

Ocular Side Effects:
    A. Systemic Administration
        1. Problems with color vision
            a. Color vision defect, blue-yellow defect
            b. Objects have yellow, green, blue, or red tinge
            c. Colored haloes around lights—mainly blue
        2. Visual sensations
            a. Flickering vision—often yellow or green
            b. Colored borders to objects
            c. Glare phenomenon—objects appear covered with brown, orange, or white snow
            d. Light flashes
            e. Scintillating scotomas
            f. Frosted appearance of objects
        3. Scotomas—central or paracentral
        4. Decreased vision
        5. Abnormal ERG or critical flicker frequency

     6. Diplopia

     7. Decreased intraocular pressure

     8. Retrobulbar neuritis

     9. Eyelids or conjunctiva

       a. Allergic reactions

       b. Angioneurotic edema

    10. Mydriasis (digoxin)

    11. Visual hallucinations (digoxin)

    12. Paresis of extraocular muscles (digitoxin)

    13. Photophobia (digitoxin)

    14. Corneal edema

    15. Pain on ocular movement

  B. Local Ophthalmic Use or Exposure—Topical Application

     1. Keratitis

     2. Corneal edema

     3. Decreased intraocular pressure

Clinical Significance: Nearly all of the ocular side effects due to the digitalis glycosides are reversible. Most studies have estimated that some ocular side effects occur in 11% to 25% of patients taking digitalis glycosides. They are most frequently seen with the long-acting agents such as digoxin or digitoxin, and least often with short-acting agents such as ouabain. The unique adverse ocular reaction to this group of drugs is the glare phenomenon or the snowy appearance of objects. While common to all the drugs in this group, it is most severe and frequent with acetyldigitoxin. Since one of the first signs of digitalis glycoside toxicity is disturbance of the yellow-blue axis of color vision, testing in this area can aid in the adjustments of therapy; however, one should not rely too heavily on this. In one series, nearly 80% of patients receiving long-term digoxin had a generalized disturbance of color vision, although most of these patients were unaware of any visual disturbance. Alterations in both light- and dark-adapted cone-mediated ERG amplitudes have been described as a retinal toxic reaction from cardiac glycosides. Individuals in whom cone dysfunction is diagnosed should be carefully questioned regarding cardiac medications, especially since digitalis glycoside toxicity can be made worse by concomitant quinidine. In addition, a decreased sensitivity to flickering light has been demonstrated due to a toxic effect of these drugs. Piltz, et al. feel that blurred vision is a more common side effect of digoxin toxicity than xanthopsia. Intraocular pressure may be decreased by deslanoside, digitoxin, digoxin, gitalin, and lanatoside C. The endothelial ion pump (sodium-potassium adenosine triphosphatase) is inhibited by digoxin and other cardiac glycosides such as ouabain. Both Johnson as well as Madreperla, Johnson, and O'Brien reported patients taking these agents with enhanced corneal edema. Mermoud, Safran, and de Stoutz reported a well-documented case of digoxin-related pain on ocular movement. Visual disturbances along with trigeminal neuralgia were reported by Johnson. Clinical use of these drugs for the treatment of glaucoma is not practical since the required therapeutic systemic dose is very near toxic levels. Topical ocular application of these agents causes keratopathy.

References:

Aronson, J.K., and Ford, A.R.: The use of colour vision measurement in the diagnosis of digoxin toxicity. Q.J. Med. *49*:273, 1980.

Closson, R.G.: Visual hallucinations as the earliest symptom of digoxin intoxication. Arch. Neurol. *40*:386, 1983.

Guignard, C., et al.: Effect of digoxin on the sensitivity to flickering light. Br. J. Clin. Pharmacol. *15*:189, 1983.

Haustein, K.O., et al.: Differences in color vision impairment caused by digoxin, digitoxin, or pengitoxin. J. Cardiovasc. Pharmacol. *4*:536, 1982.

Johnson, L.N.: Digoxin toxicity presenting with visual disturbance and trigeminal neuralgia. Neurology *40*:1469–1470, 1990.

LeSage, J.M.: Color vision deficiencies in people taking digoxin. Invest. Ophthalmol. Vis. Sci. *24*(Suppl.):59, 1983.

Madreperla, S.A., Johnson, M., and O'Brien, T.P.: Corneal endothelial dysfunction in digoxin toxicity. Am. J. Ophthalmol. *113(2)*:211–212, 1992.

Massaro, F.J., et al.: Scotomas secondary to digoxin intoxication. Drug Intell. Clin. Pharm. *17*:368, 1983.

Mermoud, A., Safran, A.B., and de Stoutz, N.: Pain upon eye movement following digoxin absorption. J. Clin. Neurol. Ophthalmol. *12(1)*:41–42, 1992.

Piltz, J.R., et al.: Digoxin toxicity. Recognizing the varied visual presentations. J. Clin. Neurol. Ophthalmol. *13*:275, 1993.

Ritebrock, N., and Alken, R.G.: Color vision deficiencies: A common sign of intoxication in chronically digoxin-treated patients. J. Cardiovasc. Pharmacol. *2*:93, 1980.

Weleber, R.G., and Shults, W.T.: Digoxin retinal toxicity. Clinical and electrophysiologic evaluation of a cone dysfunction syndrome. Arch. Ophthalmol. *99*:1568, 1981.

Generic Name: Digitalis

Proprietary Name: Digitalysat (Germ.)

Primary Use: The active constituents of digitalis are the glycosides that are effective in the control of congestive heart failure and certain arrhythmias.

Ocular Side Effects:

    A. Systemic Administration

        1. Problems with color vision

            a. Color vision defect, blue-yellow or red-green defect

            b. Objects have yellow, green, blue, or red tinge

            c. Colored haloes around lights—mainly blue

        2. Visual sensations

            a. Flickering vision—often yellow or green

        b. Colored borders to objects

        c. Glare phenomenon—objects appear covered with brown, orange, or white snow

        d. Light flashes

        e. Scintillating scotomas

        f. Frosted appearance of objects

3. Decreased vision

        a. Hemeralopia

        b. Abnormal photo stress testing

4. Visual fields

        a. Scotomas—central or paracentral

        b. Constriction

5. Photophobia

6. Abnormal ERG

7. Mydriasis

8. Visual hallucinations—especially bright floating spots

9. Diplopia

10. Ptosis

11. Paresis of extraocular muscles

12. Accommodative spasm

13. Eyelids or conjunctiva

        a. Allergic reactions

        b. Angioneurotic edema

        c. Urticaria

        d. Lupoid syndrome

14. Toxic amblyopia

15. Retrobulbar or optic neuritis

Clinical Significance: Ocular side effects are common with digitalis and are probably seen more frequently with it than with all the other digitalis glycosides combined. Most of the ocular side effects are transitory and reversible. The glare phenomenon and disturbances with color vision are the most striking and the most common adverse ocular reactions seen. Most patients receiving digitalis therapy are also taking numerous other drugs, and it may be difficult to decide which side effect is due to which medication. Since one of the first signs of digitalis toxicity is disturbance of the yellow-blue axis of color vision, testing in this area can aid in the adjustment of therapy. Patients receiving long-term digitalis therapy frequently experience red-green color defects. Although at least 25% of patients in the toxic digitalis range have ocular manifestations, color vision testing is not infallible and has limited clinical importance. In selected cases of corneal edema in already compromised endothelium, high serum levels of digitalis may enhance the edema due to a possible direct toxic effect on corneal endothelial cells.

References:

Aronson, J.K.: Digitalis intoxication. Clin. Sci. *64*:253–258, 1983.

Beller, G.A., et al.: Digitalis intoxication. N. Engl. J. Med. *284*:989–997, 1971.

Birch, J., et al.: Acquired color vision defects. *In* Pokorny, J., et al. (Eds.): Congenital and Acquired Color Vision Defects. New York, Grune & Stratton, 1979, pp. 243–350.

Bullock, R.E., and Hall, R.J.C.: Digitalis toxicity and poisoning. Adverse Drug React. Acute Poisoning Rev. *1*:201, 1982.

Duncker, G.: Ocular side effects of digitalis. Klin. Monatsbl. Augenheilkd. *178*:397, 1981.

Duncker, G., and Krastel, H.: Ocular digitalis effects in normal subjects. Lens Eye Toxicity Research *7(3&4)*:281–303, 1990.

Duzanec, Z.: Colored vision with glaucoma and digitalis intoxication. Dtsch. Med. Wochenschr. *104*:1094, 1979.

George, C.F.: Digitalis intoxication: A new approach to an old problem. Br. Med. J. *286*:1533, 1983.

Volpe, P.T., and Soave, R.: Formed visual hallucinations as digitalis toxicity. Ann. Intern. Med. *91*:865, 1979.

Wamboldt, F., et al.: Digitalis intoxication misdiagnosed as depression by primary care physicians. Am. J. Psychiatry *143*:219, 1986.

Woodcock, B.G., and Rietbrock, N.: Colour vision in clinical pharmacology. Trends Pharmacol. Sci. *4*:447, 1983.

Class: Diuretics

Generic Name: 1. Bendroflumethiazide; 2. Benzthiazide; 3. Chlorothiazide; 4. Chlorthalidone; 5. Cyclothiazide; 6. Hydrochlorothiazide; 7. Hydroflumethiazide; 8. Indapamide; 9. Methyclothiazide; 10. Metolazone; 11. Polythiazide; 12. Quinethazone; 13. Trichlormethiazide

Proprietary Name: 1. Aprinox (Austral., G.B.), Benzide (Austral.), Berkozide (G.B.), Centyl (G.B., Ire., Swed.), Esbericid (Germ.), **Naturetin** (Canad.), Naturine (Fr.), Neo-NaClex (G.B.), Pluryl (Neth.), Salures (Swed.), Sinesalin (Germ., Switz.); 2. Diurin (S. Afr.), **Exna**; 3. Azide (Austral.), Chlotride (Austral., Neth.), **Diuril**, Saluric (G.B.); 4. Axamin (S. Afr.), Higrotona (Span.), Hydro-long (Germ.), **Hygroton** (Austral., Canad., Fr., G.B., Germ., Ire., Neth., S. Afr., Swed., Switz.), Igroton (Ital.), Novothalidone (Canad.), Ödemo-Genat (Germ.), Renidone (S. Afr.), **Thalitone**, Urolin (Ital.); 6. Apo-Hydro (Canad.), Cloredema H (Span.), Dichlotride (Austral., Neth., S. Afr., Swed.), Diuchlor H (Canad.), diu-melusin (Germ.), Esidrex (Fr., G.B., Ital., Neth., Span., Swed., Switz.), **Esidrix** (Germ.), Hidrosaluretil (Span.), **HydroDiuril** (Canad.), Hydro Saluric (G.B.), Idrodiuvis (Ital.), Neo-Codema (Canad.), Novohydrazide (Canad.), **Oretic**, Thiazid-Wolff (Germ.); 7. **Diucardin**, Hydrenox (G.B.), Leodrine (Fr.), Rivosil (Ital.), **Saluron**; 8. Agelan (Ire.), Damide (Ital.), Extur (Span.), Fludex (Fr., Neth., Switz.), Indaflex (Ital.), Indamol (Ital.), Indolin (Ital.), Ipamix (Ital.),

Lozide (Canad.), **Lozol**, Millibar (Ital.), Natrilix (Austral., G.B., Germ., Ire., Ital., S. Afr.), Pressural (Ital.), Tertensif (Span.), Veroxil (Ital.); 9. **Aquatensen**, Duretic (Canad.), **Enduron** (Austral., G.B.), Endurona (Swed.), Thiazidil (Fr.); 10. Diondel (Span.), **Diulo** (Austral.), Metenix 5 (G.B.), **Mykrox**, Xuret (G.B.), **Zaroxolyn** (Canad., Germ., Ital., S. Afr., Swed.), Zaroxolyne (Switz.); 11. Drenusil (Germ.), Nephril (G.B.), Rénèse (Fr.), **Renese** (Swed.); 12. Aquamox (Austral., Ital., Neth.), **Hydromox**; 13. Esmarin (Germ.), Fluitran (Ital.), **Metahydrin, Naqua**

Primary Use: These thiazides and related diuretics are effective in the maintenance therapy of edema associated with chronic congestive heart failure, essential hypertension, renal dysfunction, cirrhosis, pregnancy, premenstrual tension, and hormonal imbalance.

Ocular Side Effects:
  A. Systemic Administration
    1. Decreased vision
    2. Myopia
    3. Problems with color vision
        a. Objects have yellow tinge (chlorothiazide)
        b. Large yellow spots on white background
    4. Retinal edema
    5. Eyelids or conjunctiva
        a. Allergic reactions
        b. Conjunctivitis—nonspecific
        c. Photosensitivity
        d. Urticaria
        e. Purpura
        f. Lupoid syndrome
        g. Erythema multiforme
        h. Stevens-Johnson syndrome
        i. Lyell's syndrome
    6. Decreased lacrimation
    7. Decreased intraocular pressure—minimal
    8. Paralysis of accommodation
    9. Visual hallucinations
    10. Subconjunctival or retinal hemorrhages secondary to drug-induced anemia

Clinical Significance: Ocular side effects due to these diuretics occur only occasionally and are usually transitory. It appears that most of these agents may cause myopia on rare occasions. This is probably caused by an increase in the anteroposterior diameter of the lens that may be reversible, even if use of the drug is continued. Sponsel and Rapoza reported a posterior subcapsular cataract after indapamide therapy but claim no causal association. Miller and Moses described a case of transient oculomotor nerve palsy associated with thiazide-induced glucose intolerance. Thiazide diuretics can also cause hypercalcemia, which may result in band keratopathy. When thiazide diuretics are used in combination with carbonic anhydrase inhibitors, one should be alert for signs of hypokalemia. These agents are photosensitizers, and Hartzer, et al. showed that in tissue culture hydrochlorothiazide will interact with UV-A radiation to produce toxic synergistic effects on human RPE cells. To date, no human data are evident to confirm this.

References:

Ashraf, N., Locksley, R., and Arieff, A.I.: Thiazide-induced hyponatremia associated with death or neurologic damage in outpatients. Am. J. Med. *70*:1163, 1981.

Beasley, F.J.: Transient myopia during trichlormethiazide therapy. Ann. Ophthalmol. *12*:705, 1980.

Bergmann, M.T., Newman, B.L., and Johnson, N.C., Jr.: The effect of a diuretic (hydrochlorothiazide) on tear production in humans. Am. J. Ophthalmol. *99*:473, 1985.

Birch, J., et al.: Acquired color vision defects. *In* Pokorny, J., et al. (Eds.): Congenital and Acquired Color Vision Defects. New York, Grune & Stratton, 1979, pp. 243–350.

Gould, L., et al.: Life-threatening reaction to thiazides. NY State J. Med. *80*:1975, 1980.

Hartzer, M., et al.: Hydrochlorothiazide: Increased human retinal epithelial cell toxicity following low-level UV-A irradiation. ARVO Invest. Ophthalmol. Vis. Sci. Annual Meeting Abstract Issue, 3633–3640, May, 1993.

Miller, N.R., and Moses, H.: Transient oculomotor nerve palsy. Association with thiazide-induced glucose intolerance. JAMA *240*:1887, 1978.

Palmer, F.J.: Incidence of chlorthalidone-induced hypercalcemia. JAMA *239*:2449, 1978.

Robinson, H.N., Morison, W.L., and Hood, A.F.: Thiazide diuretic therapy and chronic photosensitivity. Arch. Dermatol. *121*:522, 1985.

Sponsel, W.E., and Rapoza, P.A.: Posterior subcapsular cataract associated with indapamide therapy. Arch. Ophthalmol. *110*:454, 1992

Generic Name: Furosemide

Proprietary Name: Aluzine (G.B.), Aquarid (S. Afr.), Arcanamide (S. Afr.), Diural (Swed.), Diurolasa (Span.), Dryptal (G.B., Ire.), durafurid (Germ.), Frumax (G.B.), Frusid (G.B.), Fumarenid (Germ.), Furix (Swed.), furobasan (Switz.), Furo-Puren (Germ.), Furorese (Germ.), Fusid (Germ., Neth.), Hydrex (S. Afr.), Hydro-rapid (Germ.), Hydro-Rapid-Tablinen (Switz.), Impugan (Swed., Switz.), Lasiletten (Neth.), Lasilix (Fr.), **Lasix** (Austral., Canad., G.B., Germ., Ire., Ital., Neth., S. Afr., Swed., Switz.), Novosemide (Canad.), Ödemase (Germ.), Oedemex (Switz.), Puresis (S. Afr.), Rusyde (G.B.), Seguril (Span.), Sigasalur (Germ.), Uremide (Austral.), Urex (Austral.), Uritol (Canad.), Vesix (Neth.)

Primary Use: This potent sulfonamide diuretic is effective primarily in the treatment of hypertension complicated by congestive heart failure or renal impairment.

Ocular Side Effects:
    A. Systemic Administration
        1. Decreased vision
        2. Problems with color vision—objects have yellow tinge
        3. Eyelids or conjunctiva
            a. Allergic reactions
            b. Photosensitivity
            c. Urticaria
            d. Purpura
            e. Lupoid syndrome
            f. Erythema multiforme
            g. Exfoliative dermatitis
            h. Pemphigoid lesion
        4. Visual hallucinations
        5. Decreased intraocular pressure—minimal
        6. Decreased tolerance to contact lenses
        7. Subconjunctival or retinal hemorrhages secondary to drug-induced anemia

Clinical Significance: Furosemide has potent systemic side effects but is not commonly used. Ocular side effects are rare and seldom of significance. One instance of a baby born blind after the mother took 40 mg of furosemide 3 times daily during her second trimester has been reported.

References:
Castel, T., et al.: Bullous pemphigoid induced by frusemide. Clin. Exp. Dermatol. 6: 635, 1981.
Davidson, S.I.: Reports of ocular adverse reactions. Trans. Ophthalmol. Soc. U.K. 93: 495, 1973.
Peczon, J.D., and Grant, W.M.: Diuretic drugs in glaucoma. Am. J. Ophthalmol. 66: 680, 1968.
Zugerman, C., and La Voo, E.J.: Erythema multiforme caused by oral furosemide. Arch. Dermatol. 116:518, 1980.

Generic Name: Spironolactone

Proprietary Name: Aldace (Germ.), **Aldactone** (Austral., Canad., Fr., G.B., Germ., Ire., Ital., Neth., S. Afr., Span., Swed., Switz.), Aldopur (Germ.), Aquareduct (Germ.), duraspiron (Germ.), Idrolattone (Ital.), Laractone (G.B.), Melactone (Ire.), Novospiroton (Canad.), Osiren (Switz.), Osyrol (Germ.), Practon (Fr.), Sincomen (Ital.), Spiractin (S. Afr.), Spiretic (G.B.),

Spirix (Swed.), Spiroctan (Fr., G.B., Neth., Switz.), Spirolang (Ital.), Spirolone (G.B.), Spironone (Fr.), Spirospare (G.B.), Spiro-Tablinen (Germ.), Spirotone (Austral.), Tensin (S. Afr.), Uractone (Ital.), Xénalon (Switz.)

Primary Use: This aldosterone antagonist is effective in the treatment of edema associated with cirrhosis, nephrotic syndrome, congestive heart failure, and essential hypertension. It is also used in the diagnosis of hyperaldosteronism.

Ocular Side Effects:
A. Systemic Administration
1. Decreased vision
2. Myopia
3. Decreased intraocular pressure—minimal
4. Eyelids or conjunctiva
   a. Erythema
   b. Lupoid syndrome

Clinical Significance: Few significant ocular side effects due to spironolactone have been reported, and all are transitory and reversible.

References:
Belci, C.: Miopia transitoria in corso di terapia con diuretici. Boll. Oculist 47:24, 1968.
Duke-Elder, S.: System of Ophthalmology. St. Louis, C.V. Mosby, Vol. XIV, Part 2, 1972, p. 1343.
Dukes, M.N.G. (Ed.): Meyler's Side Effects of Drugs. Amsterdam, Excerpta Medica, Vol. X, 1984, pp. 379–381.
Grant, W.M.: Toxicology of the Eye. 3rd Ed., Springfield, Charles C Thomas, 1986, p. 845.

Class: Osmotics

Generic Name: Glycerin (Glycerol)

Proprietary Name: *Systemic*: Babylax (Germ., S. Afr.), Bulboïd (Switz.), Cristal (Switz.), **Fleet Babylax**, Glicerotens (Span.), Glycérotone (Fr.), Glycilax (Germ.), Microclisma Evacuante AD-BB (Ital.), Microclismi (Ital.), Practomil (Switz.), Supo Gliz (Span.), Vitrosups (Span.) *Ophthalmic*: **Ophthalgan Ophthalmic Solution**

Primary Use: *Systemic*: This trihydric alcohol is a hyperosmotic agent used to decrease intraocular pressure in various acute glaucomas and in preoperative intraocular procedures. *Ophthalmic*: This topical trihydric alcohol is a hyperosmotic used to reduce corneal edema for diagnostic procedures, increased comfort, or improved vision.

Ocular Side Effects:
   A. Systemic Administration
      1. Decreased intraocular pressure
      2. Subconjunctival or retinal hemorrhages
      3. Visual hallucinations
      4. Retinal tear
      5. Decreased vision
      6. Expulsive hemorrhage
   B. Local Ophthalmic Use or Exposure
      1. Irritation
         a. Lacrimation
         b. Hyperemia
         c. Ocular pain
         d. Burning sensation
      2. Vasodilation
      3. Subconjunctival hemorrhages
      4. Corneal endothelial damage

Systemic Side Effects:
   A. Systemic Administration
      1. Headache
      2. Nausea
      3. Vomiting
      4. Dehydration
      5. Cardiac arrhythmia
      6. Pulmonary edema
      7. Intracranial hemorrhage
      8. Hypotension
      9. Hemolysis (intravenous)
      10. Diabetic acidosis

Clinical Significance: Systemic glycerin causes decreased intraocular pressure, which is an intended ocular response, and has surprisingly few other ocular effects. However, severe vitreal dehydration with resultant shrinkage of the vitreous possibly may cause traction on the adjacent retina, resulting in a tear. This principle has been described as well with cerebral dehydration causing intracranial hemorrhages. In addition, visual hallucinations are thought to occur probably due to cerebral dehydration. There have been reports of expulsive hemorrhages occurring during intraocular surgery due to strong osmotic agents. The postulated mechanism is that a sudden drop in intraocular pressure may rupture sclerotic posterior ciliary arteries. Patients with renal, cardiovascular, or diabetic disease are more susceptible to serious systemic side effects, particularly if they are elderly and already somewhat dehydrated. Kalin, et al. report percutaneous retrogasserian glycerol injection to control intractable pain; however, in one instance inadvertent orbital injection caused proptosis and vision loss.

References:
Almog, Y., Geyer, O., and Lazar, M.: Pulmonary edema as a complication of oral glycerol administration. Ann. Ophthalmol. *18*:38, 1986.
Chang, S., Abramson, D.H., and Coleman, D.J.: Diabetic ketoacidosis with retinal tear. Ann. Ophthalmol. *9*:1507, 1977.
Goldberg, M.H., et al.: The effects of topically applied glycerin on the human corneal endothelium. Cornea *1*:39, 1982.
Havener, W.H.: Ocular Pharmacology. 5th Ed., St. Louis, C.V. Mosby, 1983, pp. 552–558.
Hovland, K.R.: Effects of drugs on aqueous humor dynamics. Int. Ophthalmol. Clin. *11(2)*:99, 1971.
Kalin, N.S., et al.: Visual loss after retrogasserian glycerol injection. Am. J. Ophthalmol. *115(3)*:396–398, 1993.

Generic Name: 1. Isosorbide; 2. Mannitol

Proprietary Name: 1. **Ismotic**; 2. Eufusol M 20 (Germ.), Isotol (Ital.), Manicol (Fr.), Mannistol (Ital.), Mede-prep (Austral.), Osmitrol (Austral., Canad.), Thomaemannit (Germ.)

Primary Use: These hyperosmotic agents are used to decrease intraocular pressure in various acute glaucomas and in preoperative intraocular procedures. Mannitol is also used in the management of oliguria and anuria.

Ocular Side Effects:
A. Systemic Administration
  1. Decreased intraocular pressure
  2. Increased cells in the aqueous
  3. Decreased vision
  4. Subconjunctival or retinal hemorrhages
  5. Visual hallucinations
  6. Eyelids or conjunctiva
     a. Edema
     b. Urticaria
  7. Retinal tear
  8. Expulsive hemorrhage

Systemic Side Effects:
A. Systemic Administration
  1. Headache
  2. Nausea
  3. Vomiting

4. Dehydration
5. Polyuria
6. Pulmonary edema
7. Intracranial hemorrhage
8. Anaphylactoid reaction

Clinical Significance: Isosorbide is excreted unchanged in the urine so that both systemic and ocular side effects are rare. Adverse ocular reactions are more frequent with mannitol, since it is administered parenterally and is a more potent agent. Increase in aqueous flare but not cells, especially in the elderly, has been caused by mannitol. Probably most other ocular side effects listed are secondary to dehydration effects. Severe vitreal dehydration with resultant shrinkage of the vitreous possibly may cause traction on the adjacent retina, resulting in a tear. This principle has been described as well with cerebral dehydration causing intracranial hemorrhage. Expulsive hemorrhages have been reported to occur during surgery in which strong osmotic agents were used. The postulated mechanism for this is a sudden decrease in intraocular pressure, which may rupture sclerotic posterior ciliary arteries. Isosorbide does not adversely affect blood glucose levels and is preferred in diabetics. Cardiovascular or renal disease may contraindicate use of isosorbide or mannitol. It has been suggested that these agents open the blood-retinal barrier and may give drugs or chemicals greater access to the retina and CNS.

References:

Chang, S., Abramson, D.H., and Coleman, D.J.: Diabetic ketoacidosis with retinal tear. Ann. Ophthalmol. *9*:1507, 1977.

Grabie, M.T., et al.: Contraindications for mannitol in aphakic glaucoma. Am. J. Ophthalmol. *91*:265, 1981.

Havener, W.H.: Ocular Pharmacology. 5th Ed., St. Louis, C.V. Mosby, 1983, pp. 550–552, 558–559.

Lamb, J.D., and Keogh, J.A.M.: Anaphylactoid reaction to mannitol. Can. Anaesth. Soc. J. *26*:435, 1979.

Mehra, K.S., and Singh, R.: Lowering of intraocular pressure by isosorbide. Arch. Ophthalmol. *86*:623, 1971.

Millay, R.H., et al.: Maculopathy associated with combination chemotherapy and osmotic opening of the blood-brain barrier. Am. J. Ophthalmol. *102*:626–632, 1986.

Miyake, Y., et al.: Increase in aqueous flare by a therapeutic dose of mannitol in humans. Acta. Soc. Ophthalmol. Jpn. *93*:1149–1153, 1989.

Quon, D. K., and Worthen, D. M.: Dose response of intravenous mannitol on the human eye. Ann. Ophthalmol. *13*:1392, 1981.

Wood, T.O., et al.: Effect of isosorbide on intraocular pressure after penetrating keratoplasty. Am. J. Ophthalmol. *75*:221, 1973.

Class: Peripheral Vasodilators

Generic Name: 1. Aluminum Nicotinate; 2. Niacin (Nicotinic Acid); 3. Niacinamide (Nicotinamide); 4. Nicotinyl Alcohol

Proprietary Name: 2. and 3. Bioglan Tri-B3 (Austral.), **Endur-acin**, **Nia-Bid**, **Niacels**, **Niacor**, **Niaplus**, Nicangin (Swed.), **Nico-400**, **Nicobid Tem-pules**, Nicobion (Fr., Germ.), **Nicolar**, Niconacid (Germ.), Nikacid (Austral.), **Slo-Niacin**, Tri-B3 (Austral.); 4. Roniacol Supraspan (Canad.), Roni-col (G.B., Germ., Ire., Ital., Neth., Swed., Switz.), Selcarbinol (Ital.)

Primary Use: Nicotinic acid and its derivatives are used as peripheral vasodilators, as vitamins, and in the treatment of hyperlipidemia.

Ocular Side Effects:
    A. Systemic Administration
        1. Decreased vision
        2. Sicca sensation
        3. Cystoid macular edema
        4. Eyelids or conjunctiva
           a. Allergic reactions
           b. Hyperpigmentation
           c. Angioneurotic edema
           d. Urticaria
           e. Loss of eyelashes or eyebrows
           f. Edema
        5. Diplopia
        6. Proptosis (minimal)
        7. Decreased lacrimation (doubtful)
        8. Increased intraocular pressure (doubtful)

Clinical Significance: All of the above signs and symptoms have been related to niacin (nicotinic acid) use. Theoretically, the other agents may cause these as well. The most serious side effect from this group of drugs is cystoid macular edema. This is primarily in patients who are taking at least 3 g/day, although it has been seen in patients taking as little as 1.5 g/day. Macular edema is most common in men in the third to fifth decades of life. The edema usually disappears upon discontinuation of the drug. Patients can have transient visual loss at lower dosages. The visual acuity can be so severe, in rare instances, that the patient is unable to function. This can occur in any age group, but is more common in males, and clears within 24 to 48 hours once the medicine is discontinued. Some patients will experience transient blurring of vision for 1 to 2 hours after taking niacin. These visual changes apparently are dose related, since one can decrease the medication and this phenomenon may not occur. In all probability, this drug is also secreted in the tears and will aggravate patients that already have a sicca-type problem. It is debatable if it can induce sicca. There is also a group of patients who will develop some lid or periorbital edema with or without minimal proptosis while taking this drug. Occasionally, a transitory, grayish discoloration of the eyelids occurs as well. There are a few cases in the

Registry of superficial punctate keratitis and two cases of eyelash or eye-brow loss. A retrospective survey showed that 7% of patients had to discontinue niacin in dosages above 3 g/day, secondary to adverse ocular effects. All of the above side effects seem to be dose related, so if the patient needs to continue therapy, he or she may consider titrating the drug. If, however, decreased vision occurs, one needs to consider macular edema on the differential diagnosis. While we have a number of cases in the Registry of a possible association between niacin and cataract formation, the data are weak. There is no specific lens pattern, and patients are predominantly in the cataract age group. Although this agent decreases lipids, and other lipid lowering agents have been linked to cataract formation, no relationship with nicotinic acid has been established. In fact, a case—control study (Leske, et al.), suggests that the anti-oxidant potential of niacin is inhibitory in the formation of cortical, nuclear, or mixed cataracts.

References:
Chazin, B.J.: Effect of nicotinic acid on blood cholesterol. Geriatrics, *15*:423, 1960.
Choice of Cholesterol-Lowering Drugs. Med. Lett. Drugs Ther. *33(835)*:2, 1991.
Fraunfelder, F.W., Fraunfelder, F.T., and Illingworth, D.R.: Adverse ocular effects associated with niacin therapy. Br. J. Ophthalmol. *79*:1995.
Gass, J.D.M.: Nicotinic acid maculopathy. Am J Ophthalmol *76*:500–510, 1973.
Harris, J.L.: Toxic amblyopia associated with administration of nicotinic acid. AJO, *55*:133, 1963.
Jampol, L.M.: Niacin Maculopathy. Authors reply R.H. Millay. Ophthalmology, *95(12)*:1704–1705, 1988.
Leske, M.C., Chylack, L.T., Suh-Yuh, W: The lens opacities case-control study. Risk factors for cataract. Arch. Ophthalmol. *109*:244–251, 1991.
Millay, R.H., Klein, M.L., and Illingworth, D.R.: Niacin maculopathy. Ophthalmology *95(7)*:930–936, 1988.
Peczon, J.D., Grant, W.M., and Lambert, B.W.: Systemic vasodilator, intraocular pressure and chamber depth in glaucoma. AJO, *72*:74–78, 1971.
Parsons, W.B., Jr., and Flinn, J.H.: Reduction in elevated blood cholesterol levels by large doses of nicotinic acid. JAMA *165*:234–238, 1957.
Zahn, K.: The effect of vasoactive drugs on the retinal circulation. Trans. Ophth. Soc. U.K., *86*:529–536, 1966.

Generic Name: Phenoxybenzamine

Proprietary Name: Dibenyline (Austral., G.B., Ire., Neth., S. Afr.), **Dibenzyline**, Dibenzyran (Germ.)

Primary Use: This alpha-adrenergic blocking agent is used in the management of pheochromocytoma and sometimes in the treatment of vasospastic peripheral vascular disease other than the obstructive types.

Ocular Side Effects:
  A. Systemic Administration
    1. Miosis
    2. Ptosis
    3. Conjunctival hyperemia
    4. Decreased intraocular pressure—minimal

Clinical Significance: Although ocular side effects due to phenoxybenzamine are frequently seen, they are seldom clinically significant. Miosis is rarely a problem, except when associated with posterior subcapsular or central lens changes. All adverse ocular reactions are reversible and transitory after discontinued drug use.

References:

Drug Evaluations. 6th Ed., Chicago, American Medical Association, 1986, pp. 491–492, 529–530, 577.

Gilman, A.G., Goodman, L.S., and Gilman, A. (Eds.): The Pharmacological Basis of Therapeutics. 6th Ed., New York, Macmillan, 1980, pp. 178–183.

Grant, W.M.: Toxicology of the Eye. 3rd Ed., Springfield, Charles C Thomas, 1986, p. 723.

Potter, D.E., and Rowland, J.M.: Adrenergic drugs and intraocular pressure. Gen. Pharmacol. *12*:1,1981.

Walsh, F.B., and Hoyt, W.F.: Clinical Neuro-Ophthalmology. 3rd Ed., Baltimore, Williams & Wilkins, Vol. 1, 1969, p. 447

Generic Name: Tolazoline

Proprietary Name: Priscol (Germ., Switz.), **Priscoline** (Canad.)

Primary Use: This alpha-adrenergic blocking agent is used in the management of spastic peripheral vascular disorders and as a diagnostic test for open-angle glaucoma.

Ocular Side Effects:
  A. Systemic Administration
    1. Intraocular pressure
      a. Increased
      b. Decreased—especially in hypertensive individuals
    2. Subconjunctival or retinal hemorrhages secondary to drug-induced anemia
  B. Local Ophthalmic Use or Exposure—Subconjunctival Injection
    1. Increased intraocular pressure—especially in open-angle glaucoma
    2. Ptosis
    3. Miosis
    4. Conjunctival hyperemia

Clinical Significance: In general, the ocular pressure response from systemic tolazoline is of little clinical significance because of its variability and small amplitude. However, in hypertensive individuals, the transient decreased intraocular pressure induced by tolazoline may be significant. Ocular side effects from subconjunctival injections are common but rarely significant. Increased intraocular pressure may be attributable in part to vasodilatation. Allergic contact dermatitis of the periorbital region has been reported in a patient receiving topical tolazoline and chloramphenicol for treatment of chalazion.

References:

Duke-Elder, S.: System of Ophthalmology. St Louis, C.V. Mosby, Vol. XIV, Part 2, 1972, p. 1046.

Frosch, P.J., Olbert, D., and Weickel, R.: Contact allergy to tolazoline. Contact Dermatitis *13*:272, 1985.

Preis, O., and Noonan, L.: Prolonged mydriatic effect of tolazoline in the premature infant. Am. J. Dis. Child. *141*:474, 1987.

Walsh, F.B., and Hoyt, W.F.: Clinical Neuro-Ophthalmology. 3rd Ed., Baltimore, Williams & Wilkins, Vol. I, 1969, p. 447.

Class: Vasopressors

Generic Name: Albuterol (Salbutamol)

Proprietary Name: Abbutamol (S. Afr.), Acrolin (G.B.), Apo-Salvent (Canad.), Apsomol (Germ.), Asmaven (G.B.), Asmaxen (Switz.), Breatheze (S. Afr.), Broncho Inhalat (Germ.), Broncho Spray (Germ.), Broncovaleas (Ital.), Buto Asma (Span.), Cyclocaps (G.B.), Ecovent (Switz.), Loftan (Germ.), Maxivent (G.B.), Novosalmol (Canad.), **Proventil**, Respolin (Austral.), Rimasal (G.B.), Salamol (G.B.), Salbulin (G.B.), Salbumol (Fr.), Salbuvent (G.B.), Salomol (Ire.), Sultanol (Germ.), Venteze (S. Afr.), Ventodisk (Canad., S. Afr., Switz.), Ventodisks (G.B., Ire.), **Ventolin** (Austral., Canad., G.B., Ire., Ital., Neth., S. Afr., Span., Switz.), Ventoline (Fr., Swed.), Volmac (Germ.), Volmax (G.B., S. Afr., Switz.)

Primary Use: This sympathomimetic amine is primarily used as a bronchodilator in the symptomatic relief of bronchospasm.

Ocular Side Effects:
    A. Systemic Administration
        1. Decreased vision
        2. Eyelids or conjunctiva
            a. Erythema
            b. Blepharoconjunctivitis
            c. Edema

        d. Angioneurotic edema
        e. Urticaria
   3. Visual hallucinations
   4. Decreased lacrimation
   5. Decreased intraocular pressure
   6. Mydriasis—may precipitate narrow-angle glaucoma

Clinical Significance: Ocular side effects following albuterol administration are seldom of clinical significance. Vivid visual hallucinations lasting for approximately 1 hour have been reported within 5 minutes following albuterol administration. One patient treated with albuterol and ipratropium developed bilateral corneal edema, limbal congestion, increased intraocular pressure, and dilatation of both pupils, consistent with closed-angle glaucoma.

References:

Khanna, P.B., and Davies, R.: Hallucinations associated with the administration of salbutamol via a nebulizer. Br. Med. J. *292*:1430, 1986.

Packe, G.E., Cayton, R.M., and Mashhoudi, N.: Nebulised ipratropium bromide and salbutamol causing closed-angle glaucoma. Lancet 2:691, 1984.

Shurman, A., and Passero, M.A.: Unusual vascular reactions to albuterol. Arch. Intern. Med. *144*:1771, 1984.

Generic Name: Ephedrine

Proprietary Name: C.A.M. (G.B.), Fedrine (Austral.), **NeoRespin**, Rino Pumilene (Ital.), Stopasthme (Mon.)

Primary Use: *Systemic*: This sympathomimetic amine is effective as a vasopressor, a bronchodilator, and a nasal decongestant. *Ophthalmic*: This topical sympathomimetic amine is used as a conjunctival vasoconstrictor.

Ocular Side Effects:
   A. Systemic Administration
       1. Mydriasis—may precipitate narrow-angle glaucoma
       2. Visual hallucinations
       3. Decreased intraocular pressure
       4. Acute macular neuroretinopathy
   B. Local Ophthalmic Use or Exposure
       1. Conjunctival vasoconstriction
       2. Decreased vision
       3. Eyelids or conjunctiva
          a. Allergic reactions
          b. Conjunctivitis—nonspecific
       4. Irritation

      a. Lacrimation
      b. Rebound hyperemia
      c. Photophobia
   5. Mydriasis—may precipitate narrow-angle glaucoma
   6. Aqueous floaters—pigment debris
   7. Decreased intraocular pressure—minimal

Clinical Significance: Ocular side effects from systemic administration of ephedrine are rare. Topical ocular ephedrine is not currently used by most ophthalmologists. The currently used concentration of ephedrine is rarely sufficient to cause significant side effects other than the intended response of vasoconstriction. Repeated use of topical ocular ephedrine, however, may cause rebound conjunctival hyperemia, or, in some instances, loss of the drug's vasoconstrictive effect. O'Brien, et al. suggest that acute macular neuroretinopathy may be due to either acute hypertension or sympathomimetic effects.

References:

Crandall, D.C., and Leopold, I.H.: The influence of systemic drugs on tear constituents. Ophthalmology 86:115, 1979.

Drug Evaluations. 6th Ed., Chicago, American Medical Association, 1986, pp. 377, 404, 574–575.

Escobar, J.I., and Karno, M.: Chronic hallucinosis from nasal drops. JAMA 247:1859, 1982.

Havener, W.H.: Ocular Pharmacology. 5th Ed., St. Louis, C.V. Mosby, 1983, p. 299.

O'Brien, D.M., et al.: Acute macular neuroretinopathy following intravenous sympathomimetics. Retina 9(4):281–286, 1989

Walsh, F.B., and Hoyt, W.F.; Clinical Neuro-Ophthalmology. 3rd Ed., Baltimore, Williams & Wilkins, Vol. I, 1969, p. 446

Generic Name: Epinephrine

Proprietary Name: *Systemic*: Adrenalin-Medihaler (Germ.), Anahelp (Fr.), Anakit (Fr.), **Bronkaid Mist Suspension**, Bronkaid Mistometer (Canad.), Dyspné-Inhal (Fr.), **Epipen** (Canad.), **Medihaler-Epi** (Austral., Canad., G.B., S. Afr.), **Primatene Mist Suspension, Sus-Phrine** *Ophthalmic*: **Epifrin** (Austral., Canad., Ire., S. Afr., Switz.), Epiglaufrin (Germ.), **Epinal, Epinephrine HCL Solution**, Eppy (G.B., Ire., Ital., Mon., Neth., S. Afr., Swed.), **Eppy/N** (Austral., Switz.), **Glaucon**, Glauposine (Fr.), Isopto Epinal (Span.), Simplene (G.B., Ire., S. Afr.)

Primary Use: *Systemic*: This sympathomimetic amine is effective as a vasopressor, a bronchodilator, and a vasoconstrictor in prolonging the action of anesthetics. *Ophthalmic*: This topical sympathomimetic amine is used in the management of open-angle glaucoma.

Ocular Side Effects:
  A. Systemic Administration
      1. Mydriasis—may precipitate narrow-angle glaucoma
      2. Problems with color vision
          a. Color vision defect, red-green defect
          b. Objects have green tinge
      3. Hemianopsia
      4. Lacrimation
      5. Acute macular neuroretinopathy
      6. Increased aqueous production
      7. Vision loss
  B. Local Ophthalmic Use or Exposure
      1. Decreased intraocular pressure
      2. Decreased vision
      3. Mydriasis—may precipitate narrow-angle glaucoma
      4. Eyelids or conjunctiva
          a. Allergic reactions
          b. Blepharoconjunctivitis—follicular
          c. Vasoconstriction
          d. Poliosis
          e. Pemphigoid lesion with symblepharon
          f. Hyperplasia of sebaceous glands
          g. Loss of eyelashes or eyebrows
      5. Irritation
          a. Lacrimation
          b. Rebound hyperemia
          c. Photophobia
          d. Ocular pain
          e. Burning sensation
      6. Adrenochrome deposits
          a. Conjunctiva (cysts)
          b. Cornea
          c. Nasolacrimal system (cast formation)
      7. Cystoid macular edema
      8. Punctate keratitis
      9. Corneal edema
      10. Narrowing or occlusion of lacrimal canaliculi
      11. Subconjunctival or retinal hemorrhages
      12. Paradoxical pressure elevation in open-angle glaucoma
      13. Scotomas
      14. Aqueous floaters—increased pigment granules in anterior
          chamber
      15. Periorbital edema
      16. Iris

      a. Iritis
      b. Cysts
  17. Black discoloration of soft contact lenses
  18. May aggravate herpes infections

Systemic Side Effects:
  A. Local Ophthalmic Use or Exposure
    1. Headache
    2. Sweat
    3. Syncope
    4. Arrhythmia
    5. Tachycardia
    6. Palpitation
    7. Hypertension
    8. Ventricular extrasystole

Clinical Significance: Ocular side effects from systemic epinephrine are uncommon; however, topical ocular application may commonly cause significant side effects other than the intended responses of decreased intraocular pressure and conjunctival vasoconstriction. In over 20% of patients receiving topical ocular application, the drug must be stopped after prolonged use because of ocular discomfort and rebound conjunctival hyperemia. Over 50% of patients develop reactive hyperemia with long-term use; concomitant timolol and epinephrine therapy occasionally has an additive effect on reactive hyperemia. While most epinephrine-induced macular edema is reversible, there are rare cases of advanced cystoid macular edema that have irreversible changes. Cystoid maculopathy may require over 6 months to clear once the medication is discontinued. Cystoid macular changes secondary to epinephrine occur more frequently in aphakic patients but have been seen in phakic eyes as well. This drug can cause a pseudo-ocular pemphigoid; it can also cause conjunctival epidermalization, loss of eyelashes, blepharitis, and meibomianitis. Most ocular adverse reactions due to epinephrine resolve or significantly improve with discontinuation of the drug. However, adrenochrome deposits in the cornea or conjunctiva may be exceedingly slow to absorb. There are data to suggest that long-term topical ocular or intracameral epinephrine may cause significant corneal edema due to a toxic response on the endothelium, resulting in increased corneal hydration. This primarily occurs in corneas with damaged epithelium, if given topically, which allows for increased penetration of this drug through the cornea. Anterior chamber injections primarily cause endothelial problems in the bisulfite form in poorly buffered systems. Systemically given epinephrine may cause transitory mydriasis, color vision difficulty, etc. Both O'Brien et al. and Desai, Sudhamathi, and Natarajan feel it is a factor in causing acute macular neuroretinopathy. Although systemic side effects are not frequently seen, topical ophthalmic epinephrine should be used with caution in patients with cardiac disease. Local anesthetics that contain epinephrine may pose a threat to patients who are also being treated with a nonselective beta blocker. In addition, patients undergoing ocular surgery with halothane anesthesia may experience tachycardia and arrhythmia from supplemental injection of local anesthetics containing epinephrine or from topical ophthalmic administration or intracameral injection of epinephrine. A slight transitory rise of diastolic blood pressure and occasional arrhythmias have also been noted in patients using concomitant topical ophthalmic epinephrine and timolol eyedrops. Savino, Burde, and Mills describe four patients with severe visual loss after intranasal anesthetic injections. Cause of the visual loss includes retinal arterial occlusion and optic nerve ischemia, both of which the authors feel were due to secondary vasospasm induced by an anesthetic with epinephrine.

References:

Bealka, N., and Schwartz, B.: Enhanced ocular hypotensive response to epinephrine with prior dexamethasone treatment. Arch. Ophthalmol. *109*:346–348, 1991.

Blondeau, P., and Cote, M.: Cardiovascular effects of epinephrine and dipivefrin in patients using timolol: A single-dose study. Can. J. Ophthalmol. *19*:29, 1984.

Brummett, R.: Warning to otolaryngologists using local anesthetics containing epinephrine: Potential serious reactions occurring in patients treated with beta-adrenergic receptor blockers. Arch. Otolaryngol. *110*:561, 1984.

Camras, C.B., et al.: Inhibition of the epinephrine-induced reduction of intraocular pressure by systemic indomethacin in humans. Am. J. Ophthalmol. *100*:169, 1985.

Desai, U.R., Sudhamathi, K., and Natarajan, S.: Intravenous epinephrine and acute macular neuroretinopathy. Arch. Ophthalmol. *111*:1026–1027, 1993.

Edelhauser, H.F., et al.: Corneal edema and the intraocular use of epinephrine. Am. J. Ophthalmol. *93*:327, 1982.

Kacere, R.D., Dolan, J.W., and Brubaker, R.F.: Intravenous epinephrine stimulates aqueous formation in the human eye. Invest. Ophthalmol. Vis. Sci. *33(10)*: 2861–2865, 1992.

Kaufman, H.E.: Chemical blepharitis following drug treatment. Am. J. Ophthalmol. *95*:703, 1983.

Kerr, C.R., et al.: Cardiovascular effects of epinephrine and dipivalyl epinephrine applied topically to the eye in patients with glaucoma. Br. J. Ophthalmol. *66*:109, 1982.

Krejci, L., Rezek, P., and Hoskovcova-Krejcova, H.: Effect of long-term treatment with antiglaucoma drugs on corneal endothelium in patients with congenital glaucoma: Contact specular microscopy. Glaucoma 7:81, 1985.

O'Brien, D.M., et al.: Acute macular neuroretinopathy following intravenous sympathomimetics. Retina 9:281–286, 1989.

Sasamoto, K., et al.: Corneal endothelial changes caused by ophthalmic drugs. Cornea *3*:37, 1984.

Savino, P.J., Burde, R.M., and Mills, R.P.: Visual loss following intranasal anesthetic injection. J. Clin. Neuro-ophthalmol. *10(2)*:140–144, 1990.

Generic Name: Hydroxyamphetamine

Proprietary Name: *Ophthalmic*: **Paredrine**

Primary Use: *Ophthalmic*: This topical sympathomimetic amine is used as a mydriatic.

Ocular Side Effects:
A. Local Ophthalmic Use or Exposure
1. Mydriasis—may precipitate narrow-angle glaucoma
2. Decreased vision
3. Irritation
   a. Lacrimation
   b. Photophobia
   c. Ocular pain
4. Palpebral fissure—increase in width
5. Paradoxical pressure elevation in open-angle glaucoma
6. Eyelids or conjunctiva—allergic reactions
7. Paralysis of accommodation—minimal
8. Problems with color vision—objects have a blue tinge

Clinical Significance: Other than precipitating narrow-angle glaucoma, ocular side effects from ocular administration of hydroxyamphetamine are insignificant and reversible. An increase in palpebral fissure width reaches a maximum 30 minutes after topical ocular application. This is secondary to stimulation of Müeller's muscle. Some feel this may be the safest mydriatic to use with a shallow anterior chamber since it is slow-acting and possibly more easily counteracted by miotics. Administration of 1% hydroxyamphetamine eyedrops causes a more pronounced mydriasis in patients with Down's syndrome.

References:

Gartner, S., and Billet, E.: Mydriatic glaucoma. Am. J. Ophthalmol. *43*:975, 1957.
Grant, W.M.: Toxicology of the Eye. 2nd Ed., Springfield, Charles C Thomas, 1974, pp. 567–568.
Kronfeld, P.C., McGarry, H.I., and Smith, H.E.: The effect of mydriatics upon the intraocular pressure in so-called primary wide-angle glaucoma. Am. J. Ophthalmol. *26*:245, 1943.
Munden, P.M., et al.: Palpebral fissure responses to topical adrenergic drugs. Am. J. Ophthalmol. *111*:706–710, 1991.
Priest, J.H.: Atropine response of the eyes in mongolism. Am. J. Dis. Child. *100*:869, 1960.
Walsh, F.B., and Hoyt, W.F.: Clinical Neuro-Ophthalmology. 3rd Ed., Baltimore, Williams & Wilkins, Vol. I, 1969, p. 446.

Generic Name: 1. Mephentermine; 2. Metaraminol; 3. Methoxamine; 4. Norepinephrine (Levarterenol)

Proprietary Name: 2. **Aramine** (Austral., G.B., Neth.), Levicor (Ital.); 3. Idasal (Span.), Vasoxine (G.B., Ire.), **Vasoxyl** (Canad.), Vasylox Junior (Austral.); 4. Adrenor (Span.), Levophed (Austral., Canad., G.B., Ire.), **Levophed Bitartrate**, Noradrec (Ital.)

Primary Use: These sympathomimetic amines are used in the management of hypotension and shock.

Ocular Side Effects:
  A. Systemic Administration
       1. Mydriasis—may precipitate narrow-angle glaucoma
       2. Horizontal nystagmus
       3. Decreased intraocular pressure (norepinephrine)
       4. Photophobia (norepinephrine)
       5. Diplopia (norepinephrine)
       6. Rebound conjunctival hyperemia (norepinephrine)
       7. Visual hallucinations (mephentermine)
  B. Local Ophthalmic Use or Exposure
       1. Decreased intraocular pressure
       2. Mydriasis—may precipitate narrow-angle glaucoma
       3. Irritation
            a. Hyperemia
            b. Photophobia
            c. Ocular pain

Clinical Significance: Ocular side effects due to these sympathomimetic amines are reversible and transitory. Seldom are adverse ocular reactions seen due to these drugs, except in overdose situations.

References:
Bigger, J.F.: Norepinephrine therapy in patients allergic to or intolerant of epinephrine. Ann. Ophthalmol. *11*:183, 1979.

Gilman, A.G., Goodman, L.S., and Gilman, A. (Eds.): The Pharmacological Basis of Therapeutics. 6th Ed., New York, Macmillan, 1980, pp. 151–153, 164–166.

McEvoy, G.K. (Ed.): American Hospital Formulary Service Drug Information 87. Bethesda, American Society of Hospital Pharmacists, 1987, pp. 592–604.

Pollack, I.P., and Rossi, H.: Norepinephrine in the treatment of ocular hypertension and glaucoma. Arch. Ophthalmol. *93*:173, 1975.

Spaeth, G.L.: The effect of autonomic agents on the pupil and the intraocular pressure of eyes treated with dexamethasone. Br. J. Ophthalmol. *64*:426, 1980.

Stewart, R., et al.: Norepinephrine dipivalylate dose-response in ocular hypertensive subjects. Ann. Ophthalmol. *13*:1279, 1981.

Generic Name: Phenylephrine

Proprietary Name: *Systemic*: **Neo-Synephrine Hydrochloride** *Ophthalmic*: **AK-Dilate** (Canad.), **AK-Nefrin Ophthalmic**, Analux (Span.), Bonnington's Junior Elixir (Austral.), Constrictor (Span.), Decongestant Eye Drops (Austral.), Decongestant Nasal Spray (Austral.), Fenox (G.B., S. Afr.), Gouttes nasales (Switz.), Isonefrine (Ital.), **Isopto Frin** (Austral., G.B.), Mydfrin (Canad.), **Mydfrin 2.5%**, Neo Lacrim (Span.), Neosynephrine (Swed.), Néo-Synéphrine (Switz.), **Neo-Synephrine** (Austral., Canad., Germ., Ital.), **Neo-Synephrine Viscous**, Neosynephrine-POS (Germ.), Novahistine (Canad.), Nycto (Fr.), Optistin (Ital.), **Phenoptic, Phenylephrine HCL**, Prefrin (Ire.), **Prefrin Liquifilm** (Austral., Canad., S. Afr.), Pulverizador Nasal (Span.), **Relief**, Spersaphrine (Canad.), **St. Joseph Measured Dose Nasal Decongestant**, Visadron (Germ., Ital., Neth., Span.), Visopt (Austral.), Vistafrin (Span.), Vistosan (Germ.), Vital Eyes (Canad.)

Primary Use: *Systemic*: This sympathomimetic amine is effective as a vasopressor and is used in the management of hypotension, shock, and tachycardia. *Ophthalmic*: This topical sympathomimetic amine is used as a vasoconstrictor and a mydriatic.

Ocular Side Effects:
    A. Systemic Administration—Nasal Application
        1. Visual hallucinations
    B. Local Ophthalmic Use or Exposure
        1. Mydriasis—may precipitate narrow-angle glaucoma
        2. Decreased vision
        3. Conjunctival vasoconstriction
        4. Rebound miosis
        5. Irritation
           a. Lacrimation
           b. Rebound hyperemia
           c. Photophobia
           d. Ocular pain
        6. Punctate keratitis
        7. Eyelids or conjunctiva
           a. Allergic reactions
           b. Erythema
           c. Conjunctivitis—nonspecific
           d. Blepharospasm
           e. Eczema
           f. Palpebral fissure—increase in width
        8. Aqueous floaters—pigment debris
        9. Corneal edema
      10. Paradoxical pressure elevation in open-angle glaucoma

Systemic Side Effects:
 A. Local Ophthalmic Use or Exposure
  1. Hypertension
  2. Myocardial infarct
  3. Tachycardia
  4. Subarachnoid hemorrhage
  5. Cardiac arrest
  6. Cardiac arrhythmia
  7. Coronary artery spasm
  8. Headache
  9. Syncope

Clinical Significance: Long-term overuse of phenylephrine nasal spray may cause visual hallucinations. Other than the possibility of precipitating narrow-angle glaucoma, the ocular side effects due to topical ocular phenylephrine are usually of little significance. While this is one of the more toxic drugs to the corneal epithelium, keratitis is seldom a problem because the drug is not used for prolonged periods. A 10% concentration of phenylephrine can cause significant keratitis and a reduction in the conjunctival PO_2, which may result in delayed wound healing by reducing aerobic metabolism of rapidly dividing cells. Pupillary dilatation lasting for prolonged periods has been reported, especially in patients taking guanethidine. Mydriasis varies with iris pigmentation and depth of the anterior chamber. Blue irides and shallow anterior chambers produce the greatest mydriasis, and dark irides or deep chambers the least. A diminished mydriatic response has been seen after subsequent use of phenylephrine. Blanching of the skin, particularly the lower eyelid, may occur secondary to phenylephrine ophthalmic solution. Following ophthalmic examination with a combination of phenylephrine and cyclopentolate in neonates, an increased risk of feeding intolerance may result, which could be due to the mydriatic drugs, the physical stress of the examination, or a combination of these factors. Data suggest that the 10% concentrations of phenylephrine should be used with caution or not at all in patients with cardiac disease, significant hypertension, aneurysms, and advanced arteriosclerosis. It also should be used with caution in the elderly and in patients taking monoamine oxidase inhibitors, tricyclic antidepressants, or atropine. In rare instances, 2.5% phenylephrine can also cause significant adverse systemic reactions, just as 10% phenylephrine can.

References:
Epstein, D.L., Boger, W.P.III, and Grant, W.M.: Phenylephrine provocative testing in the pigmentary dispersion syndrome. Am. J. Ophthalmol. *85*:43–50, 1978.
Escobar, J.I., and Karno, M.: Chronic hallucinosis from nasal drops. JAMA *247*:1859, 1982.
Fraunfelder, F.T., and Meyer, S.M.: Possible cardiovascular effects secondary to topical ophthalmic 2.5% phenylephrine. Am. J. Ophthalmol. *99*:362, 1985.

Hanna, C., et al.: Allergic dermatoconjunctivitis caused by phenylephrine. Am. J. Ophthalmol. *95*:703,1983.

Hermansen, M.C., and Sullivan, L.S.: Feeding intolerance following ophthalmologic examination. Am. J. Dis. Child. *139*:367, 1985.

Isenberg, S.J., and Green, B.F.: Effect of phenylephrine hydrochloride on conjunctival PO$_2$. Arch. Ophthalmol. *102*:1185, 1984.

Kumar, S.P.: Adverse drug reactions in the newborn. Ann. Clin. Lab. Sci. *15*:195, 1985.

Kumar, V., et al.: Systemic absorption and cardiovascular effects of phenylephrine eyedrops. Am. J. Ophthalmol. *99*:180, 1985.

Kumar, V., Packer, A.J., and Choi, W.W.: Hypertension following phenylephrine 2.5% ophthalmic drops. Glaucoma *7*:131, 1985.

Mathias, C.G.T., et al.: Allergic contact dermatitis to echothiophate iodide and phenylephrine. Arch. Ophthalmol. *97*:286–287, 1979.

Munden, P.M., et al.: Palpebral fissure responses to topical adrenergic drugs. Am. J. Ophthalmol. *111*:706–710, 1991.

Powers, J.M.: Decongestant-induced blepharospasm and orofacial dystonia. JAMA *247*:3244, 1982.

Wesley, R.E.: Phenylephrine eyedrops and cardiovascular accidents after fluorescein angiography. J. Ocular Ther. Surg. *2*:212, 1983.

VII Hormones and Agents Affecting Hormonal Mechanisms

Class: Adrenal Corticosteroids

Generic Name: 1. Adrenal Cortex Injection; 2. Aldosterone; 3. Beclomethasone; 4. Betamethasone; 5. Cortisone; 6. Desoxycorticosterone (Desoxycortone); 7. Dexamethasone; 8. Fludrocortisone; 9. Fluorometholone; 10. Fluprednisolone; 11. Hydrocortisone; 12. Medrysone; 13. Meprednisone; 14. Methylprednisolone; 15. Paramethasone; 16. Prednisolone; 17. Prednisone; 18. Triamcinolone

Proprietary Name: *Systemic*: 1. Cortelan (Ital.), Cortine Naturelle Laroche Navarron (Fr.), Supracort (Ital.); 2. Aldocorten (Germ.); 3. Aerobec (G.B.), Aldecin (Austral., Neth., Switz.), Aldécine (Fr.), Beclo Asma (Span.), Beclo Rino (Span.), Beclodisk (Canad.), Becloforte (Austral., Canad., G.B., Neth., S. Afr., Switz.), Beclorhinol (Germ.), Beclosona (Span.), Becloturmant (Germ.), **Beclovent** (Canad.), Becodisk (Switz.), Becodisks (G.B., Ire., S. Afr.), Béconase (Fr.), **Beconase** (Austral., Canad., G.B., Ire., Neth., S. Afr., Switz.), **Beconase AQ** (Austral.), Beconase Aquosum (Germ.), Beconase Dosier-Spray (Germ.), Beconasol (Switz.), Bécotide (Fr.), Becotide (Austral., G.B., Ire., Ital., Neth., S. Afr., Span., Swed., Switz.), Bronco-Turbinal (Ital.), Cleniderm (Ital.), Clenil (Ital., Neth., S. Afr.), Clenil-A (Ital.), Dereme (Span.), Dermisone Beclo (Span.), Inalone (Ital.), Menaderm Simple (Span.), Menaderm Simplex (Ital.), Propaderm (Canad., G.B., Ital., S. Afr.), Rino Clenil (Ital.), Sanasthmax (Germ.), Sanasthmyl (Germ.), Turbinal (Ital.), **Vancenase** (Canad.), **Vancenase AQ**, **Vanceril** (Canad.), Viarin (Neth.), Viarox (Germ., S. Afr.); 4. **Alphatrex**, Beben (Canad., Ital.), Bedermin (Ital.), Bentelan (Ital.), Betacort (Canad.), Betaderm (Canad.), Betagel (Canad.), Betamatil (Span.), Betapred (Swed.), **Betatrex**, Betnelan (G.B., Ire., Neth., S. Afr.), Betnelan-V (Neth.), Betnesol (Canad., Fr., G.B., Germ., Ire., Neth., S. Afr., Switz.), Betnesol-V (Germ.), Betnesol-WL (Germ.), Betneval (Fr.), Betnovat (Swed.), Betnovate (Austral., Canad., G.B., Ire., S. Afr., Span., Switz.), Betnovate RD (Ready Diluted) (G.B.), Betoid (Swed.), **B-S-P**, Celestan (Germ.), Celestan-V (Germ.), Célestène (Fr.), Célestoderm (Fr.), Celestoderm (Canad., Neth., Span.), Celestoderm-V (Ital., S.

Afr., Span., Switz.), Celeston (Swed.), Celeston valerat (Swed.), **Celestone** (Austral., Canad., Ital., Neth., S. Afr., Span., Switz.), Celestone M (Austral.), **Celestone Phosphate**, Celestone V (Austral.), Cordes Beta (Germ.), Diproderm (Span., Swed.), Diprolène (Fr., Switz.), **Diprolene** (Neth., S. Afr.), Diprolene Glycol (Canad.), Diprosis (Germ.), **Diprosone** (Austral., Canad., Fr., G.B., Germ., Ire., Ital., Neth., S. Afr., Switz.), durabetason (Germ.), Ecoval (Ital.), Ectosone (Canad.), Euvaderm (Germ.), **Maxivate**, Minisone (Ital.), Novobetamet (Canad.), Paucisone (Ital.), Persivate (S. Afr.), Prevex B (Canad.), Sclane (Span.), Topilene (Canad.), Topisone (Canad.), **Valisone** (Canad.), Vista-Methasone (G.B.); 5. Adreson (Neth.), Altesona (Span.), Cortal (Swed.), Cortate (Austral.), Cortelan (G.B.), Cortistab (G.B.), Cortisyl (G.B., Ire.), Cortogen (S. Afr.), Cortone (Canad., Swed.), **Cortone Acetate**, Cortone Acetato (Ital.); 6. Cortiron (Ital.), Syncortyl (Fr.); 7. **Aeroseb-Dex**, afpred-1 (Germ.), Ak-Dex (Canad.), Anemul Mono (Germ.), Artrosone (Span.), Auxiloson (Germ.), Auxisone (Fr.), **Baldex**, Cébédex (Fr.), Cortidexason (Germ.), Cortisumman (Germ.), **Dalalone D.P.**, **Decaderm in Estergel**, Decadran (Span.), Décadron (Fr.), **Decadron** (Austral., Canad., G.B., Germ., Ital., Neth., S. Afr., Swed., Switz.), Decadron Depot (Neth.), Decadron Phosphat (Germ.), **Decadron Phosphate** (Canad., Switz.), **Decadron-LA**, **Decaspray**, Decofluor (Ital.), Dectancyl (Fr.), Deronil (Canad.), Desalark (Ital.), Deseronil (Ital.), Dexa in der Ophtiole (Germ.), Dexabene (Germ.), Dexa-Brachialin N (Germ.), Dexa-Clinit (Germ.), Dexacortal (Swed.), Dexa-Effekton (Germ.), Dexalocal (Switz.), Dexamed (Germ.), Dexamiso (Span.), Dexamonozon (Germ.), Dexamonozon N (Germ.), Dexane (Fr.), Dexaplast (Span.), Dexapos (Germ.), Dexa-ratiopharm (Germ.), Dexa-sine (Germ.), Dexa-sine SE (Germ.), Dexasone (Canad.), **Dexasone 4**, **Dexasone 10**, **Dexasone LA**, Dexmethsone (Austral.), Etacortilen (Ital.), Firmalone (Ital.), Fortecortin (Germ., Span., Switz.), Fosfodexa (Span.), **Hexadrol** (Canad.), **Hexadrol Phosphate** (Canad.), Isopto Dex (Germ.), Isopto Maxidex (Swed.), Luxazone (Ital.), Maxidex (Austral., Canad., Fr., G.B., Neth., S. Afr., Span., Switz.), Megacort (Ital.), Mephamésone (Switz.), Millicortène (Switz.), Oradexon (Austral., Canad., Neth., S. Afr., Switz.), Predni-F-Tablinen (Germ.), Soldesam (Ital.), Solone (Span.), Soludécadron (Fr.), Spersadex (Canad., Germ., S. Afr., Switz.), Totocortin (Germ.), Tuttozem N (Germ.), Visumetazone (Ital.); 8. Florinef (Austral., Canad., G.B., Ire., S. Afr., Swed., Switz.), Florinef Acetaat (Neth.), **Florinef Acetate**; 9. Efflumidex (Germ.), Flarex (Canad., Neth., Switz.), Fluaton (Ital.), Flucon (Austral., Fr., Neth., S. Afr., Switz.), Flumetol Semplice (Ital.), FML (Ire., S. Afr., Span.), FML Forte (Canad.), FML Liquifilm (Austral., Canad., G.B., Neth., Switz.), Isopto Flucon (Germ., Span.); 11. Actocortina (Span.), Adacor (Austral.), **Aeroseb-HC**, **A-Hydrocort Univial**, Alfason (Germ.), Algicortis (Ital.), Alocort (Canad.), **Anuprep HC**, Barriere-HC (Canad.), Buccalsone (Neth.), **Carmol HC**, Colifoam (Austral, G.B., Germ., S. Afr., Switz.), Colofoam (Fr.), Cordes H (Germ.), Corlan (Austral., G.B., Ire.), Cortacet (Canad.), Cortaid (Austral., Ital.), Cortamed (Canad.), Cortate

(Canad.), **Cort-Dome**, Cortef (Austral., Canad.), **Cortenema** (Canad.), Cortic (Austral.), **Corticaine**, Corticreme (Canad.), Cortidro (Ital.), **Cortifair**, **Cortifoam** (Canad.), Cortiment (Canad.), Cortoderm (Canad.), **Cortril**, Covocort (S. Afr.), Crema Transcutan Astier (Span.), Cutaderm (S. Afr.), Dermacalm (Switz.), Dermacort (Austral., G.B.), Derm-Aid (Austral.), Dermocortal (Ital.), **Dermolate**, Dermosa Cusi Hidrocort (Span.), Dilucort (S. Afr.), Dioderm (G.B.), Efcortelan (Austral., G.B.), Efcortelan Soluble (G.B., Ire.), Efcortesol (G.B.), Egocort Cream (Austral.), Ekzesin (Germ.), Emo-Cort (Canad.), Ficortril (Germ., Swed.), Flebocortid (Ital.), Glycocortison H (Germ.), Glycocortisone H (Switz.), Hc45 (G.B.), **Hemril-HC**, Hidroaltesona (Span.), Hycor (Austral.), Hycort (Canad.), Hyderm (Canad.), Hydro-Adreson (Neth.), Hydrocortistab (G.B.), Hydrocortisyl (G.B., Ire.), **Hydrocortone** (G.B., Switz.), **Hydrocortone Acetate**, **Hydrocortone Phosphate**, Hydrosone (Austral.), Hysone (Austral.), Hysone-A (Austral.), **Hytone**, Idracemi (Ital.), Idrocortigamma (Ital.), Lanacort (G.B., Ital.), Lenirit (Ital.), Locoïd (Fr.), **Locoid** (G.B., Neth., S. Afr., Swed., Switz.), Locoidon (Ital.), Mildison (Neth., Swed.), Mildison Lipocream (G.B.), Munitren H (Germ.), Mylocort (S. Afr.), Nordicort (Austral.), Novohydrocort (Canad.), **Nutracort**, **Orabase HCA**, Oralsone (Span.), Pandel (Germ.), Paro (Ital.), **Penecort**, Prevex HC (Canad.), Procort (Austral.), Proctocort (Fr.), Procutan (S. Afr.), Rapicort (Ital.), Rectocort (Canad.), Retef (Germ.), sagittacortin (Germ.), Sanatison Mono (Germ.), Sarna HC (Canad.), Schericur (Span.), Sigmacort (Austral.), Siguent Hycor (Austral.), Sintotrat (Ital.), Skincalm (S. Afr.), **Solu-Cortef** (Austral., Canad., G.B., Ire., Ital., Neth., S. Afr., Swed., Switz.), Solu-Glyc (Swed.), Squibb-HC (Austral.), Supralef (Span.), **Synacort**, **Texacort** (Canad.), Unicort (Canad.), Uniderm (Swed.), Urecortyn (Ital.), Velopural (Germ.), **Westcort** (Canad.), Zenoxone (G.B.); 12. HMS Liquifilm (Austral., Canad., Neth., S. Afr., Switz.), Medriusar (Ital.), Ophtocortin (Germ.), Spectramedryn (Germ.); 14. **A-Methapred Univial**, Asmacortone (Ital.), Caberdelta M (Ital.), Depo-Medrate (Germ.), Dépo-Médrol (Fr.), **Depo-Medrol** (Austral., Canad., Ital., Neth., S. Afr., Switz.), Depo Moderin (Span.), Depomedrone (Swed.), **Depo-Predate**, Esametone (Ital.), Firmacort (Ital.), Medrate (Germ.), Médrol (Fr.), **Medrol** (Austral., Canad., Ital., S. Afr., Switz.), Medrol Topical (Canad.), Medrol Veriderm (Ital.), Medrone (G.B., Ire., Swed.), Mega Star (Ital.), Metilbetasone Solubile (Ital.), Metypresol (Neth.), Prednilen (Ital.), Predni-M-Tablinen (Germ.), Reactenol (Ital.), Sieropresol (Ital.), Solpredone (Fr.), Solu Moderin (Span.), Solu-Médrol (Fr.), **Solu-Medrol** (Austral., Canad., Ital., Neth., S. Afr., Switz.), Solu-Medrone (G.B., Ire., Swed.), Summicort (Ital.), Urbason (Germ., Ital., Span., Switz.), Vériderm Médrol (Fr.); 15. Cortidene (Span.), Depodillar (Neth.), Dilar (Fr.), Dillar (Neth.), **Haldrone**, Monocortin (Germ.), Monocortin Dépôt (Switz.), Monocortin Depot (Germ.), Triniol (Span.); 16. Adnisolone (Austral.), Ak-Tate (Canad.), Balpred (Canad.), Corti-Clyss (Switz.), Cortisolone (Ital.), Dacortin H (Span.), Decaprednil (Germ.), Decortin-H (Germ.), Decortin-H-KS (Germ.), Delta-Cortef (Austral.), Deltacortilen (Ital.), Deltacortril (G.B., Germ.), Deltasolone (Austral.), Deltastab (G.B.), Deltidrosol (Ital.), Di-Adreson-F (Neth.), duraprednisolon (Germ.), Estilsona (Span.), hefasolon (Germ.), Hexacortone (Switz.), **Hydeltrasol, Hydeltra-T.B.A.,** Hydrocortancyl (Fr.), Inflamase (Canad.), Inflanefran (Germ.), Itacortone (Ital.), Klismacort (Germ.), Linola-H N (Germ.), Linola-H-Fett N (Germ.), Meticortelone (Ital., S. Afr.), Normonsona (Span.), Ophtho-Tate (Canad.), Panafcortelone (Austral.), **Pediapred,** Precortalon aquosum (Swed.), Precortisyl (G.B., Ire.), Prectal (Germ.), Pred Forte (G.B., Ire., Neth., S. Afr.), Pred Forte, Mild (Canad., Switz.), Pred Mild (Ire., S. Afr.), **Predate 50, Predate S, Predate TBA,** Pred-Clysma (Swed.), Predeltilone (S. Afr.), Predenema (G.B.), Predfoam (G.B.), Prednabene (Germ.), Prednesol (G.B., Ire.), Predni-Coelin (Germ.), Prednicort (Swed.), Predni-Helvacort (Switz.), PredniHexal (Germ.), Predni-H-Injekt (Germ.), Predni-H-Tablinen (Germ.), Predsol (Austral., G.B., Ire., S. Afr.), **Prelone,** Scherisolon (Germ.), Sintisone (Austral., Swed.), Solone (Austral.), Solu Dacortin H (Span.), Solucort (Fr.), Soludacortin (Ital.), Solu-Dacortine (Switz.), Solu-Decortin-H (Germ.), Solupred (Fr.), Sterofrin (Austral.), Ultracortenol (Canad., Germ., Neth., Swed., Switz.); 17. Adasone (Austral.), Cortancyl (Fr.), Dacortin (Span.), Decortin (Germ.), Decortisyl (G.B., Ire.), Decorton (Ital.), Deltacortene (Ital.), **Deltasone** (Austral., Canad.), **Liquid Pred, Meticorten** (S. Afr.), Panafcort (Austral.), Predeltin (S. Afr.), **Prednicen-M,** Predniment (Germ.), Predni-Tablinen (Germ.), Rectodelt (Germ.), Sone (Austral.), **Sterapred,** Ultracorten (Germ.), Winpred (Canad.); 18. Adcortyl (G.B.), Adcortyl in Orabase (G.B., Ire.), Albacort Idrodispersibile (Ital.), Albicort (Neth.), **Aristocort** (Austral., Canad.), **Aristocort A,** Aristocort Acetonide (Canad.), **Aristospan** (Canad.), **Azmacort** (Canad.), **Cinalone 40, Cinonide 40,** Corticothérapique (Switz.), Delphi (Neth.), Delphicort (Germ.), Delphimix (Germ.), Extracort (Germ.), Extracort N (Germ.), Ipercortis (Ital.), **Kenacort** (Austral., Fr., Ire., Ital, Neth., Swed., Switz.), Kenacort-A (Austral., Ire., Ital., Neth., Switz.), Kenacort-A Solubile (Neth., Switz.), Kenacort-T (Swed.), **Kenalog** (Canad., G.B., Ire., Neth.), **Kenalog in Orabase** (Austral., S. Afr.), Kenalone (Austral.), Kortikoid-ratiopharm (Germ.), Ledercort (G.B., Ital., Neth., S. Afr., Span., Swed., Switz.), Lederlon (Germ.), Lederspan (G.B., Neth., S. Afr., Swed.), **Oralone Dental,** Proctosteroid (Span.), Respicort (Switz.), **Tac-3,** Taucorten (Ital.), Tédarol (Fr.), Triaderm (Canad.), **Triamcinair,** Triamhexal (Germ.), Triam-Injekt (Germ.), Triam-oral (Germ.), Tri-Anemul (Germ.), Tricortale (Ital.), Trigon Depot (Span.), **Trymex,** Volon (Germ.), Volon A (Germ.), Volonimat (Germ.) *Ophthalmic*: 4. Betnesol (Canad., S. Afr.); 5. Cortistab (G.B.); 7. **AK-Dex** (Canad.), **Decadron** (Canad., Germ., Neth., Swed.), **Decadron Phosphate,** Desalark (Ital.), **Dexamethasone Sodium Phosphate Solution and Ointment, Dexamethasone Suspension,** Isopto Maxidex (Swed.), **Maxidex** (Austral., Canad., Fr., G.B., Neth., S. Afr., Span., Switz.); 9. **Flarex, Fluor-Op, FML, FML Forte, FML Liquifilm** (Austral., Canad.,

G.B., Neth., Switz.), **FML SOP**; 11. Cortef (Austral.), Ficortril (Swed.), Idracemi (Ital.); 12. **HMS**, HMS Liquifilm (Austral., Canad., Neth., S. Afr., Switz.); 16. **AK-Pred, Econopred, Econopred Plus**, Inflamase (Canad.), **Inflamase Forte, Inflamase Mild, Pred Forte** (G.B., Ire., Neth., S. Afr.), Pred Forte, Mild (Canad., Switz.), **Pred Mild** (Ire., S. Afr.), **Prednisolone Sodium Phosphate Solution**, Predsol (Austral., G.B.), Ultracortenol (Canad., Germ., Neth., Swed., Switz.) *Topical*: 4. **Alphatrex, Betatrex**, Diprolène (Fr., Switz.), **Diprolene** (Neth., S. Afr.), **Diprosone** (Austral., Canad., Fr., G.B., Germ., Ire., Ital., Neth., S. Afr., Switz.), **Valisone** (Canad.); 7. **Aeroseb-Dex, Decaspray**; 11. **Aeroseb-HC, Alphaderm** (G.B., Ire.), **Cort-Dome**, Cortef (Austral.), **Cortril**, Dermacort (Austral., G.B.), Hydrocortistab (G.B.), **Hytone**, Locoïd (Fr.), **Locoid** (G.B., Neth., S. Afr., Swed., Switz.), **Synacort, Westcort** (Canad.); 14. **Medrol**; 18. **Aristocort** (Austral.), Kenalog (Neth.)

Primary Use: *Systemic*: These corticosteroids are effective in the replacement therapy of adrenocortical insufficiency and in the treatment of inflammatory and allergic disorders. *Ophthalmic*: These corticosteroids are effective in the treatment of ocular inflammatory and allergic disorders. *Topical*: These corticosteroids are effective for the relief of inflammatory and pruritic dermatoses.

Ocular Side Effects:
A. Systemic Administration
 1. Decreased vision
 2. Posterior subcapsular cataracts (some may be reversible)
 3. Increased intraocular pressure
 4. Decreased resistance to infection
 5. Mydriasis—may precipitate narrow-angle glaucoma
 6. Myopia
 7. Exophthalmos
 8. Papilledema secondary to pseudotumor cerebri
 9. Diplopia
 10. Myasthenic neuromuscular blocking effect
　　a. Paresis or paralysis of extraocular muscles
　　b. Ptosis
 11. Problems with color vision—color vision defect
 12. Delayed corneal wound healing
 13. Visual fields
　　a. Scotomas
　　b. Constriction
　　c. Enlarged blind spot
　　d. Glaucoma field defect
 14. Visual hallucinations
 15. Abnormal ERG or VEP

16. Retinal edema
17. Translucent blue sclera
18. Eyelids or conjunctiva
    a. Hyperemia
    b. Edema
    c. Angioneurotic edema
    d. Lyell's syndrome
19. Microcysts—nonpigment epithelium of ciliary body and pigment epithelium of iris
20. Subconjunctival or retinal hemorrhages
21. Decreased tear lysozymes
22. Toxic amblyopia
23. Retinal embolic phenomenon (injection)
24. Ocular teratogenic effect—cataracts
B. Local Ophthalmic Use or Exposure—Topical Application, Intralesional or Subconjunctival or Retrobulbar Injection
    1. Increased intraocular pressure
    2. Decreased resistance to infection
    3. Delayed healing of corneal or scleral wounds
    4. Mydriasis—may precipitate narrow-angle glaucoma
    5. Ptosis
    6. Posterior subcapsular cataracts
    7. Decreased vision
    8. Enhances lytic action of collagenase
    9. Paralysis of accommodation
    10. Visual fields
        a. Scotomas
        b. Constriction
        c. Enlarged blind spot
        d. Glaucoma field defect
    11. Problems with color vision
        a. Color vision defect
        b. Colored haloes around lights
    12. Eyelids or conjunctiva
        a. Allergic reactions
        b. Persistent erythema
        c. Telangiectasia
        d. Depigmentation
        e. Poliosis
        f. Scarring (subconjunctival injection)
        g. Fat atrophy (retrobulbar or subcutaneous injection)
        h. Skin atrophy (subcutaneous injection)
    13. Cornea
        a. Punctate keratitis
        b. Superficial corneal deposits

    14. Irritation
       a. Lacrimation
       b. Photophobia
       c. Ocular pain
       d. Burning sensation
       e. Anterior uveitis
    15. Corneal or scleral thickness
       a. Increased—initial
       b. Decreased
    16. Toxic amblyopia
    17. Optic atrophy
    18. Granulomas
    19. May aggravate the following diseases
       a. Scleromalacia perforans
       b. Corneal "melting" diseases
       c. Behcet's disease
       d. Eales' disease
       e. Presumptive ocular toxoplasmosis
    20. Retinal embolic phenomenon (injection)
    21. Enhances facultative intraocular pathogens
  C. Inadvertent Ocular Exposure—Intraocular Injection
    1. Ocular pain
    2. Decreased vision
    3. Intraocular pressure
       a. Increased—initial
       b. Decreased
    4. Retinal hemorrhages
    5. Retinal degeneration
    6. Ascending optic atrophy
    7. Toxic amblyopia
    8. Retinal detachment
    9. Global atrophy
    10. Endophthalmitis
  D. Systemic Absorption from Topical Application to the Skin or Nasal Inhalants
    1. Increased intraocular pressure (beclomethasone)
    2. Decreased resistance to infection
    3. Eyelids or conjunctiva
       a. Photosensitivity
       b. Urticaria
       c. Purpura
       d. Telangiectasia
       e. Depigmentation
       f. Skin atrophy

    4. Papilledema secondary to pseudotumor cerebri

    5. Cataracts (beclomethasone)

Clinical Significance: Ocular side effects due to systemic or ocular administration of steroids are common and have significant clinical importance. It is possible that of all the medications used by ophthalmologists, this group of drugs causes the most side effects, perhaps because of frequency of drug use. The idea of "safe" oral, subconjunctival, or topical ocular dosage is now in jeopardy, and patients must be evaluated for individual susceptibility. This is illustrated by a study in which there was no significant correlation between patients taking oral steroids and posterior subcapsular cataracts, based on total dosage, weekly dosage (intensity), duration of dosage, or age of the patients. However, in susceptible individuals, systemically these agents can clearly cause posterior subcapsular lens changes. It was shown that 50% of the patients using 800 drops of 0.1% dexamethasone developed some lens changes. Excessive use of nasal inhalation corticosteroids in susceptible individuals has also been associated with an increased incidence of posterior lens changes. Generally, steroid-induced posterior subcapsular cataracts are irreversible, but data support the reversibility of cataracts in some lenses of nephrotic children. Age may not be the prominent factor in steroids causing lens changes, because the young patient's lenses may be more susceptible to systemic steroid effects, especially topical ocular, and subconjunctival administration of fluorinated corticosteroids. In fact, the fluorinated compounds given by the periocular and topical ophthalmic routes have been implicated in the death of an infant. Race is a factor, since steroid-induced glaucoma from topical ocular medication is less frequent in blacks than in whites, and depigmentation from subcutaneous steroid injection is more frequent in blacks. Even the withdrawal of steroids possibly can cause significant adverse effects, as postulated in a 7-month-old child who developed benign intracranial hypertension with severe visual loss following withdrawal of topical cutaneous steroids. Although individual variation to steroid exposure may be marked, steroid responders with elevated intraocular pressure secondary to topical ocular corticosteroids have more field loss than steroid nonresponders.

Steroids affect changes in almost all ocular structures. This has recently been reconfirmed by reports that steroids can cause microcysts of the iris pigment epithelium and of the ciliary body nonpigment epithelium. The time required for onset of a major adverse effect from topical ocular steroids varies greatly. Effects to enhance epithelial herpes simplex may be days, while it may take years for posterior subcapsular cataracts to develop. Topical ocular corticosteroid-induced glaucoma may take a number of weeks to develop, yet most patients who receive the stronger topical steroid dosages will develop elevated intraocular pressure in months to years. Recently, beclomethasone inhalants have been shown to cause glaucoma and posterior subcapsular cataracts on long-term usage, often in higher than recommended dosages. Taravella, et al. have shown that the topical ocular phosphate preparations can cause a corneal band keratopathy, especially in patients with sicca. Cases in the Registry support that nonphosphated forms can cause this as well. The recent popularity of subconjunctival injections of steroids has brought additional drug reactions. Subconjunctival injections of steroids placed over a diseased cornea or sclera can cause a thinning, and possibly rupture, at the site of the injection. Posterior subcapsular cataracts and subconjunctival granulomas have also been induced from this mode of drug administration. Intractable glaucoma can occur after subconjunctival depot injections of steroids. The surgical removal of the subconjunctival steroids is required to normalize the ocular pressure. Inadvertent intraocular steroid injections have caused blindness, probably due to the drug vehicle since the drug itself is nontoxic to the retina and optic nerve in most cases. However, depot steroids are toxic; complications from inadvertent intraocular depot injections are numerous. While triamcinolone acetonide appears to be the least toxic with inadvertent vitreous injections, often vitrectomy may be required to remove the depot steroid, prevent tract bands, and view the penetration site. Topical use of steroid medication for the treatment of eyelid dermatitis may result in ocular contamination of accumulated amounts of medication, which is capable of causing all of the untoward effects seen with topical ocular application of steroids. A fatal reaction from complications of Cushing's syndrome following 3 months' treatment with corticosteroid eyedrops and sub-Tenon's injection occurred in an 11-month-old child. Topical ocular corticosteroids are generally not associated with any significant risk of adrenal axis suppression, although care must be exercised as to the amount prescribed in infants.

References:
Allen, M.B., et al.: Steroid aerosols and cataract formation. Br. Med. J. *299*:432, 1989.
Costagliola, C., et al: Cataracts associated with long-term topical steroids. Br. J. Dermatol. *120*:472, 1989.
Cohen, B.A., et al.: Steroid exophthalmos. J. Comput. Assist. Tomogr. *5*:907, 1981.
Donshik, P.C., et al.: Posterior subcapsular cataracts induced by topical corticosteroids following keratoplasty for keratoconus. Ann. Ophthalmol. *13*:29, 1981.
Dreyer, E.B.: Inhaled steroid use and glaucoma. To the Editor. N. Engl. J. Med. p. 1822, December 9, 1993.
Fischer, R., Henkind, P., and Gartner, S.: Microcysts of the human iris pigment epithelium. Br. J. Ophthalmol. *63*:750, 1979.
Floman, N.N., Moisseiev, J., and Blumenthal, M.: Monocular glaucomatous disc changes following bilateral topical steroid therapy. Glaucoma *5*:62, 1983.
Fraunfelder, F.T., and Meyer, S.M.: Posterior subcapsular cataracts associated with nasal or inhalation corticosteroids. Am. J. Ophthalmol. *109(4)*:489–490, 1990.
Giangiacomo, J., Dueker, D.K., and Adelstein, E.H.: Histopathology of triamcinolone in the subconjunctiva. Ophthalmology *94*:149, 1987.

Henderson, R.P., and Lander, R.: Scleral discoloration associated with long-term prednisone administration. Cutis *34*:76,1984.

Kass, M.A., et al.: Corticosteroid-induced iridocyclitis in a family. Am. J. Ophthalmol. *93*:268, 1982.

Mabry, R.L.: Visual loss after intranasal corticosteroid injection. Incidence, causes, and prevention. Arch. Otolaryngol. *107*:484, 1981.

McDonnell, P.J., and Muir, M.G.K.: Glaucoma associated with systemic corticosteroid therapy. Lancet 2:386, 1985.

Miller, J A., and Munro, D.D.: Topical corticosteroids: Clinical pharmacology and therapeutic use. Drugs *19*:119, 1980.

Mills, D.W., Siebert, L.F., and Climenhaga, D.B.: Depot triamcinolone-induced glaucoma. Can. J. Ophthalmol. *21*:150, 1986.

Petroutsos, G., et al.: Corticosteroids and corneal epithelial wound healing. Br. J. Ophthalmol. *66*:705, 1982.

Santamaria, J., II.: Steroidal agents: Their systemic and ocular complications. Ocular Inflammation Ther. *1*:19, 1983.

Taravella, M.J., et al.: Calcific band keratopathy associated with the use of topical steroid-phosphate preparations. Arch. Ophthalmol. *112*:608–613, 1994.

Class: Androgens

Generic Name: Danazol

Proprietary Name: Cyclomen (Canad.), Danatrol (Fr., Ital., Neth., Span., Switz.), Danazant (Ire.), **Danocrine** (Austral., Swed.), Danol (G.B., Ire.), Ladazol (S. Afr.), Mastodanatrol (Fr.), Winobanin (Germ.)

Primary Use: This synthetic androgen is used to treat pelvic endometriosis, fibrocystic breast disease, and hereditary angioedema.

Ocular Side Effects:
- A. Systemic Administration
  1. Decreased vision
  2. Eyelids or conjunctiva
     a. Erythema
     b. Edema
     c. Photosensitivity
     d. Urticaria
     e. Purpura
     f. Stevens-Johnson syndrome
  3. Diplopia
  4. Optic nerve
     a. Papilledema secondary to pseudotumor cerebri
     b. Pallor
     c. Atrophy
  5. Visual field defects

Clinical Significance: Decreased vision, usually associated with headaches, is the most frequent ocular side effect reported secondary to danazol. There are at least 14 cases of pseudotumor cerebri with papilledema associated with this drug that were either published or reported to the Registry. Pseudotumor cerebri may occur while taking this medication or shortly after stopping it. While pseudotumor cerebri was documented in at least half of the cases, only papilledema was mentioned in the rest. These findings resolved after stopping the drug or while receiving diuretic therapy. Causation is unknown but may be due to danazol-induced weight gain, fluid retention, or cerebral venous thrombosis. Presenile cataracts in young women treated with danazol have also been found in the absence of predisposed risk factors, but this is unsubstantiated.

References:

Fanous, M, et al.: Pseudotumor cerebri associated with danazol withdrawal. Letter to the editor. JAMA *266(9)*:1218–1219, 1991.

Hamed, L.M., et al.: Pseudotumor cerebri induced by danazol. Am. J. Ophthalmol. *107(2)*:105–110, 1989.

McEvoy, G.K. (Ed.): American Hospital Formulary Service Drug Information 87. Bethesda, American Society of Hospital Pharmacists, 1987, pp. 1616–1618.

Physicians' Desk Reference, 42nd Ed., Oradell, N.J., Medical Economics Co., 1988, pp. 2225–2226.

Pre-senile cataracts in association with the use of Danocrine (danazol). PMS News Quarterly (April-June, 1986) p. 5.

Sandercock, P.J.: Benign intracranial hypertension associated with danazol. Pseudotumour cerebri: Case report. Scottish Med. J. *35*:49, 1990.

Shah, A., et al.: Danazol and benign intracranial hypertension. Br. Med. J. *294*:1323, 1987.

Generic Name: Leuprolide Acetate

Proprietary Name: Carcinil (Germ.), Enanton Depot (Swed.), Enantone (Fr., Ital.), Lucrin (Austral., Fr., Neth., S. Afr.), **Lupron** (Canad.), Procren (Swed.), Procrin (Span.), Prostap (G.B.)

Primary Use: This gonadotropin-releasing hormone is primarily used to treat precocious puberty, control endometriosis, and as a palliative treatment for advanced prostatic cancer.

Ocular Side Effects:

    A. Systemic Administration—intramuscular
        1. Blurred vision
        2. Pseudotumor cerebri—papilledema
        3. Ocular vascular accidents
        4. Ocular pain
        5. Lid edema

Clinical Significance: This synthetic analog of a naturally occurring gonado-tropin-releasing hormone is given intramuscularly once monthly. Following injection, some patients experience transitory blurred vision, which usually lasts from 1 to 2 hours; however, it may last from 2 to 3 weeks. Blurred vision may occur after each injection or start as late as the sixth injection. This may or may not be associated with headaches or dizziness. Once the drug is discontinued, the vision reverts to pretreatment levels. Therefore, in some patients, it may be advisable to delay prescribing glasses until the medication has been discontinued. First reported by Arber, et al., pseudotumor primarily occurs in patients in the age group of idiopathic pseudotumor cerebri, so it is difficult to prove a direct cause-and-effect relationship. Regardless, in at least two instances, the pseudotumor cerebri could not be controlled without discontinuing the medication. The intraocular vascular accidents were primarily branch vein occlusions and intraocular hemor-rhages. Since this drug can also cause hemopoiesis, hematuria, phlebitis, thrombosis, and anemia, it is possible that these same effects could occur intraocularly. Lid edema and ocular pain, which have been reported, may well be due to this drug since similar findings are found elsewhere in the body secondary to this medication. Regardless, none of the above are of serious consequence, other than pseudotumor cerebri.

References:

Arber, N., et al.: Pseudotumor cerebri associated with leuprorelin acetate. Lancet *335*; 668, 1990.

Fraunfelder, F.T., Edwards, R., and Weisberg, G.: Possible ocular side effects associ-ated with leuprolide acetate injections. JAMA 273(10):773–774, 1995.

Class: Antithyroid Agents

Generic Name: 1. Carbimazole; 2. Methimazole (Thiamazole); 3. Methyl-thiouracil; 4. Propylthiouracil

Proprietary Name: 1. Basolest (Neth.), Neo Tomizol (Span.), Néo-Merca-zole (Fr., Switz.), Neo-Mercazole (Austral., G.B., Ire., S. Afr., Swed.), neo-morphazole (Germ.), Neo-Thyreostat (Germ.); 2. Antitiroide G.W. (Ital.), Favistan (Germ.), Strumazol (Neth.), **Tapazole** (Canad., Ital., S. Afr., Switz.), Thacapzol (Swed.), Thyrozol (Germ.), Tirodril (Span.); 3. Thyreo-stat (Germ.); 4. Propycil (Germ.), Propyl-Thyracil (Canad.), Thyreostat II (Germ.), Tiotil (Swed.)

Primary Use: These thioamides are effective in the treatment of hyperthyroid-ism and angina pectoris.

Ocular Side Effects:
   A. Systemic Administration
      1. Nystagmus (methylthiouracil)
      2. Keratitis

3. Eyelids or conjunctiva
    a. Allergic reactions
    b. Conjunctivitis—nonspecific
    c. Depigmentation
    d. Urticaria
    e. Lupoid syndrome
    f. Exfoliative dermatitis
    g. Lyell's syndrome (carbimazole)
4. Decreased lacrimation (methylthiouracil)
5. Exophthalmos
6. Subconjunctival or retinal hemorrhages secondary to drug-induced anemia

Clinical Significance: Ocular side effects secondary to these thioamides are rare. Nystagmus and decreased lacrimation have only been reported with methylthiouracil. Adverse ocular reactions are reversible and transitory after discontinued use of these drugs. There are three cases (Sponzilli, et al. and Taloni, et al.) of questionable drug-related retrobulbar neuritis related to methimazole use.

References:

Blankenship, M.L.: Drugs and alopecia. Aust. J. Dermatol. *24*:100, 1983.
Cooper, D.S., et al.: Agranulocytosis associated with antithyroid drugs. Effects of patient age and drug dose. Ann. Intern. Med. *98*:26, 1983.
Mikol, F., Simon, F., and Falcy, M.: Gougerot-Sjögren's syndrome and polyneuritis due to carbimazole. Rev. Neurol. *138*:259, 1982.
Sponzilli, T., et al.: Retrobulbar optic neuritis in the course of treatment with methimazole. Riv. Neurobiol. *8*:1, 1979.
Taloni, M., et al.: Clinical study of retrobulbar optic neuritis from methimazole. Boll. Oculist. *68*:913–921, 1989.
Wilkey, I.S., and McDonald, A.: A probable case of Chromobacterium violacium infection in Australia. Med. J. Aust. *2*:38, 1983.
Zurcher, K., and Krebs, A.: Cutaneous Side Effects of Systemic Drugs. Basel, S. Karger, 1980, pp. 22–23, 300–303.

Generic Name: 1. Iodide and iodine solutions and compounds; 2. Radioactive iodides

Proprietary Name: *Systemic*: 1. Bioiodine (G.B.), Essasorb (Germ.), Iodex (Austral.), Iodoflex (G.B.), Iodosan (Ital.), Iodosorb (Fr., G.B., Ital., Swed., Switz.), Jodetten (Germ.), Jodid (Germ.), Katarakton (Germ.), Leukona-Jod-Bad (Germ.), Mikroplex Jod (Germ.), Mucolitico Maggioni (Ital.), Navarroyodol (Span.), **Organidin** (Canad.), **Pima, Roma-nol, SSKI,** Strumex (Germ.), Thyro-Block (Canad.), Thyrojod depot (Germ.); 2. **Sodium Iodide (I ^{125}) U.S.P., Sodium Iodide (I ^{131}) U.S.P.** *Topical*: 1. Amyderm S (Germ.), Batticon S (Germ.), Betadermyl (Ital., Neth.), Bétadine (Fr.), **Betadine**

(Austral., Canad., G.B., Ire., Ital., Neth., S. Afr., Span., Switz.), Betaisodona (Germ.), Betasept (G.B.), Betaseptic (Ital., Span., Switz.), Betatul (Span.), Braunol (Irc., Ital., Span., Switz.), Braunol 2000 (Germ.), Braunosan (Ire., Ital.), Braunovidan (Ire.), Braunovidon (Germ., Ital., Switz.), Brush Off (G.B.), Cold Sore Lotion (Austral., Canad., G.B.), Cyderm Tinea Paint (Austral.), Destrobac (Switz.), Esoform Jod 75 (Ital.), Esoform Jod 100 (Ital.), Euroiod-Disinfettante Iodoforo Analcolico (Ital.), Freka cid (Germ.), Gammadin (Ital.), Inadine (G.B., Ital.), Iodine Tri-Test (Austral.), Iodoril (Ital.), Iodoscrub (Ital.), Iodosteril (Ital.), Isodine (Austral.), Jodocur (Ital.), Jodoplex (Switz.), **Massengill Medicated**, **Minidyne**, Orodine (Austral.), Orto Dermo "P" (Span.). Podine (S. Afr.), **Povidone-Iodine Cleansing Solution U.S.P.**, Proviodine (Canad.), Savlon Dry (Austral., G.B.), SP Betaisodona (Germ.), Stoxine (Austral.), **Summer's Eve**, Topionic (Span.), Topionic Gin (Span.), Videne (G.B.), Viodine (Austral.), Viraban (Austral.)

Primary Use: *Systemic*: Iodide and iodine are effective in the diagnosis and management of thyroid disease, in the short-term management of respiratory tract disease, and in some instances, of fungal infections. *Ophthalmic*: Topical iodide and iodine solutions are used primarily as a chemical cautery in the treatment of herpes simplex.

Ocular Side Effects:
   A. Systemic Administration—Oral
     1. Decreased vision
     2. Decreased accommodation
     3. Exophthalmos
     4. Nonspecific ocular irritation
       a. Lacrimation
       b. Ocular pain
       c. Burning sensation
     5. Eyelids or conjunctiva
       a. Allergic reactions
       b. Hyperemia
       c. Conjunctivitis—nonspecific
       d. Edema
       e. Angioneurotic edema
       f. Urticaria
       g. Exfoliative dermatitis
       h. Nodules
     6. Keratitis sicca
     7. Punctate keratitis
     8. Hemorrhagic iritis
     9. Hypopyon
    10. Vitreous opacities

　　　11. Ocular teratogenic effects (radioactive iodides)
　　　12. Scleral thinning
　B. Systemic Administration—Intravenous
　　　1. Those mentioned for oral administration
　　　2. Visual fields
　　　　a. Scotomas
　　　　b. Constriction
　　　　c. Hemianopsia
　　　3. Paralysis of accommodation
　　　4. Problems with color vision
　　　　a. Color vision defect
　　　　b. Objects have green tinge
　　　5. Visual hallucinations
　　　6. Mydriasis
　　　7. Retinal degeneration
　　　8. Retinal or macular edema
　　　9. Retinal vasoconstriction
　　　10. Retrobulbar neuritis
　　　11. Toxic amblyopia
　　　12. Optic atrophy
　C. Local Ophthalmic Use or Exposure
　　　1. Decreased vision
　　　2. Keratitis bullosa
　　　3. Eyelids or conjunctiva
　　　　a. Allergic reactions
　　　　b. Blepharoconjunctivitis
　　　　c. Edema
　　　　d. Urticaria
　　　4. Irritation
　　　　a. Lacrimation
　　　　b. Hyperemia
　　　　c. Ocular pain
　　　　d. Edema
　　　5. Brown corneal discoloration
　　　6. Corneal vascularization
　　　7. Stromal scarring
　　　8. Delayed corneal wound healing

Clinical Significance: Few serious irreversible ocular side effects secondary
to iodide have been reported, except when these agents have been given
intravenously. The severe retinal changes reported in the literature are secondary to a drug septojod (iodines and iodates) that is no longer in use;
however, it was the first drug recognized to cause retinal pigmentary degeneration (Duke-Elder and MacFaul). When currently available products are
given orally, retinal findings are probably nonexistent. Allergic reactions

to these agents are often of rapid onset and not uncommon. These may occur at small doses with responses occurring within minutes. A delayed hypersensitivity reaction may occur causing iododerma with tender pustules, vesicles, and nodular lesions. This has been associated with keratitis sicca, hemorrhagic iritis, and vitreous opacities.

References:
Balázs, G., Kincses, E., and Kósa, C.: Iatrogenic diseases caused by iodine. Orv. Hetil. *108*:407, 167.

Duke-Elder, S., and MacFaul, P.A.: System of Ophthalmology. (Eds.): Sir Stewart Duke-Elder, C.V. Mosby, Co., St. Louis, 1972, Vol. XIII, p. 957.

Gerber, M.: Ocular reactions following iodide therapy. Am. J. Ophthalmol. *43*:879, 1957.

Goldberg, H.K.: Iodism with severe ocular involvement. Report of a case. Am. J. Ophthalmol. *22*:65,1939.

Grant, W.M., and Schuman, J.S.: Toxicology of the Eye. 4th Ed. Charles C. Thomas (Ed.), Springfield, IL, 1993, pp. 833–834.

Inman, W.H.W.: Iododerma. Br. J. Dermatol. *91*:709, 1974.

Kincaid, M.C., et al.: Iododerma of the conjunctiva and skin. Ophthalmology *88*:1216, 1981.

Class: Contraceptives

Generic Name: Combination products of estrogens and progestogens.

Proprietary Name: Anovlar (Ital.), **Brevicon** (Canad.), Demulen (Canad., S. Afr.), Eugynon (Ital., Span.), Loestrin (G.B.), Loestrin 1.5/30 (Canad.), **Loestrin 21 1.5/30, Loestrin 21 1/20, Loestrin Fe 1.5/30, Loestrin Fe 1/20, Lo/Ovral, Lo/Ovral-28**, Microgynon (Austral., Ital., Neth., Span., Switz.), Microgynon 21 (Germ.), Microgynon 28 (Germ.), Microgynon 30 (G.B., Ire.), Microgynon ED (Austral.), Minovlar ED (S. Afr.), Min-Ovral (Canad.), Min-Ovral 28 (Canad.), Modicon (Neth.), **Modicon 21, Modicon 28**, Norinyl-1 (Austral., G.B.), Norinyl-1/28 (Austral., S. Afr.), Norinyl 1/50 (Canad.), **Norinyl 1 + 35, Norinyl 1 + 50, Norinyl 1 + 35 28-Day, Norinyl 1 + 50 28-Day**, Norinyl 1/50 28-Day (Canad.), Norlestrin 1/50 (Canad.), **Norlestrin 21 2.5/50, Norlestrin 28 1/50, Norlestrin 21 1/50, Norlestrin Fe 1/50, Norlestrin Fe 2.5/50**, Orlest 21 (Germ.), Orthonett Novum (Swed.), Ortho-Novin 1/50 (G.B.), **Ortho-Novum 1/35** (Fr.), **Ortho-Novum 1/50** (Austral., Canad., Germ., Neth., Switz.), **Ortho-Novum 1/35 28-Day, Ortho-Novum 1/50 28-Day** (Canad.), **Ovcon 35, Ovcon 50, Ovcon 35 28-Day, Ovcon 50 28-Day, Ovral** (Canad., S. Afr.), **Ovral 28** (Canad.), Ovran (G.B., Ire.), Ovran 30 (G.B., Ire.), Ovranet (Ital.), Ovranette (G.B., Ire.), Ovulen (Switz.), Ovulen 50 (Neth.), Ovysmen (Switz.), Ovysmen 0.5/35 (G.B., Germ.), Ovysmen 1/35 (Germ.)

Primary Use: These hormonal agents are used in the treatment of amenorrhea, dysfunctional uterine bleeding, premenstrual tension, dysmenorrhea, hypogonadism, and most commonly, as oral contraceptives.

Ocular Side Effects:
   A. Systemic Administration
      1. Decreased vision
      2. Retinal vascular disorders
         a. Occlusion
         b. Thrombosis
         c. Hemorrhage
         d. Retinal or macular edema
         e. Spasms
         f. Acute macular neuroretinopathy
         g. Periphlebitis
      3. Visual fields
         a. Scotomas—central or paracentral
         b. Constriction
         c. Quadrantanopsia or hemianopsia
         d. Enlarged blind spot
      4. Retrobulbar or optic neuritis
      5. Diplopia
      6. Papilledema secondary to pseudotumor cerebri
      7. Pupils
         a. Mydriasis—may precipitate narrow-angle glaucoma
         b. Anisocoria
      8. Decreased tolerance to contact lenses
      9. Uveitis
     10. Problems with color vision
         a. Color vision defect, red-green or yellow-blue defect
         b. Objects have blue tinge
         c. Colored haloes around lights—mainly blue
     11. Eyelids or conjunctiva
         a. Allergic reactions
         b. Edema
         c. Hyperpigmentation
         d. Photosensitivity
         e. Angioneurotic edema
         f. Urticaria
         g. Lupoid syndrome
         h. Erythema multiforme
         i. Ptosis
     12. Myopia
     13. Exophthalmos

14. Paralysis of extraocular muscles
15. Nystagmus

Clinical Significance: A higher incidence of migraine, thrombophlebitis, and pseudotumor cerebri occurs in women taking oral contraceptives than in a comparable population. A higher incidence of ocular side effects associated with these three entities is therefore probable. There is some evidence that combination oral contraceptives that contain more progestins have fewer side effects than those that contain mainly estrogens. There may be a relationship between women taking oral contraceptives and a decreased tolerance to wearing contact lenses. Most of the other ocular side effects listed are based on clinical reports of possible adverse reactions. Probably many of these are true ocular side effects, but at present, most must be assumed to be only possible and await further documentation. With long-term use, there are data that suggest that these agents cause decreased color perception, mainly blue and yellow, and prolonged photostress recovery times. If a patient has a transient ischemic attack, the oral contraceptive may need to be discontinued since the incidence of strokes is significantly increased. In the Registry and the literature, there are cases that implicate these drugs in causing macular edema. A number of these patients have been rechallenged with recurrence of the edema. Rait and O'Day state that most patients with acute macular neuroretinopathy have been taking oral contraception medication in addition to other possible causative factors. They postulate the "pill" as a possible cofactor. There is a suggestion without definite proof that pregnancy causes progression of retinitis pigmentosa. Since these oral contraceptives cause a "pseudo-pregnancy," there is a question whether they may also cause progression of this retinal disease. However, there is no proof of this and, in all probability, these agents are safe for the retinitis pigmentosa patient to use. In a few cases, the courts have ruled that a cause-and-effect relationship between the use of oral contraceptives and retinal vascular abnormalities exists. Therefore, some patients with retinal vascular abnormalities probably should give informed consent before receiving these medications. If retinal vascular abnormalities develop, the use of these drugs in that patient may need to be re-evaluated. The Registry has received numerous case reports of cataracts possibly related to the administration of oral contraceptives; however, recent data by Klein, Klein, and Ritter show no evidence to support this. In fact, oral contraceptives may even have a modest protective effect on the lens. Tucker, et al. postulate that these hormonal factors have a limited role in the causation of ocular malignancies.

References:
Byrne, E.: Retinal migraine and the pill. Med. J. Aust. 2:659, 1979.
Chakrapani, K., et al.: Ovulation-associated uveitis. Br. J. Ophthalmol. 66:320, 1982.

Chilvers, E., and Rudge, P.: Cerebral venous thrombosis and subarachnoid haemorrhage in users of oral contraceptives. Br. Med. J. *292*:524, 1986.

Hartge, P., et al.: Case-control study of female hormones and eye melanoma. KEY Ophthalmol. *5(1)*:18, 1990.

Klein, B.E.K., Klein, R., and Ritter, L.L.: Is there evidence of an estrogen effect on age-related lens opacities? Arch. Ophthalmol. *112*:85–91, 1994.

Lalive d'Epinay, S.P., and Trub, P.: Retinale vaskulare Komplicationen bei oralen Kontrazeptiva. Klin. Monatsbl. Augenheilkd. *188*:394, 1986.

Perry, H.D., and Mallen, F.J.: Cilioretinal artery occlusion associated with oral contraceptives. Am. J. Ophthalmol. *84*:56, 1977.

Petursson, G.J., Fraunfelder, F.T., and Meyer, S.M.: 6. Oral contraceptives. Ophthalmology *88*:368, 1981.

Rait, J.L., and O'Day, J.: Acute macular neuroretinopathy. Aust. N. Z. J. Ophthalmol. *15*:337–340, 1987.

Rock, T., Dinar, Y., and Romen, M.: Retinal periphlebitis after hormonal treatment. Ann. Ophthalmol. *21*:75–76, 1989.

Snir, M., et al.: Retinal manifestations of thrombotic thrombocytopenic purpura (TTP) following use of contraceptive treatment. Ann. Ophthalmol. *17*:109, 1985.

Stowe, G.C., III, Zakov, Z.N., and Albert, D.M.: Central retinal vascular occlusion associated with oral contraceptives. Am. J. Ophthalmol. *86*:798, 1978.

Tagawa, H., Yoshida, A., and Takahashi, M.: A case of bilateral branch vein occlusion due to long-standing use of oral contraceptives. Folia Ophthalmol. Jpn. *32*:1951, 1981.

Takahashi, H., Sakai, F., and Sakuragi, S.: A case of retinal branch vein occlusion associated with oral contraceptives. Folia Ophthalmol. Jpn. *34*:2670, 1983

Generic Name: Levonorgestrel

Proprietary Name: Follistrel (Swed.), Microlut (Austral., Germ., Ire., Ital., Switz.), Microval (Austral, Fr., G.B., Ire., S. Afr.), Mikro-30 (Germ.), Neogest (G.B.), Norgeston (G.B.), **Norplant** (Swed.), **Ovrette**

Primary Use: Synthetic progestin given as an intradermal implant that acts as a long-term contraceptive agent.

Ocular Side Effects:
A. Subdermal Implantation
   1. Blurred vision
   2. Papilledema—pseudotumor cerebri
   3. Diplopia

Clinical Significance: A recent publication by Alder, Fraunfelder, and Buchhalter suggests that 57 cases of pseudotumor cerebri or papilledema have been reported from a spontaneous reporting system, possibly due to levonorgestrel. All patients were female with a mean age of 23 years (range, 16 to 34 years), with a mean levonorgestrel treatment of 175 days (range, 9 to 616 days) before the onset of pseudotumor. Visual field defects were present in at least 12 cases, which were primarily enlarged blind spots. Diplopia, usually due to sixth nerve paresis, was present in 16 cases. However, there were at least 140 cases of blurred vision reported with patients taking this agent. The problem, of course, with this type of data is that pseudotumor cerebri occurs in this age group of persons without obesity at a rate of approximately 3.3 per hundred thousand per year. Therefore, a report of 57 cases, much of the data incomplete, is suspect. Regardless, this is an abnormally high number of cases. This drug first came on the market in 1991, and in 1994 the manufacturer first released the possible association of this drug with pseudotumor cerebri. In fact, they state that in patients who have vision disturbances or headaches, especially headaches that change in frequency, pattern, severity, or persistence, it is particularly important to view the optic nerves of these patients. Also, they suggest that patients who develop papilledema or pseudotumor cerebri have the implants removed. There are cases in this series in which pseudotumor cleared after removal of the implant, but then recurred months later.

References:

Alder, J.B., Fraunfelder, F.T., and Buchhalter, J.R.: Levonorgestrel implants and idiopathic intracranial hypertension. Submitted to the New Engl. J. of Med., 1995.

Physicians' Desk Reference, 48th Ed., Medical Economics Data Publication Company, Montvale, New Jersey, 1994, pp. 2564-2568.

Class: Ovulatory Agents

Generic Name: Clomiphene (Clomifene)

Proprietary Name: **Clomid** (Austral., Canad., Fr., G.B., Ital., Neth., S. Afr., Switz.), Clomivid (Swed.), Dyneric (Germ.), **Milophene**, Omifin (Span.), Pergotime (Fr., Germ., Swed.), Prolifen (Ital.), **Serophene** (Canad., G.B., Neth., S. Afr., Switz.)

Primary Use: This synthetic nonsteroidal agent is effective in the treatment of anovulation.

Ocular Side Effects:

    A. Systemic Administration
        1. Visual sensations
           a. Flashing lights
           b. Scintillating scotomas
           c. Distortion of images secondary to sensations of waves or glare
           d. Various colored lights—mainly silver
           e. Phosphene stimulation

      f. Prolongation of after image

      g. Entoptic phenomenon

   2. Decreased vision

   3. Mydriasis

   4. Visual fields

      a. Scotomas—central, paracentral, centrocecal

      b. Constriction

   5. Photophobia

   6. Diplopia

   7. Eyelids or conjunctiva

      a. Allergic reactions

      b. Urticaria

      c. Loss of eyelashes or eyebrows

   8. Decreased tolerance to contact lenses

   9. Ocular teratogenic effects

      a. Retinal aplasia

      b. Cyclopia

      c. Nystagmus

Clinical Significance: Clomiphene appears to have a unique effect on the retina that may occur in up to 10% of patients. This consists of any or all of the following: flashing lights, glare, various colored lines (often silver), multiple images, prolonged after-images, "like looking through heat waves," objects have "comet" tails, phosphene stimulation, and scintillating scotomas identical to migraine. These effects may occur as early as 48 hours after taking this agent and are reversible after stopping the medication. Transitory and prolonged decreased vision have also been reported. With prolonged use (years), vision loss in the 20/40-60 range may occur (etiology unknown), which may be slow to recover. Cases in the Registry of irreversibility are not well documented. Bilateral acute reversible loss of vision, even in the light perception range, is a rare event. Mydriasis is common, but of a mild degree and reversible. Of major clinical significance are the unilateral or bilateral scotomas and visual field constriction. In general, this side effect requires discontinuing the medication. Usually, the patient refuses to take further medication and the long-term sequelae, if the drug is continued, is unclear. Decreased contact lens wear may be due to clomiphene's ability to inhibit mucus production. Monocular and binocular diplopia has been reported but is not well documented. While the literature contains references to cataractogenic potential of this agent, in part, due to its chemical structure, as with retinal spasms and phlebitis, a drug-related cause has not been proven. It is of interest, however, that classic scintillating scotoma occurs secondary to clomiphene. While we have a few cases of retrobulbar and optic neuritis in the Registry, these are in females in the multiple sclerosis age group and a cause-and-effect relationship is conjecture. There is only one well-documented case in the Registry of this agent

causing bilateral elevated intraocular pressure. This drug has ocular teratogenic effects. It has been reported that about 1% of patients are forced to
stop taking it secondary to ocular side effects.

References:

Asch, R.H., and Greenblatt, R.B.: Update on the safety and efficacy of clomiphene
citrate as a therapeutic agent. J. Reprod. Med. *17*:175, 1976.

Kistner, R.W.: The use of clomiphene citrate in the treatment of anovulation. Semin.
Drug Treatment *3(2)*: 159, 1973.

Kurachi, K., et al.: Congenital maliformations of newborn infants after clomiphene-
induced ovulation. Fertility and Sterility. *40(2)*:187-189, 1983.

Laing, I.A., et al.: Clomiphene and congenital retinopathy. Lancet 2:1107, 1981.

Piskazeck, V.K., and Leitsmann, H.: Über die Behandlung der funktionellen Sterilität
mit Clostylbegyt. Zentralbl. Gynaekol. *98*:904, 1976.

Roch, L.M., II, et al.: Visual changes associated with clomiphene citrate therapy. Arch.
Ophthalmol. *77*:14, 1967.

Rock, T., Dinar, Y., Romen, M.: Retinal periphlebitis after hormonal treatment. Ann.
Ophthalmol. *21*:75-76, 1989.

Van Der Merwe, J.V.: The effect of clomiphene and conjugated oestrogens on cervical
mucus. SA Medical Journal *60(9)*:347-349, 1981.

Class: Thyroid Hormones

Generic Name: 1. Dextrothyroxine; 2. Levothyroxine; 3. Liothyronine; 4.
Liotrix; 5. Thyroglobulin; 6. Thyroid

Proprietary Name: 1. **Choloxin** (Canad.), Dynothel (Germ.), Eulipos
(Germ.), Lisolipin (Ital.); 2. Dexnon (Span.), Eferox (Germ.), Eltroxin
(Canad., G.B., Ire., S. Afr., Switz.), Euthyrox (Germ., Neth.), Eutirox (Ital.),
Lévothyrox (Fr.), Levaxin (Swed.), **Levothroid** (Span.), Levotirox (Ital.),
Levoxine, Oroxine (Austral.), **Synthroid** (Canad.), Thevier (Germ.),
Thyrax (Neth., Span.); 3. Cynomel (Fr.), **Cytomel** (Canad., Neth.), Ter-
troxin (Austral., G.B., Ire., S. Afr.), Ti-Tre (Ital.), Triiodothyronine Injection
(G.B.), **Triostat**; 4. **Euthroid, Thyrolar**; 5. Proloid (Canad., S. Afr.), Pro-
loide (Span.); 6. Cinetic (Ital.), **S-P-T (pork)**, Thyranon (Span.), Thyreoid-
Dispert (Germ.)

Primary Use: These thyroid hormones are effective in the replacement therapy of thyroid deficiencies such as hypothyroidism and simple goiter. Dextrothyroxine is also effective in the management of hypercholesterolemia.

Ocular Side Effects:
   A. Systemic Administration
      1. Decreased vision
      2. Eyelids or conjunctiva
         a. Hyperemia

      b. Edema

      c. Blepharospasm

  3. Photophobia

  4. Myasthenic neuromuscular blocking effect

      a. Paralysis of extraocular muscles

      b. Ptosis

      c. Diplopia

  5. Exophthalmos

  6. Visual hallucinations

  7. Papilledema secondary to pseudotumor cerebri (levothyroxine)

Clinical Significance: Serious CNS adverse effects, including psychosis with hallucinations, have appeared soon after initiation of thyroid replacement therapy in hypothyroid patients with an underlying psychiatric disorder. Prepubertal and peripubertal hypothyroid children may be susceptible to pseudotumor cerebri when beginning levothyroxine-replacement therapy. Petit mal status epilepticus with rapid rhythmic eyelid fluttering and blinking occurred in a patient approximately 1 week after starting levothyroxine therapy. Generally, all these eye symptoms clear within a few months after discontinuing the medication.

References:

Hymes, L.C., Warshaw, B.L., and Schwartz, J.F.: Pseudotumor cerebri and thyroid-replacement therapy. N. Engl. J. Med. *309*:732, 1983.

Josephson, A.M., and MacKensie, T.B.: Thyroid-induced mania in hypothyroid patients. Br. J. Psychiatry *137*:222, 1980.

Kaeser, H.E.: Drug-induced myasthenic syndromes. Acta Neurol. Scand. *70*(Suppl. 100):39,1984.

McVie, R.: Pseudotumor cerebri and thyroid-replacement therapy. N. Engl. J. Med. *309*:731, 1983.

Sundaram, M.B.M., Hill, A., and Lowry, N.: Thyroxine-induced petit mal status epilepticus. Neurology *35*:1792, 1985.

Van Dop, C., et al.: Pseudotumor cerebri associated with initiation of levothyroxine therapy for juvenile hypothyroidism. N. Engl. J. Med. *308*:1076, 1983.

VIII Agents Affecting Blood Formation and Coagulability

Class: Agents Used to Treat Deficiency Anemias

Generic Name: Cobalt

Proprietary Name: None

Primary Use: This agent is used in the treatment of iron-deficiency anemia and as a dye in tattoos.

Ocular Side Effects:
   A. Systemic Administration
      1. Decreased vision
      2. Eyelids or conjunctiva
         a. Allergic reactions
         b. Photosensitivity
         c. Urticaria
      3. Uveitis (skin tattoo)

Clinical Significance: Cobalt is now only occasionally used since significant systemic side effects occur and safer drugs are currently available. Only rarely are ocular side effects due to cobalt therapy seen, and decreased vision is the most common complaint. One case of possible cobalt-induced optic atrophy with retinal and choroidal changes has been reported. Rorsman, et al. reported three cases of uveitis associated with cobalt skin tattooing. The tattoos were removed in two patients, with improvement of the uveitis.

References:
Camarasa, J.G., and Alomar, A.: Photosensitization to cobalt in a bricklayer. Contact Dermatitis 7:154, 1981.
Gilman, A.G., Goodman, L.S., and Gilman, A. (Eds.): The Pharmacological Basis of Therapeutics. 6th Ed., New York, Macmillan, 1980, pp. 1326–1327.
Hjorth, N.: Contact dermatitis in children. Acta Derm. Venereol. 95(Suppl.):36, 1981.

Light, A., Oliver, M., and Rachmilewitz, E.A.: Optic atrophy following treatment with cobalt chloride in a patient with pancytopenia and hypercellular marrow. Isr. J. Med. Sci. 8:61, 1972.

Rorsman, H., et al.: Tattoo granuloma and uveitis. Lancet 2:27–28, 1969.

Smith, J.D., Odom, R.B., and Maibach, H.I.: Contact urticaria from cobalt chloride. Arch. Dermatol. 111:1610, 1975.

Walsh, F.B., and Hoyt, W.F.: Clinical Neuro-Ophthalmology. 3rd Ed., Baltimore, Williams & Wilkins, Vol. III, 1969, pp. 2686–2687.

Generic Name: Erythropoietin

Proprietary Name: Epogen, Epoxitin (Ital.), Eprex (Fr., G.B., Ital., Neth., Swed., Switz.), Globuren (Ital.), **Procrit**, Recormon (G.B., Germ., Neth., Swed.)

Primary Use: Recombinant human erythropoietin is widely used in the treatment of anemia in chronic renal failure in dialysis patients.

Ocular Side Effects:
   A. Systemic Administration
       1. Visual hallucinations

Clinical Significance: Patients on hemodialysis receiving erythropoietin develop visual hallucinations. Hallucinations consist of moving objects, such as people, cartoon figures, animals, or birds. These are friendly hallucinations, not terrifying, and occur in patients within 2 to 13 months after starting this drug. Dosages range from 2000 units/week to 4000 units up to 3 times a week. There were instances of positive challenge, rechallenge. A report by Stead from the manufacturer noted they had 11 such reports out of 85,000 patients. They were reluctant, however, to accept a clear-cut cause-and-effect relationship, in part because the patients often were elderly, taking multiple medications, and had multiple other medical problems, some of which could also cause hallucinations. In addition, this agent has not been shown to directly cause any other CNS side effect. Therefore, one must state that this is a possible, but not necessarily a probable, cause-and-effect relationship.

References:
Stead, R.: Erythropoietin and visual hallucinations (reply). N. Engl. J. Med. 325(July 25):285, 1991.

Steinberg, H.: Erythropoietin and visual hallucinations (letter). N. Engl. J. Med. 325: 285, 1991

Generic Name: 1. Ferrocholinate; 2. Ferrous Fumarate; 3. Ferrous Gluconate; 4. Ferrous Succinate; 5. Ferrous Sulfate; 6. Iron Dextran; 7. Iron Sorbitex; 8. Polysaccharide-Iron Complex

Proprietary Name: 1. Emofer (Ital.); 2. Erco-Fer (Swed.), **Feostat**, Ferrocap (G.B.), ferrolande (Germ.), Ferrum (Switz.), Ferrum Hausmann (Germ.), Ferrum Klinge (Germ.), Fersaday (G.B., Ire.), Fersamal (G.B., S. Afr.), Ferumat (Neth.), Fumafer (Fr.), Galfer (G.B.), **Hemocyte**, Neo-Fer (Canad.), Novofumar (Canad.), Palafer (Canad.), Rulofer (Germ.); 3. **Fergon** (Austral., G.B., Ire.), **Ferralet**, Ferrominerase (Germ.), Fertinic (Canad.), Lösferron (Germ.), Novoferrogluc (Canad.); 4. Cerevon (Canad.), Ferrlecit 2 (Germ.), Ferromyn (G.B., Ire.), Ferromyn S (Swed.), Wellcofer (Fr.); 5. Ce-Ferro forte (Germ.), Dreisafer (Germ.), Duroferon (Swed.), Eisen-Diasporal (Germ.), Eisendragees-ratiopharm (Germ.), Eryfer (Germ., Ital., Neth.), Feosol, Feospan (G.B., Ire.), **Feratab**, Fer-In-Sol (Canad., Ire.), Feritard (Austral.), Fero-Grad (Canad.), **Fero-Gradumet** (Neth., Span.), Ferro 66 DL (Germ.), Ferrograd (G.B., Ire.), Ferro-Grad (Ital.), Ferro-Gradumet (Austral., Switz.), Fesofor (S. Afr.), Fespan (Austral.), Haemoprotect (Germ.), Ironorm (G.B.), Liquifer (Neth.), Novoferrosulfa (Canad.), Plastufer (Germ.), Plexafer (Neth.), Resoferix (Germ.), Resoferon (Neth.), **Slow-Fe** (Austral., Canad., G.B., Ire.), Tardyferon (Germ.); 6. Ferrum (Switz.), Imferdex (Switz.), Imferon (Austral., Canad., G.B., Neth.); 7. Jectofer (Canad., Fr., G.B., Germ., Ire., Neth., Swed.), Yectofer (Span.); 8. **Niferex** (G.B., Ire., Span.), **Nu-Iron**

Primary Use: These iron preparations are effective in the prophylaxis and treatment of iron-deficiency anemias.

Ocular Side Effects:
   A. Systemic Administration
      1. Decreased vision (iron dextran)
      2. Yellow-brown discoloration
         a. Sclera
         b. Choroid
      3. Eyelids or conjunctiva (iron dextran)
         a. Erythema
         b. Edema
         c. Angioneurotic edema
         d. Urticaria
      4. Retinal degeneration
   B. Inadvertent Ocular Exposure
      1. Irritation
         a. Hyperemia
         b. Photophobia
         c. Edema
      2. Yellow-brown discoloration or deposits
         a. Eyelids
         b. Conjunctiva

    c. Cornea
    d. Sclera
  3. Hypopyon
  4. Ulceration
    a. Eyelids
    b. Conjunctiva
    c. Cornea

Clinical Significance: Systemically administered iron preparations seldom cause ocular side effects. Adverse ocular reactions have been reported after multiple blood transfusions (over 100), with unusually large amounts of iron in the diet, or with markedly prolonged iron therapy. A few cases of retinitis pigmentosa-like fundal degeneration have been reported. Direct ocular exposure to acidic ferrous salts can cause ocular irritation, but significant ocular side effects rarely occur.

References:
Appel, I., and Barishak, Y.R.: Histopathologic changes in siderosis bulbi. Ophthalmologica *176*:205, 1978.
Brunette, J.R., Wagdi, S., and Lafond, G.: Electroretinographic alterations in retinal metallosis. Can. J. Ophthalmol. *15*:176, 1980.
Declerc, S.S.: Desferrioxamine in ocular siderosis. Br. J. Ophthalmol. *64*:626, 1980.
Kearns, M., and McDonald, R.: Generalized siderosis from an iris foreign body. Aust. J. Ophthalmol. *8*:311, 1980.
Salminen, L., Paasio, P., and Ekfors, T.: Epibulbar siderosis induced by iron tablets. Am. J. Ophthalmol. *93*:660, 1982.
Syversen, K.: Intramuscular iron therapy and tapetoretinal degeneration. Acta Ophthalmol. *57*:358, 1979.
Wolter, J.R.: The lens as a barrier against foreign body reaction. Ophthalmic Surg. *12*: 42, 1981.

Generic Name: Methylene Blue (Methylthionine)

Proprietary Name: Desmoidpillen (Germ.), **Urolene Blue**, Vitableu (Fr.)

Primary Use: *Systemic*: Methylene blue is a weak germicidal agent used in the treatment of methemoglobinemia and "cyanosis anemia" and as a urinary or gastrointestinal antiseptic. It is also used as a dye to demonstrate cerebrospinal fluid fistulae or blocks. *Ophthalmic*: Methylene blue is used as a tissue marker during ocular or lacrimal surgery and has been applied to the conjunctiva to decrease glare during microsurgery.

Ocular Side Effects:
  A. Systemic Administration
    1. Decreased vision
    2. Decreased accommodation

    3. Mydriasis
    4. Papilledema
    5. Diplopia
    6. Paresis of extraocular muscles
    7. Accommodative spasm
    8. Optic atrophy
    9. Blue-gray discoloration of ocular tissue—especially vitreous
       and retina
   10. Problems with color vision—objects have blue tinge
   11. Subconjunctival or retinal hemorrhages secondary to drug-
       induced anemia
   B. Local Ophthalmic Use or Exposure
    1. Irritation
       a. Lacrimation
       b. Edema
       c. Burning sensation
    2. Blue discoloration or staining
       a. Eyelid margins
       b. Conjunctiva
       c. Corneal nerves and epithelium

Clinical Significance: Severe ocular side effects due to methylene blue have only been reported with intrathecal or intraventricular injections. The most common ocular side effects after intravenous administration, other than cyanopsia or blue-gray discoloration of ocular tissue, are decreased vision, mydriasis, and decreased accommodation. Infrequent use of topical ocular application in low concentrations (1%) is almost free of ocular side effects; however, irritation may be so severe that a local anesthetic may be required for the patient's comfort.

References:
Evans, J.P., and Keegan, H.R.: Danger in the use of intrathecal methylene blue. JAMA *174*:856, 1960.
Lubeck, M.J.: Effects of drugs on ocular muscles. Int. Ophthalmol. Clin. *11(2)*:35, 1971.
Morax, S., Limon, S., and Forest, A.: Exogenous conjunctival pigmentation by methylene blue. Arch. Ophthalmol. *37*:708A, 1977.
Norn, M.S.: Methylene blue (Methylthionine) vital staining of the cornea and conjunctiva. Acta Ophthalmol. *45*:347, 1967.
Pasticier-Florquin, B., et al.: Ocular tattooing from abuse of methylene blue collyrium. Bull. Soc. Ophthalmol. Fr. *77*:147, 1977.
Walsh, F.B., and Hoyt, W.F.: Clinical Neuro-Ophthalmology. 3rd Ed., Baltimore, Williams & Wilkins, Vol III, 1969, pp. 2706–2707.

Class: Anticoagulants

Generic Name: 1. Acenocoumarol; 2. Dicumarol (Dicoumarol); 3. Ethyl Biscoumacetate; 4. Phenprocoumon; 5. Warfarin

Proprietary Name: 1. Sinthrome (G.B., Ire.), Sintrom (Canad., Fr., Germ., Ital., Neth., Span., Switz.); 2. Apekumarol (Swed.); 3. Tromexane (Fr.); 4. Marcoumar (Neth., Switz.), Marcumar (Germ., Span.); 5. Aldocumar (Span.), **Coumadin** (Austral., Canad., Germ., Ital., S. Afr.), Coumadine (Fr.), Marevan (Austral., G.B.), **Panwarfarin**, **Sofarin**, Waran (Swed.), Warfilone (Canad.)

Primary Use: These coumarin derivatives are used as anticoagulants in the prophylaxis and treatment of venous thrombosis.

Ocular Side Effects:
 A. Systemic Administration
  1. Subconjunctival or retinal hemorrhages
   a. Secondary to drug-induced anticoagulation
   b. Secondary to drug-induced anemia
  2. Eyelids or conjunctiva
   a. Allergic reactions
   b. Conjunctivitis—nonspecific
   c. Urticaria
   d. Necrosis
   e. Bleeding
  3. Hyphema
  4. Problems with color vision—color vision defect (acenocoumarol)
  5. Lacrimation (dicumarol, warfarin)
  6. Decreased vision (dicumarol, warfarin)
  7. Ocular teratogenic effect (warfarin)
   a. Optic atrophy
   b. Cataracts
   c. Microphthalmia
   d. Blindness

Clinical Significance: Ocular side effects due to coumarin anticoagulants are uncommon. Massive retinal hemorrhages have been reported, especially in diseased tissue with possible capillary fragility (diabetic disciform degeneration of the macula). In addition, spontaneous hyphema developed with or without iris fixed lenses. A potentially dangerous association between herpes zoster infection and oral anticoagulant therapy has also been found. Even so, as extensively as this group of agents has been used, only a few major adverse ocular side effects have been reported. These drugs may be discontinued before ocular surgery to prevent increased hemorrhaging in patients with diabetes or hypertension; however, it is now questioned if this is necessary for most other patients. There are data to suggest that this group of drugs can cause teratogenic effects. Although the teratogenic effects appear to be most severe when warfarin is taken during the first trimester, the effects can occur anytime during gestation. Conradi-Hunermann syndrome or chondrodysplasia punctata and Dandy-Walker syndrome with their associated ocular defects have been reported in offspring of patients receiving warfarin therapy throughout their pregnancies.

References:
Blumenkopf, B., and Lockhart, W.S.,Jr.: Herpes zoster infection and use of oral anticoagulants. A potentially dangerous association. JAMA 250:936, 1983.

Gainey, S.P., et al.: Ocular surgery on patients receiving long-term warfarin therapy. Am. J. Ophthalmol. 108:142–146, 1989.

Hall, D.L., Steen, W.H., Jr., and Drummond, J.W.: Anticoagulants and cataract surgery. Ann. Ophthalmol. 12:759, 1980.

Harrod, M.J.E., and Sherrod, P.S.: Warfarin embryopathy in siblings. Obstet. Gynecol. 57:673, 1981.

Kaplan, L.C.: Congenital Dandy Walker malformation associated with first trimester warfarin: A case report and literature review. Teratology 32:333, 1985.

Kleincbrecht, J.: Zur Teratogenitat von Cumarin-Derivaten. Dtsch. Med. Wochenschr. 107:1929, 1982.

Koehler, M.P., and Sholiton, D.B.: Spontaneous hyphema resulting from warfarin. Ann. Ophthalmol. 15:858–859, 1983.

Leath, M.C.: Coumarin skin necrosis. Texas Med. 79:62, 1983.

Lewis, H., Sloan, S.H., and Foos, R.Y.: Massive intraocular hemorrhage associated with anticoagulation and age-related macular degeneration. Graefe's Arch. Clin. Exp. Ophthalmol. 226:59–64, 1988.

Robinson, G.A., and Nylander, A.: Warfarin and cataract extraction. Br. J. Ophthalmol 73:702–703, 1989.

Schiff, F.S.: Coumadin related spontaneous hyphemas in patients with iris fixated pseudophakos. Ophthalmic Surg. 16:172–173, 1985.

Taylor, R.H., and Gibson, J.M.: Warfarin, spontaneous hyphaemas, and intraocular lenses. Lancet 1:762–763, 1988.

Generic Name: 1. Anisindione; 2. Diphenadione; 3. Phenindione

Proprietary Name: 1. **Miradon**; 3. Dindevan (Austral., G.B.), Pindione (Fr.)

Primary Use: These indandione derivatives are used as anticoagulants in the prophylaxis and treatment of venous thrombosis.

Ocular Side Effects:
    A. Systemic Administration
        1. Subconjunctival or retinal hemorrhages
          a. Secondary to drug-induced anticoagulation
          b. Secondary to drug-induced anemia
        2. Decreased vision
        3. Problems with color vision—color vision defect (phenindione)
        4. Paralysis of accommodation

5. Eyelids or conjunctiva
   a. Allergic reactions
   b. Conjunctivitis—nonspecific
   c. Urticaria
   d. Exfoliative dermatitis
   e. Necrosis

Clinical Significance: The most common adverse ocular reaction due to these indandione anticoagulants is ocular hemorrhage, which is just an extension of the intended pharmacologic activity of these drugs. This is probably more common in ocular conditions with associated capillary fragility, such as disciform macular degeneration. Most other ocular side effects are uncommon, insignificant, and reversible. To date, no ocular teratogenic effects have been reported with this group of anticoagulants.

References:
Gilman, A.G., Goodman, L.S., and Gilman, A. (Eds.): The Pharmacological Basis of Therapeutics. 6th Ed., New York, Macmillan, 1980, p. 1359.

Laroche, J., and Laroche, C.: Nouvelles recherches sur la modification de la vision des couleurs sous l'action des medicaments dose thrapeutique. Ann. Pharm. Fr. *35*: 173, 1977.

McEvoy, G.K. (Ed.): American Hospital Formulary Service Drug Information 87. Bethesda, American Society of Hospital Pharmacists, 1987, p. 679.

Renick, A.M., Jr.: Anticoagulant-induced necrosis of skin and subcutaneous tissues: Report of two cases and review of the English literature. South. Med. J. *69*:775, 1978.

Reynolds, J.E.F. (Ed.): Martindale: The Extra Pharmacopoeia. 28th Ed., London, Pharmaceutical Press, 1982, pp. 770–774

Generic Name: Heparin

Proprietary Name: Ateroclar (Ital.), Calcihep (Austral.), Calcilean (Canad.), Calciparin (Germ.), Calciparina (Ital.), Calciparina Choay (Span.), **Calciparine** (Austral., Canad., Fr., G.B., S. Afr., Switz.), Calparine (Neth.), Canusal (G.B.), Caprin (Austral.), Chemyparin (Ital.), Clarisco (Ital.), Croneparina (Ital.), Disebrin (Ital.), Ecasolv (Ital.), Eparical (Ital.), Eparinovis (Ital.), HpaGel (Switz.), Hepalean (Canad.), Hepalean-Lok (Canad.), Hep-Flush (G.B.), **Hep-Lock**, **Hep-Lock U/P (Preservative-Free)**, Heplok (G.B., Ire.), **Hep-Pak**, Hep-Rinse (Ire.), Hepsal (G.B.), Lioton (Ital.), **Liquaemin Sodium**, Liquemin (Ital., Neth.), Liquemin N (Germ.), Liqumine (Fr., Switz.), Liquemine (Span.), Minihep (G.B., Ire., Neth.), Minihep Calcium (G.B., Ire.), Monoparin (G.B.), Monoparin-Calcium (G.B.), Multiparin (G.B.), Noparin (Swed.), Percase (Fr.), Praecivenin (Germ.), Pularin (S. Afr.), Pump-Hep (G.B., Ire.), Thrombareduct (Germ.), Thrombophob (Germ., Switz.), Thrombo- Vetren (Germ.), Tromboliquine (Neth.), Unihep

(G.B., Ire.), Uniparin (Austral., G.B.), Uniparin-Ca (Austral.), Uniparin-Calcium (G.B.), Vetren (Germ.), Zuk Hepagel/salbe (Germ.)

Primary Use: This complex organic acid inhibits the blood-clotting mechanism and is used in the prophylaxis and treatment of venous thrombosis.

Ocular Side Effects:
  A. Systemic Administration
      1. Subconjunctival or retinal hemorrhages
          a. Secondary to drug-induced anticoagulation
          b. Secondary to drug-induced anemia
      2. Eyelids or conjunctiva
          a. Allergic reactions
          b. Conjunctivitis—nonspecific
          c. Angioneurotic edema
          d. Urticaria
          e. Lyell's syndrome
          f. Necrosis
      3. Decreased vision
      4. Lacrimation
      5. Hyphema
  B. Local Ophthalmic Use or Exposure—Subconjunctival Injection
      1. Subconjunctival or periocular hemorrhages
      2. Subconjunctival scarring
      3. Exacerbation of primary disease
      4. Decreased intraocular pressure—minimal

Clinical Significance: Ocular side effects due to systemic heparin are few and usually of little consequence. Ocular hemorrhage is the most serious adverse reaction and is probably more common in ocular conditions with increased capillary fragility. Subconjunctival or periocular hemorrhage is the most common adverse reaction due to subconjunctival heparin injections. It is more common after the third or fourth injection and seldom prevents continuation of this mode of heparin therapy. Reports of decreased vision are rare, and the cause of such is unknown. A single case of sudden onset severe keratoconjunctivitis sicca associated with the use of intravenous and subcutaneous heparin injections has been received by the Registry. Hyphema in an otherwise normal eye was seen 1 hour after 10,000 units of heparin were administered intravenously.

References:
Aronson, S.B., and Elliott, J.H.: Ocular Inflammation. St. Louis, C.V. Mosby, 1972, pp. 91–92.
Leung, A.: Toxic epidermal necrolysis associated with maternal use of heparin. JAMA 253:201, 1985.

Levine, L.E., et al.: Heparin-induced cutaneous necrosis unrelated to injection sites. Arch. Dermatol. *119*:400, 1983.

Lipson, M.L.: Toxicity of systemic agents. Int. Ophthalmol. Clin. *11(2)*:159, 1971.

Slusher, M.M., and Hamilton, R.W.: Spontaneous hyphema during hemodialysis. N. Engl. J. Med. *293*:561, 1975.

Zurcher, K., and Krebs, A.: Cutaneous Side Effects of Systemic Drugs. Basel, S. Karger, 1980, pp. 18–19, 300–303

Generic Name: Streptokinase

Proprietary Name: Kabikinase (Austral., Fr., G.B., Germ., Ire., Ital., S. Afr., Span., Swed., Switz.), **Streptase** (Austral., Canad., Fr., G.B., Germ., Ire., Ital., Neth., S. Afr., Span.)

Primary Use: This protein is used to dissolve thrombi in patients with myocardial infarction, pulmonary embolism, and other thrombo-embolic occlusions of veins and arteries.

Ocular Side Effects:
A. Systemic Administration
  1. Intraocular hemorrhage
  2. Total hyphema
  3. Choroidal hematoma
  4. Vitreous hemorrhage
  5. Periorbital swelling
  6. Eyelids
    a. Urticaria
    b. Rash
    c. Angioneurotic edema
  7. Uveitis
  8. Postoperative ocular bleeding

Clinical Significance: There are a number of reports of streptokinase causing intraocular bleeding, such as hyphemas, vitreous hemorrhages, or choroidal hematomas. Patients who were given this agent have had myocardial infarcts, previous ocular surgery, diabetic retinopathy, telangectatic intraocular vessels, or were elderly. This drug, when administered intravenously, has been well documented in causing cerebral hemorrhages. Marcus and Frederick describe a case of streptokinase-induced tenon's hemorrhage following a retinal detachment surgery. The patient received intravenous streptokinase 2 hours after surgery when he developed a myocardial infarct. Proctor and Joondeph reported bilateral anterior uveitis as an early feature in a patient who developed serum sickness caused by streptokinase. Up to 6% of patients develop serum sickness secondary to streptokinase exposure. Anterior chamber injections of this agent for dissolution of fibrin exudates have had no detectable adverse intraocular effects (Cherfan, et al.). Berger stated that there was intraocular irritation secondary to streptokinase, but it is possible that the drug used was not in as purified a form as is available now. Up to one-third of patients who have received repeat injections of this drug have become hypersensitive to it. This may present itself by periorbital swelling or angioneurotic edema.

References:

Berger, B.: The effect of streptokinase irrigation on experimentally clotted blood in the anterior chamber of human eyes. Acta Ophthalmol. *40*:373–378, 1962.

Boyer, H.K., et al.: Studies on simulated vitreous hemorrhages. Arch. Ophthalmol. *59*: 333–336, 1958.

Cahane, M., et al.: Total hyphaema following streptokinase administration eight days after cataract extraction. Br. J. Ophthalmol. *74*:447, 1990.

Caramelli, B., et al.: Retinal haemorrhage after thrombolytic therapy. Lancet *337*: 1356–1357, 1991.

Cherfan, G.M., et al.: Dissolution of intraocular fibrinous exudate by streptokinase. Ophthalmology *98(6)*:870–874, 1991.

Glikson, M., et al.: Thrombolytic therapy for acute myocardial infarction following recent cataract surgery. Am. Heart J. *121*:1542–1543, 1991.

Marcus, D.M., and Frederick Jr., A.R.: Streptokinase-induced tenon's hemorrhage after retinal detachment surgery. Am. J. Ophthalmol. *118(6)*:815–816, 1994.

Pick, R., et al.: Acute renal failure following repeated streptokinase therapy for pulmonary embolism. West. J. Med. *138*:878–880, 1983.

Proctor, B.D., and Joondeph, B.C.: Bilateral anterior uveitis. A feature of streptokinase-induced serum sickness. N. Engl. J. Med. *330*:576, 1994.

Steinemann, T., et al.: Acute closed-angle glaucoma complicating hemorrhagic choroidal detachment associated with parenteral thrombolytic agents. Am. J. Ophthalmol. *106*:752–753, 1988.

Sunderraj, P.: Intraocular hemorrhage associated with intravenously administered streptokinase. Am. J. Ophthalmol. *112(6)*:734–735, 1991.

Class: Blood Substitutes

Generic Name: Dextran

Proprietary Name: Dextraven (G.B.), Dialens (Fr., Switz.), Eudextran (Ital.), Fisiodex 40 & Fisiodex 70 (Span.), Gentran 40 & Gentran 70 (G.B.), Hmodex (Fr.), **Hyskon** (Canad., G.B., Swed.), Lomodex 40 & Lomodex 70 (G.B.), Longasteril 40 & Longasteril 70 (Germ.), **Macrodex** (Austral., Canad., G.B., Ital., S. Afr., Span., Swed., Switz.), Macrodex RL (Germ.), Onkovertin & Onkovertin N (Germ.), Parenteral D 40 (Germ.), Perfadex (Swed.), Plander & Plander R (Ital.), Plasmacair (Fr.), Plasmodex (Fr.), Promit (Austral., Fr., Germ., Switz.), Promiten (Swed.), Rheofusin (Germ.), Rhomacrodex (Fr.), **Rheomacrodex** (Austral., Canad., G.B., Germ., Ital., S. Afr., Span., Swed., Switz.), Saviosol (Jap.), Solplex 40 & Solplex 70 (Ital.), Thomaedex 40 & Thomaedex 60 (Germ.)

Primary Use: This water-soluble glucose polymer is used for early fluid replacement and for plasma volume expansion in the adjunctive treatment of certain types of shock.

Ocular Side Effects:
A. Systemic Administration
  1. Eyelids or conjunctiva
    a. Erythema
    b. Conjunctivitis—nonspecific
    c. Angioneurotic edema
    d. Urticaria
  2. Nonspecific ocular irritation
    a. Lacrimation
    b. Photophobia
    c. Edema
    d. Burning sensation
  3. Keratitis

Clinical Significance: The most common adverse ocular reaction due to dextran is ocular irritation. An allergic keratitis, which disappeared when the drug was discontinued, has also been reported in several patients.

References:
Blake, J., and Cassidy, H.: Ocular hypersensitivity to dextran. Ir. J. Med. Sci. *148*: 249, 1979.
Fothergill, R., and Heaney, G.A.: Reactions to dextran. Br. Med. J. 2:1502, 1976.
Krenzelok, E.P., and Parker, W.A.: Dextran 40 anaphylaxis. Minn. Med. 58:454, 1975.
Ledoux-Corbusier, M.: L'urticaire medicamenteuse. Brux. Med. 55:629, 1975.
Richter, W., et al.: Adverse reactions to plasma substitutes: Incidence and pathomechanisms. *In* Watkins, J., and Wand, A. (Eds.): Adverse Response to Intravenous Drugs. New York, Grune & Stratton, 1978, pp. 49–70.

Class: Oxytocic Agents

Generic Name: Ergot

Proprietary Name: None

Primary Use: This drug is used to control postpartum and illegal abortion hemorrhages.

Ocular Side Effects:
A. Systemic Administration
  1. Decreased vision
  2. Paralysis of accommodation

 3. Hypermetropia
 4. Pupils
   a. Mydriasis
   b. Miosis
   c. Decreased reaction to light
 5. Toxic amblyopia
 6. Visual fields
   a. Scotomas
   b. Constriction
   c. Enlarged blind spot
 7. Retinal edema
 8. Retinal vasoconstriction
 9. Scintillating scotomas (convulsive form of ergotism)
 10. Diplopia (convulsive form of ergotism)
 11. Nystagmus (convulsive form of ergotism)
 12. Cataracts (convulsive form of ergotism)

Clinical Significance: Ergot preparations have caused numerous ocular side effects, primarily in overdose situations for attempted abortions. In general, these adverse ocular reactions are usually transitory and rarely permanent. While amblyopia may occur, it is reversible in most instances. To date, no solid data have incriminated medically administered ergot in causing lens changes. A convulsive form of ergotism described by Pentschew and reviewed by Grant and Schuman describes cataracts, diplopia, nystagmus, and scintillating scotomas in an epidemic ergot intoxication due to contaminated grain. A single case of optic atrophy has been reported by Kravitz.

References:
Kohn, B.A.: The differential diagnosis of cataracts in infancy and childhood. Am. J. Dis. Child. *130*:184, 1976.
Kravitz, D.: Neuroretinitis associated with symptoms of ergot poisoning. Report of a case. Arch. Ophthalmol. *13*:201, 1935.
Grant, W.M., and Schuman, J.S.: Toxicology of the Eye. Charles C. Thomas, Springfield, IL. 1993, pp. 640–641.
Pentschew, A.: Intoxikationen. Handbuch der speziellen pathologischen Anatomie und Histologie. *In* Lubarsch O., Henke F., Rossle R. (Eds.): Erkrankungen des zentralen Nervensystems. Berlin, Springer, 1958, vol. 12, pp. 1907–2502.
Reynolds, J.E.F. (Ed.): Martindale: The Extra Pharmacopoeia. 28th Ed., London, Pharmaceutical Press, 1982, pp. 662–663.
Schneider, P.: Beiderseitige Ophthalmoplegia interna, hervorgerufen durch Extractum Secalis cornuti. Munch. Med. Wochenschr. *49*:1620, 1902.
Scott, J.G.: Does ergot cause cataract? Med. Proc. *8*:4, 1962.

IX　Homeostatic and Nutrient Agents

Class: Agents Used to Treat Hyperglycemia

Generic Name: 1. Acetohexamide; 2. Chlorpropamide; 3. Glyburide (Glibenclamide); 4. Tolazamide; 5. Tolbutamide

Proprietary Name: 1. Dimelor (Canad., Ital., S. Afr.), **Dymelor**; 2. Diabemide (Ital.), Diabexan (Ital.), Diabines (Swed.), Diabinese (Fr., Switz.), **Diabinese** (Austral., Canad., G.B., Ital., S. Afr., Span.), Gliconorm (Ital.), Glymese (G.B.), Hypomide (S. Afr.), Normoglic (Ital.), Novopropamide (Canad.); 3. Abbenclamide (S. Afr.), Azuglucon (Germ.), Bastiverit (Germ.), Calabren (G.B.), Daonil (Austral., Fr., G.B., Ire., Ital., Neth., S. Afr., Span., Swed., Switz.), Dia Basan (Germ.), **DiaBeta** (Canad.), Diabetamide (G.B.), Duraglucon N (Germ.), Euglucan (Fr.), Euglucon (Austral., Canad., G.B., Ire., Ital., Neth., S. Afr., Span., Swed., Switz.), Euglucon N (Germ.), Gli-basan (Switz.), Gliben (Ital.), Glibenhexal (Germ.), Gliben-Puren N (Germ.), Gliboral (Ital.), Glimel (Austral.), Glimidstada (Germ.), Glucolon (Span.), Gluconorm (Germ.), Gluco-Tablinen (Germ., Switz.), Glukoreduct (Germ.), Glukovital (Germ.), Glyben (S. Afr.), Glycolande (Germ.), Glycomin (S. Afr.), **Glynase**, Hemi-Daonil (Fr., Neth.), Libanil (G.B.), Malix (G.B.), Melbetese (Ire.), Melix (S. Afr., Switz.), **Micronase**, Miglucan (Fr.), Norglicem (Span.), Orabetic (Germ.), Praeciglucon (Germ.), Semi-Daonil (G.B., Ire., S. Afr., Switz.), Semi-Euglucon (Neth., Switz.), Semi-Euglucon N (Germ.), Semi-Gliben-Puren N (Germ.); 4. Diabewas (Ital.), Norglycin (Germ.), Tolanase (G.B., Ire.), **Tolinase** (Austral., Neth., Swed.); 5. Aglycid (Ital.), Artosin (Germ., Neth.), Diabeton Metilato (Ital.), Dolipol (Fr.), Glyconon (G.B.), Guabeta N (Germ.), Mobenol (Canad.), Novobutamide (Canad.), **Orinase** (Canad.), Rastinon (Austral., G.B., Germ., Ire., Ital., Neth., S. Afr., Span., Swed., Switz.)

Primary Use: These oral hypoglycemic sulfonylureas are effective in the management of selected cases of diabetes mellitus.

Ocular Side Effects:
A. Systemic Administration
1. Decreased vision
2. Paresis of extraocular muscles
3. Diplopia
4. Eyelids or conjunctiva
   a. Allergic reactions
   b. Hyperemia
   c. Conjunctivitis—nonspecific
   d. Edema
   e. Photosensitivity
   f. Purpura
   g. Lupoid syndrome (tolazamide)
   h. Erythema multiforme
   i. Stevens-Johnson syndrome
   j. Exfoliative dermatitis
5. Photophobia
6. Problems with color vision—color vision defect, red-green defect
7. Subconjunctival or retinal hemorrhages secondary to drug-induced anemia
8. Scotomas—central or centrocecal (chlorpropamide, tolbutamide)
9. Retrobulbar or optic neuritis
10. May aggravate Wernicke's syndrome
11. Cataracts
12. Decreased accommodation (glibenclamide)
13. Myopia (glibenclamide)

Clinical Significance: As with other hypoglycemics, the sulfonylureas have few documented toxic effects on the eyes. Adverse ocular reactions are mainly due to drug-induced hypoglycemic attacks. Overall, chlorpropamide has a 6% incidence of untoward reactions, while the incidence of acetohexamide, tolazamide, and tolbutamide is around 3%. Cutaneous reactions due to these drugs are not unusual. While optic nerve disease has been reported in the literature and to the Registry, differentiation of which changes are due to diabetes and which are due to a toxic drug effect is difficult and may be impossible. Regardless, these changes are usually reversible. In susceptible individuals who have low thiamine reserves, hypoglycemic agents can induce Wernicke's encephalopathy, including oculomotor disturbances such as ophthalmoplegia, ptosis, and nystagmus. The transient refractory changes seen secondary to tolbutamide are presumed due to a variation in the water content of the crystalline lens. An increased incidence of posterior subcapsular lens changes was observed in diabetic patients treated with oral hypoglycemics compared with diabetics controlled with diet and insulin. Isaac et al., found an increased risk of cataracts in patients who have used antibiotic agents. Transient myopia and decreased accommodation have been seen due to glibenclamide.

References:

Birch, J., et al.: Acquired color vision defects. *In* Pokorny, J., et al. (Eds.): Congenital and Acquired Color Vision Defects. New York, Grune & Stratton, 1979, p. 243.

George, C.W.: Central scotomata due to chlorpropamide (Diabenese). Arch. Ophthalmol. *69*:773, 1963.

Isaac, N.E., et al.: Exposure to phenothiazine drugs and risk of cataract. Arch. Ophthalmol. *109*:256–260, 1991.

Kanefsky, T.M., and Medoff, S.J.: Stevens-Johnson syndrome and neutropenia with chlorpropamide therapy. Arch. Intern. Med. *140*:1543, 1980.

Kapetansky, F.M.: Refractive changes with tolbutamide. Ohio State Med. J. *59*:275, 1963.

Kwee, I.L., and Nakada, T.: Wernicke's encephalopathy induced by tolazamide. N. Engl. J. Med. *309*:599, 1983.

Paice, B.J., Paterson, K.R., and Lawson, D.H.: Undesired effects of the sulphonylurea drugs. Adverse Drug React. Acute Poisoning Rev. *4*:23, 1985.

Skalka, H.W., and Prchal, J.T. The effect of diabetes mellitus and diabetic therapy on cataract formation. Ophthalmology *88*:117, 1981.

Teller, J., Rasin, M., and Abraham, F.A.: Accommodation insufficiency induced by glybenclamide. Ann. Ophthalmol. *21*:275–276, 1989.

Transient myopia from glibenclamide: Short-sightedness with glibenclamide. International Pharmacy Journal *3*:221–222, 1989.

Wymore, J., and Carter, J.E.: Chlorpropamide-induced optic neuropathy. Arch. Intern. Med. *142*:381, 1982

Generic Name: Insulin

Proprietary Name: Actrap MC (Span.), Actraphane HM (Austral., Fr., Germ., Ital., S. Afr., Switz.), Actraphane MC (Austral.), Actrapid (Swed.), Actrapid HM (Austral., Fr., Germ., Ital., S. Afr., Span., Switz.), Actrapid MC (Austral.), Basal-H-Insulin (Germ.), Bio-Insulin I (Ital.), Bio-Insulin R (Ital.), Depot-H15-Insulin (Germ.), Depot-H-Insulin (Germ.), Depot-Insulin (Germ.), Depot-Insulin Horm (Germ.), Depot-Insulin S (Germ.), Durasuline (Fr.), Endopancrine (Fr.), Endopancrine Zinc Protamine (Fr.), H-Insulin (Germ.), H-Tronin (Germ.), Human Actraphane (G.B., Ire.), Human Actrapid (G.B., Ire.), Human Initard 50/50 (G.B., Ire.), Human Insulatard (G.B., Ire.), Human Mixtard 30/70 (G.B., Ire.), Human Monotard (G.B., Ire.), Human Protaphane (G.B., Ire.), Human Ultratard (G.B., Ire.), Human Velosulin (G.B., Ire.), Huminsulin (Germ.), Huminsulin Basal (Germ.), Huminsulin Basal (NPH) (Switz.), Huminsulin Long (Switz.), Huminsulin Normal (Switz.), Huminsulin Profil (Germ.), Huminsulin Profil I (Switz.), Huminsulin Profil II (Switz.), Huminsulin Profil III (Switz.), Huminsulin Profil IV ((Switz.), Huminsulin Ultralong (Switz.), Humulin 20/80 (S. Afr.),

Humulin 30/70 (Canad., S. Afr.), Humulin 40/60 (S. Afr.), Humulin 70/30, Humulin BR, Humulin I (G.B., Ital.), Humulin L (Austral., Canad., S. Afr.), Humulin Lente (G.B.), Humulin M1 (G.B.), Humulin M2 (G.B.), Humulin M3 (G.B.), Humulin M4 (G.B.), Humulin mix 30/70 (Swed.), Humulin N (Canad., S. Afr.), Humulin NPH (Austral., Swed.), Humulin R (Austral., Canad., Ital., S. Afr.), Humulin Regular (Swed.), Humulin S (G.B.), Humulin U (Canad., S. Afr.), Humulin U Ultralente, Humulin UL (Austral.), Humulin Zn (G.B.), Humulina 10:90 (Span.), Humulina 20:80 (Span.), Humulina 30:70 (Span.), Humulina Lenta (Span.), Humulina NPH (Span.), Humulina Regular (Span.), Humulina Ultralente (Span.), Humuline 10/90 (Neth.), Humuline 20/80 (Neth.), Humuline 30/70 (Neth.), Humuline 40/60 (Neth.), Humuline NPH (Neth.), Humuline Regular (Neth.), Humuline Zink (Neth.), Humutard (Swed.), Hypurin Isophane (Austral., G.B.), Hypurin Lente (G.B.), Hypurin Neutral (Austral., G.B.), Hypurin Protamine Zinc (G.B.), Initard (Switz.), Initard 50/50 (Canad., G.B.), Initard Humaine (Switz.), Initard Human (Austral.), Insulatard (G.B., Germ., Swed., Switz.), Insulatard Huma (Span.), Insulatard Humaine (Fr., Switz.), Insulatard Human (Austral., Germ., Swed.), Insulatard Nordisk (Fr.), Insulatard NPH (Canad., Span.), Insulatard NPH Human (Canad.), Insulatard Pen Set (Swed.), Insulin (Germ.), Insulin 2 (Austral.), Insulin S (Germ.), Insuline N.P.H. (Fr.), Insuline Semi Tardum (Fr.), Insuline Tardum MX (Fr.), Insuline Ultra Tardum (Fr.), Insulin-Toronto (Regular) (Canad.), Isotard MC (Austral.), Isuhuman Basal (Neth., Swed.), Isuhuman Comb 15 (Neth.), Isuhuman Comb 25 (Neth.), Isuhuman Comb 25/75 (Swed.), Isuhuman Comb 50 (Neth.), Isuhuman Comb 50/50 (Swed.), Isuhuman Infusat (Neth., Swed.), Isuhuman Rapid (Neth., Swed.), Komb-H-Insulin (Germ.), Komb-Insulin (Germ.), Komb-Insulin S (Germ.), Lenta MC (Ital.), Lentard MC (G.B.), Lente (Germ.), Lente Iletin (Canad.), Lente Iletin I, Lente Iletin II Pork (Canad.), Lente Insulin (Canad.), Lente MC (Austral., Fr., Span., Switz.), Meztardia Huma (Span.), Meztardia Nordi (Span.), Mixtard (Fr., Germ., Span., Switz.), Mixtard 15/85 (Canad.), Mixtard 20/80 (Swed.), Mixtard 30/70 (Canad., G.B., Swed.), Mixtard 50/50 (Canad.), Mixtard 10 HM (Switz.), Mixtard 20 HM (Switz.), Mixtard 40 HM (Switz.), Mixtard 50 HM (Switz.), Mixtard Humaine (Fr., Switz.), Mixtard Human (Austral., Germ., Swed.), Mixtard Human 70/30, Mixtard Humana (Span.), Monotard (Swed.), Monotard HM (Austral., Fr., Germ., Ital., S. Afr., Span., Switz.), Neulente (Ire.), Neuphane (Ire.), Novolin-30/70 (Canad.), Novolin 70/30, Novolin L, Novolin N, Novolin R, Novolin-Lente (Canad.), Novolin-NPH (Canad.), Novolin-Toronto (Regular) (Canad.), Novolin-Ultralente (Canad.), NPH Iletin (Canad.), NPH Iletin I, NPH Iletin II Pork (Canad.), NPH Insulin (Canad.), Orgasuline (Fr.), Orgasuline N.P.H. (Fr.), PenMix 10/90 (G.B.), PenMix 20/80 (G.B.), PenMix 30/70 (G.B.), PenMix 40/60 (G.B.), PenMix 50/50 (G.B.), Protamine Zinc Iletin (Canad.), Protamine Zinc Insulin MC (Austral.), Protaphan HM (Germ.), Protaphane HM (Austral., Fr., Ital., S. Afr., Switz.), Pur-in Isophane (G.B.), Pur-in Mix 15/85

(G.B.), Pur-in Mix 25/75 (G.B.), Pur-in Mix 50/50 (G.B.), Pur-in Neutral (G.B.), Rapitar MC (Span.), Rapitard (Germ.), Rapitard MC (Austral., Fr., G.B., Ital., Switz.), Regular Iletin I, Regular Iletin II, Regular Iletin II Pork (Canad.), Regular Iletin (Neutral) (Canad.), Semilen MC (Span.), Semilente (Canad., Germ.), Semilente Iletin (Canad.), Semilente Iletin I, Semilente MC (Austral., Fr., Switz.), Semitard MC (G.B.), Ultrale MC (Span.), Ultralente (Germ.), Ultralente Iletin (Canad.), Ultralente Iletin I, Ultralente Insulin (Canad.), Ultralente MC (Austral., Fr., Switz.), Ultratard (Swed.), Ultratard HM (Austral., Fr., Germ., Ital., S. Afr., Span., Switz.), Umuline Profil 20 (Fr.), Umuline Profil 30 (Fr.), Umuline Profil 40 (Fr.), Umuline Protamine Isophane (N.P.H.) (Fr.), Umuline Rapide (Fr.), Velasulin (Germ.), Velasulin human (Germ.), Velasulin PP (Germ.), Velosulin (Austral., G.B., Ire., Span., Swed., Switz.), Velosulin Huma (Span.), Velosulin Humaine (Switz.), Velosulin Human, Velosulin (Regular) (Canad.), Vlosuline (Fr.), Vlosuline Humaine (Fr.)

Primary Use: This hypoglycemic agent is effective in the management of diabetes mellitus.

Ocular Side Effects:
  A. Systemic Administration
     1. Decreased vision
     2. Nystagmus
     3. Paresis of extraocular muscles
     4. Diplopia
     5. Pupils
        a. Mydriasis
        b. Absence of reaction to light
     6. Eyelids or conjunctiva
        a. Allergic reactions
        b. Erythema
        c. Blepharoconjunctivitis
        d. Angioneurotic edema
        e. Urticaria
     7. Decreased tear lysozymes
     8. Strabismus
     9. Intraocular pressure
        a. Increased
        b. Decreased
    10. Immunogenic retinopathy

Clinical Significance: Since most of the adverse ocular effects attributed to insulin normally occur with diabetes mellitus, the condition for which insulin is used, it is most difficult to state a cause-and-effect relationship. Generally, if an adverse insulin-related event occurs, it is reversible and primarily due to a drug-related hypoglycemic attack. In some cases, the reversibility is delayed and may take many weeks to resolve. It has recently been suggested that some diabetic retinopathy is insulin-induced and immunogenic in nature. While data in primates support this, it will be difficult to prove in humans. A separate report has also suggested that insulin caused or aggravated lipemic retinitis in a patient with possible hyperlipoproteinemia type V. Chiou, Chuang, and Chang suggest applying topical ocular insulin to lower glucose concentrations. Bartlett, et al. have shown insulin applied to the human eye in concentrations up to 100 u/mL is not toxic.

References:
Bartlett, J.D., et al.: Toxicity of insulin administered to the human eye in vivo. Invest. Ophthalmol. Vis. Sci. ARVO Annual Abstract Issue. 3916–3930, May, 1993.
Chiou, G.C.Y., Chuang, C.Y., and Chang, M.S.: Systemic delivery of insulin through eyes to lower the glucose concentration. J. Ocul. Pharmacol. 5:81, 1989.
Gralnick, A.: The retina and intraocular tension during prolonged insulin coma with autopsy eye findings. Am. J. Ophthalmol. 24:1174, 1941.
Moses, R.A. (Ed.): Adler's Physiology of the Eye. 6th Ed., St. Louis, C.V. Mosby, 1975, p. 21.
Shabo, A.L., and Maxwell, D.S.: Insulin-induced immunogenic retinopathy resembling the retinitis proliferans of diabetes. Trans. Am. Acad. Ophthalmol. Otolaryngol. 81:497, 1976.
Vermeer, B.J., and Polano, M.K.: A case of xanthomatosis and hyperlipoproteinemia type V probably induced by overdosage of insulin. Dermatologica 151:43, 1975.
Walsh, F.B., and Hoyt, W.F.: Clinical Neuro-Ophthalmology. 3rd Ed., Baltimore, Williams & Wilkins, Vol. III, 1969, pp. 2684–2685.

Class: Vitamins

Generic Name: Vitamin D. The following preparations contain Vitamin D as a single entity: 1. Calcifediol; 2. Calcitriol; 3. Dihydrotachysterol (DHT); 4. Ergocalciferol (Calciferol)

Proprietary Name: 1. **Calderol**; 2. **Calcijex** (Swed.), **Rocaltrol** (Austral., Canad., Fr., G.B., Germ., Ire., Ital., Neth., S. Afr., Span., Swed., Switz.); 3. Hytakerol (Canad.); 4. Drisdol (Canad.)

Primary Use: Vitamin D is used as a dietary supplement and in the management of vitamin D-deficient states and hypoparathyroidism.

Ocular Side Effects:
    A. Systemic Administration
        1. Strabismus
        2. Epicanthus
        3. Calcium deposits or band keratopathy
            a. Conjunctiva

b. Cornea
c. Sclera
4. Nystagmus
5. Decreased pupillary reaction to light
6. Narrowed optic foramina
7. Papilledema
8. Optic atrophy
9. Small optic discs
10. Visual hallucinations
11. Subconjunctival or retinal hemorrhages secondary to drug-induced anemia

Clinical Significance: Severe adverse ocular reactions due to vitamin D are either caused by a direct toxicity or an unusual sensitivity and are primarily seen in infants. Calcium deposits in or around the optic canal cause narrowing of the optic foramina, which may in turn cause papilledema. If the vitamin intake is not discontinued, optic atrophy may result. Children with these toxic effects often have elfin-like faces and prominent epicanthal folds. In adults, the toxic effects are few and the calcium deposits in ocular tissue appear to be the main adverse reaction. One case of a presumed basilar artery insufficiency with hemianopsia due to vitamin D intake has been reported.

References:
Baxi, S.C., and Dailey, G.E.: Hypervitaminosis. A cause of hypercalcemia. West. J. Med. *137*:429, 1982.
Cogan, D.G., Albright, F., and Bartter, F.C.: Hypercalcemia and band keratopathy. Arch. Ophthalmol. *40*:624, 1948.
Cohen, H.N., et al.: Deafness due to hypervitaminosis D. Lancet *1*:973, 1978.
Dukes, M.N.G. (Ed.): Meyler's Side Effects of Drugs. Amsterdam, Excerpta Medica, Vol. X, 1984, pp. 721–723.
Gartner, S., and Rubner, K.: Calcified scleral nodules in hypervitaminosis D. Am. J. Ophthalmol. *39*:658, 1955.
Harley, R.D., et al.: Idiopathic hypercalcemia of infancy: Optic atrophy and other ocular changes. Trans. Am. Acad. Ophthalmol. Otolaryngol. *69*:977, 1965.
Wagener, H.P.: The ocular manifestations of hypercalcemia. Am. J. Med. Sci. *231*: 218, 1956.

Generic Name: Vitamin A (Retinol)

Proprietary Name: A 313 (Fr.), Amirale (Ital.), A-Mulsin (Germ.), Aquasol A (Canad.), Arovit (Fr., Ital., S. Afr., Span., Swed., Switz.), Auxina A Masiva (Span.), Avibon (Fr.), A-Vicotrat (Germ.), Avitina (Ital.), Axrol (Switz.), Biominol A (Span.), Biovit-A (G.B.), Dagravit A (Neth.), Davitamon A (Neth.), Dif Vitamin A Masivo (Span.), Euvitol (Ital.), Ido A 50 (Span.), Idrurto A (Ital.), Ledovit A (Span.), Micelle A (Austral.), Mulsal

A Megadosis (Span.), Oculotect (Germ., Switz.), Ophtosan (Germ.), **Pedi-Vit A**, Primavit (Ital.), Ro-A-Vit (G.B.), Vit-A-N (Ital.)

Primary Use: Vitamin A is used as a dietary supplement and in the management of vitamin A-deficient states and in the treatment of acne.

Ocular Side Effects:
  A. Systemic Administration
    1. Nystagmus
    2. Eyelids or conjunctiva
      a. Conjunctivitis—nonspecific
      b. Yellow or orange discoloration
      c. Exfoliative dermatitis
      d. Loss of eyelashes or eyebrows
    3. Paresis or paralysis of extraocular muscles
    4. Diplopia
    5. Papilledema secondary to pseudotumor cerebri
    6. Miosis
    7. Exophthalmos
    8. Strabismus
    9. Decreased intraocular pressure
    10. Visual fields
      a. Scotomas
      b. Enlarged blind spot
    11. Problems with color vision
      a. Objects have yellow tinge
      b. Improves red dyschromatopsia
    12. Subconjunctival or retinal hemorrhages
    13. Optic atrophy
    14. Ocular irritation—drug found in tears

Clinical Significance: With increased interest in diet and popularization of vitamin therapy, an increased incidence of vitamin intoxication is occurring. Ocular manifestations from hypervitaminosis A are varied and dose-related. While some direct effects, such as loss of eyelashes, are evident, many of the central effects, such as diplopia and strabismus, are due to increased intracranial pressure. Simultaneous use of vitamin A and tetracyclines may increase the incidence of pseudotumor cerebri. To date, the mechanism of how excess vitamin A causes intracranial hypertension is not known. Ocular side effects due to hypervitaminosis A are much more frequent and extensive in infants and children than in adults. Nearly all ocular side effects are rapidly reversible if recognized early and the vitamin therapy is discontinued; however, in some instances, it may be several months before these effects are completely resolved. Papilledema, if untreated, may progress to permanent optic atrophy. The prolonged effect of vitamin A probably occurs because of the extensive storage of vitamin A in the liver. If exophthalmos is present, it may be secondary to thyroid changes since vitamin A has antithyroid activity. Hypercalcemia due to vitamin A is infrequent; although no reports of band keratopathy have been received, the potential for such exists. Dryness and irritation of the eyes have been reported in patients taking high doses of vitamin A, which has been found to be present in tears.

References:

Baadsgaard, O., and Thomsen, N.H.: Chronic vitamin A intoxication. Dan. Med. Bull. *30*:51, 1983.

Baxi, S.C., and Dailey, G.E.: Hypervitaminosis. A cause of hypercalcemia. West. J. Med. *137*:429, 1982.

LaMantia, R.S., and Andrews, C.E.: Acute vitamin A intoxication. South. Med. J. *74*: 1012, 1981.

Marcus, D.F., et al.: Optic disk findings in hypervitaminosis A. Ann. Ophthalmol. *17*: 397, 1985.

Morrice, G., Havener, W.H., and Kapetansky, F.: Vitamin A intoxication as a cause of pseudotumor cerebri. JAMA *173*:1802–1805, 1960.

Oliver, T.K., and Havener, W.H.: Eye manifestations of chronic vitamin A intoxication. Arch. Ophthalmol. *60*:19–22, 1958.

Pasquariello, P.S., Jr.: Benign increased intracranial hypertension due to chronic vitamin A overdosage in a 26-month-old child. Clin. Pediatr. *16*:379–382, 1977.

Pearson, M.G., Littlwood, S.M., and Bowden, A.N.: Tetracycline and benign intracranial hypertension. Br. Med. J. *1*:292, 1981.

Stirling, H.F., Laing, S.C., and Barr, D.G.D.: Hypercarotenaemia and vitamin A overdose from proprietary baby food. Lancet *1*:1089, 1986.

Ubels, J.L., and MacRae, S.M.: Vitamin A is present as retinol in the tears of humans and rabbits. Curr. Eye Res. *3*:815, 1984.

Van Dyk, H.J.L., and Swan, K.C.: Drug-induced pseudotumor cerebri. *In* Symposium on ocular therapy. *4*:71–77, 1969, Edited by I.H. Leopold, St. Louis, CV Mosby.

Wason, S., and Lovejoy, F.H., Jr: Vitamin A toxicity. Am. J. Dis. Child. *136*:174, 1982.

White, J.M.: Vitamin-A-induced anaemia. Lancet 2:573, 1984.

X   Agents Used to Treat Allergic and Neuromuscular Disorders

Class: Agents Used to Treat Myasthenia Gravis

Generic Name: 1. Ambenonium; 2. Edrophonium; 3. Pyridostigmine

Proprietary Name: 1. Mytelase (Fr., Swed.); 2. **Enlon** (Canad.), **Reversol**, **Tensilon** (Canad., G.B., Ire., S. Afr.); 3. **Mestinon** (Austral., Canad., Fr., G.B., Germ., Ire., Ital., Neth., S. Afr., Span., Swed., Switz.), **Regonol** (Canad.)

Primary Use: These anticholinesterase agents are effective in the treatment of myasthenia gravis. Edrophonium is primarily used as an antidote for curariform agents and as a diagnostic test for myasthenia gravis.

Ocular Side Effects:
   A. Systemic Administration
      1. Miosis
      2. Decreased vision
      3. Diplopia
      4. Lacrimation
      5. Blepharoclonus—toxic states
      6. Paradoxical response (ptotic eye up and nonptotic eye down)
      7. Oculogyric crisis (edrophonium HCL)

Systemic Side Effects:
   A. Systemic Administration—Edrophonium
      1. Perspiration
      2. Asthma
      3. Apnea
      4. Bradycardia
      5. Cardiac arrest
      6. Hypotension
      7. GI disorder
      8. Incontinence

Clinical Significance: Ocular side effects due to these anticholinesterase agents are rare and seldom of clinical significance. All adverse ocular reactions are reversible with discontinued drug use. Blepharoclonus is only seen in overdose situations. In rare instances, edrophonium may cause a paradoxical response when used in myasthenia gravis testing. In these cases, the ptotic eyelid goes up, while the normal eyelid goes down. Serious systemic side effects from the edrophonium test for myasthenia gravis are relatively uncommon, especially if a preliminary test dose is performed to detect hypersensitive patients. Patients without myasthenia gravis are more likely to experience systemic side effects, such as sweating and mild sensations of gastrointestinal motility. Bowel and bladder side effects are minimal. Bronchospasm may follow the use of edrophonium in asthmatic patients. Nucci and Brancato recently reported an episode of oculogyric crisis within a few minutes after performing a "Tensilon test" (edrophonium hydrochloride).

References:

Drug Evaluations. 6th Ed., Chicago, American Medical Association, 1986, pp. 224–226, 450.

Dukes, M.N.G. (Ed.): Meyler's Side Effects of Drugs. Amsterdam, Excerpta Medica, Vol. X, 1984, p. 246.

Field, L.M.: Toxic alopecia caused by pyridostigmine bromide. Arch. Dermatol. *116*: 1103, 1980.

Havener, W.H.: Ocular Pharmacology. 5th Ed., St. Louis, C.V. Mosby, 1983, pp. 347–349.

McEvoy, G.K. (Ed.): American Hospital Formulary Service Drug Information 87. Bethesda, American Society of Hospital Pharmacists, 1987, pp. 520–521, 528–530, 1206–1208.

Nucci, P., and Brancato, R.: Oculogyric crisis after the Tensilon test. Graefe's Arch. Clin. Exp. Ophthalmol. *228*:382–385, 1990.

Van Dyk, H.J.L., and Florence L.: The Tensilon test. A safe Procedure. Ophthalmology *87*:210–216, 1980.

Class: Antihistamines

Generic Name: 1. Antazoline; 2. Pyrilamine (Mepyramine); 3. Tripelennamine

Proprietary Name: *Systemic*: 2. Antemesyl (Ital.), Anthisan (Austral., G.B., Ire., S. Afr.), **Medacote**, Pyriped (S. Afr.), Relaxa-Tabs (Austral.); 3. **PBZ**, Pyribenzamine (Canad.) *Ophthalmic*: Antazoline and Pyrilamine are available in multi-ingredient preparations. 1. Visuphrine N in der Ophtiole (Germ.) *Topical*: 1. Insect Ointment (G.B.); 2. Histamed (S. Afr.); 3. Azaron (Germ., Neth.), **PBZ**

Primary Use: *Systemic*: These ethylenediamines are indicated for the treatment of allergic or vasomotor rhinitis, allergic conjunctivitis, and allergic skin manifestations of urticaria and angioneurotic edema. *Ophthalmic*: Antazoline is used in the treatment of ocular irritation or congestion of allergic or inflammatory origin.

Ocular Side Effects:
A. Systemic Administration
   1. Decreased vision
   2. Pupils
      a. Mydriasis—may precipitate narrow-angle glaucoma
      b. Decreased or absent reaction to light
      c. Anisocoria
   3. Decreased accommodation
   4. Decreased tolerance to contact lenses
   5. Diplopia
   6. Decreased lacrimation
   7. Eyelids or conjunctiva
      a. Erythema
      b. Photosensitivity
      c. Urticaria
      d. Blepharospasm
   8. Visual hallucinations
   9. Nystagmus (tripelennamine)—toxic states
  10. Strabismus (tripelennamine)—toxic states
  11. Subconjunctival or retinal hemorrhages secondary to drug-induced anemia
  12. Constriction of visual fields—variable
  13. May aggravate keratoconjunctivitis sicca
B. Local Ophthalmic Use or Exposure
   1. Conjunctival vasoconstriction
   2. Irritation
      a. Lacrimation
      b. Reactive hyperemia
      c. Photophobia
      d. Ocular pain
      e. Edema
      f. Burning sensation
   3. Mydriasis—may precipitate narrow-angle glaucoma
   4. Decreased vision
   5. Decreased intraocular pressure
   6. Punctate keratitis
   7. Eyelids or conjunctiva
      a. Allergic reactions
      b. Conjunctivitis—nonspecific
   8. Decreased tolerance to contact lenses

Systemic Side Effects:
A. Local Ophthalmic Use or Exposure
   1. Nausea
   2. Somnolence
   3. Dizziness
   4. Headache
   5. Hypertension
   6. Cardiac arrhythmia
   7. Hyperglycemia
   8. Asthenia
   9. Nervousness
   10. Hypothermia
   11. Anaphylactic reaction

Clinical Significance: Ocular side effects due to these antihistamines are uncommon and frequently disappear even if the use of the drug is continued. These antihistamines have a weak atropine action that accounts for pupillary changes. However, with long-term use, these effects may accumulate so that unilateral or bilateral signs such as anisocoria, decreased accommodation, and blurred vision may occur. These drugs seem to cause a decrease in mucoid or lacrimal secretions, which possibly accounts for decreased contact lens tolerance and aggravation or induction of keratoconjunctivitis sicca. These drugs in large dosages or with chronic therapy can produce facial dyskinesia that may start as a unilateral or bilateral blepharospasm. Total lack of pupillary responses and visual hallucinations usually only occur in toxic states. There is, however, a report of visual hallucinations occurring in a 5-year-old child after only the third oral dose of tripelennamine. Topical ophthalmic antazoline is a strong contact sensitizer and the only antihistamine known to cause a decrease in intraocular pressure. Untoward systemic reactions due to ocular use of antihistamines are infrequent, with nausea and somnolence the most common.

References:

Abelson, M.B., Allansmith, M.R., and Friedlaender, M.H.: Effects of topically applied ocular decongestant and antihistamine. Am. J. Ophthalmol. *90*:254, 1980.

Dukes, M.N.G. (Ed.): Meyler's Side Effects of Drugs. Amsterdam, Excerpta Medica, Vol. X, 1984, pp. 286–287, 883.

Grant, W.M., and Loeb, D.R.: Effect of locally applied antihistamine drugs on normal eyes. Arch. Ophthalmol. *39*:553–554, 1948.

Hays, D.P., Johnson, B.F., and Perry, R.: Prolonged hallucinations following a modest overdose of tripelennamine. Clin. Toxicol. *16*:331, 1980.

Rinker, J.R., and Sullivan, J.H.: Drug reactions following urethral instillation of tripelennamine (Pyribenzamine). J. Urol. *91*:433, 1964.

Schipior, P.G.: An unusual case of antihistamine intoxication. J. Pediatr. *71*:589, 1967.

Generic Name: 1. Azatadine; 2. Cyproheptadine

Proprietary Name: 1. Idulian (Fr., Ital.), Lergocil (Span.), **Optimine** (Canad., G.B., Germ., Ire., Neth., S. Afr.), Zadine (Austral.); 2. Klarivitina (Span.), Nuran (Germ.), **Periactin** (Austral., Canad., G.B., Ital., Neth., S. Afr., Span., Swed., Switz.), Périactine (Fr.), Periactinol (Germ.)

Primary Use: These chemically related antihistamines are used in the symptomatic relief of allergic or vasomotor rhinitis, allergic conjunctivitis, and allergic skin manifestations.

Ocular Side Effects:
   A. Systemic Administration
      1. Decreased vision
      2. Mydriasis—may precipitate narrow-angle glaucoma
      3. Decreased tolerance to contact lenses
      4. Diplopia
      5. Decreased lacrimation
      6. Eyelids or conjunctiva
         a. Erythema
         b. Edema
         c. Photosensitivity
         d. Urticaria
      7. May aggravate keratoconjunctivitis sicca
      8. Visual hallucinations
      9. Subconjunctival or retinal hemorrhages secondary to drug-induced anemia

Clinical Significance: Ocular side effects due to these agents are rare and frequently disappear even if use of the drug is continued. Both agents have atropine-like effects, such as mydriasis and decreased secretions. Possible decreased lacrimal or mucoid secretion has been suggested as the cause of decreased tolerance to contact lenses and aggravation of keratoconjunctivitis sicca.

References:
Drugs that cause photosensitivity. Med. Lett. Drugs Ther. 28:51, 1986.
Gilman, A.G., Goodman, L.S., and Gilman, A. (Eds.): The Pharmacological Basis of Therapeutics. 6th Ed., New York, Macmillan, 1980, p. 639.
McEvoy, G.K. (Ed.): American Hospital Formulary Service Drug Information 87. Bethesda, American Society of Hospital Pharmacists, 1987, pp. 5–6, 14–15.
Miller, D.: Role of the tear film in contact lens wear. Int. Ophthalmol. Clin. 13(1): 247, 1973.

Generic Name: 1. Brompheniramine; 2. Chlorpheniramine; 3. Dexbrompheniramine; 4. Dexchlorpheniramine; 5. Dimethindene; 6. Pheniramine; 7. Triprolidine

Proprietary Name: 1. Antial (Ital.), **Bromarest**, Dimégan (Fr.), Dimegan (Germ.), Dimetane (Austral., Canad.), Dimetane prolongatum (Swed.), Dimotane (G.B., Ire.), Gammistin (Ital.); 2. **Aller-Chlor**, Allergex (Austral., S. Afr.), Allerhist (S. Afr.), Antihista (Span.), Chlortrimeton (S. Afr.), **Chlor-Trimeton**, Chlor-Tripolon (Canad.), Clorten (Ital.), Contac Allergy Formula (Canad.), Histamed (S. Afr.), Lentostamin (Ital.), Methyrit (Neth.), Novopheniram (Canad.), **Pedia Care Allergy Formula**, Piriton (Austral., G.B., Ire.), **Teldrin**, Trimeton (Ital.); 3. See No. 1.; 4. Polaramin (Ital., Swed.), **Polaramine** (Austral., Canad., Fr., Neth., S. Afr., Span., Switz.), Polaronil (Germ.); 5. Fengel (Ital.), Fenistil (Germ., Ital., Neth., Span., Swed., Switz.), Fenistil Topico (Span.), Fenostil (G.B.), Fenostil Retard (Ire.); 6. Aller-G (Austral.), Avil (Austral., Germ.), Avil Retard (S. Afr.), Aviletten (Germ.), Avilettes (Austral.), Daneral SA (G.B., Ire.), Fenamine (Austral.), Inhiston (Ital.); 7. Actidil (Ire., Ital.), Actidilon (Fr.), Pro-Actidil (G.B., Germ., Ire., Neth., S. Afr., Span., Switz.)

Primary Use: These alkylamine antihistamines are used in the symptomatic relief of allergic or vasomotor rhinitis, allergic conjunctivitis, and allergic skin manifestations.

Ocular Side Effects:
    A. Systemic Administration
        1. Decreased vision
        2. Pupils
           a. Mydriasis—may precipitate narrow-angle glaucoma
           b. Decreased or absent reaction to light—toxic states
           c. Anisocoria
        3. Decreased tolerance to contact lenses
        4. Diplopia
        5. Decreased lacrimation
        6. Eyelids or conjunctiva
           a. Erythema
           b. Photosensitivity
           c. Urticaria
           d. Blepharospasm
        7. Nonspecific ocular irritation
           a. Ocular pain
           b. Burning sensation
         8. Punctate keratitis
        9. May aggravate keratoconjunctivitis sicca
      10. Visual hallucinations
      11. Subconjunctival or retinal hemorrhages secondary to drug-induced anemia

12. Constriction of visual fields—variable
13. Abnormal critical flicker fusion (triprolidine)

Clinical Significance: Ocular side effects due to these antihistamines are rare and frequently disappear even if use of the drug is continued. These antihistamines have a weak atropine action that accounts for the pupillary changes. With chronic use, anisocoria, decreased accommodation, and blurred vision can also occur. Chlorpheniramine has been found to decrease tear production, which may account for decreased contact lens tolerance and aggravation or even induction of keratoconjunctivitis sicca in some patients. Antihistamines in large dosages or with chronic therapy can produce facial dyskinesia, which may start with unilateral or bilateral blepharo spasms. Lack of pupillary responses occurs only in toxic states. The alkylamines seem to have a lower incidence of ocular side effects than do other antihistamines, with dexchlorpheniramine having the fewest reported side effects.

References:
Davis, W.A.: Dyskinesia associated with chronic antihistamine use. N. Engl. J. Med. *294*:113, 1976.
Farber, A.S.: Ocular side effects of antihistamine-decongestant combinations. Am. J. Ophthalmol. *94*:565, 1982.
Granacher, R.P., Jr.: Facial dyskinesia after antihistamines. N. Engl. J. Med. *296*:516, 1977.
Halperin, M., Thorig, L., and van Haeringen, N.J.: Ocular side effects of antihistamine-decongestant combinations. Am. J. Ophthalmol. *95*;563, 1983.
Koffler, B.H., and Lemp, M.A.: The effect of an antihistamine (chlorpheniramine maleate) on tear production in humans. Ann. Ophthalmol. *12*:217, 1980.
Miller, D.: Role of the tear film in contact lens wear. Int. Ophthalmol. Clin. *13(1)*: 247, 1973.
Nicholson, A.N., Smith, P.A., and Spencer, M.B.: Antihistamines and visual function: Studies on dynamic acuity and the pupillary response to light. Br. J. Clin. Pharmacol. *14*:683, 1982.
Schuller, D.E., and Turkewitz, D.: Adverse effects of antihistamines. Postgrad. Med. *79*:75, 1986.
Soleymanikashi, Y., and Weiss, N.S.: Antihistaminic reaction: A review and presentation of two unusual examples. Ann. Allergy *28*:486, 1970.
Sovner, R.D.: Dyskinesia associated with chronic antihistamine use. N. Engl. J. Med. *294*:113, 1976.

Generic Name: 1. Carbinoxamine; 2. Clemastine; 3. Diphenhydramine; 4. Diphenylpyraline; 5. Doxylamine

Proprietary Name: 1. Allergefon (Fr.), Polistin Päd (Germ.), Polistin T-Caps (Germ.); 2. Aller-eze (G.B.), Tavegil (G.B., Germ., Ire., Ital., Neth., Span.), Tavégyl (Fr.), Tavegyl (Austral., S. Afr., Swed., Switz.), **Tavist** (Canad.), **Tavist-1**; 3. **Allerdryl** (Canad.), Allergan (Ital.), Allergina (Ital.), **Benadryl** (Austral., Canad., Span., Switz.), Benadryl N (Germ.), Benocten (Switz.), Bénylin (Fr.), Benylin (Neth., S. Afr., Span., Switz.), Betasleep

(S. Afr.), Butix (Fr.), Dihydral (Neth., S. Afr.), **Diphenhist**, Dobacen (Switz.), **Dytuss**, **Genahist**, Histergan (G.B.), Insomnal (Canad.), Lupovalin (Germ.), Nautamine (Fr.), nervo-OPT-N (Germ.), Pheramin N (Germ.), S.8 (Germ.), Sediat (Germ.), Sedopretten (Germ.), Sedovegan Novo (Germ.), Sekundal-D (Germ.), Sleep-Eze D (Canad.), **Uni-Bent Cough**; 4. Histalert (Austral.), Histryl (G.B., Ire.), Lergoban (G.B.); 5. Alsadorm (Germ.), Donormyl (Fr., Span.), Doxised (Ital.), **Doxysom**, Gittalun (Germ.), Hoggar N (Germ.), Méréprine (Fr.), Mereprine (Germ., Switz.), Restaid (Austral.), Restavit (Austral.), Sanalepsi-N (Switz.), Sedaplus (Germ.), Somnil (S. Afr.), Unisom (Span.), **Unisom Nighttime Sleep-Aid**

Primary Use: These ethanolamine antihistamines are used in the symptomatic relief of allergic or vasomotor rhinitis, allergic conjunctivitis, and allergic skin manifestations.

Ocular Side Effects:
 A. Systemic Administration
   1. Decreased vision
   2. Pupils
      a. Mydriasis—may precipitate narrow-angle glaucoma
      b. Decreased or absent reaction to light
      c. Anisocoria
   3. Decreased tolerance to contact lenses
   4. Eyelids or conjunctiva
      a. Erythema
      b. Photosensitivity
      c. Urticaria
      d. Blepharospasm
   5. Decreased lacrimation
   6. Diplopia
   7. Visual hallucinations
   8. Decrease or paralysis of accommodation
   9. Nystagmus
   10. Subconjunctival or retinal hemorrhages secondary to drug-induced anemia
   11. Constriction of visual fields—variable
   12. May aggravate keratoconjunctivitis sicca

Clinical Significance: Ocular side effects due to these antihistamines are rare and frequently disappear even if use of the drug is continued. These ethanolamines have a weak atropine action that accounts for the pupillary and ciliary body changes. However, with chronic long-term use, these effects can build so that unilateral or bilateral signs such as anisocoria, loss of accommodation, and decreased vision can occur. A suspected decrease in mucoid and lacrimal secretions may account for contact lens intolerance and aggravation or induction of keratoconjunctivitis sicca in some patients. Recently, it has been shown that these drugs in large dosages or with chronic therapy can produce facial dyskinesia. Many of these cases started with unilateral or bilateral blepharospasm. Lack of pupillary responses, visual hallucinations, and nystagmus usually only occur in toxic states. Most of the ocular side effects in this group are attributed to diphenhydramine, which is the most commonly used drug. There are reports by both Walsh and Nigro of comas secondary to diphenhydramine ingestion in infants and teenagers where, upon awaking, cortical blindness was evident. Over time, however, this reverted to normal vision. The Registry has received two case reports of possible ocular teratogenic effects secondary to diphenhydramine or doxylamine.

References:
Delaney, W.V., Jr.: Explained unexplained anisocoria. JAMA *244*:1475, 1980.
Drugs that cause photosensitivity. Med. Lett. Drugs Ther. *28*:51, 1986.
Miller, D.: Role of the tear film in contact lens wear. Int. Ophthalmol. Clin. *13(1)*: 247, 1973.
Nigro, S.A.: Toxic psychosis due to diphenhydramine hydrochloride. JAMA *203*: 301–302, 1968.
Seedor, J.A., et al.: Filamentary keratitis associated with diphenhydramine hydrochloride (Benadryl). Am. J. Ophthalmol. *101*:376, 1986.
Walsh, F.B.: Clinical Neuro-Ophthalmology. Baltimore, Williams and Wilkins, 1957.

Class: Antiparkinsonism Agents

Generic Name: Amantadine

Proprietary Name: Antadine (Austral., S. Afr.), Contenton (Germ.), Mantadan (Ital.), Mantadix (Fr.), Mantaviral (Span.), PK-Merz (Germ., Switz.), Protexin (Span.), **Symadine**, **Symmetrel** (Austral., Canad., G.B., Germ., Ire., Neth., S. Afr., Swed., Switz.), Virofral (Swed.)

Primary Use: This synthetic antiviral agent is used in the treatment of Parkinson's disease, tardive dyskinesia, and in the prophylaxis of influenza A_2 (Asian) virus infections.

Ocular Side Effects:
   A. Systemic Administration
      1. Decreased vision
      2. Visual hallucinations
      3. Cornea
         a. Edema
         b. Punctate keratitis
         c. Subepithelial opacities

4. Oculogyric crises
5. Eyelids or conjunctiva
   a. Photosensitivity
   b. Purpura
   c. Eczema
   d. Loss of eyelashes or eyebrows
6. Mydriasis—may precipitate narrow-angle glaucoma

Clinical Significance: Ocular side effects due to amantadine are rare except for decreased vision, which is transitory and seldom significant. All ocular effects appear to be dose-related and are reversible with discontinued amantadine usage. Visual hallucinations are often lilliputian and colored. The Registry has nine case reports of corneal lesions associated with the use of oral amantadine hydrochloride. The patterns are diffuse, white punctate subepithelial opacities, more prominent inferonasally, occasionally associated with a superficial punctate keratitis, corneal epithelial edema, and markedly reduced visual acuity. This usually occurs within 1 to 2 weeks after starting the drug and clears between 2 and 6 days after stopping it. Amantadine was reinstituted in two patients, and the corneal deposits recurred. Blanchard has reported one case, and there are six similar cases of corneal edema associated with amantadine usage. The edema is more prominent in the palpebral aperture and involves the full thickness of the cornea including epithelial blebs. This can occur anytime between a few weeks to a few years into therapy, and is reversible after the drug is discontinued. If this drug-related ocular side effect goes unrecognized, vision can go to light perception. One case of sudden bilateral loss of vision in otherwise normal eyes has been reported secondary to amantadine; this sudden loss of vision was reversible after discontinuing the drug for several weeks.

References:

Blanchard D.L.: Amantadine caused corneal edema. Letter to the Editor. Cornea *9(2)*: 181, 1990.

Drugs that cause psychiatric symptoms. Med. Lett. Drugs Ther. *28*:81, 1986.

Fraunfelder F.T., and Meyer S.M.: Amantadine and corneal deposits. Am. J. Ophthalmol. *110(1)*:96–97, 1990.

Pearlman, J.T., Kadish, A.H., and Ramseyer, J.C.: Vision loss associated with amantadine hydrochloride use. JAMA *237*:1200, 1977.

Postma, J.U., and Van Tilburg, W.: Visual hallucinations and delirium during treatment with amantadine (Symmetrel). J. Am. Geriatr. Soc. *23*:212, 1975.

Selby, G.: Treatment of Parkinsonism. Drugs *11*:61, 1976.

van den Berg, W.H.H.W., and van Ketel, W.G.: Photosensitization by amantadine (Symmetrel). Contact Dermatitis *9*:165, 1983.

Wilson, T.W., and Rajput, A.H.: Amantadine-Dyazide interaction. Can. Med. Assoc. J. *129*:974, 1983

Generic Name: 1. Benztropine; 2. Biperiden; 3. Chlorphenoxamine; 4. Procyclidine; 5. Trihexyphenidyl

Proprietary Name: 1. **Cogentin** (Austral., Canad., G.B., Neth., Swed.), Cogentinol (Germ.); 2. **Akineton** (Austral., Canad., Fr., G.B., Germ., Ire., Ital., Neth., S. Afr., Span., Swed., Switz.), Akineton Retard (Germ., Ire., Span., Switz.); 3. Systral (Germ.); 4. Arpicolin (G.B.), Kemadren (Span.), **Kemadrin** (Austral., Canad., G.B., Ire., Ital., Neth., Swed., Switz.), Kémadrine (Fr.), Osnervan (Germ.), Procyclid (Canad.); 5. Anti-Spas (Austral.), Apo-Trihex (Canad.), **Artane** (Austral., Canad., Fr., G.B., Germ., Ital., Neth., S. Afr., Span., Switz.), Bentex (G.B.), Broflex (G.B.), Novohexidyl (Canad.), Pargitan (Swed.), Parkinane (Fr.)

Primary Use: These anticholinergic agents are used in the management of Parkinson's disease and in the control of extrapyramidal disorders due to central nervous system drugs, such as reserpine or the phenothiazines.

Ocular Side Effects:
  A. Systemic Administration
    1. Pupils
       a. Mydriasis—may precipitate narrow-angle glaucoma
       b. Decreased reaction to light
    2. Decreased vision
    3. Decrease or paralysis of accommodation
    4. Visual hallucinations

Clinical Significance: The degree of anticholinergic activity of these drugs that induces ocular side effects varies with each agent. With benztropine, adverse ocular reactions are common; while with biperiden, they are rare. In the younger age groups, decreased accommodation may cause considerable inconveniences that may be partially reversed by topical ocular application of a weak, long-acting anticholinesterase. There are cases in the literature and Registry of these drugs precipitating glaucoma in patients taking recommended dosages. Hallucinations in patients taking these drugs are primarily of people, normal in size, in color, which disappear if the dosage of the drug is reduced. Retinal pigmentary changes have been seen in patients taking these medications, but this has not been proven as a drug-related event.

References:
Acute drug abuse reactions. Med. Lett. Drugs Ther. *27*:77, 1985.
Anticholinergic drugs are abused. Int. Drug Therapy Newsletter *20*:1, 1985.
Friedman, Z., and Neumann, E.: Benzhexol induced blindness in Parkinson's disease. Br. Med. J. *1*:605, 1972.
Gilbert, G.J.: Hallucinations from levodopa. JAMA *235*:597, 1976.
McGucken, R.B., Caldwell, J., and Anthon, B.: Teenage procyclidine abuse. Lancet *1*:1514, 1985.
Selby, G.: Treatment of Parkinsonism. Drugs *11*:61, 1976.

Thaler, J.S.: Effects of benztropine mesylate (Cogentin) on accommodation in normal volunteers. Am. J. Optom. Physiol. Optics *59*:918, 1982.
Thaler, J.S.: The effect of multiple psychotropic drugs on the accommodation of prepresbyopes. Am. J. Optom. Physiol. Optics *56*:259, 1979.

Generic Name: Caramiphen

Proprietary Name: None

Primary Use: This anticholinergic agent is used in the treatment of Parkinson's disease.

Ocular Side Effects:
    A. Systemic Administration
        1. Mydriasis—may precipitate narrow-angle glaucoma
        2. Paralysis of accommodation
        3. Retrobulbar neuritis
        4. Scotomas

Clinical Significance: Significant ocular side effects due to caramiphen are very rare. Only one case of retrobulbar neuritis has been reported; however, it was well documented. The retrobulbar neuritis occurred each time caramiphen therapy was restarted.

References:
Bruckner, R.: Über pharmakologische Beeinflussung des Augendruckes bei verschiedenen Körperlagen. Ophthalmologica *116*:200, 1948.
Hermans, G.: Le système moteur. Bull. Soc. Belge Ophtalmol. *160*:97, 1972.
Leibold, J.E.: Drugs having toxic effect on the optic nerve. Int. Ophthalmol. Clin. *11(2)*:137, 1971.
Lubeck, M.J.: Effects of drugs on ocular muscles. Int. Ophthalmol. Clin. *11(2)*:35, 1971.
Walsh, F.B., and Hoyt, W.F.: Clinical Neuro-Ophthalmology. 3rd Ed., Baltimore, Williams & Wilkins, Vol. III, 1969, p. 2664.

Generic Name: Levodopa

Proprietary Name: Brocadopa (G.B.), Eldopal (Neth.), **Larodopa** (Austral., Canad., Fr., G.B., Ire., Ital., S. Afr.), Rigakin (Neth.)

Primary Use: This beta-adrenergic blocking agent is used in the management of Parkinson's disease.

Ocular Side Effects:
    A. Systemic Administration
        1. Pupils

      a. Mydriasis—may precipitate narrow-angle glaucoma
      b. Miosis
  2. Widening of palpebral fissure
  3. Decreased vision
  4. Diplopia
  5. Blepharospasm
  6. Horner's syndrome
      a. Miosis
      b. Ptosis
  7. Extraocular muscles
      a. Paresis
      b. Abnormal involuntary movement
  8. Blepharoclonus
  9. Visual hallucinations
10. Oculogyric crises
11. Amblyopia
      a. Increases visual acuity
      b. Decreases binocular suppression
12. Eyelids or conjunctiva
      a. Allergic reactions
      b. Edema
      c. Lupoid syndrome
13. Subconjunctival or retinal hemorrhages secondary to drug-induced anemia
14. Stimulation of malignant melanoma

Clinical Significance: While numerous ocular side effects due to levodopa are known, they appear to be dose-dependent and reversible. Pupillary side effects are variable. Initially, mydriasis may occur and has been reported to precipitate narrow-angle glaucoma. After a few weeks of levodopa therapy, miosis is not uncommon. Lid responses also appear to be variable and may be painful. In some patients, levodopa produces ptosis, sometimes unilateral, while blepharospasm is reported in other patients. Visual hallucinations are menacing and primarily of normal-size people and in color. These hallucinations can be stopped or decreased in frequency by reducing the drug dosage and appear to occur more commonly in the elderly. Oculogyric crises have been precipitated by levodopa, primarily in patients with a history of encephalitis. Gottlob, Charlier, and Reinecke have reported that levodopa has improved contrast sensitivity, decreased the size of scotomas, and improved vision in up to 70% of amblyopic eyes. This improvement is said to persist. Leguire, et al. reported that after a single dose, vision improved by 1.5 Snellen visual acuity lines and pattern-visual evoked potential by 41%. One case of drug-induced pseudotumor cerebri occurred in a patient taking carbidopa and levodopa. Since levodopa is an intermediate in melanin synthesis, there is a question whether it might induce or stimulate the growth of melanomas. Although there are no proven data to support this, alternate forms of anti-Parkinsonian therapy have been suggested for some patients.

References:

Abramson, D.H., and Rubenfeld, M.R.: Choroidal melanoma and levodopa. JAMA 252:1011, 1984.

Barbeau, A.: L-Dopa therapy in Parkinson's disease: A critical review of nine years' experience. Can. Med. Assoc. J. 101:791–800, 1969.

Barone, D.A., and Martin, H.L.: Causes of pseudotumor cerebri and papilledema. Arch. Intern. Med. 139:830, 1979.

Cotzias, G.C., Papavasilliou, P.S., and Gellene, R.: Modifications of Parkinsonism-chronic treatment with L-dopa. N. Engl. J. Med. 280:337–345, 1969.

Glantz, R., et al.: Drug-induced asterixis in Parkinson disease. Neurology 32:553, 1982.

Gottlob, I., Charlier, J., and Reinecke, R.D.: Visual acuities and scotomas after one week levodopa administration in human amblyopia. Invest. Ophthalmol. Vis. Sci. 33(9):2722–2728, 1992.

Leguire, L.E., et al.: Levodopa treatment for childhood amblyopia. Invest. Ophthalmol. Vis. Sci. 32(Suppl):820, 1991.

Martin, W.E.: Adverse reactions during treatment of Parkinson's disease with levodopa. JAMA 216:1979–1983, 1971.

Shimizu, N., et al.: Ocular dyskinesias in patients with Parkinson's disease treated with levodopa. Ann. Neurol. 1:167–171, 1977.

van Rens, G.H., et al.: Uveal maligninant melanoma and levodopa therapy in Parkinson's disease. Ophthalmololgy 89:1464, 1982.

Weiner, W.J., and Nausieda, P.A.: Meige's syndrome during long-term dopaminergic therapy in Parkinson's disease. Arch. Neurol. 39:451, 1982.

Generic Name: Selegiline

Proprietary Name: Eldéprine (Fr.), **Eldepryl** (G.B., Neth., S. Afr., Swed.), Jumex (Ital.), Jumexal (Switz.), Movergan (Germ.), Plurimen (Span.)

Primary Use: This is a selective inhibitor of monoamine oxidase type B that enhances the effects of levodopa and is used in the management of Parkinson's disease.

Ocular side effects:
   A. Systemic Administration
      1. Blurred vision
      2. Photophobia
      3. Chromatopsia
      4. Blepharospasm
      5. Photosensitivity
      6. Visual hallucinations

Clinical Significance: This fairly recently released drug has had only a few ocular adverse events associated with its use. It is an agent that increases dopaminergic activity, thereby acting as a sympathomimetic. To date, all of the above side effects are reversible once the drug is discontinued. Rarely are any of the above side effects in themselves a reason to discontinue the drug, except in patients with diplopia or severe blepharospasm.

References:

Physicians Desk Reference Medical Economics Data, Montvale, NJ, 47th Edition, 1993, pp. 2351–2353.

Reynolds, J.E.F. (Ed.): Martindale: The Extra Pharmacopoeia. 30th Ed., London, Pharmaceutical Press, 1993, pp. 849–850.

Class: Cholinesterase Reactivators

Generic Name: Pralidoxime

Proprietary Name: Contrathion (Fr., Ital.), **Protopam Chloride** (Canad.)

Primary Use: This cholinesterase reactivator is used as an antidote for poisoning due to organophosphate pesticides or other chemicals that have anticholinesterase activity. It is also of value in the control of overdosage by anticholinesterase agents used in the treatment of myasthenia gravis.

Ocular Side Effects:
A. Systemic Administration
  1. Decreased vision
  2. Diplopia
  3. Decreased accommodation
B. Local Ophthalmic Use or Exposure—Subconjunctival Injection
  1. Irritation
    a. Hyperemia
    b. Burning sensation
  2. Subconjunctival hemorrhages
  3. Iritis
  4. Reverses miosis
  5. Reverses accommodative spasms

Clinical Significance: Pralidoxime commonly causes adverse ocular reactions after systemic administration. These effects are of rapid onset, last from a few minutes to a few hours, and are completely reversible. In one series, up to 60% of patients using the agent complained of misty vision, heaviness of the eye, blurred near vision, or decreased accommodation, especially after sudden head movement. Ocular side effects from subconjunctival injection are also transitory and reversible.

References:

Bryon, H.M., and Posner, H.: Clinical evaluation of Protopam. Am. J. Ophthalmol. *57*:409, 1964.

Dekking, H.M.: Stopping the action of strong miotics. Ophthalmologica *148*:428, 1964.

Drug Evaluations. 6th Ed., Chicago, American Medical Association, 1986, pp. 1647–1648.

Holland, P., and Parkes, D.C.: Plasma concentrations of the oxime pralidoxime mesylate (P2S) after repeated oral and intramuscular administration. Br. J. Ind. Med. *33*:43, 1976.

Jager, B.V., and Stagg, G.N.: Toxicity of diacetyl monoxime and of pyridine-2-aldoxime methiodide in man. Bull. Johns Hopkins Hosp. *102*:203, 1958.

Taylor, W.J.R., et al.: Effects of a combination of atropine, metaraminol and pyridine aldoxime methanesulfonate (AMP therapy) on normal human subjects. Can. Med. Assoc. J. *93*:957, 1965.

Class: Muscle Relaxants

Generic Name: Baclofen

Proprietary Name: Baclospas (G.B.), Liorésal (Fr., Switz.), **Lioresal** (Austral., Canad., G.B., Germ., Ire., Ital., Neth., S. Afr., Span., Swed.), Neurospas (S. Afr.)

Primary Use: This chlorophenyl derivative of gamma-aminobutyric acid is useful for alleviation of spasticity symptoms resulting from multiple sclerosis and other disorders of the spinal cord.

Ocular Side Effects:
   A. Systemic Administration
       1. Decreased vision
       2. Decreased accommodation
       3. Diplopia
       4. Visual hallucinations
       5. Pupils
           a. Mydriasis—may precipitate narrow-angle glaucoma
           b. Miosis
           c. Decreased reaction to light
       6. Nystagmus
       7. Strabismus

Clinical Significance: Ocular side effects from baclofen are rare and transient. Usually, the adverse effects can be abolished by reduction of the dosage of baclofen without loss of benefit. Hallucinations have sometimes occurred with treatment but usually after abrupt withdrawal of this drug. Therefore, except for serious adverse reactions, the dose should be reduced slowly when the drug is discontinued. Accommodative disorders have been reported in overdosage situations.

References:
Blankenship, J.M.K., and Moses, E.S..: Baclofen overdose in a child resulting in respiratory arrest. Vet. Human Toxicol. *25*(Suppl. 1):45, 1983.
Garabedian-Ruffalo, S.M., and Ruffalo, R.L.: Adverse effects secondary to baclofen withdrawal. Drug Intell. Clin. Pharm. *19*:304, 1985.
Haubenstock, A., et al.: Baclofen (Lioresal) intoxication report of 4 cases and review of the literature. J. Toxicol. Clin. Toxicol. *20*:59, 1983.
Sandyk, R.: Orofacial dyskinesia induced by baclofen in a patient with hypothyroidism. Clin. Pharm. *5*:109, 1986.
Terrence, C.F., and Fromm, G.H.: Complications of baclofen withdrawal. Arch. Neurol. *38*:588, 1981

Generic Name: Dantrolene

Proprietary Name: Danlene (Ital.), Dantamacrin (Germ., Switz.), Dantralen (Span.), **Dantrium** (Austral., Canad., Fr., G.B., Ital., Neth., S. Afr.)

Primary Use: This skeletal muscle relaxant is effective in controlling the manifestations of clinical spasticity resulting from serious chronic disorders, such as spinal cord injury, stroke, cerebral palsy, or multiple sclerosis.

Ocular Side Effects:
A. Systemic Administration
  1. Decreased vision
  2. Eyelids or conjunctiva
    a. Photosensitivity
    b. Urticaria
  3. Diplopia
  4. Lacrimation
  5. Visual hallucinations

Clinical Significance: Ocular side effects due to dantrolene are transient and seldom of clinical significance. Decreased vision, diplopia, and excessive lacrimation are the most common adverse ocular effects. Visual hallucinations associated with the use of this drug usually subside upon drug withdrawal; however, several days may be required.

References:
Andrews, L.G., Muzumdar, A.S., and Pinkerton, A.C. Hallucinations associated with dantrolene sodium therapy. Can. Med. Assoc. J. *112*:148, 1975.
McEvoy, G.K. (Ed.): American Hospital Formulary Service Drug Information 87. Bethesda, American Society of Hospital Pharmacists, 1987, pp. 652–655.
Pembroke, A.C., et al.: Acne induced by dantrolene. Br. J. Dermatol. *104*:465, 1981.

Reynolds, J.E.F. (Ed.): Martindale: The Extra Pharmacopoeia. 28th Ed., London, Pharmaceutical Press, 1982, pp. 989–990.

Silverman, H.I., and Harvie, R.J.: Adverse effects of commonly used systemic drugs on the human eye—Part III. Am. J. Optom. Physiol. Optics 52:275, 1975.

Generic Name: 1. Mephenesin; 2. Methocarbamol

Proprietary Name: 1. Décontractyl (Fr.), Relaxar (Ital.), Reoxyl (Germ.); 2. Lumirelax (Fr.), Miowas (Ital., Span.), **Robaxin** (Austral., Canad., G.B., S. Afr., Span., Swed.), Traumacut (Germ.)

Primary Use: These centrally acting muscle relaxants are used in the treatment of acute musculoskeletal disorders. Mephenesin has also been used as an adjunct to anesthesia and in the treatment of Parkinson's disease and tetanus.

Ocular Side Effects:
   A. Systemic Administration
      1. Decreased vision
      2. Nystagmus—horizontal, vertical, or rotary
      3. Diplopia
      4. Ptosis (mephenesin)
      5. Ciliary hyperemia (mephenesin)
      6. Decreased intraocular pressure (mephenesin)
      7. Paresis of extraocular muscles (mephenesin)
      8. Eyelids or conjunctiva (methocarbamol)
         a. Erythema
         b. Conjunctivitis—nonspecific
         c. Urticaria

Clinical Significance: Ocular side effects due to these muscle relaxants are much more common after intravenous administration than when given orally. Adverse ocular reactions are transitory and usually of little consequence. Ptosis, ciliary hyperemia, decreased intraocular pressure, and paresis of extraocular muscles are only seen with mephenesin, while nonspecific conjunctivitis, erythema, and urticaria have been reported only with methocarbamol. Erythema multiforme-like eruptions associated with contact dermatitis have been associated with topical application of mephenesin.

References:
Degreef, H., et al.: Mephenesin contact dermatitis with erythema multiforme features. Contact Dermatitis 10:220, 1984.

Gilman, A.G., Goodman, L.S., and Gilman, A. (Eds.): The Pharmacological Basis of Therapeutics. 6th Ed., New York, Macmillan, 1980, pp. 488–489.

Hunter, A.R., and Waterfall, J.M.: Myanesin in hyperkinetic states. Lancet *1*:366–367, 1948.

Schlesinger, E.B., Drew, A.L., and Wood, B.: Clinical studies in the use of myanesin. Am. J. Med. *4*:365–372, 1948.

Stephen, C.R., and Chandy, J.: Clinical and experimental studies with myanesin. Can. Med. Assoc. J. *57*:463–468, 1947.

Walsh, F.B., and Hoyt, W.F.: Clinical Neuro-Ophthalmology. 3rd Ed., Baltimore, Williams & Wilkins, Vol. III, 1969, p. 2648.

Generic Name: Orphenadrine

Proprietary Name: Biorphen (G.B.), Disipal (Austral., Canad., Fr., G.B., Ital., Neth., S. Afr., Swed., Switz.), Disipaletten (Neth.), **Myotrol, Norflex** (Austral., Canad., G.B., Germ., S. Afr., Swed., Switz.)

Primary Use: This antihistaminic agent is used in the treatment of skeletal muscle spasm and the associated pain of Parkinsonism.

Ocular Side Effects:
  A. Systemic Administration
    1. Pupils
      a. Mydriasis—may precipitate narrow-angle glaucoma
      b. Absence of reaction to light
    2. Decreased vision
    3. Decrease or paralysis of accommodation
    4. Diplopia
    5. Visual hallucinations
    6. Subconjunctival or retinal hemorrhages secondary to drug-induced anemia
    7. Decreased tolerance to contact lenses

Clinical Significance: Ocular side effects due to orphenadrine are transient and probably the result of its weak anticholinergic effect. These are seldom a significant clinical problem, although narrow-angle glaucoma has been precipitated secondary to drug-induced mydriasis. Nonreactive dilated pupils are only seen in overdose situations.

References:
Bennett, N.B., and Kohn, J.: Case report: Orphenadrine overdose. Cerebral manifestations treated with physostigmine. Anaesth. Intensive Care *4*:67, 1976.

Davidson, S.I.: Reports of ocular adverse reactions. Trans. Ophthalmol. Soc. U.K. *93*: 495–510, 1973.

Drug Evaluations. 6th Ed., Chicago, American Medical Association, 1986, pp. 208, 235.

Furlanut, M., et al.: Orphenadrine serum levels in a poisoned patient. Hum. Toxicol. *4*:331, 1985.

Gilman, A.G., Goodman, L.S., and Gilman, A. (Eds.): The Pharmacological Basis of Therapeutics. 6th Ed., New York, Macmillan, 1980, pp. 485–487.

Heinonen, J., et al.: Orphenadrine poisoning. A case report supplemented with animal experiments. Arch. Toxicol. *23*:264, 1968.

Selby, G.: Treatment of Parkinsonism. Drugs *11*:61, 1976.

Stoddart, J.C., Parkin, J.M., and Wynne, N.A.: Orphenadrine poisoning. A case report. Br. J. Anaesth. *40*:789, 1968.

XI   Oncolytic Agents

Class: Antineoplastic Agents

Generic Name: 1. Bleomycin; 2. Cactinomycin; 3. Dactinomycin; 4. Daunorubicin; 5. Doxorubicin; 6. Mitomycin

Proprietary Name: 1. **Blenoxane** (Austral., Canad., S. Afr.), Bleo-S (Jap.), Oil Bleo (Jap.); 3. **Cosmegen** (Austral., Canad., Ital., S. Afr., Swed., Switz.), Cosmegen, Lyovac (G.B.), Lyovac Cosmegen (Neth.), Lyovac-Cosmegen (Germ.); 4. Cerubidin (Austral., S. Afr., Swed.), Cérubidine (Fr., Switz.), **Cerubidine** (Canad., Neth.), Daunoblastin (Germ.), Daunoblastina (Ital., Span.); 5. Adriblastin (Germ.), Adriblastina (Ital., S. Afr.), Adriblastine (Fr., Switz.), Farmiblastina (Span.), **Rubex**; 6. Amétycine (Fr.), **Mutamycin** (Canad., Neth., Swed., Switz.)

Primary Use: *Systemic:* These antibiotics are used in a variety of malignant conditions. Bleomycin is a polypeptide antibiotic used in the management of squamous cell carcinomas, lymphomas, and testicular carcinomas. Cactinomycin and dactinomycin are antibiotics used in the management of choriocarcinoma, rhabdomyosarcoma, Wilms' tumor, testicular neoplasms, and carcinoid syndrome. Daunorubicin is used in the treatment of acute leukemia, and doxorubicin is used in sarcomas, lymphomas, and leukemia. Mitomycin is useful in the therapy of disseminated adenocarcinoma of the stomach or pancreas. *Ophthalmic:* Mitomycin is used as an adjunct in the surgical treatment of pterygia and glaucoma. It has also been used as a modulator of corneal wound healing after excimer laser refractive surgery.

Ocular Side Effects:
A. Systemic Administration
1. Eyelids or conjunctiva
   a. Allergic reactions
   b. Erythema
   c. Conjunctivitis

349

        d. Edema
        e. Hyperpigmentation
        f. Angioneurotic edema
        g. Urticaria
        h. Erythema multiforme
        i. Loss of eyelashes or eyebrows
    2. Decreased vision
    3. Subconjunctival or retinal hemorrhages secondary to drug-induced anemia
    4. Lacrimation
    5. May aggravate herpes infections
    6. Alopecia
    7. Cataracts
    8. Ocular teratogenic effects
  B. Local Ophthalmic Use or Exposure—Mitomycin
    1. Irritation
        a. Lacrimation
        b. Hyperemia
        c. Photophobia
        d. Ocular pain
    2. Eyelids or conjunctiva
        a. Allergic or irritative reactions
        b. Hyperemia
        c. Erythema
        d. Blepharitis
        e. Conjunctivitis
        f. Edema
        g. Granuloma
        h. Avascularity
        i. Symblepharon
    3. Cornea
        a. Punctate keratitis
        b. Edema
        c. Delayed wound healing
        d. Erosion (epithelial and stromal)
        e. Perforation
        f. Crystalline epithelial deposits
        g. Recurrence of herpes simplex
    4. Sclera
        a. Erosion
        b. Delayed wound healing
        c. Perforation
        d. Avascularity
        e. Necrotizing scleritis

    f. Calcium deposits
    g. Yellowish plaques
  5. Uvea
    a. Iridocyclitis
    b. Hypopigmentation of iris
    c. Hyperemia
  6. Glaucoma
  7. Punctal occlusion
  8. Hypotony—persistent

Clinical Significance: Systemic chemotherapeutic agents in the main are secreted via the lacrimal gland, which initially results in ocular and lid irritation. Conjunctivitis or blepharoconjunctivitis are the most common adverse events. Frequently, the patient has so many significant systemic side effects, the ocular symptomatology is overlooked. In the main, the ocular side effects are reversible and transitory. Most antimetabolites may be co-factors in causing lens opacities. Nystagmus has been seen, but it is difficult to prove if it was due to the drug. Since most systemic chemotherapy is used only in short-pulsed dosage schedules, ocular side effects are seldom of significant clinical importance. The exception is intracarotid administration proximal to the ophthalmic artery. In this instance, disastrous ocular toxicity may occur, including permanent blindness. If these agents have direct inadvertent contact with the eye, a superficial punctate keratitis with or without iritis may occur. To our knowledge, no long-term sequelae have occurred. Mitomycin has gained the most exposure in ophthalmology because of its use in glaucoma and pterygium surgery. The popularity of topical ocular mitomycin has peaked because of a number of publications of adverse ocular side effects. Some ophthalmologists are still using this agent; however, it is at lower dosages, less frequently, and for a shorter duration. Mitomycin action on ocular tissue mimics that of ionizing radiation with the resultant lifelong effects on tissue. As with radiation, side effects increase along with increased cumulative doses. A major characteristic of this chemical is that some side effects are immune-mediated and may manifest themselves months after exposure. Irritative signs and symptoms are usually short-lived and seldom last more than a few weeks. The most serious side effects are probably immune-mediated. Although these include many factors, some may have a long-term effect on both fibroblast activity and vascular endothelial cells. This could account for severe, unresponsive corneal and scleral melts that may mimic scleromalacia perforans and/or necrotizing scleritis. Cases in the literature report perforation, and in some instances, the loss of the eye. Porcelainization of the conjunctiva and sclera (avascularity) has been permanent. As with systemic exposure, local recurrence of herpes simplex and calcification of tissue in direct contact with mitomycin can occur. If the drug is given intraocularly, uveitis with or without secondary glaucoma can occur. In animal studies, this agent is highly toxic to all uveal and retinal tissue. McDermott, Wang, and Shin, using human donor tissue, showed undiluted mitomycin to cause prompt destruction of the endothelial cells. Exposure to 20 μg/mL of mitomycin (levels exceeding normal clinical use) were nontoxic to human endothelial cells.

References:

Imperia, P.S., Lazarus, H.M., and Lass, J.H.: Ocular complications of systemic cancer chemotherapy. Surv. Ophthalmol. *34(3)*:209–230, 1989.

Knowles, R.S., and Virden, J.E.: Handling of injectable antineoplastic agents. Br. Med. J. *2*:589, 1980.

McDermott, M.L., Wang, J., and Shin, D.H.: Mitomycin and the human corneal endothelium. Arch. Ophthalmol. *112*:533–537, 1994.

Nuyts, R.M.M., et al.: Histopathologic effects of mitomycin C after trabeculectomy in human glaucomatous eyes with persistent hypotony. Am. J. Ophthalmol. *118(2)*: 225–237, 1994.

Oram, O., et al.: Necrotizing keratitis following trabeculectomy with mitomycin. Arch. Ophthalmol. *113*:19–20, 1995.

Oster, M.W.: Ocular side effects of cancer chemotherapy. *In* Perry, M.C., and Yarbro, J.W. (Eds.): Toxicity of Chemotherapy. New York, Grune & Stratton, 1984, pp. 181–197.

Rubinfeld, R.S., et al: Serious complications of topical mitomycin-C after pterygium surgery. Ophthalmology *99(11)*:1647–1654, 1992.

Singh, G., Wilson, M.R., and Foster, C.S.: Mitomycin eyedrops as treatment for pterygium. Ophthalmology *95(6)*:813–821, 1988.

Skuta, G.L., et al: Intraoperative mitomycin versus postoperative 5-fluorouracil in high-risk glaucoma filtering surgery. Ophthalmology *99(3)*:438–444, 1992.

Vizel, M., and Oster, M.W.: Ocular side effects of cancer chemotherapy. Cancer *49*: 1999, 1982.

Generic Name: 1. Busulfan; 2. Carmustine (BCNU); 3. Chlorambucil; 4. Cyclophosphamide; 5. Dacarbazine (DIC); 6. Lomustine (CCNU); 7. Mechlorethamine; 8. Melphalan; 9. Semustine; 10. Streptozocin (Streptozotocin); 11. Triethylenemelamine (Tretamine); 12. Uracil Mustard (Uramustine)

Proprietary Name: 1. Misulban (Ital., Mon.), **Myleran** (Austral., Canad., G.B., Germ., Ital., Neth., S. Afr., Swed., Switz.); 2. Becenun (Swed.), **BiCNU** (Austral., Canad., Fr., G.B.), Carmubris (Germ.), Nitrumon (Ital.); 3. **Leukeran** (Austral., Canad., G.B., Germ., Ital., Neth., S. Afr., Span., Swed., Switz.), Linfolysin (Ital.); 4. Cicloxal (Span.), Cycloblastin (Austral., S. Afr.), Cyclostin (Germ.), **Cytoxan** (Canad.), Endoxan (Austral., Germ., Ital., Neth., S. Afr., Switz.), Endoxana (G.B.), Genoxal (Span.), **Neosar**, Procytox (Canad.), Sendoxan (Swed.); 5. Déticène (Fr.), Deticene (Germ., Ital., Neth.), DTIC (Canad., Swed.), **DTIC-DOME** (G.B., S. Afr.); 6. Bélustine (Fr.), Belustine (Ital., Span.), CCNU (G.B., Span.), Cecenu (Germ.),

CeeNU (Austral., Canad., S. Afr.), CiNU (Switz.), Lomeblastin (Germ.), Lucostine (Swed.); 7. Caryolysine (Fr.), **Mustargen** (Canad., Switz.); 8. Alkéran (Fr.), **Alkeran** (Austral., Canad., G.B., Germ., Ital., Neth., S. Afr., Swed., Switz.); 10. **Zanosar** (Canad., Fr.)

Primary Use: These alkylating agents are used in the treatment of Hodgkin's disease, lymphomas, multiple myeloma, leukemia, neuroblastoma, and retinoblastoma. Chlorambucil, cyclophosphamide, mechlorethamine, melphalan, and uracil mustard are nitrogen mustards, and carmustine, lomustine, semustine, and streptozocin are nitrosureas. Busulfan is an alkyl sulfonate, dacarbazine is a triazene, and triethylenemelamine is an ethylenimine derivative.

Ocular Side Effects:
  A. Systemic Administration
    1. Eyelids or conjunctiva
      a. Allergic reactions
      b. Hyperemia (carmustine)
      c. Erythema
      d. Blepharoconjunctivitis (cyclophosphamide, mechlorethamine, melphalan)
      e. Edema (chlorambucil)
      f. Hyperpigmentation (busulfan, carmustine, chlorambucil, cyclophosphamide, mechlorethamine, uracil mustard)
      g. Photosensitivity (cyclophosphamide, dacarbazine)
      h. Angioneurotic edema (melphalan)
      i. Urticaria (busulfan, chlorambucil, cyclophosphamide, dacarbazine, melphalan)
      j. Erythema multiforme (busulfan, mechlorethamine)
      k. Exfoliative dermatitis (chlorambucil, cyclophosphamide, mechlorethamine)
      l. Loss of eyelashes or eyebrows
    2. Decreased vision
    3. Subconjunctival or retinal hemorrhages secondary to drug-induced anemia
    4. Nonspecific ocular irritation (cyclophosphamide)
      a. Lacrimation
      b. Hyperemia
      c. Photophobia
      d. Ocular pain
      e. Edema
      f. Burning sensation
    5. Cataracts (busulfan)
    6. Keratoconjunctivitis sicca (busulfan, chlorambucil, cyclophosphamide)

7. Decreased lacrimation (busulfan)
8. Corneal edema (melphalan)
9. Increased intraocular pressure (carmustine)
10. Pupils
    a. Absence of pupillary reaction to light (carmustine)
    b. Pinpoint pupils (cyclophosphamide)
11. Visual hallucinations (chlorambucil)
12. Optic neuritis (carmustine)
13. Papilledema secondary to pseudotumor cerebri (chlorambucil)
14. Retinal vascular disorders (carmustine)
    a. Occlusion
    b. Thrombosis
    c. Hemorrhages
15. May aggravate the following diseases
    a. Herpes infections
    b. Sjögren's syndrome
16. Myopia (cyclophosphamide)
17. Maculopathy (carmustine)
18. Ocular teratogenic effects
    a. Microphthalmia (busulfan)
    b. Retinal degeneration (busulfan)

Clinical Significance: In general, ocular side effects due to these alkylating agents are uncommon, transitory, and seldom of major significance. However, depending on long-term use or the method of administration, significant ocular side effects can occur. The overview paper by Imperia, Lazarus, and Lass is the most complete review on this group of agents and their possible ocular side effects. Busulfan has caused posterior subcapsular cataracts and keratoconjunctivitis sicca. Reversible hyperpigmentation of the skin and mucous membranes seen with some of these agents may be an indication for discontinuing the drug. Loss of eyelashes or eyebrows is almost always seen only with severe drug-induced alopecia. In up to 20% of cases, the regrowth of hair is a different color. Secondary glaucoma, internal ophthalmoplegia, optic neuroretinitis, cilioretinal artery occlusion, and choroidal thrombus have been reported with carmustine chemotherapy. Intra-arterially administered cisplatin and intravenous carmustine in combination caused severe macular pigmentary changes. This was a direct toxic effect and not on the basis of vascular changes as with other carmustine ocular side effects. Reversible pseudotumor cerebri with papilledema while being treated with chlorambucil has occurred. Herpes infections, which commonly occur in patients with lymphomas, may be precipitated by the immunosuppressive effect of these agents. Acute leukemia has been seen following cyclophosphamide treatment in patients with Sjögren's syndrome. Many antineoplastic agents may be found in lacrimal secretions, causing conjunctival, corneal, punctal, lacrimal outflow, and lid irritation. Since most of these agents are used only for short periods, low concentrations of topical ophthalmic corticosteroids may be used to alleviate these symptoms. Ocular teratogenic effects seen with busulfan include microphthalmia and atypical tapetoretinal degeneration. Inadvertent topical ocular exposure with these agents has caused severe conjunctival irritation and has been suspected of causing corneal opacities.

References:

Council on Scientific Affairs. Guidelines for handling parenteral antineoplastics. JAMA *253*:1590, 1985.

Fraunfelder, F.T., and Meyer, S.M.: Ocular toxicity of antineoplastic agents. Ophthalmology *90*:1, 1983.

Griffin, J.D., and Garnick, M.B.: Eye toxicity of cancer chemotherapy. A review of the literature. Cancer *48*:1539, 1981.

Imperia, P.S., Lazarus, H.M., and Lass, J.H.: Ocular complications of systemic cancer chemotherapy. Surv. Ophthalmol. *34(3)*:209–230, 1989.

Jack, M.K., and Hicks, J.D.: Ocular complications in high-dose chemoradiotherapy and marrow transplantation. Ann. Ophthalmol. *13*:709, 1981.

Kupersmith, M.J., et al: Maculopathy caused by intra-arterially administered cisplatin and intravenously administered carmustine. Am. J. Ophthalmol. *113*:435–438, 1992.

Louie, A.C., et al.: Letter to the editor. Med. Pediatr. Oncol. *5*:245, 1978.

McLennan, R., and Taylor, H.R. · Optic neuroretinitis in association with BCNU and procarbazine therapy. Med. Pediatr. Oncol. *4*:43, 1978.

Millay, R.H., et al: Maculopathy associated with combination chemotherapy and osmotic opening of the blood-brain barrier. Am. J. Ophthalmol. *102*:626–632, 1986.

Miller, D.F., et al.: Ocular and orbital toxicity following intracarotid injection of BCNU (carmustine) and cisplatinum for malignant gliomas. Ophthalmology *92*:402, 1985.

Shingleton, B.J., et al: Ocular toxicity associated with high-dose carmustine. Arch. Ophthalmol. *100*:1766, 1982.

Vizel, M., and Oster, M.W.: Ocular side effects of cancer chemotherapy. Cancer *49*: 1999, 1982.

Weiss, R.B., and Bruno, S.: Hypersensitivity reactions to cancer chemotherapeutic agents. Ann. Intern. Med. *94*:66, 1981.

Generic Name: Cisplatin (Cisplatinum)

Proprietary Name: Abiplatin (Neth., S. Afr.), Cisplatyl (Fr.), Citoplatino (Ital.), Lederplatin (Swed.), Neoplatin (Span.), Norplatin (S. Afr.), Placis (Span.), Platamine (Austral., Ital., S. Afr.), Platibastin (Germ.), Platiblastine (Switz.), Platinex (Germ., Ital.), **Platinol** (Canad., Neth., Swed., Switz.), Platistil (Span.), Platistin (Swed.), Platosin (Neth.), Pronto Platamine (Ital.), Randa (Jap.)

Primary Use: This platinum-containing antineoplastic agent is used for the treatment of metastatic testicular or ovarian tumors, advanced bladder carcinoma, and a wide variety of other neoplasms.

Ocular Side Effects:
  A. Systemic Administration
      1. Decreased vision
      2. Eyelids or conjunctiva
          a. Erythema
          b. Conjunctivitis—nonspecific
          c. Edema
          d. Urticaria
          e. Loss of eyelashes or eyebrows
      3. Retrobulbar or optic neuritis
      4. Papilledema
      5. Myasthenic neuromuscular blocking effect
          a. Paralysis of extraocular muscles
          b. Ptosis
          c. Diplopia
      6. Abnormal ERG, EOG, or VEP
      7. Hemianopsia
      8. Cortical blindness
      9. Subconjunctival or retinal hemorrhages secondary to
         drug-induced anemia
     10. Oculogyric crises
     11. Retinal pigmentary changes
          a. Mild perimacular (intravenous)
          b. Severe—total retinal (intracarotid)
     12. Orbital pain
     13. May aggravate herpes infections
     14. Color vision defect

Clinical Significance: Well-documented serious side effects have been associated with cisplatin, which is a commonly used anti-cancer agent. It appears
   that the intracarotid infusion adverse ocular effects are dose-related and
   have caused ipsilateral visual loss with associated retinal and optic nerve
   ischemia. While it has been reported that the serious side effects can be
   prevented if the infusion catheter is advanced beyond the ophthalmic artery,
   Margo and Murtagh recently showed that this is not necessarily true. Their
   case had uveal effusion, exudative retinal detachment, enlarged rectus muscles, and inflammation of orbital and periorbital soft tissue. Ophthalmoplegia also occurred, and complete visual loss was permanent. Intravenous cisplatin adverse ocular effects are more neuroretinal and consist of
   ERG changes, blurred vision, color blindness, disc edema, retrobulbar neuritis, and cortical blindness. Alteration of color vision is usually in the blue-
   green axis, and retinal toxicity is mainly that of cone dysfunction. Vision
   rarely gets worse than 20/25, and central field constriction has been documented. Retinal changes are usually mild, irregular macular pigmentary
   changes; while most visual acuities return to normal after therapy is com-

pleted, color vision may take as long as 16 months to resolve. Ozols, et al. believe that ocular toxicity seems to be more common in the older age group and in females. An accumulative dose-toxicity relationship seems to occur. Retrobulbar neuritis and disc edema have been shown to be more common in patients with a high cerebral spinal fluid level of cisplatin. This may lead to a segmental demyelination similar to that with other heavy metals. It is interesting that retrobulbar neuritis, cortical blindness, and papilledema have been found with no evidence of elevated intracranial pressure. A myasthenic-like syndrome characterized by ptosis and diplopia has been associated with cisplatin. Most antineoplastic agents may be found in lacrimal secretion causing conjunctival and corneal abnormalities, punctal constriction, and lid irritation. Probably the best review of cisplatin, along with other anticancerous agents since they are often used in combination, is that by Imperia, Lazarus, and Lass.

References:

Cohen, R.J., et al.: Transient left homonymous hemianopsia and encephalopathy following treatment of testicular carcinoma with cisplatinum, vinblastine, and bleomycin. J. Clin. Oncol. *1*:392, 1983.

Diamond, S.B., et al.: Cerebral blindness in association with cis-platinum chemotherapy for advanced carcinoma of the fallopian tube. Obstet. Gynecol. *59*:84S, 1982.

Feun, L.G., et al.: Intracarotid infusion of cis-diammine-dichloroplatinum in the treatment of recurrent malignant brain tumors. Cancer *54*:794, 1984.

Imperia, P.S., Lazarus, H.M., and Lass, J.H.: Ocular complications of systemic cancer chemotherapy. Surv. Ophthalmol. *34(3)*:209–230, 1989.

Margo, C.E., and Murtagh, F.R.: Ocular and orbital toxicity after intracarotid cisplatin therapy. Am. J. Ophthalmol. *116(4)*:508–509, 1993.

Miller, D.F., et al.: Ocular and orbital toxicity following intracarotid injection of BCNU (carmustin) and cisplatinum for malignant gliomas. Ophthalmology *92*:402, 1985.

Ozols, R.F., et al.: Treatment of poor prognosis nonseminomatous testicular cancer with a ''high dose'' platinum combination chemotherapy regimen. Cancer *51*: 1803–1807, 1983.

Pollera, C.F., et al.: Sudden death after acute dystonic reaction to high-dose metoclopramide. Lancet *2*:460, 1984.

Tang, R.A., et al.: Ocular toxicity and cis-platin. Invest. Ophthalmol. Vis. Sci. *24*(Suppl.):284, 1983.

Walsh, T.J., et al.: Neurotoxic effects of cisplatin therapy. Arch. Neurol. *39*:719, 1982.

Wilding, G., et al.: Retinal toxicity after high-dose cisplatin therapy. J. Clin. Oncol. *3*:1683–1689, 1985.

Generic Name: Cytarabine (Ara-C, Cytosine Arabinoside)

Proprietary Name: Alexan (Austral., G.B., Germ., Ital., Neth., Switz.), Aracytin (Ital.), Aracytine (Fr.), Cytarbel (Fr.), Cytosar (Canad., G.B., Neth., S. Afr., Swed., Switz.), **Cytosar-U** (Austral.), Erpalfa (Ital.), Udicil (Germ.)

Primary Use: *Systemic*: This antimetabolite is effective in the management of acute granulocytic leukemia, polycythemia vera, and malignant neoplasms.

Ophthalmic: This topical pyrimidine nucleoside is used in the treatment of herpes simplex keratitis.

Ocular Side Effects:
  A. Systemic Administration
      1. Eyelids or conjunctiva
          a. Allergic reactions
          b. Erythema
          c. Conjunctivitis—hemorrhagic
          d. Hyperpigmentation
          e. Urticaria
          f. Purpura
      2. Nonspecific ocular irritation
          a. Lacrimation
          b. Hyperemia
          c. Photophobia
          d. Ocular pain
          e. Burning sensation
      3. Decreased vision
      4. Cornea
          a. Keratitis
          b. Opacities
      5. Subconjunctival or retinal hemorrhages secondary to drug-induced anemia
      6. Extraocular muscles—intrathecal
          a. Paresis
          b. Diplopia
          c. Nystagmus
      7. May aggravate herpes infections
  B. Local Ophthalmic Use or Exposure
      1. Ocular pain
      2. Iritis
      3. Corneal opacities
      4. Corneal ulceration
      5. Delayed corneal wound healing
      6. Decreased resistance to infection

Clinical Significance: Conjunctivitis and ocular irritation are commonly seen in patients receiving high-dose (> 3 g/m^2) systemic cytarabine chemotherapy. Many antineoplastic agents have been found in lacrimal secretions, which may be the cause for the conjunctival, corneal, eyelid, or lacrimal outflow system irritation. In addition, fine, punctate corneal epithelial opacities and refractile microcysts associated with systemic cytarabine are transitory and reversible usually within 1 to 2 weeks after discontinuation of therapy. These symptoms usually appear 5 to 7 days after initiation of therapy and may be minimized or prevented by prophylaxis with short-term use of topical ocular corticosteroids. Adverse effects associated with high-dose intravenous regimens may also include cerebral or cerebellar dysfunction, which is usually reversible. Ocular manifestations of this CNS toxicity may include lateral gaze nystagmus, diplopia, and lateral rectus palsy. Neurotoxicity following intrathecal injection of cytarabine has been associated with diluents containing preservatives. Blindness occurred in two leukemic patients in remission who had received systemic combination chemotherapy, prophylactic CNS irradiation, and intrathecal cytarabine. Because topical cytarabine causes significant corneal toxicity, it has been replaced by equally effective and less toxic antiviral agents.

References:

Gressel, M.G., and Tomsak, R.L.: Keratitis from high dose intravenous cytarabine. Lancet 2:273, 1982.

Hwang, T.-L., et al.: Central nervous system toxicity with high-dose Ara-C. Neurology 35:1475, 1985.

Lass, J.H., et al.: Topical corticosteroid therapy for corneal toxicity from systemically administered cytarabine. Am. J. Ophthalmol. 94:617, 1982.

Lazarus, H.M., et al.: Comparison of the prophylactic effects of 2-deoxycytidine and prednisolone for high-dose intravenous cytarabine-induced keratitis. Am. J. Ophthalmol. 104:476, 1987.

Lopez, J.A., and Agarwal, R.P.: Acute cerebellar toxicity after high-dose cytarabine associated with CNS accumulation of its metabolite, uracil arabinoside. Cancer Treat. Rep. 68:1309, 1984.

Ritch, P.S., Hansen, R.M., and Heuer, D.K.: Ocular toxicity from high-dose cytosine arabinoside. Cancer 51:430, 1983.

Spaeth, G.S., Nelson, L.B., and Beaudoin, A.E.: Ocular teratology. In Jakobiec, F.A. (Ed.): Ocular Anatomy, Embryology and Teratology. Philadelphia, J.B. Lippincott, 1982, pp. 955–975.

Winkelman, M.D., and Hines, J.D.: Cerebellar degeneration caused by high-dose cytosine arabinoside: A clinicopathological study. Ann. Neurol. 14:520, 1983.

Generic Name: 1. Floxuridine; 2. Fluorouracil (5-FU)

Proprietary Name: *Systemic*: 1. **FUDR**; 2. **Adrucil** (Canad.), Cytosafe (Germ.), **5-FU**, Fluroblastin (Austral., Germ., S. Afr.), Fl_uroblastine (Switz.) *Topical*: 2. **Efudex** (Canad.), Efudix (Austral., Fr., G.B., Germ., Ital., Neth., S. Afr., Span., Switz.), **Fluoroplex** (Austral.)

Primary Use: These fluorinated pyrimidine antimetabolites are used in the management of carcinoma of the colon, rectum, breast, stomach, and pancreas. Fluorouracil is also used topically for actinic keratoses and intradermally for skin cancer. It is also used topically and subconjunctivally to enhance glaucoma filtration surgery.

Ocular Side Effects:
A. Systemic Administration
    1. Nonspecific ocular irritation
        a. Lacrimation
        b. Hyperemia
        c. Photophobia
        d. Ocular pain
        e. Edema
        f. Burning sensation
        g. Contact lens intolerance
    2. Decreased vision
    3. Eyelids or conjunctiva
        a. Cicatricial ectropion
        b. Occlusion of lacrimal canaliculi or punctum
        c. Erythema
        d. Blepharoconjunctivitis
        e. Edema
        f. Hyperpigmentation
        g. Photosensitivity
        h. Erythema multiforme
        i. Ulceration
        j. Loss of eyelashes or eyebrows
        k. Keratinization lid margin
    4. Cornea
        a. Superficial punctate keratitis
        b. Ulceration
        c. Opacity
    5. Nystagmus (coarse)
    6. Decreased convergence or divergence
    7. Diplopia
    8. Decreased accommodation
    9. Blepharospasm
  10. Subconjunctival or retinal hemorrhages secondary to drug-induced anemia
  11. May aggravate herpes infections
  12. Optic neuritis
  13. Ocular teratogenic effects
B. Local Ophthalmic Use or Exposure—Subconjunctival or Intradermal Injection (Fluorouracil)
    1. Irritation
        a. Lacrimation
        b. Ocular pain
        c. Edema
        d. Burning sensation

    2. Eyelids or conjunctiva
      a. Cicatricial ectropion
      b. Allergic reactions
      c. Erythema
      d. Edema
      e. Hyperpigmentation
      f. Keratinization
      g. Urticaria
      h. Pemphigoid lesion
      i. Loss of eyelashes or eyebrows
      j. Subconjunctival hemorrhages
      k. Delayed wound healing
    3. Periorbital edema
    4. Cornea
      a. Superficial punctate keratitis
      b. Ulceration
      c. Scarring—stromal
      d. Keratinized plaques
      e. Delayed wound healing
      f. Striate melanokeratosis
      g. Endothelial damage

Clinical Significance: Fluorouracil is one of the most commonly used cyto-toxic drugs in the palliative treatment of solid tumors. Since its therapeutic dose is often close to its toxic level, between 25% and 35% of patients receiving systemic therapy have some ocular side effects. The listed side effects are primarily related to fluorouracil use, since it is more commonly used than floxuridine. The most common adverse ocular effects are a low-grade blepharitis and conjunctival irritation, with symptoms well out of proportion to the clinical findings. These reactions occur within the first few weeks of therapy and are transitory, but discontinuation of the drug may be required in some patients. On long-term systemic therapy, the drug has been found in tears, which possibly causes a local irritation resulting in cicatricial reaction in the conjunctiva, punctum, canaliculi, and lacrimal sac. If recognized early, some cases have been reversed; however, in most cases, the scarring is irreversible with epiphora resulting. Neurotoxicity, which possibly affects the brain stem and causes oculomotor disturbances, can occur. Several cases of possible optic toxicity secondary to fluorouracil have been reported. Ointments containing fluorouracil that are used in the treatment of skin lesions near the eye have caused significant ocular irritation requiring discontinuation of this form of therapy. Ocular side effects due to local therapy are usually reversible if the eye had only limited exposure. Direct injection of fluorouracil into the eyelids for the treatment of basal cell carcinoma can also cause cicatricial ectropion and hyperpigmentation. This drug should be used with caution in patients with pre-existent corneal pathology, including some diabetics. Lid necrosis has been reported in one case with cryotherapy for trichiasis when the patient was also taking 5-FU. Fluorouracil has had increased popularity in the management of difficult glaucoma patients requiring filtration surgery. This is most commonly given as a subconjunctival injection that enhances a bleb formation. However, adverse ocular effects, most of which are reversible, occur in up to 50% of cases. The most common is a superficial keratitis that may rarely become ulcerated. Hayashi, Ibaraki, and Tsuru reported a permanent corneal opacity requiring a lamellar keratoplasty when this agent was used after a trabeculectomy. Other defects include conjunctival wound leaks, excessive filtration with shallow to flat anterior chambers, and conjunctival or corneal keratinization.

References:

Adams, J.W., et al.: Recurrent acute toxic optic neuropathy secondary to 5-FU. Cancer Treat. Rep. *68*:565, 1984.

Alward, W.L.M., et al.: Fluorouracil filtering surgery study one-year follow-up. Am. J. Ophthalmol. *108(6)*:625–635, 1989.

Caravella, L.P., Jr., Burns, J.A, and Zangmeister, M.: Punctal-canalicular stenosis related to systemic fluorouracil therapy. Arch. Ophthalmol. *99*:284, 1981.

Forbes, J.E., Brazier, D.J., and Spittle, M.: 5-Fluorouracil and ocular toxicity. Letters to the editor. Br. J. Ophthalmol. *77(7)*:465–466, 1993.

Galentine, P., et al.: Bilateral cicatricial ectropion following topical administration of 5-fluorouracil. Ann. Ophthalmol. *13*:575, 1981.

Goette, D.K.: Topical chemotherapy with 5-fluorouracil. A review. J. Am. Acad. Dermatol. *4*:633, 1981.

Hayashi, M., Ibaraki, N., and Tsuru, T.: Lamellar keratoplasty after trabeculectomy with 5-fluorouracil. Am. J. Ophthalmol. *117(2)*:268–269, 1994.

Hickey-Dwyer, M., and Wishart, P.K.: Serious corneal complication of 5-fluorouracil. Br. J. Ophthalmol. *77*:250–251, 1993.

Knapp, A., et al.: Serious corneal complications of glaucoma filtering surgery with postoperative 5-fluorouracil. Am. J. Ophthalmol. *103*:183, 1987.

Kondo, M., and Araie, M.: Concentration change of fluorouracil in the external segment of the eye after subconjunctival injection. Arch. Ophthalmol. *106*:1718–1721, 1988.

Mannis, M.J., Sweet, E.H., and Lewis, R.A.: The effect of fluorouracil on the corneal endothelium. Arch. Ophthalmol. *106*:816–817, 1988.

Imperia, P.S., Lazarus, H.M., and Lass, J.H.: Ocular complications of systemic cancer chemotherapy. Surv. Ophthalmol. *34(3)*:209–230, 1989.

Sato, K., et al.: Clinical investigation of corneal damage induced by 5-fluorouracil. Folia. Ophthalmol. *39(1)*:1754–1760, 1988.

Solomon, L.M.: Plastic eyeglass frames and topical fluorouracil therapy. JAMA *253*:3166, 1985.

Stank, T.M., Krupin, T., and Feitl, M.E.: Subconjunctival 5-fluorouracil-induced transient striate melanokeratosis. Arch. Ophthalmol. *108*:1210, 1990.

Generic Name: Hydroxyurea

Proprietary Name: Hydréa (Fr.), **Hydrea** (Austral., Canad., G.B., Neth., S. Afr.), Litalir (Germ.), Onco-Carbide (Ital.)

Primary Use: This substituted urea preparation is used in the management of chronic granulocytic leukemia, carcinoma of the ovary, and malignant melanoma.

Ocular Side Effects:
A. Systemic Administration
1. Ocular pain
2. Subconjunctival or retinal hemorrhages secondary to drug-induced anemia
3. Eyelids or conjunctiva
a. Erythema
b. Hyperpigmentation
c. Atrophy
d. Scaling
4. Visual hallucinations
5. May aggravate herpes infections

Clinical Significance: Adverse ocular reactions due to hydroxyurea are quite rare. A number of cases of ocular pain only while taking the medication have been reported to the Registry. Ocular side effects other than teratogenic effects are reversible and transitory after the drug is discontinued. Ocular teratogenic effects are possible, but a cause-and-effect relationship has not yet been proven.

References:
Apt, L., and Gaffney, W.L.: Congenital eye abnormalities from drugs during pregnancy. *In* Leopold, I.H. (Ed.): Symposium on Ocular Therapy. St. Louis, C.V. Mosby, Vol. VII, 1974, pp. 1–22.

Dunigan, W.G.: Dermatologic toxicity. *In* Perry, M.C., and Yarbro, J.W. (Eds.): Toxicity of Chemotherapy. New York, Grune & Stratton, 1984, pp. 125–154.

Gilman, A.G., Goodman, L.S., and Gilman, A. (Eds.): The Pharmacological Basis of Therapeutics. 6th Ed., New York, Macmillan, 1980, p. 1299.

Kennedy, B.J., Smith, L.R., and Goltz, R.W.: Skin changes secondary to hydroxyurea therapy. Arch. Dermatol. *111*:183, 1975.

Generic Name: Interferon

Proprietary Name: Intron A (Austral., Canad., G.B., Germ., Ital., Neth., S. Afr., Span., Switz.), Introna (Fr., Swed.), **Roferan-A** (Austral., Canad., G.B., Germ., Neth., Span.), Wellferon (Canad., G.B., Ital., Span., Swed.)

Primary Use: This protein product is used in the treatment of hairy cell leukemia.

Ocular Side Effects:
A. Systemic Administration
1. Decreased vision

2. Ocular pain
3. Eyelids or conjunctiva
    a. Conjunctivitis—nonspecific
    b. Increased growth of eyelashes
    c. Urticaria
    d. Purpura
4. Papilledema—minimal
5. Abnormal VEP
6. Visual hallucinations
7. Subconjunctival or retinal hemorrhages secondary to
   drug-induced anemia
8. May aggravate herpes infections

Clinical Significance: Human leukocyte interferon is usually given by intravenous or intramuscular infusion, and various untoward adverse reactions are not uncommon. As interferon becomes more purified, one would expect that many of these suspected drug-related events will become less common. Visual complaints are minimal and transitory. Ocular pain of unexplained origin can occur but is seldom a significant problem. A number of reports of growth of thick, curly long eyelashes that can range in length from 2.0 to 6.5 cm have been well documented as secondary to interferon. This may require biweekly trimming. This side effect may persist for a few years. In patients taking high-dose interferon, mild disc edema may occur, cause unknown, although some suspect venostasis. This is reversible when therapy is discontinued. Visuospatial disorientation has been reported in some patients receiving interferon therapy. To our knowledge, all adverse ocular effects are reversible and are not threats to vision.

References:

Adams, F., Quesada J.R., and Gutterman, J.U.: Neuropsychiatric manifestations of human leukocyte interferon therapy in patients with cancer. JAMA *252(7)*:938–941, 1984.

Farkkila, M., et al.: Neurotoxic and other side effects of high-dose interferon in amyotrophic lateral sclerosis. Acta Neurol. Scand. *70*:42, 1984.

Foon, K.A.: Increased growth of eyelashes in a patient given leukocyte A interferon. N. Engl. J. Med. *311*:1259, 1984.

Rohatiner, A.Z.S., et al.: Central nervous system toxicity of interferon. Br. J. Cancer *47*:419, 1983.

Scott, G.M., et al: Toxicity of interferon. Br. Med. J. *282(25)*:1345–1348, 1981.

Generic Name: Interleukin 2

Proprietary Name: Proleukin (Germ.)

Primary Use: This lymphokine is used in the treatment of various neoplasms, notably metastatic renal cell carcinoma and malignant melanomas.

Ocular Side Effects:

A. Systemic Administration
1. Scintillating scotoma
2. Binocular negative scotoma
3. Diplopia
4. Palinopsia
5. Eyelids
   a. Pruritus
   b. Macular erythema
   c. Desquamative rash
   d. Angioneurotic edema
   e. Urticaria
   f. Subcutaneous lymphomas (transient)
6. Amaurosis fugax
7. Visual hallucinations
8. Visual field defects (transient)
   a. Quadrantic defects
   b. Total loss

Clinical Significance: The most striking effects of this agent are neural ophthalmic complications. They appear to be dose-related and in the main are prevented by nonsteroidal anti-inflammatory agents. The cause of transient migraine-like symptoms may well be hypotensive episodes that may be prolonged. It has also been suggested that there is alteration in the permeability of the blood-brain barrier by interleukin 2, which may be responsible for some of these side effects. It is not apparent that any of the visual ophthalmic side effects prevent the continued use of this agent. Palinopsia is an object seen in the functioning visual area that is drawn to a nonfunctioning (blind) area and may be persistently visible.

References:

Bernard, J.T., et al.: Transient focal neurologic deficits complicating interleukin-2 therapy. Neurology *40*:154–155, 1990.

Friedman, D.I., Hu, E.H., and Sadun, A.A.: Neuro-ophthalmic complications of interleukin 2 therapy. Arch. Ophthalmol. *109*:1679–1680, 1991.

Gaspari, A.A., et al.: Dermatologic changes associated with interleukin 2 administration. JAMA *258(12)*:1624–1629, 1987.

Whittington, R., and Faulds, D.: Interleukin 2: A review of its pharmacological properties and therapeutic use in patients with cancer. Drugs *46(3)*:446–514, 1993.

Generic Name: 1. Mercaptopurine; 2. Thioguanine

Proprietary Name: 1. Ismipur (Ital.), Purinéthol (Fr.), **Purinethol** (Austral., Canad., Ital.), Puri-Nethol (G.B., Germ., Neth., S. Afr., Swed., Switz.); 2. Lanvis (Austral., Canad., G.B., Neth., S. Afr., Swed., Switz.)

Primary Use: These purine analogs are used in the treatment of acute and some forms of chronic leukemias.

Ocular Side Effects:
A. Systemic Administration
   1. Eyelids or conjunctiva
      a. Hyperpigmentation
      b. Icterus
   2. Subconjunctival or retinal hemorrhages secondary to drug-induced anemia
   3. Problems with color vision—color vision defect, red-green defect
   4. May aggravate herpes infections

Clinical Significance: Ocular side effects due to these antimetabolites are seldom of clinical importance. Between 10% and 40% of patients with acute leukemia receiving mercaptopurine may develop conjunctival icterus.

References:

Apt, L., and Gaffney, W.L.: Congenital eye abnormalities from drugs during pregnancy. *In* Leopold, I.H. (Ed.): Symposium on Ocular Therapy. St. Louis, C.V. Mosby, Vol. VII, 1974, pp. 1–22.

Birch, J., et al.: Acquired color vision defects. *In* Pokorny, J., et al. (Eds.): Congenital and Acquired Color Vision Defects. New York, Grune & Stratton, 1979, pp. 243–350.

Buscema, J., Stern, J.L., and Johnson, T.R.B., Jr.: Antineoplastic drugs and pregnancy. *In* Niebyl, J.R.: Drug Use in Pregnancy. Philadelphia, Lea & Febiger, 1988, pp. 89–108.

Gilman, A.G., Goodman, L.S., and Gilman, A. (Eds.): The Pharmacological Basis of Therapeutics. 6th Ed., New York, Macmillan, 1980, pp. 1285–1287.

McEvoy, G.K. (Ed.): American Hospital Formulary Service Drug Information 87. Bethesda, American Society of Hospital Pharmacists, 1987, pp. 482–484, 505–506.

Generic Name: Methotrexate

Proprietary Name: Abitrexate (S. Afr.), Brimexate (Ital.), Emthexat (Swed.), Emthexate (Neth.), Farmitrexat (Germ.), **Folex**, Ledertrexate (Austral., Fr., Neth.), Maxtrex (G.B.), Methoblastin (Austral., S. Afr.), **Rheumatrex**, Tremetex (Swed.)

Primary Use: This folic acid antagonist is effective in the treatment of certain neoplastic diseases and in the management of psoriasis.

Ocular Side Effects:
A. Systemic Administration
   1. Eyelids or conjunctiva

      a. Allergic reactions
      b. Erythema
      c. Blepharoconjunctivitis
      d. Depigmentation
      e. Hyperpigmentation
      f. Photosensitivity
      g. Urticaria
      h. Lyell's syndrome
      i. Loss of eyelashes or eyebrows
      j. Erythema multiforme
  2. Decreased vision
  3. Nonspecific ocular irritation
      a. Lacrimation
      b. Hyperemia
      c. Photophobia
      d. Ocular pain
      e. Burning sensation
  4. Periorbital edema
  5. Subconjunctival or retinal hemorrhages secondary to drug-induced anemia
  6. Keratitis
  7. Decreased lacrimation
  8. Drug found in tears
  9. Paralysis of extraocular muscles (intrathecal or carotid artery infusion)
10. Retinal pigmentary changes (intrathecal or carotid artery infusion)
11. Optic atrophy (intrathecal or carotid artery infusion)
12. May aggravate herpes infections

Clinical Significance: Both systemic and ocular side effects due to methotrexate are common. In the opinion of some oncologists, about 25% of patients taking this drug will develop periorbital edema, blepharitis, conjunctival hyperemia, increased lacrimation, or photophobia. Despite minimal blepharoconjunctivitis, occasional patients have marked subjective complaints. This also appears to be associated with a pronounced temporary tear production impairment. Methotrexate drug levels were measured in tears and found to be equivalent to plasma levels 48 hours after therapy in both symptomatic and asymptomatic patients. O'Neill, et al. reported small vessel vasculitis in the skin after low-dose methotrexate. A case of transient bilateral ophthalmoplegia with exotropia has been reported from intrathecal administration of methotrexate in combination with irradiation for the treatment of lymphoma. Millay, et al. reported that retinal pigmentary epithelial changes developed ipsilateral to the carotid arterial infusion of mannitol and methotrexate in patients with intracranial malignant neoplasms; these changes may have been potentiated by a mannitol-induced "opening" of the blood-retina barrier. In children with acute leukemia, intrathecal methotrexate in conjunction with radiation therapy has been associated with reports of optic nerve atrophy at radiation therapy doses below those usually associated with such toxicity. Boogerd, Moffie, and Smets reported extensive degeneration and demyelination of the optic nerve and chasm in a 35-year-old woman who received intrathecal methotrexate.

References:

Boogerd, W., Moffie, D., and Smets, L.A.: Early blindness and coma during intrathecal chemotherapy for meningeal carcinomatosis. Cancer 65:452–457, 1990.

Doroshow, J.H., et al.: Ocular irritation from high-dose methotrexate therapy: Pharmacokinetics of drug in the tear film. Cancer 48:2158, 1981.

Fishman, M.L., Bean, S.C., and Cogan, D.G.: Optic atrophy following prophylactic chemotherapy and cranial radiation for acute lymphocytic leukemia. Am. J. Ophthalmol. 82:571, 1976.

Fraunfelder, F.T.: Interim report: National Registry of Drug-Induced Ocular Side Effects. Ophthalmology 87:87, 1980.

Hussain, M.I.: Ocular irritation from low-dose methotrexate therapy. Cancer 50:605, 1982.

Imperia, P.S., Lazarus, H.M., and Lass, J.H.: Ocular complications of systemic cancer chemotherapy. Surv. Ophthalmol. 34(3):209–230, 1989.

Knowles, R.S., and Virden, J.E.: Handling of injectable antineoplastic agents. Br. Med. J. 281:589, 1980.

Lepore, F.E., and Nissenblatt, M.J.: Bilateral internuclear ophthalmoplegia after intrathecal chemotherapy and cranial irradiation. Am. J. Ophthalmol. 92:851, 1981.

Margileth, D.A., et al.: Blindness during remission in two patients with acute lymphoblastic leukemia. A possible complication of multimodality therapy. Cancer 39:58, 1977.

Millay, R.H., et al.: Maculopathy associated with combination chemotherapy and osmotic opening of the blood-brain barrier. Am. J. Ophthalmol. 102:626, 1986.

Nelson, R.W., and Frank, J.T.: Intrathecal methotrexate-induced neurotoxicities. Am. J. Hosp. Pharm. 38:65, 1981.

O'Neill, T., et al.: Porphyria cutanea tarda associated with methotrexate therapy. Br. J. Rheumatol. 32:411–412, 1993.

Oster, M.W.: Ocular side effects of cancer chemotherapy. In Perry, M.C., and Yarbro, J.W. (Eds.): Toxicity of Chemotherapy. New York, Grune & Stratton, 1984, pp. 181–197.

Generic Name: Mitotane

Proprietary Name: Lysodren (Canad.)

Primary Use: This adrenal cytotoxic agent is used in the treatment of inoperable adrenocortical carcinoma.

Ocular Side Effects:
  A. Systemic Administration
    1. Decreased vision
    2. Diplopia
    3. Eyelids or conjunctiva
      a. Erythema
      b. Hyperpigmentation
    4. Cataracts
    5. Retinal pigmentary changes
    6. Papilledema
    7. Retinal hemorrhages
    8. May aggravate herpes infections

Clinical Significance: While systemic side effects due to mitotane occur commonly, adverse ocular reactions occur infrequently. Significant ocular side effects do occur, but seldom require discontinued drug use because of the seriousness of the underlying disease.

References:
Apt, L., and Gaffney, W.L.: Congenital eye abnormalities from drugs during pregnancy. *In* Leopold, I.H. (Ed.): Symposium on Ocular Therapy. St. Louis, C.V. Mosby, Vol. VII, 1974, pp. 1–22.

Colliard, M., et al.: Troubles de l'acuite visuelle imputables a l'Op'DDD? Nouv. Presse Med. 9:631, 1980.

Fraunfelder, F.T., and Meyer, S.M.: Ocular toxicity of antineoplastic agents. Ophthalmology 90:1–3, 1983.

Hoffman, D.L., and Mattox, V.R.: Treatment of adrenocortical carcinoma with o,p-DDD. Med. Clin. North. Am. 56:999–1012, 1972.

Vizel, M., and Oster, M.W.: Ocular side effects of cancer chemotherapy. Cancer 49: 1999, 1982.

Generic Name: Mitoxantrone (Mitozantrone)

Proprietary Name: Novantron (Germ., Switz.), **Novantrone** (Austral., Canad., Fr., G.B., Ital., Neth., S. Afr., Span., Swed.)

Primary Use: This is a synthetic anthracycline derivative used for its antineoplastic properties to treat acute leukemias and various malignant neoplasms of the breast and ovary.

Ocular Side Effects:
  A. Systemic administration
    1. Conjunctivitis
    2. Sclera
      a. Blue pigmentation
      b. Blue-green pigmentation

    3. Eyelids
      a. Edema
      b. Blue or blue-green pigmentation
    4. Alopecia primarily in areas of white hair

Clinical Significance: As with most antineoplastic drugs, this agent is probably secreted via the lacrimal gland. This drug is present in the tears, as shown by color changes in the conjunctiva, eyelid, and sclera. The drug, either mechanically or chemically, is the probable reason for conjunctivitis. The conjunctivitis is self-limiting and resolves once the therapy is stopped. The pigmentation of the sclera and eyelids is transitory and secondary to the deposition of the drug, which is a dark blue. All ocular side effects are transitory and of no major clinical significance.

References

Leyden, M.J., et al.: Unusual side effect of mitoxantrone. Med. J. Australia. 2:514, 1983.
Kumar, K., and Kochipillai, V.: Mitoxantrone induced hyperpigmentation. N. Z. Med. J. *103*:55, 1990.
Reynolds, J.E.F. (Ed.): Martindale: The Extra Pharmacopoeia. 30th Ed., London, Pharmaceutical Press, 1993, p. 494.

Generic Name: Nilutamide

Proprietary Name: Anandron (Fr., Neth., Swed.)

Primary Use: This antiandrogen is used in the treatment of prostatic cancer.

Ocular Side Effects:
    A. Systemic Administration
        1. Photostress—slow recovery
        2. Decreased dark adaptation
        3. Chromatopsia

Clinical Significance: The most common adverse drug-related effects of nilutamide are visual. Multiple, well-controlled clinical trials state that, after roughly 2 weeks, anywhere from 12% to 65% of patients receiving this drug had the onset of delayed adaptation to darkness after exposure to bright illumination (sun, television, or bright light). In general, photostress recovery time values were from 9 to 25 minutes depending on the study. In one double-blind placebo control trial, 30% of patients had this adverse event versus 6% of those taking placebos. In all patients, this adverse event discontinued on cessation of therapy, although some patients recovered on dosage reduction. Some patients took up to a year before recovery was complete. Theoretically, this may be due to a delayed regeneration of the visual pigments. In a randomized double-blind study, Namer, et al. showed a 3% incidence of chromatopsia, 1% incidence of diplopia, and 1% incidence of abnormal accommodation in which the placebo group showed none of these adverse events. This visual phenomenon is rarely an indication for discontinuing the drug.

References:

Harris, M.G., et al.: Nilutamide: A review of its pharmacodynamic and pharmacokinetic properties, and therapeutic efficacy in prostate cancer. Drugs & Aging *3(1)*:9–25, 1993.

Harnois, C., et al.: Ocular toxicity of Anandron in patients treated for prostatic cancer. Br. J. Ophthalmol. *70*:471–473, 1986.

Kuhn, J.-M., et al.: Prevention of the transient adverse effects of a gonadotropin-releasing hormone analogue (buserelin) in metastatic prostatic carcinoma by administration of an antiandrogen (nilutamide). N. Engl. J. Med. *321*:413–418, 1989.

Migliari, R., et al.: Evaluation of efficacy and tolerability of nilutamide and buserelin in the treatment of advanced prostate cancer. Arch. It. Urol. *63*:147–153, 1991.

Namer, M., et al.: A randomized double-blind study evaluating anandron associated with orchiectomy in stage D prostate cancer. J. Steroid Biochem. Molec. Biol. *37(6)*: 909–915, 1990.

Generic Name: Plicamycin (Mithramycin)

Proprietary Name: Mithracin (Austral., G.B., Neth.), **Mithracine** (Fr., Switz.)

Primary Use: This cytostatic antibiotic is used primarily in the treatment of testicular neoplasms.

Ocular Side Effects:

A. Systemic Administration
   1. Subconjunctival or retinal hemorrhages
   2. Periorbital pallor
   3. May aggravate herpes infections
   4. Inhibits wound healing

Clinical Significance: The main adverse reaction to plicamycin is severe thrombocytopenia, which causes a bleeding diathesis that may also affect the eye. A striking periorbital pallor may occur in patients taking this drug, as reported by Oster. Further documentation of this adverse event, however, is needed. Other antineoplastic agents causing this unusual reaction have not been reported.

References:

Drug Evaluations. 6th Ed., Chicago, American Medical Association, 1986, p. 1203.

Lee, D.A., et al.: Effects of mithramycin, mitomycin, daunorubicin, and bleomycin on human subconjunctival fibroblast attachment and proliferation. Invest. Ophthalmol. Vis. Sci. *31(10)*:2136–2144, 1990.

Oster, M.W.: Ocular side effects of cancer chemotherapy. *In* Perry, M.C., and Yarbro, J.W. (Eds.): Toxicity of Chemotherapy. New York, Grune & Stratton, 1984, pp. 181–197.

Reynolds, J.E.F. (Ed.): Martindale: The Extra Pharmacopoeia. 28th Ed., London, Pharmaceutical Press, 1982, p. 220.

Generic Name: Procarbazine

Proprietary Name: Matulane, Natulan (Austral., Canad., Fr., G.B., Germ., Ital., Neth., S. Afr., Span., Switz.), Natulanar (Swed.)

Primary Use: This methylhydrazine derivative is used in the management of generalized Hodgkin's disease.

Ocular Side Effects:
  A. Systemic Administration
      1. Subconjunctival or retinal hemorrhages secondary to drug-induced anemia
      2. Eyelids or conjunctiva
          a. Erythema
          b. Hyperpigmentation
          c. Photosensitivity
          d. Urticaria
          e. Purpura
          f. Exfoliative dermatitis
          g. Lyell's syndrome
      3. Nystagmus
      4. Photophobia
      5. Diplopia
      6. Decreased accommodation
      7. Papilledema
      8. May aggravate herpes infections

Clinical Significance: Numerous adverse ocular reactions have been caused by procarbazine, with the most frequent secondary to drug-induced hematologic disorders. Most ocular side effects are transitory and reversible with discontinued drug use and seldom are of major clinical significance. Bilateral optic neuritis developed in a patient treated with carmustine, procarbazine, prednisolone, and cyclophosphamide for multiple myeloma and plasma cell leukemia; both carmustine and procarbazine were suspected as possible causes of the optic neuropathy because they are known to cross the blood-brain barrier. A cause-and-effect relationship has not been established.

References:

Batist, G., and Andrews, J.L., Jr.: Pulmonary toxicity of antineoplastic drugs. JAMA *246*:1449, 1981.

Drug Evaluations. 6th Ed., Chicago, American Medical Association, 1986, pp. 1208–1209.

Gilman, A.G., Goodman, L.S., and Gilman, A. (Eds.): The Pharmacological Basis of Therapeutics. 6th Ed., New York, Macmillan, 1980, pp. 1299–1300.

McLennan, R., and Taylor, H.R.: Optic neuroretinitis in association with BCNU and procarbazine therapy. Med. Pediatr. Oncol. *4*:43, 1978.

Spaeth, G.L., Nelson, L.B., and Beaudoin, A.R.: Ocular teratology. *In* Jakobiec, F.A. (Ed.): Ocular Anatomy, Embryology and Teratology. Philadelphia, J.B. Lippincott, 1982, pp. 955–975.

Vizel, M., and Oster, M.W.: Ocular side effects of cancer chemotherapy. Cancer *49*: 1999, 1982.

Generic Name: Tamoxifen

Proprietary Name: Apo-Tamox (Canad.), Dignotamoxi (Germ.), Emblon (G.B.), Kessar (Fr., Germ., S. Afr., Switz.), Ledertam (Swed.), Noltam (G.B.), **Nolvadex** (Austral., Canad., Fr., G.B., Germ., Ire., Ital., Neth., S. Afr., Span., Swed., Switz.), Nolvadex D (Span.), Nourytam (Germ.), Oestrifen (G.B.), Tamaxin (Swed.), Tamofen (Canad., G.B., Germ), Tamofène (Fr.), Tamone (Canad.), Tamoplex (Neth.), Tamoxasta (Germ.), Tamoxigenat (Germ.), Zemide (Germ.)

Primary Use: This antiestrogen is used primarily in the palliative treatment of advanced breast carcinoma in postmenopausal women.

Ocular Side Effects:
  A. Systemic Administration
    1. Decreased vision
    2. Corneal opacities
      a. Whorl-like, subepithelial
      b. Calcium
    3. Retina or macula
      a. Yellow-white refractile opacities
      b. Edema
      c. Degeneration
      d. Pigmentary changes
      e. Hemorrhages
    4. Visual fields
      a. Constriction
      b. Paracentral scotoma
    5. Papilledema
    6. Optic neuritis
    7. ERG changes

Clinical Significance: Tamoxifen has been in use for almost 25 years with fewer than 3% of patients unable to tolerate the drug. Nausea and vomiting are the predominant causes for discontinuing the drug, and only in rare instances is progressive, irreversible vision loss the reason. In a prospective study by Pavlidis, et al., 6.3% of patients developed keratopathy or retinopathy due to tamoxifen. At lower dosages, this incidence level will probably be in the 1% to 2% range. Based on data in the literature and the Registry, there appear to be two forms of posterior segment involvement. An acute form, which is not well defined and is debatable, may occur after only a few weeks of therapy with any or all of the following: vision loss, retinal edema, retinal hemorrhage, and optic disc swelling. These findings are reversible with discontinuation of tamoxifen. This may be associated with other systemic changes, and it has been postulated that this has an immune basis or is an idiosyncratic response. Typical tamoxifen retinopathy, i.e., striking white-to-yellow refractile bodies perimacular and temporal to the macula, most commonly occur after 1 + years of therapy with at least 100 + grams of the drug. There are, however, a number of cases in the Registry of minimal retinal pigmentary changes occurring after a few months and only a few grams of tamoxifen. This may be associated with cystoid macular edema, punctate macular retinal pigment epithelial changes, parafoveal hemorrhages, and peripheral reticular pigment changes. The refractile bodies are located in the inner retina and histologically are the products of axonal degeneration. These lesions do not appear to regress if the drug is discontinued. Retinopathy due to tamoxifen can be seen without refractile bodies being present. Loss of visual acuity in this chronic form is often progressive, dose-dependent, and often irreversible unless the CME or hemorrhage is the cause of the visual loss. The corneal deposits are seldom of major clinical significance and are the typical white, whorl-like subepithelial corneal deposits. These deposits are similar to other amphiphilic-like compounds (chloroquine, amiodarone, etc.), and appear to be reversible. In rare patients, hypercalcemia developed with associated corneal calcific changes. A recent case of possible Goldenhar's syndrome in the offspring of a mother taking this drug during pregnancy was reported by Cullins, et al. Optic neuritis has been reported in the literature and the Registry. Patients to be started on tamoxifen therapy should have a baseline ophthalmic examination. If the acute form occurs, stopping the drug may be necessary to allow vision to return to normal. However, in general this is not necessary; but if it is, the drug may be restarted and the patient monitored closely. If the more chronic form occurs, close follow-up is necessary since the possibility of discontinuing tamoxifen needs to be discussed with the oncologist. In rare instances, decreasing the dosage has slowed the progression of the retinopathy and this form may be irreversible.

References:

Ashford, A.R., et al: Reversible ocular toxicity related to tamoxifen therapy. Cancer *61*:33, 1988.

Cullins, S.L., et al: Goldenhar's syndrome associated with tamoxifen given to the mother during gestation. JAMA *271(24)*:1905–1906, 1994.

Griffiths, M.F.P.: Tamoxifen retinopathy at low dosage. Am. J. Ophthalmol. *104*: 185–186, 1987.

Heier, J.S., et al.: Screening for ocular toxicity in asymptomatic patients treated with tamoxifen. Am. J. Ophthalmol. *117*:772–775, 1994.

Imperia, P.S., Lazarus, H.M., and Lass, J.H.: Ocular complications of systemic cancer chemotherapy. Survey of Ophthalmol. *34(3)*:209–230, 1989.

Kaiser-Kupfer, M.I., Kupfer, C., and Rodrigues, M.M.: 1. Tamoxifen retinopathy. A clinicopathologic report. Ophthalmology *88*:89, 1981.

McKeown, C.A., et al.: Tamoxifen retinopathy. Br. J. Ophthalmol. *65*:177, 1981.

Pavlidis, N.A., et al.: Clear evidence that long-term, low-dose tamoxifen treatment can induce ocular toxicity. A prospective study of 63 patients. Cancer *69(12)*:2961–2964, 1992.

Pugesgaard, T., and von Eyben, F.: Bilateral optic neuritis evolved during tamoxifen treatment. Cancer *58*:383, 1986.

Vinding, T., and Nielsen, N.V.: Retinopathy caused by treatment with tamoxifen in low dosage. Acta Ophthalmol. *61*:45, 1983.

Generic Name: Thiotepa

Proprietary Name: Ledertepa (Neth.), Tespamin (Jap.)

Primary Use: *Systemic*: This ethylenimine derivative is used in the management of carcinomas of the breast and ovary, lymphomas, Hodgkin's disease, and various sarcomas. *Ophthalmic*: This topical agent is used to inhibit pterygium recurrence and possibly to prevent corneal neovascularization after chemical injuries.

Ocular Side Effects:
  A. Systemic Administration
      1. Eyelids or conjunctiva
          a. Erythema
          b. Angioneurotic edema
          c. Urticaria
          d. Loss of eyelashes or eyebrows
          e. Hyperpigmentation
      2. Subconjunctival or retinal hemorrhages secondary to drug-induced anemia
      3. May aggravate herpes infections
      4. Acute fibrinous uveitis
  B. Local Ophthalmic Use or Exposure
      1. Irritation
      2. Eyelids or conjunctiva
          a. Allergic reactions
          b. Conjunctivitis—nonspecific

   c. Depigmentation
   d. Poliosis
  3. Delayed corneal wound healing
  4. Keratitis
  5. Corneal edema
  6. Occlusion of lacrimal punctum
  7. Corneal ulceration

Clinical Significance: Intravenous thiotepa has resulted in hyperpigmentation. This probably caused the excretion of the drug from sweat glands with accumulation caused by adjacent occlusive adhesive material. Horn, et al. reported five cases of hyperpigmentation in females treated for metastatic adenocarcinoma of the breast. In Grant's textbook, Himelfarb reported bilateral acute plastic uveitis secondary to systemic thiotepa. Ocular side effects due to topical ophthalmic thiotepa application are rare. While ocular irritation and allergic reactions are the most common, depigmentation of the eyelids may be the most disturbing periocular reaction. Eyelid depigmentation has been reported to occur 6 years after topical ocular use of thiotepa. Depigmentation due to thiotepa is probably enhanced by excessive exposure to sunlight. In some patients, depigmentation returns in a few months to years, but in rare instances it may be permanent. Use of thiotepa for many months in dosages of 4 to 6 times daily has caused keratitis and conjunctivitis. There are reports in the literature and in the Registry of punctal occlusion due to topical ocular use of this drug. Corneal ulcerations have been attributed to thiotepa when it was used in alkaline injuries; however, this is difficult to substantiate due to the coexisting alkaline injury.

References:

Asregadoo, E.R.: Surgery, thio-tepa, and corticosteroid in the treatment of pterygium. Am. J. Ophthalmol. *74*:960, 1972.

Cooper, J.C.: Pterygium: Prevention of recurrence by excision and post-operative thiotepa. Eye Ear Nose Throat Monthly *45*:59–61, 1966.

Dunigan, W.G.: Dermatologic toxicity. *In* Perry, M.C., and Yarbro, J.W. (Eds.): Toxicity of Chemotherapy. New York, Grune & Stratton, 1984, pp. 125–154.

Grant, W.M., and Schuman, J.S.: Toxicology of the Eye. Charles C. Thomas (Ed.), 4th Edition, Springfield, IL, pp. 1412–1415, 1993.

Greenspan, E.M., Jaffrey, I., and Bruckner, H.: Thiotepa, cutaneous reactions, and efficacy. JAMA *237*:2288, 1977.

Harben, D.J., Cooper, P.H., and Rodman, O.G.: Thiotepa-induced leukoderma. Arch. Dermatol. *115*:973, 1979.

Horn, T.D., et al.: Observations and proposed mechanism of N, N′, N″-triethylenethiophosphoramide (thiotepa)-induced hyperpigmentation. Arch. Dermatol. *125*: 524–527, 1989.

Hornblass, A., et al.: A delayed side effect of topical thiotepa. Ann. Ophthalmol. *6*: 1155, 1974.

Olander, K., Haik, K.G., and Haik, G.M.: Management of pterygia. Should thiotepa be used? Ann. Ophthalmol. *10*:853, 1978.

Weiss, R.B., and Bruno, S. Hypersensitivity reactions to cancer chemotherapeutic agents. Ann. Intern. Med. *94*:66, 1981.

Generic Name: Urethan

Proprietary Name: None

Primary Use: This carbamic acid ester is used in the management of multiple myeloma and leukemia.

Ocular Side Effects:
  A. Systemic Administration
    1. Subconjunctival or retinal hemorrhages secondary to drug-induced anemia
    2. Decreased vision
    3. Nystagmus
    4. Pupils
      a. Mydriasis
      b. Absence of reaction to light
    5. May aggravate herpes infections

Clinical Significance: Adverse ocular reactions due to urethan are rare and seldom of major significance. Nystagmus and pupillary changes have only been seen in extreme toxic states and are probably central in origin. While corneal crystals, iritis, ciliary body cysts, and corneal foreign body sensations have been attributed to urethan, these are more likely due to multiple myeloma and not the drug. Urethan-induced retinopathy has been induced in various animals, but to date, no human cases have been reported.

References:
Aronson, S.B., and Shaw, R.: Corneal crystals in multiple myeloma. Arch. Ophthalmol. *61*:541, 1959.
Ashton, N.: Cystic changes and urethane (Correspondence). Arch. Ophthalmol. *78*: 416, 1967.
Handley, G.J., and Arney, G.K.: Plasma cell myeloma and associated amino acid disorder: Case with crystalline deposition in the cornea and lens. Arch. Intern. Med. *120*:353, 1967.
Reynolds, J.E.F. (Ed.): Martindale: The Extra Pharmacopoeia. 28th Ed., London, Pharmaceutical Press, 1982, p. 230.
Spaeth, G.L., Nelson, L.B., and Beaudoin, A.R.: Ocular teratology. In Jakobiec, F.A. (Ed.): Ocular Anatomy, Embryology and Teratology. Philadelphia, J.B. Lippincott, 1982, pp. 955–975.
Tyler, N.K., and Burns, M.S.: Alterations in glial cell morphology and glial fibrillary acidic protein expression in urethane-induced retinopathy. Invest. Ophthalmol. Vis. Sci. *32(2)*:246–256, 1991.

Generic Name: 1. Vinblastine; 2. Vincristine

Proprietary Name: 1. Periblastine (S. Afr.), **Velban**, Velbé (Fr.), Velbe (Austral., Canad., G.B., Germ., Ital., Neth., Swed., Switz.), **Velsar**; 2. Norcristine (S. Afr.), **Oncovin** (Austral., Canad., Fr., G.B., Neth., S. Afr., Swed., Switz.), Pericristine (S. Afr.), **Vincasar PFS**, Vincrisul (Span.)

Primary Use: These vinca alkaloids are often used in conjunction with other antineoplastic agents. Vinblastine is primarily used in inoperable malignant neoplasms of the breast, female genital tract, lung, testis, and gastrointestinal tract. Vincristine is primarily used in Hodgkin's disease, lymphosarcoma, reticulum cell sarcoma, rhabdomyosarcoma, neuroblastoma, and Wilms' tumor.

Ocular Side Effects:
    A. Systemic Administration—Vincristine
        1. Eyelids
            a. Ptosis
            b. Photosensitivity
            c. Loss of eyelashes or eyebrows
        2. Extraocular muscles
            a. Paresis or paralysis
            b. Diplopia
            c. Nystagmus
        3. Visual hallucinations
        4. Photophobia
        5. Decreased accommodation
        6. Decreased corneal reflex
        7. Problems with color vision—color vision defect, red-green defect
        8. Decreased dark adaptation
        9. Visual fields
            a. Scotomas—central or centrocecal
            b. Constriction
            c. Hemianopsia
      10. Retrobulbar or optic neuritis
      11. Abnormal ERG
      12. May aggravate herpes infections
      13. Subconjunctival or retinal hemorrhages secondary to drug-induced anemia
      14. Cortical blindness
      15. Optic atrophy
      16. Ocular signs of gout
    B. Inadvertent Ocular Exposure—Vinblastine
        1. Irritation

        a. Lacrimation
        b. Hyperemia
        c. Photophobia
        d. Edema
    2. Cornea
        a. Keratitis
        b. Superficial gray opacities
        c. Edema
        d. Decreased corneal reflex
        e. Ulceration
    3. Blepharospasm
    4. Decreased vision
    5. Astigmatism

Clinical Significance: All the above possible systemic side effects are reported due to vincristine. The best overall review of vincristine is by Imperia, Lazarus, and Lass. The local effects of inadvertently splashed vinblastine are reported under "B," which are reversible with time. The accidental splashing of vinblastine on patient eyes caused corneal clouding, with vision reduced to seeing hand movements. Vision returned to near normal after a number of weeks with a correcting lens. Prolonged or high-dose vincristine therapy can cause cranial nerve abnormalities, including ptosis, diplopia, ophthalmoplegia, oculomotor disturbances, and corneal hypesthesia. Nystagmus has been reported in a patient treated with vincristine and bleomycin chemotherapy for non-Hodgkin's lymphoma. Optic neuropathy and retinal injury have also been suspected with vincristine use. A depressed b-wave potential of the ERG has been found in a patient who developed night blindness after treatment with vincristine and other antineoplastic agents. Transient cortical blindness, lasting from 24 hours to 14 days, and permanent bilateral blindness with optic atrophy have been reported as complications of vincristine therapy. The ocular signs of gout that may occur include conjunctival hyperemia, uveitis, scleritis, and corneal deposits or ulcerations.

References:

Albert, D.M., Wong, V., and Henderson, E.S.: Ocular complications of vincristine therapy. Arch. Ophthalmol. *78*:709–713, 1967.

Awidi, A.S.: Blindness and vincristine. Ann. Intern. Med. *93*:781, 1980.

Birch, J., et al.: Acquired color vision defects. *In* Pokorny, J., et al. (Eds.): Congenital and Acquired Color Vision Defects. New York, Grune & Stratton, 1979, pp. 243–350.

Byrd, R.L., et al.: Transient cortical blindness secondary to vincristine therapy in childhood malignancies. Cancer *47*:37, 1981.

Cohen, R.J., et al.: Transient left homonymous hemianopsia and encephalopathy following treatment of testicular carcinoma with cisplatinum, vinblastine, and bleomycin. J. Clin. Oncol. *1*:392, 1983.

Elomaa, I., Pajunen, M., and Virkkunen, P.: Raynaud's phenomenon progressing to gangrene after vincristine and bleomycin therapy. Acta Med. Scand. *216*:323, 1984.

Imperia, P.S., Lazarus, H.M., and Lass, J.H.: Ocular complications of systemic cancer chemotherapy. Surv. Ophthalmol. *34(3)*:209–230, 1989.

Kaplan, R.S., and Wiernik, P.H.: Neurotoxicity of antineoplastic drugs. Semin. Oncol. *9*:103, 1982.

McLendon, B.F., and Bron, A.J.: Corneal toxicity from vinblastine solution. Br. J. Ophthalmol. *62*:97, 1978.

Norton, S.W., and Stockman, J.A., III: Unilateral optic neuropathy following vincristine chemotherapy. J. Pediatr. Ophthalmol. Strabismus *16*:190, 1979.

Ripps, H., et al.: Functional abnormalities in vincristine-induced night blindness. Invest. Ophthalmol. Vis. Sci. *25*:787, 1984.

Shurin, S.B., Rekate, H.L., and Annable, W.: Optic atrophy induced by vincristine. Pediatrics *70*:288, 1982.

Spaeth, G.L., Nelson, L.B., and Beaudoin, A.R.: Ocular teratology. *In* Jakobiec, F.A. (Ed.): Ocular Anatomy, Embryology and Teratology. Philadelphia, J.B. Lippincott, 1982, pp. 955–975.

Teichmann, K.D., and Dabbagh, N.: Severe visual loss after a single dose of vincristine in a patient with spinal cord astrocytoma. J. Ocular Pharmacol. *4*:149–151, 1988; Surv. Ophthalmol. *34*:149–150, 1989.

XII   Heavy Metal Antagonists and Miscellaneous Agents

Class: Agents Used to Treat Alcoholism

Generic Name: Disulfiram

Proprietary Name: Antabus (Germ., Neth., Span., Swed., Switz.), **Antabuse** (Austral., Canad., G.B., Ital., S. Afr.), Espéral (Fr.), Etiltox (Ital.), Refusal (Neth.)

Primary Use: This thiuram derivative is used as an aid in the management of chronic alcoholism.

Ocular Side Effects:
   A. Systemic Administration
      1. Decreased vision
      2. Retrobulbar or optic neuritis
      3. Scotomas—central or centrocecal
      4. Problems with color vision—color vision defect, red-green defect
      5. Eyelids or conjunctiva
         a. Allergic reactions
         b. Erythema
         c. Urticaria
      6. Visual hallucinations
      7. Extraocular muscles
         a. Paresis or paralysis
      8. Toxic amblyopia

Clinical Significance: Adverse ocular side effects due to disulfiram are uncommon. Retrobulbar neuritis has been well documented by numerous authors; when the drug was restarted, the optic neuritis, often bilateral, would recur. In general, the vision lost during retrobulbar or optic neuritis returned within a few weeks after disulfiram was discontinued. This ocular side effect may be more common in higher dosages, the elderly, or patients with impaired hepatic function. There are a few reports of optic disc hyperemia and optic pallor. Other ocular side effects are reversible and seldom of importance.

References:

Acheson, J.F., and Howard, R.S.: Reversible optic neuropathy associated with disulfiram. A clinical and electrophysiological report. Neuro-Ophthalmol. *8*:175–177, 1988.

Birch, J., et al.: Acquired color vision defects. *In* Pokorny, J. et al. (Eds.): Congenital and Acquired Color Vision Defects. New York, Grune & Stratton, 1979, pp. 243–350.

Gardner, R.J.M., and Clarkson, J.E.: A malformed child whose previously alcoholic mother had taken disulfiram. N Z Med. J. *93*:184, 1981.

Graveleau, J., Ecoffet, M., and Villard, A.: Les neuropathies peripheriques dues au disulfirame. Nouv. Presse Med. *9*:2905, 1980.

Mokri, B., Ohnishi, A., and Dyck, P.J.: Disulfiram neuropathy. Neurology *31*:730, 1981.

Morcamp, D., Boudin, G., and Mizon, J.P.: Complications neurologiques inhabituelles du disulfirame. Nouv. Presse Med. *10*:338, 1981.

Class: Calcium Regulating Agents

Generic Name: 1. Disodium Clodronate; 2. Disodium Etidronate; 3. Disodium Pamidronate

Proprietary Name: 1. Bonefos (G.B., Swed., Switz.), Clasteon (Ital.), Difosfonal (Ital.), Loron (G.B.), Ossiten (Ital.), Ostac (Germ., Swed., Switz.); 2. Didronate (Swed.), **Didronel** (Austral., Canad., Fr., G.B., Ire., Neth., S. Afr., Switz.), Difosfen (Span.), Diphos (Germ.), Etidron (Ital.), Osteum (Span.); 3. Aredia (G.B., S. Afr., Swed.), **Aredin**

Primary Use: These biphosphonate calcium regulating agents are used primarily in the management of hypercalcemia of malignancy, metastatic bone pain, osteoporosis, and Paget's disease of bone.

Ocular Side Effects:

A. Systemic Administration (Disodium Pamidronate)
    1. Blurred vision
    2. Conjunctiva—transitory
       a. Lacrimation
       b. Hyperemia
       c. Ocular pain
       d. Burning sensation
       e. Gritty sensation
       f. Irritation
    3. Anterior uveitis

4. Episcleritis
5. Scleritis

Clinical Significance: The above data are for disodium pamidronate, and it is unclear if the other drugs have any of these visual side effects. Seven reports of anterior uveitis (six of seven bilateral) occurring within 24 to 48 hours of exposure to this calcium regulating agent have been reported by Macarol and Fraunfelder. Five of these patients were rechallenged, and bilateral uveitis recurred in four of them. The severity of the uveitis varied from clearing within 24 hours to requiring hospitalization in two patients. There were three reports involving unilateral episcleritis or scleritis occurring within 3 to 6 days after exposure. The episcleritis case was rechallenged and recurred in the same eye 6 months later. Thirteen patients developed nonspecific conjunctivitis within 6 to 48 hours after drug exposure. There was a positive rechallenge in six of eight of these patients. This conjunctivitis was transitory and seldom required treatment. The cause of the uveitis, scleritis, and episcleritis is conjecture; however, since this is a high molecular weight drug, the potential for an immune complex formation has been suggested. The cause for the nonspecific conjunctivitis is also unknown, but in all reasonable probability, the pattern suggests that the drug has been secreted by the lacrimal gland, and that the drug then causes transitory irritation to the mucous membranes. This drug has been used for over 5 years, and there are surprisingly few reports. Therefore, these events are rare. Regardless, if patients start to develop an anterior uveitis, episcleritis, or scleritis, one needs to monitor these patients more closely, and in some cases discontinue the drug. Xanthopsia has occurred within 2 hours after drug exposure, but this is still only a possible drug-related event.

References:
Macarol, V., and Fraunfelder, F.T.: Pamidronate disodium and possible ocular adverse drug reactions. Am. J. Ophthalmol. *118*:220–224, 1994.
Morton, A.R., et al: Disodium pamidronate (APD) for the management of single-dose versus daily infusions and of infusion duration. *In* Disodium pamidronate (APD) in the treatment of malignancy-related disorders. Hans Huber Publishers, Toronto, 1989, pp. 85–100.
Siris, E.S.: Biphosphonates and iritis. Lancet *342*:436–437, 1993.

Class: Chelating Agents

Generic Name: Deferoxamine

Proprietary Name: Desféral (Fr., Switz.), **Desferal** (Austral., Canad., G.B., Germ., Ital., Neth., S. Afr., Swed.), Desferin (Span.)

Primary Use: *Systemic*: This chelating agent is used in the treatment of iron-storage diseases and acute iron poisoning. *Ophthalmic*: This topical agent is used in the treatment of ocular siderosis and hematogenous pigmentation of the cornea.

Ocular Side Effects:
  A. Systemic Administration
    1. Eyelids or conjunctiva
      a. Allergic reactions
      b. Erythema
      c. Urticaria
    2. Decreased vision
    3. Photophobia
    4. Problems with color vision—color vision defect, red-green defect
    5. Visual fields
      a. Scotomas—central or centrocecal
      b. Constriction
    6. Decreased dark adaptation
    7. Retrobulbar or optic neuritis
    8. Retinal or macular
      a. Degeneration
      b. Pigmentary changes
      c. Abnormal ERG, EOG, or VEP
    9. Optic nerve
      a. Disc pallor
      b. Translucent swelling
      c. Atrophy
  B. Local Ophthalmic Use or Exposure
    1. Eyelids or conjunctiva
      a. Allergic reactions
      b. Hyperemia

Clinical Significance: Long-term intravenous, continuous, or multiple single injections of subcutaneous deferoxamine may cause acute visual loss, color vision abnormalities, and night blindness. Toxic retrobulbar optic neuropathy with central or centrocecal scotomas and peripheral constriction of visual fields has also been reported in patients receiving deferoxamine. Various symmetrical or asymmetrical disc changes have been described. Diffuse retinal damage has been evidenced by pigmentary degeneration and abnormal ERG, EOG, and dark adaptation. These adverse ocular side effects are rare and usually due to high doses of deferoxamine. Following cessation of therapy, vision usually improves but may not attain pretreatment levels. Progressive pigmentary changes may be seen months after discontinuation of deferoxamine. Bene, et al. observed irreversible vision loss to 20/100 and 20/200 in each eye on a small rechallenge dose of deferoxamine in a renal compromised patient. The cause was optic nerve, macular, and posterior pole pigmentary changes. Reversible lens opacities have been described in patients receiving intramuscular or intravenous deferoxamine over prolonged periods, but there is no hard data as to this agent being cataractogenic, except in animals.

References:

Arden, G.B., and Wonke, B.: Desferrioxamine (DFX) and ocular toxicity. Invest. Ophthalmol. Vis. Sci. 25(Suppl.):336, 1984.

Bene, C., et al.: Irreversible ocular toxicity from single "challenge" dose of deferoxamine. Clin. Nephrol. 31(1):45–48, 1989.

Bentur, Y., McGuigan, M., and Koren, G.: Deferoxamine (Desferrioxamine) new toxicities for an old drug. Drug Safety 6(1):37–46, 1991.

Blake, D.R., et al.: Cerebral and ocular toxicity induced by desferrioxamine. Q. J. Med. 56:345, 1985.

Borgna-Pignatti, C., de Stefano, P., and Broglia, A.M.: Visual loss in patient on high-dose subcutaneous desferrioxamine. Lancet 1:681, 1984.

Davies, S.C., et al.: Ocular toxicity of high-dose intravenous desferrioxamine. Lancet 2:181, 1983.

Lakhanpal, V., Schocket, S.S., and Jiji, R.: Deferoxamine (Desferal)-induced toxic retinal pigmentary degeneration and presumed optic neuropathy. Ophthalmology 91:443, 1984.

Mehta, A.M., Engstrom, R.E., and Kreiger, A.E.: Deferoxamine-associated retinopathy after subcutaneous injection. Am. J. Ophthalmol. 118(2):260–262, 1994.

Olivieri, N.F., et al.: Visual and auditory neurotoxicity in patients receiving subcutaneous deferoxamine infusions. N. Engl. J. Med. 314:869, 1986.

Orton, R.B., de Veber, L.L., and Sulh, H.M.B.: Ocular and auditory toxicity of long-term, high-dose subcutaneous deferoxamine therapy. Can. J. Ophthalmol. 20:153, 1985.

Rubinstein, M., et al.: Ocular toxicity of desferrioxamine. Lancet 1:817,1985.

Simon, P., et al.: Desferrioxamine, ocular toxicity, and trace metals. Lancet 2:512, 1983.

Generic Name: Dimercaprol

Proprietary Name: Sulfactin Homburg (Germ.)

Primary Use: This chelating agent is effective in the treatment of arsenic, gold, or mercury poisonings.

Ocular Side Effects:

A. Systemic Administration
  1. Nonspecific ocular irritation
    a. Lacrimation
    b. Edema
    c. Burning sensation
  2. Eyelids or conjunctiva
    a. Allergic reactions

      b. Conjunctivitis—nonspecific
      c. Blepharospasm
      d. Chemosis
   3. Subconjunctival or retinal hemorrhages secondary to
      drug-induced anemia
B. Inadvertent Ocular Exposure
   1. Irritation
      a. Lacrimation
      b. Photophobia
      c. Burning sensation
   2. Blepharospasm

Clinical Significance: Approximately 50% of patients receiving intramuscular injections of dimercaprol experience a burning sensation around their eyes within 15 to 20 minutes. This persists for 1 to 2 hours and is completely reversible. Other ocular manifestations to systemic dimercaprol are also of little consequence, transitory, and reversible. Direct ocular contact with this drug causes significant local irritation that lasts for a few hours but without apparent ocular damage.

References:

Acalovschi, M.: Anemii hemolitice induse medicamentos. Med. Intern. *31*:217, 1979.
Dimercaprol. Council on pharmacy and chemistry. ''Bal'' (British anti-lewisite) in the treatment of arsenic and mercury poisoning. JAMA *131*:824, 1946.
Grant, W.M. (Personal observation): Toxicology of the Eye, 1st Ed. Springfield, Thomas, 1962.
Peters, R.A., Stocken, L.A., and Thompson, R.H.S.: British anti-lewisite (BAL). Nature *156*:616, 1945.
Reynolds, J.E.F. (Ed.): Martindale: The Extra Pharmacopoeia. 28th Ed., London, Pharmaceutical Press, 1982, pp. 382–383.
Scherling, S.S., and Blondis, R.R.: The effect of chemical warfare agents on the human eye. Milit. Surg. *96*:70, 1945.

Generic Name: Penicillamine

Proprietary Name: Cuprimine (Canad., Neth., Swed.), Cupripen (Span.), **Depen** (Canad.), Distamine (G.B., Neth.), D-Penamine (Austral.), Gerodyl (Neth.), Kelatin (Neth.), Mercaptyl (Switz.), Metalcaptase (Germ., S. Afr.), Pendramine (G.B.), Sufortan (Ital.), Sufortanon (Span.), Trolovol (Fr., Germ.)

Primary Use: This amino acid derivative of penicillin is a potent chelating agent effective in the management of Wilson's disease, cystinuria, and copper, iron, lead, or mercury poisonings.

Ocular Side Effects:
  A. Systemic Administration
    1. Myasthenic neuromuscular blocking effect
       a. Paresis or paralysis of extraocular muscles
       b. Ptosis
       c. Diplopia
    2. Visual changes—variable myopia—hypermetropia
    3. Extraocular muscles
       a. Decreased convergence
       b. Nystagmus
    4. Nonspecific ocular irritation
       a. Lacrimation
       b. Hyperemia
       c. Photophobia
       d. Edema
    5. Retina
       a. Pigmentary changes
       b. Hemorrhages
       c. Serous detachment
    6. Eyelids or conjunctiva
       a. Blepharoconjunctivitis
       b. Urticaria
       c. Lupoid syndrome
       d. Lyell's syndrome
       e. Pemphigoid lesion with symblepharon
       f. Trichomegaly
       g. Yellowing and wrinkling
       h. Chalazion
    7. Retrobulbar or optic neuritis
    8. Visual fields
       a. Scotomas—centrocecal
       b. Constriction
    9. Problems with color vision—color vision defect, red-green
       defect

Clinical Significance: Adverse ocular reactions to the three isomers of penicillamine (D, DL, and L) are rare. Most side effects are probably due to
  penicillamine-pyridoxine antagonism. This is most common with the DL
  or L isomers, and only rarely with the D form. Unfortunately, most of the
  literature does not differentiate which isomer was prescribed, although now
  only the D form is used. To date, myopia and papilledema have not been
  reported with the D isomer form of penicillamine. Myasthenia gravis symptoms associated with penicillamine therapy are common. It appears that this
  drug can cause antistriational and antiacetylcholine receptor antibodies. Not
  infrequently, the first signs of this drug-related myasthenia involve the eyes,

with ptosis, diplopia, or extraocular muscle paresis. This drug is associated with a number of skin disorders with ocular-related abnormalities. Penicillamine has possibly been implicated in delayed corneal wound healing, proliferation of connective tissue, and corneal superficial punctate keratitis. Retinal pigment epithelial defects, serous detachment of the macula, and subretinal or choroidal hemorrhages have also been reported. Penicillamine-induced zinc deficiency may be the cause of keratitis, blepharitis, and loss of eyelashes, but this is unproven to date. Both in the literature and Registry, there are cases suggesting that this drug can cause an ocular pemphigoid clinical picture.

References:

Atcheson, S.G., and Ward, J.R.: Ptosis and weakness after start of D-penicillamine therapy. Ann. Intern. Med. 89:939, 1978.

Birch, J., et al.: Acquired color vision defects. In Pokorny, J., et al. (Eds.): Congenital and Acquired Color Vision Defects. New York, Grune & Stratton, 1979, pp. 243–350.

Delamere, J.P., et al.: Penicillamine-induced myasthenia in rheumatoid arthritis: Its clinical and genetic features. Ann. Rheum. Dis. 42:500, 1983.

Dingle, J., and Havener, W.H.: Ophthalmoscopic changes in a patient with Wilson's disease during long-term penicillamine therapy. Ann. Ophthalmol. 10:1227, 1978.

Fenton, D.A.: Hypertrichosis. Semin. Dermatol. 4:58, 1985.

George, J., and Spokes, E.: Myasthenic pseudo-internuclear ophthalmoplegia due to penicillamine. J. Neurol. Neurosurg. Psychiatry 47:1044, 1984.

Kimbrough, R.L., Mewis, L., and Stewart, R.H.: D-Penicillamine and the ocular myasthenic syndrome. Ann. Ophthalmol. 13:1171, 1981.

Klepach, G.L., and Wray, S.H.: Bilateral serous retinal detachment with thrombocytopenia during penicillamine therapy. Ann. Ophthalmol. 13:201, 1981.

Loffredo, A.,et al.: Hepatolenticular degeneration. Acta Ophthalmol. 61:943, 1983.

Marti-Huguet, T., Quintana, M., and Cabiro, I.: Cicatricial pemphigoid associated with D-penicillamine treatment. Arch. Ophthalmol. 107:115, 1989.

Moore, A.P., Williams, A.C., and Hillenbrand, P.: Penicillamine induced myasthenia reactivated by gold. Br. Med. J. 288:192, 1984.

Peyri, J., et al.: Cicatricial pemphigoid in a patient with rheumatoid arthritis treated with d-penicillamine. J. Am. Acad. Dermatol. 14:681, 1986.

Generic Name: Canthaxanthin

Proprietary Name: Available as multi-ingredient preparations only.

Primary Use: This carotenoid is used in cosmetics, as a food color, and to produce an artificial suntan.

Ocular Side Effects:

A. Systemic Administration
  1. Retina

      a. Extracellular yellow or gold-like particles
      b. Predisposed to macular area
      c. Decreased retinal sensitivity
2. Blurred vision
3. Decreased dark adaptation
4. ERG
      a. Hypernormal scotopic amplitudes (low doses)
      b. Increased scotopic latencies (higher doses)
      c. Depressed photopic activity

Clinical Significance: There is a significant amount of data in the literature on canthaxanthin, especially in the European medical literature. In essence, it is clear that the deposition of this agent in a crystalline form can be found in all layers of the retina, primarily superficially, with a predisposition for the macular area. It can also be found in the equatorial area, peripheral retina, and the ciliary body. There may be a predisposition of its deposition in diseased areas of the retina. These deposits are dose-related, reversible, and while they have a startling clinical appearance, rarely cause visual symptoms. Clinical tests of color vision, visual fields, dark adaptations, and ERGs, etc. are all near normal. While there has been canthaxanthin retinopathy without direct intake of canthaxanthin, some postulate that this may be due to deposits from food coloring (Oosterhuis, et al.). The most complete overall review of this subject is by Arden and Barker.

References:

Arden, G.B., et al.: Monitoring of patients taking canthaxanthin and carotene: An electroretinographic and ophthalmological survey. Hum. Toxicol. 8:439–450, 1989.

Arden, G.B., and Barker, F.M.: Canthaxanthin and the eye: A critical ocular toxicologic assessment. J. Toxicol. Cut. Ocul. Toxicol. 10(1&2):115–155, 1991.

Barker, F.M.: Canthaxanthin retinopathy. J. Toxicol. Cut. Ocul. Toxicol. 7:223–236. 1988.

Cortin, P., et al.: Gold sequin maculopathy. Can. J. Ophthalmol. 17:103–106, 1982. (French)

Harnois, C., et al.: Static perimetry in canthaxanthin maculopathy. Arch. Ophthalmol. 106:58–60, 1988.

Harnois, C., et al.: Canthaxanthin retinopathy. Anatomic and functional reversibility. Arch. Ophthalmol. 107:538–540, 1989.

Leyon, H., et al.: Reversibility of canthaxanthin within the retina. Acta. Ophthalmol. 68:607–611, 1990.

Lonn, L.I.: Canthaxanthin retinopathy. Arch. Ophthalmol. 105:1590, 1987.

Oosterhuis, J.A., et al: Canthaxanthin retinopathy without intake of canthaxanthin. Klin. Monatsbl. Augenheilkd. 194:110–116, 1989.

Generic Name: 1. Etretinate; 2. Isotretinoin

Proprietary Name: 1. **Tegison** (Canad.), Tigason (Austral., Fr., G.B., Germ., Ire., Ital., S. Afr., Span., Swed., Switz.); 2. **Accutane** (Canad.), Isotrex

(G.B.), Roaccutan (Germ., Ital.), Roaccutane (Austral., Fr., G.B., Ire., Neth., S. Afr., Switz.), Roacutan (Span.)

Primary Use: These retinoids are used in the treatment of psoriasis, cystic acne, and various other disorders of the skin.

Ocular Side Effects:
A. Systemic Administration
   1. Eyelids or conjunctiva
      a. Erythema
      b. Blepharoconjunctivitis
      c. Edema
      d. Hyperpigmentation
      e. Photosensitivity
      f. Urticaria
   2. Decreased lacrimation
   3. Decreased vision
   4. Decreased tolerance to contact lenses
   5. Papilledema secondary to pseudotumor cerebri
   6. Cornea
      a. Opacities
      b. Keratitis
      c. Ulceration
   7. Myopia
   8. Abnormal ERG (scopic)
   9. Decreased dark adaptation—night blindness
  10. Ocular teratogenic effects
      a. Microphthalmia
      b. Optic nerve hypoplasia
      c. Orbital hypertelorism
      d. Cortical blindness
  11. Optic neuritis

Clinical Significance: Ocular side effects are among the more frequent adverse reactions associated with these drugs. Blepharoconjunctivitis is the most common ocular side effect, along with subjective complaints of dry eyes and transient blurred vision. The drug is probably secreted in the tears via the lacrimal gland. Mathers, et al. believe that these signs and symptoms are secondary to the isotretinoin effect to decrease meibomian gland function with the resultant increased tear evaporation and osmolarity. Reversible changes in refraction have been documented in several patients, including significant shifts in myopia. Fine, rounded subepithelial opacities found in the central and peripheral corneas of patients occur but seldom interfere with vision. These are reversible with discontinuation of the drug. Excessive amounts of retinoids have been implicated in papilledema secondary to pseudotumor cerebri, which may suggest hypervitaminosis A. This is confusing, in part since other antibiotics are often used (tetracycline, minocycline), which may cause pseudotumor cerebri as well. The role of isotretinoin as a cataractogenic agent is not yet defined. Even though there are a number of reports of cataracts in the Registry, as well as a publication by Herman and Dyer, there is little hard data to say that isotretinoin is a cataractogenic agent. To date, over 500,000 people have been exposed to this agent and very few cataracts have been reported, which suggests that this agent is at worst a very weak cataractogenic agent. This drug exposure is often short-term, i.e., a number of months, and most reported cataracts came on shortly after exposure to this drug, indicating a chance event or a subset of individuals whose lenses are highly sensitive to the drug. This is unlikely because there is no apparent pattern to these lens changes. Based on the above, there is probably no association, but this area is still debatable. Decreased dark adaptation including true night blindness can be marked in some patients. This retinal dysfunction is probably due to the competition for binding sites between retinoic acid and retinol (vitamin A). The risk of a photosensitizing drug, such as isotretinoin, enhancing the effects of light on the macula is unclear. Optic neuritis, unilateral and bilateral, has been seen shortly after starting isotretinoin. Since most of these patients are in the multiple sclerosis age group, it is difficult to be confident as to a cause-and-effect relationship. To our knowledge, no case has been rechallenged to the drug. Regardless, there are cases that suggest a probable relationship; therefore, the manufacturer recommends stopping the drug if this occurs. Offspring of mothers exposed to these drugs during pregnancy may have numerous congenital abnormalities involving the eyes. Etretinate probably can cause the same side effects as isotretinoin; however, fewer cases have been reported, in part due to its later release and less-frequent usage.

References:

Brown, R.D., and Grattan, C.E.H.: Visual toxicity of synthetic retinoids. Br. J. Ophthalmol. 73:286–288, 1989.

Fraunfelder, F.T., LaBraico, J.M., and Meyer, S.M.: Adverse ocular reactions possibly associated with isotretinoin. Am. J. Ophthalmol. 100:534, 1985.

Gold, J.A., Shupack, J.L., and Nemec, M.A. Ocular side effects of the retinoids. Int. J. Dermatol. 28:218–225, 1989.

Hazen, P.G., et al.: Corneal effect of isotretinoin: Possible exacerbation of corneal neovascularization in a patient with the keratitis, ichthyosis, deafness ("KID") syndrome. J. Am. Acad. Dermatol. 14:141, 1986.

Herman, D.C., and Dyer, J.A.: Anterior subcapsular cataracts as a possible adverse ocular reaction to isotretinoin. Am. J. Ophthalmol. 103:236, 1987.

Lammer, E.J., Chen, D.T., and Hoar, R.M.: Retinoic acid embryopathy. N. Engl. J. Med. 313(14):837–841, 1985.

Mathers, W.D., et al.: Meibomian gland morphology and tear osmolarity: Changes with accutane therapy. Cornea 10(4):286–290, 1991.

Palestine, A.J.: Transient acute myopia resulting from isotretinoin (Accutane) therapy. Ann. Ophthalmol. *16*:661, 1984.

Rismondo, V., and Ubels, J.L.: Isotretinoin in lacrimal gland fluid and tears. Arch. Ophthalmol. *105*:416, 1987.

Weleber, R.G., et al.: Abnormal retinal function associated with isotretinoin therapy for acne. Arch. Ophthalmol. *104*:831, 1986.

Generic Name: Hexachlorophene

Proprietary Name: (Multi-Ingredient Preparations): Acerbine (Switz.), Acnestrol (Fr.), Aknefug-Emulsion N (Germ.), Cresophene (Span.), Dermalex (G.B.), Eskamel (S. Afr.), Mediphon (Germ.), Neo Visage (Span.), **pHiso-Hex** (Canad., Ital.), Pulvicrus (Germ.), Robusanon (Germ.), S 13 (Span.), Scheriproct (S. Afr.), Solarcaine (Span.), Solfofil (Ital.), Thrombophob (S. Afr.), Ultraproct (Austral., Neth.), Varecort (Switz.)

Primary Use: This chlorinated biphenol is a topical germicide with high bacteriostatic activity that is commonly used to degerm the skin.

Ocular Side Effects:
  A. Systemic Administration—Inadvertent Oral Ingestion
      1. Decreased vision
      2. Pupils
          a. Miosis
          b. Absence of reaction to light
      3. Optic atrophy
      4. Toxic amblyopia
  B. Systemic Absorption from Topical Application to the Skin
      1. Eyelids
          a. Erythema
          b. Photosensitivity
      2. Extraocular muscles
          a. Paresis
          b. Diplopia
      3. Mydriasis—may precipitate narrow-angle glaucoma
      4. Papilledema secondary to pseudotumor cerebri
      5. Retinal hemorrhages
  C. Local Ophthalmic Use or Exposure—Inadvertent Ocular Exposure
      1. Irritation
          a. Conjunctivitis
          b. Lacrimation
          c. Hyperemia
          d. Photophobia
          e. Burning sensation
      2. Decreased vision

3. Cornea
   a. Keratitis
   b. Edema

Clinical Significance: Hexachlorophene is toxic by the oral route. Case reports, both published and unpublished, confirm a predilection of the toxic effect on the optic nerve. Systemic toxicity can also occur from chronic dermatologic use of the drug in underweight, premature infants, in infants with excoriated skin, or in adults if applied several times a day to the skin or vagina. Hexachlorophene may enter the fetal circulation by maternal vaginal exposure, and the neonate may experience hexachlorophene neurotoxicity, including diplopia. Inadvertent ocular exposure of this agent can produce a severe keratitis involving all layers of the human cornea. A marked reduction of visual acuity has been reported to occur initially, but seldom are these changes irreversible.

References:

Dormans, J.A.M.A., and van Logten, M.J.: The effects of ophthalmic preservatives on corneal epithelium of the rabbit: A scanning electron microscopical study. Toxicol. Appl. Pharmacol. 62:251, 1982.

Goutieres, F., and Aicardi, J.: Accidental percutaneous hexachlorophene intoxication in children. Br. Med. J. 2:663, 1977.

Leopold, I.H., and Wong, E.K., Jr.: The eye: Local irritation and topical toxicity. In Drill, V.A., and Lazar, P. (Eds.): Cutaneous Toxicity. New York, Raven Press, 1984, pp. 99–108.

MacRae, S.M., Brown, B., and Edelhauser, H.F.: The corneal toxicity of presurgical skin antiseptics. Am. J. Ophthalmol. 97:221, 1984.

Martin-Bouyer, G., et al.: Outbreak of accidental hexachlorophene poisoning in France. Lancet 1:91, 1982.

Martinez, A.J., Boehm, R., and Hadfield, M.G.: Acute hexachlorophene encephalopathy: Clinico-neuropathological correlation. Acta Neuropathol. 28:93, 1974.

Slamovits, T.L., Burde, R.M., and Klingele, T.G.: Bilateral optic atrophy caused by chronic oral ingestion and topical application of hexachlorophene. Am. J. Ophthalmol. 89:676, 1980.

Strickland, D., et al.: Vaginal absorption of hexachlorophene during labor. Am. J. Obstet. Gynecol. 147:769, 1983

Generic Name: 1. Methoxsalen; 2. Trioxsalen

Proprietary Name: 1. **8-Mop**, Deltasoralen (Ire.), Geroxalen (Neth.), Méladinine (Fr., Switz.), Meladinine (Germ., Neth.), **Oxsoralen** (Austral., Canad., Ital., Neth., S. Afr., Span.), Puvasoralen (G.B.), Ultramop (Canad.); 2. **Trisoralen** (Austral., Canad., Ital., S. Afr.)

Primary Use: These psoralens are administered orally or topically for the treatment of psoriasis and vitiliginous lesions. The drugs are administered before long-wave (320 to 400 nm) ultraviolet light source exposure (PUVA therapy).

Ocular Side Effects: PUVA Therapy
  A. Systemic Administration or Systemic Absorption from Topical Application to the Skin
     1. Eyelids or conjunctiva
        a. Hyperpigmentation
        b. Erythema
        c. Photosensitivity
        d. Increased incidence of skin cancers
        e. Phytodermatitis
        f. Hypertrichosis
     2. Keratitis
     3. Photophobia
     4. Decreased lacrimation
     5. Lens changes (if UV blocking lens not used)
     6. Eyelids and periocular skin—increased incidence of malignancies

Clinical Significance: PUVA therapy usually consists of oral psoralens administered while the patient is wearing UV-blocking goggles during irradiation and wraparound UV-blocking spectacles for at least 12 hours from the time of initial drug ingestion. To date, this regimen has had little to no ocular side effect other than a photosensitizing effect on the periocular skin. Most all ocular signs are transitory and reversible, and adverse ocular effects have been due to inadvertent light exposure or not wearing protective lenses as described above. Other than the typical photosensitivity reaction of the anterior segment (conjunctival hyperemia, keratitis photophobia), occasionally a patient may also complain of sicca-like symptoms for 48 to 72 hours following therapy. Reported visual field changes (Fenton and Wilkinson) are transitory and in the main are probably functional rather than drug related. There are a few case reports of pigmentary glaucoma after PUVA therapy in the Registry, but to date this is not a proven drug-related event. Since this therapy causes proliferation of pigment epithelial cells, this association may not be coincidental. The increased incidence of skin cancers of all types is well documented. The area of greatest controversy is whether PUVA therapy causes cataracts. It has been shown in animals without UV ocular protection that systemic psoralens can cause anterior inferior cortical cataracts. Orally administered psoralens have been found in human lenses, both cataractous and noncataractous. These drugs are photobound in the lens and may be cumulative with additional therapy. There is a report of punctiform opacities in the nucleus and cortex of patients undergoing PUVA treatment. These opacities were transitory in four of five patients (Van Deenen and Lamers). There have been numerous reports both supporting and denying lens changes in patients with proper eye protection after long-term PUVA therapy. The most complete review, with the addition of a series of patients undergoing PUVA therapy followed up to 14 years, was recently reported by Glew and Nigra. With proper UV-blocking lenses, they found no evidence that there is a higher incidence of lens changes, even with long-term therapy, versus that expected with normal aging change. A review of the literature, the FDA data, and more than 30 cases in the Registry of lens changes associated with psoralen use have helped us reach the following conclusions. To date, with or without UV-blocking lenses, no characteristic human lens abnormalities have been associated with psoralen use. Few, if any, lens changes with proper UV-blocking lenses can be definitely associated with PUVA therapy. Theoretically, PUVA therapy without UV-blocking lenses could cause cataracts in humans, but a definite cause-and-effect relationship has not been proven.

References:

Farber, E.M., Abel, E.A., and Cox, A.J.: Long-term risks of psoralens and UV-A therapy for psoriasis. Arch. Dermatol. *119*:426, 1983.

Fenton, D.A., and Wilkinson, J.D.: Dose-related visual-field defects in patients receiving PUVA therapy. Lancet *1*:1106, 1983.

Glew, W.B., and Nigra, T. P.: PUVA and the Eye. Photochemotherapy in Dermatology, (Ed.). Elizabeth A. Abel, M.D., Stanford, California. IGAKU-SHOIN Medical Publishers, Inc., 1992, pp. 241–253.

Lafond, G., Roy, P.E., and Grenier, R.: Lens opacities appearing during therapy with methoxsalen and long-wavelength ultraviolet radiation. Can. J. Ophthalmol. *19*: 173, 1984.

Stern, R.S., Parrish, J.A., and Fitzpatrick, T.B.: Ocular findings in patients treated with PUVA. J. Invest. Dermatol. *85*:269, 1985.

Van Deenen, W.L., and Lamers, W.P.M.A.: PUVA therapy and the lens reconsidered. Documenta Ophthalmologica *70*:179–184, 1988.

Woo, T.Y., et al.: Lenticular psoralen photoproducts and cataracts of a PUVA-treated psoriatic patient. Arch. Dermatol. *121*:1307, 1985

Generic Name: Tretinoin (Retinoic Acid, Vitamin A Acid)

Proprietary Name: Retin-A

Primary Use: *Ocular*: Primarily used as a topical ocular medication for xerophthalmia. *Skin*: For treatment of various forms of acne vulgaris and aging changes.

Ocular Side Effects:
    A. Topical Ocular or Periocular Administration
        1. Conjunctiva
          a. Injection
          b. Edema

2. Cornea
   a. Vascularization
   b. Scarring
   c. Opacities in band or ring pattern
   d. Enhanced epithelial healing
3. Eyelids
   a. Irritation
   b. Edema
   c. Hypopigmentation
   d. Hyperpigmentation
   e. Contact allergy

Clinical Significance: The cream form of isotretinoin is highly irritating to the eye, and it is contraindicated to use it in this area. There have been reports of bleeding from mucous membranes if isotretinoin comes in contact with this tissue. Tretinoin cream has caused hypopigmentation and hyperpigmentation of the skin. Topical ocular application of this medication is usually in a vegetable oil or petroleum-based ointment. The amount of ocular irritation is directly proportional to the concentration of the drug and the frequency of application. This product has few side effects if it is used at lower concentrations. Avisar, Deutsch, and Savir noted that with topical ocular tretinoin and sicca patients, calcium-like deposits can appear in the epithelium of the cornea. This is not unlike topical ocular steroids in sicca patients. In one case, the calcium did not improve after discontinuing the drug; in the other case, the calcium disappeared over a 2-month period.

References:
Avisar, R., Deutsch, D., and Savir, H.: Corneal calcification in dry eye disorders associated with retinoic acid therapy. Am. J. Ophthalmol. *106*:753–755, 1988.
Smolin, G., and Okumoto, M.: Vitamin A acid and corneal epithelial wound healing. Ann. Ophthalmol. *13*:563–566, 1981.
Smolin, G., Okumoto, M., and Friedlaender, M.: Tretinoin and corneal epithelial wound healing. Arch. Ophthalmol. 97:545–546, 1979.
Sommer, A., and Ennran, N.: Topical retinoic acid in the treatment of corneal xerophthalmia. Am. J. Ophthalmol. 86:615–617, 1978.
Sommer, A.: Treatment of corneal xerophthalmia with topical retinoic acid. Am. J. Ophthalmol. *95*:349–352, 1983.
Soong, H.K., et al.: Topical retinoid therapy for squamous metaplasia of various ocular surface disorders. A multicenter, placebo-controlled double-masked study. Ophthalmology *95(10)*:1442–1446, 1988.
Stonecipher, K.G., et al.: Topical application of all-trans-retinoic acid, a look at the cornea and limbus. Graefes Arch. Clin. Exp. Ophthalmol. 226:371–376, 1988.
Wright, P.: Topical retinoic acid therapy for disorders of the outer eye. Trans. Ophthalmol. Soc. U.K. *104*:869–874, 1985.

Class: Diagnostic Aids

Generic Name: Diatrizoate Meglumine and/or Sodium

Proprietary Name: Angiografin (Germ., Ital., Neth.), Angiografine (Fr.), Hypaque (Canad., G.B.), Hypaque-M (Canad.), Radialar 280 (Span.), Reno-M (Canad.), Uro Angiografin (Span.), Urografin 310M (G.B.), Urovist (Germ.)

Primary Use: This organic iodide is used in excretion urography, aortography, pediatric angiocardiography, and peripheral arteriography.

Ocular Side Effects:
A. Systemic Administration
1. Decreased vision
2. Eyelids or conjunctiva
   a. Allergic reactions
   b. Hyperemia
   c. Erythema
   d. Conjunctivitis—follicular
   e. Edema
   f. Angioneurotic edema
   g. Urticaria
3. Nonspecific ocular irritation
   a. Lacrimation
   b. Photophobia
   c. Ocular pain
   d. Burning sensation
4. Corneal infiltrates
5. Cortical blindness
6. Acute macular neuroretinopathy
7. Visual fields
   a. Scotomas—paracentral
   b. Hemianopsia
8. Retinal vascular disorders
   a. Hemorrhages
   b. Thrombosis
   c. Occlusion

Clinical Significance: Ocular complications associated with radiopaque contrast media arteriography have been well documented. These complications usually result either from the toxic, irritative, or hypersensitivity responses on the vessel or the production of emboli. A number of hypersensitivity responses have occurred with these agents, especially perilimbal corneal infiltrates not unlike those seen with staphylococcal hypersensitivity reactions. These infiltrates clear on topical ocular steroids without complication. These drugs have also been reported to layer out in the anterior chamber, like a hypopyon, in a patient 2 weeks after cataract surgery. In the absence of pathologic confirmation, retinal or cerebral emboli with resultant secondary complications have been variously interpreted as cholesterol crystals, fat, air, dislodged atheromatous plaques, and the injected contrast media. Lantos describes four cases of acute cortical blindness after the use of these agents, either hemianopic or complete visual loss. All cases reverted to normal in hours or days. Guzak, Kalina, and Chenoweth describe one case of acute macular neuroretinopathy in a young woman after intravenous diatrizoate. Findings included swollen macules and subtle opacification of the parafoveal retina. Deep retinal lesions developed later. They reported an additional case of this same entity possibly associated with the intravenous contrast agent, iothalamate.

References:

Baum, J.L., and Bierstock S.R.: Peripheral corneal infiltrates following intravenous injection of diatrizoate meglumine. Am. J. Ophthalmol. 85:613, 1978.

Guzak, S.V., Kalina, R.E., and Chenoweth, R.G.: Acute macular neuroretinopathy following adverse reaction to intravenous contrast media. Retina 3:312–317, 1983.

Junck, L., and Marshall, W.H.: Neurotoxicity of radiological contrast agents. Ann. Neurol. 13:469, 1983.

Lantos, G.: Cortical blindness due to osmotic disruption of the blood-brain barrier by angiographic contrast material: CT and MRI studies. Neurology 39:567–571, 1989.

McMahon, K.A., et al.: Adverse reactions to drugs: A 12-month hospital survey. Aust. N. Z. J. Med. 7:382, 1977.

Priluck, I.A., Buettner, H. and Robertson, D.M.: Acute macular neuroretinopathy. Am. J. Ophthalmol. 86:775, 1978.

Generic Name: Iodipamide Meglumine

Proprietary Name: Cholografin (Canad.), Transbilix (Fr.)

Primary Use: This radiographic contrast medium is used for intravenous cholecystography and cholangiography.

Ocular Side Effects:

    A. Systemic Administration

        1. Eyelids or conjunctiva

            a. Allergic reactions

            b. Erythema

            c. Edema

            d. Angioneurotic edema

            e. Urticaria

        2. Corneal infiltrates

Clinical Significance: Adverse ocular reactions to intravenous cholangiography or cholecystography with iodipamide meglumine are rare. One patient has been reported to have developed corneal infiltrates following intravenous iodipamide meglumine; the corneal lesion disappeared with corticosteroid treatment. These changes are not unlike those documented for another contrast agent, diatrizoate meglumine.

References:
McEvoy, G.K. (Ed.): American Hospital Formulary Service Drug Information 86. Bethesda, American Society of Hospital Pharmacists, 1986, pp. 1253–1255.

McMahon, K.A., et al.: Adverse reactions to drugs: A 12-month hospital survey. Aust. N. Z. J. Med. 7:382, 1977.

Neetans, A., and Buroenich, H.: Anaphylactic marginal keratitis. Bull. Soc. Belge Ophtalmol. 186:69, 1979.

Reynolds, J.E.F. (Ed.): Martindale: The Extra Pharmacopoeia. 28th Ed., London, Pharmaceutical Press, 1982, pp. 439–440.

Generic Name: 1. Iopamidol; 2. Metrizamide

Proprietary Name: 1. Gastromiro (Ital.), Iopamiro (Germ., Ital., Neth., Span., Swed., Switz.), Iopamiron (Fr.), **Isovue** (Canad.), Niopam (G.B.), Solutrast (Germ.); 2. Amipaque (Austral., Canad., Fr.)

Primary Use: This radiopaque contrast medium is used in lumbar, thoracic, cervical, and total columnar myelography as well as in computer tomography to enhance images of intercranial spaces.

Ocular Side Effects:
- A. Systemic Administration
  1. Decreased vision
  2. Visual hallucinations
  3. Extraocular muscles
     a. Paresis or paralysis
     b. Diplopia
     c. Nystagmus—horizontal, vertical or downbeat
     d. Strabismus
  4. Eyelids or conjunctiva
     a. Allergic reactions
     b. Edema
     c. Angioneurotic edema
     d. Urticaria
     e. Stevens-Johnson syndrome
  5. Problems with color vision—color vision defect, red-green defect
  6. Photophobia

7. Scotomas—central
8. Cortical blindness
9. Subconjunctival or retinal hemorrhages secondary to drug-induced anemia

Clinical Significance: Visual disturbances, including unilateral and bilateral loss of vision, may last for hours following administration of iopamidol and metrizamide. Most of the data in the literature and in the Registry are for metrizamide. It is evident, however, that the ocular side effects for these two agents are similar. Visual hallucinations frequently occur 8 to 12 hours after metrizamide injection and may last up to 36 hours. Bilateral sixth nerve palsy, nystagmus, and diplopia are usually mild, transitory ocular side effects. An aseptic meningitis, sometimes with oculomotor signs, has also been reported, but this is rare. Prolonged cortical blindness has been seen in several instances following metrizamide myelography; it is unknown whether this adverse ocular reaction is secondary to the direct neurotoxic effect of metrizamide injection or the procedure itself.

References:

Bachman, D.M.: Formed visual hallucinations after metrizamide myelography. Am. J. Ophthalmol. *97*:78, 1984.

Bell, J.A., et al.: Postmyelographic abducent nerve palsy in association with the contrast agent iopamidol. J. Clin. Neuro-Ophthalmol. *10*:115–117, 1990.

Bell, J.A., and McIlwaine, G.G.: Postmyelographic lateral rectus palsy associated with iopamidol. Br. Med. J. *300*:1343, 1990.

Bendel, C.J.A., and Hoogland, P.H.: Quincke oedema following intrathecal administration of metrizamide. Neuroradiology *26*:415, 1984.

Perlman, E.M., and Barry, D.: Bilateral sixth-nerve palsy after water-soluble contrast myelography. Arch. Ophthalmol. *102*:968, 1984.

Rodman, M.D., and White, W.B.: Accelerated hypertension associated with the central nervous system toxicity of metrizamide. Drug Intell. Clin. Pharm. *20*:62, 1986.

Savill, J.S., et al.: (Depts. Med. & Radiol. Royal Postgrad. Med. Sch. Hammersmith Hosp. Du Cane Rd. London W12 OHS UK) Fatal Stevens-Johnson syndrome following urography with iopamidol in systemic lupus erythematosus. Postgrad. Med. J. *64*:392–394, 1988.

Smirniotopoulos, J.G., et al.: Cortical blindness after metrizamide myelography. Report of a case and proposed pathophysiologic mechanism. Arch. Neurol. *41*:224, 1984.

Vollmer, M.E., et al.: Prolonged confusion due to absence status following metrizamide myelography. Arch. Neurol. *42*:1005, 1985.

Wagner, J.H., Jr.: Another report of nonconvulsive status epilepticus after metrizamide myelography. Ann. Neurol. *18*:369, 1985

Generic Name: Iophendylate

Proprietary Name: None

Primary Use: This radiographic contrast medium is used for lumbar, thoracic, cervical, and total columnar myelography.

Ocular Side Effects:
A. Systemic Administration
  1. Decreased vision
  2. Ocular pain
  3. Abnormal visual sensations—flashing lights
  4. Eyelids—urticaria
  5. Extraocular muscles
    a. Paresis or paralysis
    b. Nystagmus

Clinical Significance: An unusual complication occurred in a case following the dissection of iophendylate along the optic nerves during a cervical myelogram. There was transient pain and flashes of light in the eye. A month later, temporary loss of vision with renewed periorbital pain was attributed to residual contrast material. The condition responded to systemic steroids. Other rarely reported ocular effects following iophendylate myelography may include cranial nerve palsies, extraocular muscle paralysis, nystagmus, and aseptic meningitis.

References:
Baker, R.A.: Bilateral sixth-nerve palsy. Arch. Ophthalmol. *100*:1974, 1982.
Lieberman, P., et al.: Chronic urticaria and intermittent anaphylaxis: Reaction to iophendylate. JAMA *236*:1495, 1976.
McEvoy, G. K. (Ed.): American Hospital Formulary Service Drug Information 87. Bethesda, American Society of Hospital Pharmacists, 1987, pp. 1257–1258.
Miller, E.A., Savino, P.J., and Schatz, N.J.: A rare complication of water soluble contrast myelography. Arch. Ophthalmol. *100*:603, 1982.
Reynolds, J.E.F. (Ed.): Martindale: The Extra Pharmacopoeia. 28th Ed., London, Pharmaceutical Press, 1982, p. 442.
Tabaddor, K.: Unusual complication of iophendylate injection myelography. Arch. Neurol. *29*:435–436, 1973.

Generic Name: 1. Iothalamate Meglumine and/or Sodium; 2. Iothalamic Acid

Proprietary Name: Angio-Conray (Ital.), Conray 24 (Ital.), Conray 30 (Canad., Germ., Neth.), Conray 36 (Ital.), Conray 43 (Canad.), Conray 60 (Canad., Germ., Ital., Neth.), Conray 80 (Germ.), Conray 280 (Austral., G.B.), Conray 325 (Austral., Canad., G.B.), Conray 400 (Canad., Ital.), Conray 420 (Austral., G.B.), Conray FL (Germ.), Contrix (Fr.), Cysto-Conray (Canad.), Gastro-Conray (Austral.), Sombril (Span.), Sombril-400 (Span.)

Primary Use: This radiopaque contrast medium is used for excretion urography, contrast enhancement of CT of the brain, aortography, selective renal arteriography, angiocardiography, and selective coronary arteriography.

Ocular Side Effects:
  A. Systemic Administration
    1. Decreased vision
    2. Myasthenic neuromuscular blocking effect
       a. Paralysis of extraocular muscles
       b. Ptosis
       c. Diplopia
       d. Divergent strabismus
    3. Eyelids or conjunctiva
       a. Allergic reactions
       b. Erythema
       c. Conjunctivitis—nonspecific
       d. Edema
       e. Angioneurotic edema
       f. Urticaria
    4. Cornea
       a. Superficial, cloudy infiltrates
    5. Nonspecific ocular irritation
       a. Lacrimation
       b. Photophobia
    6. Scotomas—paracentral
    7. Retina or macula
       a. Edema
       b. Wedge-shaped lesions
    8. Lowers intraocular pressure
    9. Cortical blindness

Clinical Significance: Potential complications of cerebral angiography may include temporary disturbances in vision and neuromuscular disorders. Visual field losses are usually transient, although permanent changes have been reported after intravenous iothalamate. Acute macular neuroretinopathy associated with scotoma, metamorphopsia, macular swelling, and typical wedge-shaped retinal lesions has also been reported following intravenous iothalamate. A rapid onset of corneal perilimbal superficial marginal infiltrates, which clear in a few days, was reported by Neetens and Buroenich. Smith and Carlson reported a 20% to 45% decrease in intraocular pressure after intravenous iothalamate sodium. The peak effect is at 30 minutes and returns to baseline in 120 minutes. Lantos reported four cases of cortical blindness secondary to this agent, all recovering within 1 month.

References:

Canal, N., and Franceschi, M.: Myasthenic crisis precipitated by iothalamic acid. Lancet *1*:1288, 1983.

Guzak, S.V., Kalina R E., and Chenoweth, R.G.: Acute macular neuroretinopathy following adverse re ction to intravenous contrast media. Retina *3*:312, 1983.

Junck, L., and Marshall, W.H.: Neurotoxicity of radiological contrast agents. Ann. Neurol. *13*:469, 1983.

Lantos, G.: Cortical blindness due to osmotic disruption of the blood-brain barrier by angiographic contrast material. CT and MRI studies. Neurology *39*:567–571, 1989.

McEvoy, G.K. (Ed.): American Hospital Formulary Service Drug Information 87. Bethesda, American Society of Hospital Pharmacists, 1987, pp. 1258–1270.

Neetens, A., and Buroenich, H.: Anaphylactic marginal keratitis. Bull. Soc. Belge. Ophtalmol. *186*:69–72, 1979.

Reynolds, J.E.F. (Ed.): Martindale: The Extra Pharmacopoeia. 28th Ed., London, Pharmaceutical Press, 1982, pp. 442–443.

Smith, R.E., and Carlson, D.W.: Intravenous pyelography contrast media acutely lowers intraocular pressure. Invest. Ophthalmol. Vis. Sci. *35(4)*:1387, 1994.

Class: Immunosuppressants

Generic Name: Azathioprine

Proprietary Name: Azamune (G.B.), Azapress (S. Afr.), Berkaprine (G.B.), Immunoprin (G.B.), **Imuran** (Austral., Canad., G.B., Ire., Ital., Neth., S. Afr.), Imurek (Germ., Switz.), Imurel (Fr., Span., Swed.), Thioprine (Austral.)

Primary Use: This imidazolyl derivative of mercaptopurine is used as an adjunct to help prevent rejection in homograft transplantation and to treat various possible autoimmune diseases.

Ocular Side Effects:
A. Systemic Administration
   1. Decreased resistance to infection
   2. May aggravate herpes infections
   3. Delayed corneal wound healing
   4. Retinal pigmentary changes
   5. Subconjunctival or retinal hemorrhages secondary to drug-induced anemia
   6. Ocular teratogenic effects

Clinical Significance: Ocular side effects due to azathioprine are uncommon and, except for teratogenic effects, are usually reversible on drug withdrawal. However, there are data that this agent can decrease resistance to infection or even activate some virus infections, such as vaccinia, cytomegalic inclusion disease, and possibly herpes. Inadvertent ocular exposure of the drug will cause irritation.

References:
Drug Evaluations. 6th Ed., Chicago, American Medical Association, 1986, pp. 1074–1075, 1151–1152.

Havener, W.H.: Ocular Pharmacology. 5th Ed., St. Louis, C.V. Mosby, 1981, p. 236.
Knowles, R.S., and Virden, J.E.: Handling of injectable antineoplastic agents. Br. Med. J. 2:589, 1980.
Lawson, D.H., et al.: Adverse effects of azathioprine. Adverse Drug React. Acute Poisoning Rev. 3:161, 1984.
Reynolds, J.E.F. (Ed.): Martindale: The Extra Pharmacopoeia. 28th Ed., London, Pharmaceutical Press, 1982, pp. 190–192.
Speerstra, F., et al.: Side-effects of azathioprine treatment in rheumatoid arthritis: Analysis of 10 years of experience. Ann. Rheum. Dis. 41(Suppl.):37, 1982.

Generic Name: Cyclosporine (Cyclosporin A)

Proprietary Name: Sandimmun (Austral., Fr., G.B., Germ., Ire., Ital., S. Afr., Span., Swed., Switz.), **Sandimmune** (Canad., Neth.)

Primary Use: This immunosuppressive agent is used for the prevention of kidney, liver, or heart allografts. Disorders of the skin, blood, gastrointestinal tract, liver, neurologic system, and kidney as well as collagen vascular diseases have been treated with this agent. This has also been used in the management of uveitis, Behcet's syndrome, corneal disease, scleritis, and various severe conjunctivitis cases.

Ocular Side Effects:
   A. Systemic Administration
      1. Decreased vision
      2. Eyelids or conjunctiva
         a. Erythema
         b. Conjunctivitis—nonspecific
         c. Urticaria
      3. Visual hallucinations
      4. Cortical blindness
      5. Subconjunctival or retinal hemorrhages secondary to drug-induced anemia
      6. Optic disc edema
      7. Trichomegaly
      8. Ocular pain
      9. Eyelids—edema
   B. Local Ophthalmic Use or Exposure
      1. Irritation
         a. Burning sensation
         b. Pain (with or without hyperemia)
         c. Itching
      2. Corneal—superficial punctate keratitis
      3. Conjunctival hyperemia

Clinical Significance: Cyclosporine has become increasingly popular. It has become the standard treatment for Behcet's syndrome, endogenous uveitis, psoriasis, atopic dermatitis, rheumatoid arthritis, Crohn's disease, and nephrotic syndromes. With systemic administration, severe ocular pain may occur for unexplained reasons with or without the evidence of an ocular abnormality. This may occur while taking the drug or when the drug is discontinued. The cause is unknown, but most likely it is an idiosyncratic response. It may also cause various irritative reactions around the eye that are seldom of major significance. Visual hallucinations may be so severe that they may require cyclosporine to be discontinued. Reversible cortical blindness has been reported in a number of cases. There is a question that it may also enhance malignant skin melanomas, but this is unproven. Of significant interest is a report by Avery, et al. of eight cases of optic disc edema in patients taking cyclosporine after allogenic bone marrow transplants. The optic disc edema resolves after discontinuing or decreasing the dosage of the drug. Optic disc edema due to cyclosporine may be a direct toxic effect of the drug, or papilledema secondary to increased intracranial pressure. Topical ocular 2% solution of cyclosporine seems to be fairly well tolerated; however, patients occasionally experience eyelid irritation, superficial punctate keratitis, and ocular pain with or without hyperemia. There is no evidence that cyclosporine in an eyedrop form will impede corneal wound healing. There is an unanswered question as to the systemic absorption of topical ocular cyclosporine with the low potential risk of nephrotoxicity. There is a question that cyclosporine may activate stromal herpes simplex but not corneal epithelial herpes disease (Meyers-Elliott, Chitjian, and Billups). It has been documented that this drug can cause eyelash proliferation.

References:

Ahern, M.J., et al.: A randomized double-blind trial of cyclosporin and azathioprine in refractory rheumatoid arthritis. Aust. N. Z. J. Med. *21*:844–849, 1991.

Avery, R., et al.: Optic disc edema after bone marrow transplantation. Ophthalmology *98*:1294–1301, 1991.

Beaman, M., et al.: Convulsions associated with cyclosporin A in renal transplant recipients. Br. Med. J. *290*:139, 1985.

BenEzra, D., et al.: Cyclosporine eyedrops for the treatment of severe vernal keratoconjunctivitis. Am. J. Ophthalmol. *101*:278, 1986.

Benitez del Castillo, J.M., et al.: Influence of topically applied cyclosporine A in olive oil on corneal epithelium permeability. Cornea *13*:136–140, 1994.

Filipec, M., et al.: Topical cyclosporine A and corneal wound healing. Cornea *11*: 546–552, 1992.

Ghalie, R., et al.: Cortical blindness: A rare complication of cyclosporine therapy. Bone Marrow Transpl. *6*:147–149, 1990.

Katirji, M.B.: Visual hallucinations and cyclosporine. Transplantation *43*:768, 1987.

Laibovitz, R.A., et al.: Pilot trial of cyclosporine 1% ophthalmic ointment in the treatment of keratoconjunctivitis sicca. Cornea *12*:315–323, 1993.

Merot, Y., et al.: Cutaneous malignant melanomas occurring under cyclosporin A therapy: a report of two cases. Br. J. Dermatol. *123*:237–239, 1990.

Meyers-Elliott, R.H., Chitjian, P.A., and Billups, C.B.: Effects of cyclosporine A on clinical and immunological parameters in herpes simplex keratitis. Invest. Ophthalmol. Vis. Sci. *28*:1170–1180, 1987.

Noll, R.B., and Kulkarni, R.: Complex visual hallucinations and cyclosporine. Arch. Neurol. *41*:329, 1984.

Ptachcinski, R.J., et al.: Anaphylactic reaction to intravenous cyclosporin. Lancet *1*: 636, 1985.

Rubin, A.M., and Kang, H.: Cerebral blindness and encephalopathy with cyclosporin A toxicity. Neurology *37*:1072, 1987.

Weaver, D.T., and Bartley, G.B.: Cyclosporine-induced trichomegaly. Am. J. Ophthalmol. *109*:239, 1990.

Wilson, S.E., et al.: Cyclosporin A-induced reversible cortical blindness. J. of Clin. Neuro-Ophthamol. *8*:215–220, 1988.

Class: Irrigating Solutions

Generic Name: Glycine

Proprietary Name: Gyn-Hydralin (Fr.)

Primary Use: This is a commonly used irrigating solution for transurethral resection of the prostate (TURP).

Ocular Side Effects:
   A. Irrigating Solution—TURP
      1. Decreased vision
      2. ERG
         a. Loss of oscillatory potentials
         b. Loss of 30 hertz flicker-following
         c. Increase of b-wave latency
      3. Visual evoked potential—latency suppression
      4. Pupils
         a. Mydriasis
         b. Sluggish response to light
         c. Nonresponsive to light
      5. Visual fields—various defects
      6. Cortical blindness

Clinical Significance: This commonly used, naturally occurring amino acid causes a unique ocular side effect, the exact mechanism of which is still unknown. This adverse response is a transitory loss of vision varying from a slight decrease in visual acuity to total loss of light perception lasting from a few hours to 24 hours, and rarely, 48 hours. In general, the pupils respond normally; however, in rare cases a sluggish response to light or even a nonresponse to light is found. Various visual field defects have been reported to the Registry with no clear pattern. Abnormalities of ERGs and visual-evoked potential have been well documented. The level of serum glycine concentrations alone do not explain the degree of visual symptomatology. Factors such as a decrease in serum sodium are important because rapid restoration of vision after normalization of serum sodium by intravenous furosemide and sodium chloride may be striking. Theories as to causation also include a direct retinal effect or occipital cortical edema. Animal data show that glycine can act as an inhibitory transmitter in the retina. TURP can cause many other central nervous system and cardiovascular aberrations, so there are many variables, but clearly glycine can cause this unique reversible ocular side effect.

References:

Creel, D.J., Wang, J.M., and Wong, K.C.: Transient blindness associated with transurethral resection of the prostate. Arch. Ophthalmol. *105*:1537–1539, 1987.

Defalque, R., and Miller, D.: Visual disturbance during transurethral resection of the prostate. Can. J. Ophthalmol. *22*:620–621, 1975.

Mei-Li Wang, J., Creel, D.J., and Wong, K.C.: Transurethral resection of the prostate, serum glycine levels, and ocular evoked potentials. Anesthesiology *70(1)*:36–41, 1989.

Mizutani, A.R., et al.: Visual disturbances, serum glycine levels and transurethral resection of the prostate. J. Urol. *144*:697–699, 1990.

Ovasappian, A., Joshi, C.W., and Brunner, E.A.: Visual disturbances: An unusual symptom of transurethral prostatic resection reaction. Anesthesiology *57*:332–334, 1982.

Still, J.A., and Modell, J.H.: Acute water intoxication during transurethral resection of the prostate, using glycine solution for irrigation. Anesthesiology *38*:98–99, 1973.

Class: Solvents

Generic Name: Dimethyl Sulfoxide, DMSO

Proprietary Name: Kemsol (Canad.), **Rimso** (Canad., G.B.)

Primary Use: This is an exceptional solvent with controversial medical therapeutic indications. It is also often used in the treatment of musculoskeletal pain, as a solvent for antivirals or anti-cancer drugs, and as an anti-inflammatory agent.

Ocular Side Effects:

A. Systemic Administration or Systemic Absorption from Topical Application to the Skin
   1. Potentiates the adverse effects of any drug with which it is combined
   2. Problems with color vision—color vision defect
   3. Photophobia
   4. Eyelids or conjunctiva

        a. Allergic reactions
        b. Erythema
        c. Urticaria
     5. Subconjunctival or retinal hemorrhages secondary to
       drug-induced anemia
  B. Local Ophthalmic Use or Exposure
     1. Irritation
        a. Hyperemia
        b. Burning sensation
     2. Eyelids
        a. Erythema
        b. Photosensitivity

Clinical Significance: DMSO may enhance the ocular side effects of other drugs by increasing the speed and volume of systemic absorption. Although lens opacities and changes in refractive errors have been detected in animals after prolonged administration of large amounts of dimethyl sulfoxide, no cases of lens changes have been reported in humans due to systemic, topical, or local ophthalmic exposure. A series of patients are currently being followed by Sasaki and Kojima from Kanazawa Medical University, Japan, using the Scheimpflug camera. To date, no definitive data have been released. Although color visual defects are reported, they are only of a transient nature. Topical ocular dimethyl sulfoxide in high concentrations commonly causes ocular irritation and may be associated with foul oyster-type breath because the drug drains down the nasolacrimal ducts directly into the oral cavity; however, this is now less of a problem with more refined dimethyl sulfoxide.

References:

Dimethyl sulfoxide (DMSO). Med. Lett. Drugs Ther. *22*:94, 1980.

Garcia, C.A.: Ocular toxicology of dimethyl sulfoxide and effects on retinitis pigmentosa. Ann. NY Acad. Sci. *411*:48, 1983.

Hanna, C., Fraunfelder, F.T., and Meyer, S.M.: Effects of dimethylsulfoxide on ocular inflammation. Ann. Ophthalmol. *9*:61, 1977.

Kluxen, G., and Schmitz, U.: Comparison of human nuclear cataracts with cataracts induced in rabbits by dimethylsulfoxide. Lens Res. *3*:161, 1986.

Rubin, L.F.: Toxicologic update of dimethyl sulfoxide. Ann. NY Acad. Sci. *411*:6, 1983.

Use of DMSO for unapproved indications. FDA Drug Bull. *10*:20, 1980.

Yellowless, P., Greenfield, C., and McIntyre, N.: Dimethylsulphoxide-induced toxicity. Lancet 2:1004, 1980

Generic Name: Methyl Alcohol (Methanol, Rubbing Alcohol, Wood Alcohol)

Proprietary Name: None

Primary Use: This agent is widely used industrially as a solvent. It is also used as an adulterant to "denature" the ethyl alcohol that is used for cleaning purposes, paint removal, and a variety of other uses.

Ocular Side Effects:

A. Systemic Administration
1. Decreased vision
2. Pupils
   a. Mydriasis
   b. Decreased reaction to light
3. Photophobia
4. Extraocular muscles
   a. Paresis
   b. Diplopia
   c. Horizontal nystagmus
5. Ptosis
6. Problems with color vision—color vision defect, red-green or blue-yellow defect
7. Visual fields
   a. Scotomas—central, centrocecal, or paracentral
   b. Constriction
8. Papilledema
9. Retinal vascular disorders
   a. Edema
   b. Hemorrhages
   c. Engorgement
10. Retrobulbar neuritis—toxic states
11. Optic atrophy
12. Toxic amblyopia

Clinical Significance: Methyl alcohol is highly poisonous, and oral consumption often leads to a rapid loss of vision. Ophthalmoscopically, the first sign of toxicity is hyperemia of discs, followed by peripapillary retinal edema and engorgement of the retinal veins. The more severe the retinal edema, the more likely permanent visual loss will follow. Pupillary dilatation and horizontal nystagmus are common. The earliest changes in the visual fields are due to loss of sensitivity to color. Initially, this occurs for green, followed by red, yellow, and finally blue. Prompt treatment is essential if the toxic effects of methyl alcohol are to be minimized. An excellent review of this subject was recently published by Grant and Schuman.

References:

Birch, J., et al.: Acquired color vision defects. *In* Pokorny, J., et al. (Eds.): Congenital and Acquired Color Vision Defects. New York, Grune & Stratton, 1979, pp. 243–348.

Carroll, F.D.: Toxicology of the optic nerve. *In* Srinivasan, B.D. (Ed.): Ocular Therapeutics. New York, Masson, 1980, pp. 139–144.

Dethlefs, R., and Naraqi, S.: Ocular manifestations and complications of acute methyl alcohol intoxication. Med. J. Aust. 2:483, 1978.

Grant, W.M., and Schuman, J.S.: Toxicology of the Eye. (Eds.) Charles C. Thomas, Publisher, Springfield, IL. 4th Ed. pp. 940–951, 1993.

Havener, W.H.: Ocular Pharmacology. 5th Ed., St. Louis, C.V. Mosby, 1981, pp. 501–503.

Saus, J., et al.: Recovery after potentially lethal amount of methanol. Lancet *1*:158, 1984.

Scrimgeour, E.M., Dethlefs, R.F., and Kevau, I.: Delayed recovery of vision after blindness caused by methanol poisoning. Med. J. Aust. 2:481, 1982.

Sekkat, A., et al.: Neuropathies optiques au cours d'une intoxication aigue par le methanol. J. Fr. Ophtalmol. 5:797, 1982.

Sharpe, J.A., et al.: Methanol optic neuropathy: A histopathological study. Neurology *32*:1093, 1982.

Class: Vaccines

Generic Name: BCG Vaccine

Proprietary Name: Monovax (Fr.)

Primary Use: BCG vaccine is used for active immunization against tuberculosis and in the treatment of various malignant diseases.

Ocular Side Effects:
    A. Systemic Administration
        1. Decreased vision
        2. Eyelids or conjunctiva
            a. Erythema
            b. Urticaria
            c. Purpura
            d. Lupoid syndrome
            e. Erythema multiforme
            f. Eczema
        3. Uveitis
        4. Subconjunctival or retinal hemorrhages secondary to drug-induced anemia

Clinical Significance: Ocular complications following the BCG vaccine are generally rare. Although eye disorders have been described in connection with BCG vaccination, it has not always been certain that the patients were previously in normal health. A single report noted two melanoma patients treated with BCG vaccine who developed uveitis associated with vitiligo. Bilateral cataracts have also been reported in a patient receiving BCG therapy following excision of a cutaneous melanoma. Reports to the Registry suggest that in some patients a conjunctivitis may occur, often lasting through the injection series, that can be controlled with topical ocular steroids. Two reports of choroiditis with secondary depigmentation have also been received by the Registry.

References:
Bouchard, R., Bogert, M., and Tinthoin, J.F.: Eczematides post-B.C.G. Bull. Soc. Fr. Dermatol. Syph. 72:126, 1965.
Dogliotti, M.: Erythema multiforme-An unusual reaction to BCG vaccination. S. Afr. Med. J. 57:332, 1980.
Donaldson, R.C., et al.: Uveitis and vitiligo associated with BCG treatment for malignant melanoma. Surgery 76:771, 1974.
Imperia, P.S., Lazarus, H.M., and Lass, J.H.: Ocular complications of systemic cancer chemotherapy. Surv. Ophthalmol. 34(3):209–230, 1989.
Krebs, W., and Schumann, M.: Allgenerkrankkung nach B.C.G.-Impfung. Monatsschr. Tuberk.-Bekampf. 14:80, 1971.
Vogt, D.: Die Tuberkuloseschutz-Impfung. Die Komplikationen der B.C.G.- Impfung. In Herrlich, A. (Ed.): Handbuch der Schutzimpfungen. Berlin, Springer-Verlag, 1965, p. 345

Generic Name: 1. Diphtheria (D) Toxoid Adsorbed; 2. Diphtheria and Tetanus (DT) Toxoids Adsorbed; 3. Diphtheria and Tetanus Toxoids and Pertussis (DPT) Vaccine Adsorbed

Proprietary Name: 1. H-Adiftal (Ital.), **Diphtheria Toxoid Adsorbed**; 2. Anatoxal Di Te (Switz.), Anatoxal Dite (Ital.), CDT Vaccine (Austral.), Dif-Tet-All (Ital.), D.T. Vax (Fr.), DT-Impfstoff (Germ.), DT-Rix (Germ.), DT-Vaccinol (Germ.), DT-Wellcovax (Germ.), H-Adiftetal (Ital.), Td-Impfstoff (Germ.), Td-Rix (Germ.), Td-Vaccinol (Germ.), Vaccin D.T. (Fr.), **Diphtheria and Tetanus Toxoids Adsorbed**; 3. Anatoxal Di Te Per (Switz.), Anatoxal Diteper (Ital.), Dif-Per-Tet-All (Ital.), DPT-Impfstoff (Germ.), D.T. Coq (Fr.), **Tri-Immunol**, Triple Antigen (Austral.), Trivax-AD (G.B., Ire.), **Diphtheria and Tetanus Toxoids and Pertussis Vaccine Adsorbed**

Primary Use: These combinations of diphtheria and tetanus toxoids with pertussis vaccine are the recommended preparations for routine primary immunizations and recall injections in children younger than 7 years of age.

Ocular Side Effects:
  A. Systemic Administration
    1. Eyelids or conjunctiva
       a. Allergic reactions
       b. Erythema
       c. Conjunctivitis—nonspecific (DPT)

      d. Angioneurotic edema

      e. Urticaria

      f. Eczema (DT)

  2. Decrease or paralysis of accommodation

  3. Extraocular muscles

      a. Paresis or paralysis

      b. Ptosis (DPT)

  4. Pupils

      a. Mydriasis (D)

      b. Decreased reaction to light (D)

  5. Decreased vision

  6. Uveitis (DPT)

  7. Papilledema secondary to pseudotumor cerebri (DPT)

  8. Visual field defects (DT)

  9. Optic neuritis

 10. Subconjunctival or retinal hemorrhages secondary to drug-induced anemia (DPT)

 11. Corneal graft rejection (tetanus toxoid booster)

Clinical Significance: Adverse ocular reactions secondary to this preparation are rare and transitory. Generalized urticarial reactions have been reported to occur immediately or several hours after injection. Allergic reactions due to preservatives or contaminants of the antigens are seen, although rarely. Neurologic complications, including papilledema, optic neuritis, and decreased vision, have been reported as transient adverse effects, sometimes accompanying encephalitis. Steinemann, Koffler, and Jennings reported a 33-year-old woman with a graft rejection requiring a repeat graft after receiving a tetanus toxoid booster.

References:

Dolinova, L.: Bilateral uveoretinoneuritis after vaccination with Ditepe (diphtheria, tetanus, and pertussis vaccine). Cs. Oftal. *30*:114, 1974.

Dukes, M.N.G. (Ed.): Meyler's Side Effects of Drugs. Amsterdam, Excerpta Medica, Vol. X, 1984, p. 607.

McReynolds, W.U., Havener, W.H., and Petrohelos, M.A.: Bilateral optic neuritis following smallpox vaccination and diphtheria-tetanus toxoid. Am. J. Dis. Child. *86*:601, 1953.

Pembroke, A.C., and Marten, R.H.: Unusual cutaneous reactions following diphtheria and tetanus immunization. Clin. Exp. Dermatol. *4*:345, 1979.

Steinemann, T.L., Koffler, B.H., and Jennings, C.D.: Corneal allograft rejection following immunization. Am. J. Ophthalmol. *106*:575–578, 1988.

Walsh, F.B., and Hoyt, W.F.: Clinical Neuro-Ophthalmology. 3rd Ed., Baltimore, Williams & Wilkins, Vol. III, 1969, pp. 2709–2710

Generic Name: Influenza Virus Vaccine

Proprietary Name: Agrippal (Ital.), Alorbat (Germ., Switz.), Begrivac (Germ., Swed.), Begrivac-F (Ire.), Biaflu (Ital.), Biaflu-Zonale S.U. (Ital.), **Flu-Imune, Fluogen,** Fluvax (Austral.), Fluviral (Canad.), Fluvirin (G.B.), Fluzone (Canad., G.B., Swed.), Imuvac (Span.), Inflexal (Ital., S. Afr., Span., Switz.), Influmix (Ital.), Influpozzi (Ital.), Influvac (G.B., Germ., Ire., Ital., Neth., S. Afr., Swed., Switz.), Influvirus (Ital.), Isiflu Zonale (Ital.), MFV-Ject (G.B.), Miniflu (Ital.), Mutagrip (Fr., Germ., Neth., Span.), Vaxigrip (Austral., Fr., Ital., Neth., S. Afr., Swed.)

Primary Use: Influenza virus vaccines are used to provide active immunity to influenza virus strains contained in the vaccines.

Ocular Side Effects:
A. Systemic Administration
   1. Decreased vision
   2. Eyelids or conjunctiva
      a. Allergic reactions
      b. Erythma
      c. Blepharoconjunctivitis
      d. Urticaria
      e. Purpura
   3. Extraocular muscles—paresis or paralysis
   4. Horner's syndrome
      a. Miosis
      b. Ptosis
   5. Ocular pain
   6. Problems with color vision—color vision defect, red-green defect
   7. Visual fields
      a. Scotomas—central or paracentral
      b. Constriction
   8. Papilledema
   9. Optic neuritis
   10. Posterior multifocal placoid pigment epitheliopathy
   11. Optic atrophy
   12. Subconjunctival or retinal hemorrhages secondary to drug-induced anemia
   13. Corneal graft rejection

Clinical Significance: Adverse ocular reactions due to influenza virus vaccine are rare and generally transitory. The extraocular muscle abnormalities and uveitis usually occur 2 to 8 days following the inoculation and last from 1 to 7 days. Neurologic reactions due to influenza virus vaccine range from polyneuropathy to encephalitis and Guillain-Barre syndrome. Optic neuritis ranging from reversible blindness to optic atrophy secondary to influenza virus vaccine have been described. It has been suggested that patients who have had a demyelinating disease should not receive vaccines. Patients with corneal grafts may be at risk. Most patients usually only have mild reactions that are controlled with topical ocular steroids. However, severe reactions requiring re-grafts have occurred. In addition to the Steinemann, Koffler, and Jennings report, the Registry has six cases.

References:

Cangemi, F.E., and Bergen, R.L.: Optic atrophy following swine flu vaccination. Ann. Ophthalmol. *12*:857, 1980.

Ehrengut, W.: Nebenwirkungen von Influenzaschutzimpfungen. Dtsch. Med. Wochenschr. *104*:1836, 1979.

Hara, Y., Wakano, R., and Sakaguchi, K.: A case of optic neuritis after influenza vaccination. Folia Ophthalmol. Jpn. *34*:1980, 1983.

Hector, R.E.: Acute posterior multifocal placoid pigment epitheliopathy. Notes, Cases and Instruments, Letterman Army Medical Ctr., San Francisco, CA. *86(3)*:424–425, 1978.

Knight, R.S.G., et al.: Influenza vaccination and Guillain-Barre syndrome. Lancet *1*: 394, 1984.

Macoul, K.L.: Bilateral optic nerve atrophy and blindness following swine influenza vaccination. Ann. Ophthalmol. *14*:398, 1982.

Perry, H.D., et al.: Reversible blindness in optic neuritis associated with influenza vaccination. Ann. Ophthalmol. *11*:545, 1979.

Poser, C. M.: Neurological complications of swine influenza vaccination. Acta Neurol. Scand. *66*:413, 1982.

Saito, H., et al.: Acute disseminated encephalomyelitis after influenza vaccination. Arch. Neurol. *37*:564, 1980.

Steinemann, T.L., Koffler, B.H., and Jennings, C.D.: Corneal allograft rejection following immunization. Am. J. Ophthal. *106*:575–578, 1988.

Generic Name: 1. Measles and Rubella Virus Vaccine Live; 2. Measles, Mumps, and Rubella Virus Vaccine Live; 3. Measles Virus Vaccine Live; 4. Mumps Virus Vaccine Live; 5. Rubella and Mumps Virus Vaccine Live; 6. Rubella Virus Vaccine Live.

Proprietary Name: 1. Morubel (Ital.), **M-R Vax II**, Rudi-Rouvax (Fr.); 2. Inmunivirus Triple (Span.), **M-M-R II** (Canad., G.B., Ire., Switz.), MMR II (S. Afr.), M-M-RVax (Germ.), Pluserix (Austral., Germ., Ire., Ital., Span., Switz.), R.O.R. (Fr.), Trimovax (Switz.), Triviraten (Switz.), Trivirix (Canad.), Vac Anti Sar-Rub Par (Span.), Virivac (Swed.); 3. **Attenuvax** (Austral., Ital., Neth., Switz.), Measavax (G.B.), Mevilin-L (G.B.), Moraten (Ital., Span., Switz.), Morbilvax (Ital.), Rimevax (Austral., Ital., S. Afr., Switz.), Rouvax (Fr., Ital., Span.); 4. Mumaten (Switz.), **Mumpsvax** (Austral., Canad., G.B., Germ., Neth., Switz.), Pariorix (Austral., Switz.), Pariorix Vac (Span.); 5. **Biavax II**; 6. Almevax (G.B., Ire., Swed.), Cendevax (Austral.), Ervevax (Austral., G.B., Germ., Ire., Ital., Neth., Switz.), Gunevax (Ital.), **Meruvax II** (Austral., G.B., Ital., Neth., Switz.), Rosovax

(Ital.), Röt-Wellcovax (Germ.), Rubavax (G.B.), Rubeaten (Ital., S. Afr., Span., Switz.), Rubellovac (Germ.), Rudivax (Fr., Ital.)

Primary Use: These vaccines are used to provide active immunity to measles, mumps, and rubella.

Ocular Side Effects:
A. Systemic Administration
  1. Decreased vision
  2. Eyelids or conjunctiva
     a. Allergic reactions
     b. Hyperemia
     c. Erythema
     d. Conjunctivitis—nonspecific
     e. Ptosis (measles)
     f. Angioneurotic edema
     g. Urticaria
     h. Purpura
     i. Eczema
  3. Extraocular muscles
     a. Paresis or paralysis
     b. Strabismus
  4. Ocular pain
  5. Mydriasis
  6. Scotomas—centrocecal (rubella)
  7. Papilledema
  8. Optic neuritis (rubella)
  9. Subconjunctival or retinal hemorrhages secondary to drug-induced anemia
B. Inadvertent Ocular Exposure—Rubella
  1. Keratitis
  2. Conjunctival edema

Clinical Significance: Adverse ocular reactions due to these viral vaccines are rare and usually transient. The most common is a transient conjunctivitis that has been reported to occur in 6% of patients receiving the measles vaccine. Ocular palsies generally occur 3 to 24 days following vaccination, with a few being reported as permanent. Neurologic reactions, including optic neuritis, papillitis, or retinitis, occur rarely. They usually start within 3 to 7 days after inoculation. They are often bilateral, and cases have included bilateral blindness or bare light perception. Vision may take many months to return since remyelination must occur. Some residual loss has remained in cases reported to the Registry. Cases of direct ocular exposure to live measles virus vaccine resulted in keratoconjunctivitis, which resolved within 2 weeks. Cases of transitory uveitis following inoculation are in the Registry, but a cause-and-effect relationship has not been proven.

References:

Behan, P.O.: Diffuse myelitis associated with rubella vaccination. Br. Med. J. *1*:166, 1977.

Chan, C.C., Sogg, R.L., and Steinman, L.: Isolated oculomotor palsy after measles immunization. Am. J. Ophthalmol. *89*:446, 1980.

Herman, J.J., Radin, R., and Schneiderman, R.: Allergic reactions to measles (rubeola) vaccine in patients hypersensitive to egg protein. J. Pediatr. *102*:196, 1983.

Kazarian, E.L., and Gager, W.E.: Optic neuritis complicating measles, mumps and rubella vaccination. Am. J. Ophthalmol. *86*:544, 1978.

Kline, L.B., Margulies, S.L., and Oh, S.J.: Optic neuritis and myelitis following rubella vaccination. Arch. Neurol. *39*:443, 1982.

Marshall, G.S., et al.: Diffuse retinopathy following mumps and rubella vaccination. Pediatrics *76*:989, 1985.

Maspero, A., Sesana, B., and Ferrante, P.: Adverse reactions to measles vaccine. Boll. 1st. Sieroter. Milan. *63(2)*:125, 1984.

Miller, C.L.: Surveillance after measles vaccination in children. Practitioner *226*:535, 1982.

Preblud, S.R., et al.: Fetal risk associated with rubella vaccine. JAMA *246*:1413, 1981.

Generic Name: Poliovirus Vaccine

Proprietary Name: IPOL, Opvax (Span.), Oral-Virelon (Germ.), **Orimune**, Polioral (Ital.), Polio-Vaccinol (Germ.), Poloral (Switz.), Virelon C (Germ.)

Primary Use: Poliovirus vaccine is used to provide immunity to poliomyelitis caused by poliovirus types 1, 2, and 3.

Ocular Side Effects:
A. Systemic Administration
   1. Decreased vision
   2. Eyelids or conjunctiva
      a. Erythema
      b. Edema
      c. Angioneurotic edema
      d. Urticaria
      e. Lyell's syndrome
   3. Paresis of extraocular muscles
   4. Exophthalmos
   5. Subconjunctival or retinal hemorrhages secondary to drug-induced anemia
B. Inadvertent Ocular Exposure
   1. Decreased vision

Clinical Significance: Ocular side effects due to poliovirus vaccine are generally rare. Incidental reports refer to swelling of the eyelids, exophthalmos, and sixth nerve palsy. Immunocompromised patients are more likely to develop poliomyelitis following polio vaccination. The Registry has received one report of decreased vision in a patient who was accidentally splashed in the eye with a live poliovirus vaccine.

References:
Lennartz, H., and Seeleman, K.: Wirksamkeit und Vertraglichkeit eines trivalenten Schluckimpfstoffes gegen Poliomyelitis. Munch. Med. Wochenschr. *108*:1459, 1966.

Mathias, R.G., and Routley, J.V.: Paralysis in an immunocompromised adult following oral polio vaccination. Can. Med. Assoc. J. *132*:738, 1985.

Zurcher, K., and Krebs, A: Cutaneous Side Effects of Systemic Drugs. Basel, S. Karger, 1980, pp. 22–23

Generic Name: 1. Rabies Immune Globulin; 2. Rabies Vaccine

Proprietary Name: 1. Berirab S (Germ.), **Hyperab** (Austral., Canad., Germ.), Imogam (Canad.), Imogam Rabia (Span.), **Imogam Rabies**, Lyssuman (Span.), Rabuman (Ital., Switz.), Tollwutglobulin (Germ.); 2. **Imovax Rabies**, **Imovax Rabies I.D.**, Lyssavac N (Ital., Switz.), Merieux Inactivated Rabies Vaccine (G.B.), Rabies-Imovax (Swed.), Rabipur (Germ.), Rabivac (Germ.), Rasilvax (Ital.), Tollwut-Impfstoff (HDC) (Germ.)

Primary Use: Rabies immune globulin is used to provide passive immunity to rabies for postexposure prophylaxis of individuals exposed to the disease or virus. Rabies vaccine is used to promote active immunity to rabies in individuals exposed to the disease or virus.

Ocular Side Effects:
    A. Systemic Administration
        1. Decreased vision
        2. Eyelids or conjunctiva
            a. Allergic reactions
            b. Erythema
            c. Angioneurotic edema
            d. Urticaria
        3. Diplopia
        4. Photophobia
        5. Scotomas—centrocecal
        6. Optic neuritis

Clinical Significance: Neurologic adverse reactions were much more common with the earlier preparations of rabies vaccine made from infected rabbit brain tissue than from later-generation vaccines.

References:
Cormack, H.S., and Anderson, L.A.P. Bilateral papillitis following antirabic inoculation: Recovery. Br. J. Ophthalmol. *18*:167, 1934.

Cremieux, G., Dor, J.F., and Mongin; M.: Paralysies faciales peripheriques et polyradiculoneurites post-vaccino-rabiques. Acta Neurol. Belge *78*:279, 1978.

Francois, J., and Van Lantschoot, G.: Optic neuritis and atrophy due to drugs. T. Geneesk. *32*:151, 1976.

Srisupan, V., and Konyama, K.: Bilateral retrobulbar optic neuritis following antirabies vaccination. Siriraj Hosp. Gaz. *23*:403, 1971.

Van der Meyden, C.H., Van den Ende, J., and Uys, M.: Neurological complications of rabies vaccines. S. Afr. Med. J. *53*:478, 1978.

Generic Name: 1. Tetanus Immune Globulin; 2. Tetanus Toxoid

Proprietary Name: 1. Alcangama Antitetanica (Span.), Beriglobina Antitet (Span.), Gamma Tétanos (Fr.), Gamma-Tet (Ital.), Glogama Antitetanica (Span.), Haima-Tetanus (Ital.), Humotet (G.B., Ire.), Hypertet (Germ.), Immunotetan (Ital.), Imogam Tetanos (Span.), Noviserum Antitet (Span.), Tétavenine (Switz.), Tetabulin (Ital.), Tetabuline (Switz.), Tetagam (Germ.), Tetagamma (Ital.), Tetaglobulin (Germ.), Tetanobulin (Germ.), Tetanobulina (Span.), Tetanus-Gamma (Ital.), Tetaven (Ital.), Tetuman (Ital., Span., Switz.), TIG Horm (Germ.), Torlanbulina Antitenani (Span.), WellcoTIG (Germ.); 2. Alutoxoide T Prevent (Span.), Anatelall (Ital.), Anatoxal Te (Span., Switz.), Clostet (G.B.), H-Atetal (Ital.), Tet-Aktiv (Germ.), Tetanibys (Span.), Tetanol (Germ., Ital.), Tetatox (Ital.), Tétavax (Fr.), Tetavax (G.B., Germ.), T-Immun (Germ.), T-Rix (Germ.), T-Vaccinol (Germ.), T-Wellcovax (Germ.)

Primary Use: Tetanus immune globulin is used prophylactically for wound management in patients not completely immunized. Tetanus toxoid is used for active immunization against tetanus.

Ocular Side Effects:
    A. Systemic Administration
          1. Eyelids or conjunctiva
               a. Allergic reactions
               b. Erythema
               c. Conjunctivitis—nonspecific
               d. Angioneurotic edema
               e. Urticaria
               f. Purpura
          2. Decrease or paralysis of accommodation
          3. Horizontal nystagmus
          4. Visual hallucinations
          5. Decreased pupillary response to light
          6. Corneal graft rejection
          7. Photophobia

Clinical Significance: Except for local reactions, such as erythema or urticaria, adverse ocular reactions following tetanus immunization are rare.

Neurologic complications are extremely rare. Nystagmus, accommodative paresis, and possibly optic neuritis have been reported as adverse ocular symptoms following tetanus vaccine. Steinemann, Koffler, and Jennings reported a 33-year-old woman who developed a severe graft rejection within 4 days after receiving a tetanus toxoid booster. This required a repeat graft. A similar case, with a corneal graft reaction after a tetanus immunization, is in the Registry.

References:

Harrer, V.G., Melnizky, U., and Wendt, H.: Akkommodationsparese und Schlucklähmung nach Tetanus-Toxoid-Auffrischungsimpfung. Wien. Med. Wochenschr. *15*: 296, 1971.

Jacobs, R.L., Lowe, R.S., and Lanier, B.Q.: Adverse reactions to tetanus toxoid. JAMA *247*:40, 1982.

McReynolds, W.U., Havener, W.H., and Petrohelos, M.A.: Bilateral optic neuritis following smallpox vaccination and diphtheria-tetanus toxoid. Am. J. Dis. Child. *86*:601, 1953.

Quast, U., Hennessen, W., and Widmark, R.M.: Mono- and polyneuritis after tetanus vaccination (1970–1977). Dev. Biol. Stand. *43*:25, 1979.

Schlenska, G.K.: Unusual neurological complications following tetanus toxoid administration. J. Neurol. *215*:299, 1977.

Steinemann, T.L., Koffler, B.H., and Jennings, C.D.: Corneal allograft rejection following immunization. Am. J. Ophthalmol *106*:575–578, 1988.

XIII   Drugs Used Primarily in Ophthalmology

Class: Agents Used to Treat Glaucoma

Generic Name: Apraclonidine

Proprietary Name: Iopidine

Primary Use: This ophthalmic topical ocular alpha adrenergic antagonist is used in the control of elevated ocular pressure, both acute and chronic.

Ocular Side Effects:

A. Local Ophthalmic Use or Exposure
1. Eyelids or conjunctiva (allergic reactions)
   a. Lid retraction
   b. Pruritus
   c. Edema
   d. Pain
   e. Conjunctivitis—may be follicular
   f. Microhemorrhages
   g. Hyperemia
2. Blurred vision
3. Vasoconstriction blood vessels of anterior segment
4. Mydriasis
5. Sicca
6. Photophobia
7. Conjunctival hypoxia

Systemic Side Effects:

A. Local Ophthalmic Use or Exposure
1. Dry nose and mouth
2. Taste perversion
3. Headache
4. Asthenia
5. Transient lightheadedness

Clinical Significance: The side effects of apraclonidine are significantly less than its parent drug, clonidine. Yet, up to more than 40% of patients cannot tolerate topical ocular application of apraclonidine for more than a year. The primary reason for discontinuing this drug is a local "allergic" reaction consisting of any or all of the following: hyperemia, pruritus, epiphora, lid edema, chemosis, and a foreign body sensation. This typically occurs 1 to 2 months after starting therapy and completely resolves after discontinuation of the drug. It seems to be dose-related and concentration-related, and a significant "hyperreaction" may occur on rechallenge. This agent stimulates Müller's muscle so eyelid elevation occurs in most patients. Apraclonidine is a strong vasoconstrictor, so blanching of conjunctival blood vessels occurs with conjunctival hypoxia. Wilkerson, Lewis, and Shields confirmed that follicular conjunctivitis can be caused by this agent. Jampel reported a case of hypotony following topical ocular apraclonidine for elevated intraocular pressure after trabeculoplasty. Tachyphylaxis has been seen with this drug. Systemic side effects from topical ocular application are only rarely the cause of discontinuing ocular use; however, dry mouth and/or nose, headaches, taste perversions, asthma, and transient lightheadedness may be found. Bradycardia, arrhythmia, and hypotension have been reported to the Registry but are not proven as drug-related events. Other nonproven and less-common side effects include somnolence, dizziness, nervousness, depression, insomnia, paresthesia, nausea, constipation, rhinitis, dyspnea, pharyngitis, asthma, and dermatitis.

References:

Coleman, A.L., Robin, A.L., and Pollack, I.P.: Cardiovascular and intraocular pressure effects and plasma concentrations of apraclonidine. Arch. Ophthalmol. *108*: 1264–1267, 1990.

Jampel, H.D.: Discussion: Apraclonidine. Ophthalmology *100(9)*:1323, 1993.

Jampel, H.D.: Hypotony following instillation of apraclonidine for increased intraocular pressure after trabeculoplasty. Am. J. Ophthalmol. *108*:191–192, 1989.

King, M.H., and Richards, D.W.: Near syncope and chest tightness after administration of apraclonidine before argon laser iridotomy. Am. J. Ophthalmol. *110(3)*:308–309, 1990.

Munden, P.M., et al.: Palpebral fissure responses to topical adrenergic drugs. Am. J. Ophthalmol. *111*:706–710, 1991.

Nagasubramanian, S., et al.: Comparison of apraclonidine and timolol in chronic open-angle glaucoma. A Three-Month Study. Ophthalmol. *100(9)*:1318–1323, 1993.

Samples, J.R.: New drugs in ophthalmology. Apraclonidine for ophthalmic use. J. Toxicol. Cut. Ocular Toxicol. *8*:249–252, 1989.

Serdahl, C.L., Galustian, J., and Lewis, R.A.: The effects of apraclonidine on conjunctival oxygen tension. Arch. Ophthalmol. *107*:1777–1779, 1989.

Siegel, M.J., et al.: Effect of flurbiprofen on the reduction of intraocular pressure after administration of 1% apraclonidine in patients with glaucoma. Arch. Ophthalmol. *110*:598–599, 1992.

Vocci, M.J., Robin, A.L., and Wahl, J.C.: Reformulation and drop size of apraclonidine hydrochloride. Am. J. Ophthalmol. *113*:154–160, 1992.

Wilkerson, M., Lewis, R.A., and Shields, M.B.: Follicular conjunctivitis associated with apraclonidine. Am. J. Ophthalmol. *111(1)*:105–106, 1991.

Generic Name: 1. Betaxolol; 2. Levobunolol; 3. Timolol

Proprietary Name: *Systemic*: 3. Bioptome (G.B., Neth., Scand.), Blocadren, Blocanol (Fin.), Protlax (Arg.), Temserin (Germ.), Timacor (Denm., Fr.). *Ophthalmic:* 1. **Betoptic**; 2. **Betagan**; 3. **Timoptic**, Timoptol (Austral., Fr., G.B., Neth., N.Z., S. Afr.)

Primary Use: *Systemic*: Timolol is effective in the management of hypertension and myocardial infarction. *Ophthalmic*: These beta-adrenergic blockers are used in the treatment of glaucoma.

Ocular Side Effects:
  A. Systemic Administration—Timolol
      1. Decreased vision
      2. Eyelids or conjunctiva
          a. Allergic reactions
          b. Erythema
          c. Hyperpigmentation
          d. Loss of eyelashes or eyebrows
      3. Decreased intraocular pressure
      4. Visual hallucinations
      5. Decreased lacrimation
      6. Myasthenic neuromuscular blocking effect
          a. Paralysis of extraocular muscles
          b. Ptosis
          c. Diplopia
  B. Local Ophthalmic Use or Exposure
      1. Decreased intraocular pressure
      2. Irritation
          a. Hyperemia
          b. Photophobia
          c. Ocular pain
          d. Burning sensation
      3. Decreased vision
      4. Punctate keratitis
      5. Eyelids or conjunctiva
          a. Allergic reactions
          b. Erythema
          c. Blepharoconjunctivitis
          d. Urticaria
          e. Purpura
          f. Erythema multiforme

      g. Pemphigoid-like lesion with symblepharon

      h. Loss of eyelashes or eyebrows

6. Myopia
7. Visual hallucinations
8. Corneal anesthesia
9. Myasthenic neuromuscular blocking effect
      a. Paralysis of extraocular muscles
      b. Ptosis
      c. Diplopia
10. Contact lens intolerance
      a. Corneal erosion
      b. Unable to wear
11. Tear film break-up time—decreased
12. Tear secretion—mild decrease

Systemic Side Effects:

A. Local Ophthalmic Use or Exposure

1. Asthma
2. Bradycardia
3. Dyspnea
4. Depression
5. Cardiac arrhythmia
6. Headache
7. Congestive heart failure
8. Asthenia
9. Dizziness
10. Cerebral vascular accident
11. Hypotension
12. Syncope
13. Nausea
14. Impotence
15. Rhinitis
16. Bronchospasm
17. Aggravation of chronic obstructive pulmonary disease
18. Apnea—children
19. Suppression of heart rate and blood pressure elevation
20. Rebound increased blood pressure on beta blocker withdrawal
21. Increase in high-density lipoprotein
22. Hyperkalemia
23. Raynaud's syndrome
24. Arthralgia
25. Alopecia
26. Confusion
27. Psoriasis
28. Nail pigmentation

29. Skin disease
30. Heart block
31. Respiratory failure
32. Palpitation
33. Cardiac arrest
34. Hypoglycemia
35. Cerebral ischemia

Clinical Significance: The above-mentioned potential side effects from the various beta blockers are all based on timolol. The other nonselective beta blockers should have basically these same side effects; the more selective beta blockers, such as betaxolol, in all probability have fewer side effects, especially on the respiratory system. Regardless, any of the beta blockers seem to have the potential for causing many, if not all, of the above side effects. The topical ocular administration of timolol usually has its peak systemic blood level between 30 and 90 minutes following application. The adverse effects from this drug may occur shortly after application, or may not occur for many weeks, months, or even years on therapy. It should be noted that all adverse reactions reported due to systemic beta blockers have been seen secondary to topical ocular beta blockers. Examples include fingernail and toenail pigmentation, myasthenia gravis neuroblocking effects, psoriasis, and impotency. The local ocular effects from ophthalmic use are seldom of major consequence and rarely are an indication to discontinue the drug. Newer formulations and vehicles have decreased some of the initial burning associated with some of these agents. However, if one sees superficial punctate keratitis or erosions, the possibility that this patient is one of a rare group who gets a local anesthetic effect from the medication must be considered. Long-term ocular medications, either due to the drug or its preservative, can cause pemphigoid-like lesions, especially in the inferior cul-de-sac. To date, there is no clear-cut evidence that any of the beta blockers can enhance sicca, although we do know that any drug used long-term can affect the microvilli and possibly decrease tear film break-up time. The suspicion that timolol decreases tear production is real, but it is of such a mild nature that it is unlikely to be of major clinical importance in most patients. The area in which the beta blockers cause greatest concern is their systemic side effects from topical ocular application. Grant's most recent edition of "Toxicology of the Eye," as well as a review by Akingbehin and Raj, contain complete reviews. The most severe side effects affect the cardiovascular system and the respiratory system. Cardiovascular side effects include bradycardia, which in rare individuals is an indication for stopping the drug. It is of greatest importance, however, in diabetic patients whose insulin use is dependent on the patient realizing that his or her heart rate has increased, i.e., in a hypoglycemic attack. The beta blocker may mask the increase in heart rate. It is also of importance in exertion because some patients are unable to increase their heart rate. Additional problems include arrhythmia, syncope, congestive heart failure, and possible increase in cerebral vascular accidents, especially in patients with carotid insufficiency with drug-induced decreased blood pressure or pulse rate. In rare instances, this may be associated with a fatality. Since the nonselective beta blockers decrease heart rate in a different location than the calcium channel blockers, there have been some unproven reports of sudden death in patients who are taking both drugs.

The adverse respiratory effects are equally perplexing. It has been well documented that these agents have caused bronchospasm and status asthmaticus with death reported shortly following the use of topical ocular beta blockers. In approximately two-thirds of patients with a significant bronchospastic attack, there was a previous history of asthma. This group of drugs may especially cause problems in patients with chronic, obstructive lung disease. The patient clearly recognizes that he or she can breathe easier after discontinuing these drugs, especially the nonselective beta blockers. Approximately 33% of patients who develop bronchospasm recognize the problem with the beta blockers within the first week, and 23% within the first day. It seems that patients with chronic pulmonary disease taking these drugs may suffer a decrease in their forced expiratory volume as measurable by spirometry. There have been reports of apnea in infants who received topical ocular timolol. The central nervous system may also be affected. Clearly, the beta blockers can cause depression in some patients, and in the younger age group there have been reports of increased incidence of suicide attempts. The elderly suffer increased emotional lability, vivid dreams, and increased anxiety, which may improve after discontinuation of the medication. There have been numerous reports of sexual dysfunction in both men and women while taking timolol. Skin changes from timolol are rare. However, there are well-documented reports of psoriasis, various rashes, increased pigmentation of fingernails and toenails, and male pattern baldness in men and women. This baldness is interesting because it usually does not occur until at least 4 months after the medication is started; in fact, it may take many years for it to occur. Once it is recognized and the drug discontinued, it usually takes 4 to 8 months for recovery. This has now been reported with all topical ocular beta blockers. Myasthenia has been associated with the beta blockers, as has Raynaud's phenomena, arthralgias, and one well-documented case with rechallenge of recurrent hyperkalemia. Only with timolol is there data as to interaction between topical ocular medication and oral medication. Timolol and quinine enhance bradycardia. Timolol and halothane also enhance bradycardia and hypotension. As previously mentioned, timolol and the calcium channel blockers, such as verapamil, possibly cause arrhythmia.

Topical ocular beta blockers are possibly one of the more potent topical drugs used by ophthalmologists with significant systemic adverse effects. These adverse effects can probably be decreased by only using 1 drop, and closing the eyelids for at least 3 to 5 minutes following administration of the drop to prevent the lacrimal pump from pushing the medication into the nose. In selected cases, patients can be taught to use lacrimal sac occlusion by local pressure, but this is often difficult. However, before patients open their eyes, if they are given a tissue to absorb any excess fluid in the inner canthus, this may prevent additional medication from being pumped into the nose by blinking when the lacrimal pump is allowed to function again.

References:

Akingbehin T., and Raj, P.S.: Ophthalmic topical beta blockers: review of ocular and systemic adverse effects. J. Toxicol. Cut. Ocular Toxicol. 9:131–147, 1990.

Bright, R.A., and Everitt, D.E.: Beta blockers and depression. JAMA 267:1783–1787, 1992.

Busin, M., et al.: Overcorrected visual acuity improved by antiglaucoma medication after radial keratotomy. Am. J. Ophthalmol. 101:374, 1986.

Coleman, A.L., et al.: Topical timolol decreases plasma high-density lipoprotein cholesterol level. Arch. Ophthalmol. 106:1260–1263, 1990.

Gorlich, W.: Experience in clinical research with beta blockers in glaucoma. Glaucoma 9:21, 1987.

Harris, L.S., Greenstein, S.H., and Bloom, A.F.: Respiratory difficulties with betaxolol. Am. J. Ophthalmol. 102:274, 1986.

Fraunfelder, F.T.: Ocular beta blockers and systemic effects. Arch. Intern. Med. 146: 1073, 1986.

Fraunfelder, F.T., and Meyer, S.M.: Sexual dysfunction secondary to topical ophthalmic timolol. JAMA 253:3092, 1985.

Fraunfelder, F.T., and Meyer, S.M.: Systemic side effects from ophthalmic timolol and their prevention. J. Ocular Pharmacol. 3:177, 1987.

Grant, W.M., and Schuman, J.S.(Eds.): Toxicology of the Eye. 4th Ed., Springfield, Charles C. Thomas, 1993, pp. 242–262.

Hannaway, P.J., and Hopper, G.D.K.: Severe anaphylaxis and drug-induced beta-blockade. N. Engl. J. Med. 308:1536, 1983.

Kaufman, H.S.: Timolol-induced vasomotor rhinitis: A new iatrogenic syndrome. Arch. Ophthalmol. 104:967, 1986.

Nelson, W.L., et al.: Adverse respiratory and cardiovascular events attributed to timolol ophthalmic solution, 1978-1985. Am. J. Ophthalmol. 102:606, 1986.

Orlando, R.G.: Clinical depression associated with betaxolol. Am. J. Ophthalmol. 102: 275, 1986.

Palmer, E.A.: How safe are ocular drugs in pediatrics? Ophthalmology 93:1038, 1986.

Schwab, I.R., et al.: Foreshortening of the inferior conjunctival fornix associated with chronic glaucoma medications. Ophthalmology 99:197–202, 1992.

Sharir, M., Nardin G.F., and Zimmerman, T.J.: Timolol maleate associated with phalangeal swelling. Arch. Ophthalmol. 109:1650, 1991.

Shore, J.H., Fraunfelder, F.T., and Meyer, S.M.: Psychiatric side effects from topical ocular timolol, a beta-adrenergic blocker. J. Clin. Psychopharmacol. 7:264, 1987.

Verkijk, A.: Worsening of myasthenia gravis with timolol maleate eyedrops. Ann. Neurol. 17:211, 1985.

Vogel, R.: Topical timolol and serum lipoproteins (letter). Arch. Ophthalmol. *109*: 1341, 1991.
Wilhelmus, K.R., McCulloch, R.R., and Gross, R.L.: Dendritic keratopathy associated with beta-blocker eyedrops. Cornea 9:335–337, 1990

Generic Name: Carteolol

Proprietary Name: Arteolol (Span.), Arteoptic (Germ., G.B.), Carteol (Fr., Ital.), **Cartrol** (G.B., U.S.A.), Endak (Germ.), Mikelan (Fr., Jap., S. Afr., Span.), **Ocupress**, Teoptic

Primary Use: *Systemic*: Carteolol is a nonselective beta blocker that is used in the management of hypertension and angina pectoris. *Ophthalmic*: Carteolol is used in the management of glaucoma.

Ocular Side Effects:
  A. Local Ophthalmic Use or Exposure
    1. Decreased intraocular pressure
    2. Irritation
      a. Ocular pain
      b. Burning sensation
      c. Epiphora
      d. Hyperemia
      e. Photophobia
    3. Decreased vision
    4. Eyelids or conjunctiva
      a. Allergic reactions
      b. Erythema
      c. Blepharoconjunctivitis
    5. Corneal anesthesia

Systemic Side Effects:
  A. Local Ophthalmic Use or Exposure
    1. Asthma
    2. Bradycardia
    3. Dyspnea
    4. Depression
    5. Cardiac arrhythmia
    6. Headache
    7. Congestive heart failure
    8. Asthenia
    9. Dizziness
    10. Cerebral vascular accident
    11. Hypotension
    12. Syncope

13. Rhinitis
14. Bronchospasm
15. Aggravation of chronic obstructive pulmonary disease
16. Suppression of heart rate and blood pressure elevation
17. Increase in high-density lipoprotein
18. Confusion
19. Skin disease
20. Heart block
21. Taste perversion
22. Respiratory failure
23. Palpitation
24. Cerebral ischemia

Clinical Significance: Carteolol has not been used as extensively as timolol, but in general, it is compared with timolol as to clinical and adverse effects. Clearly, it is better tolerated with regard to stinging and irritation; in fact, these symptoms usually decrease with time. Ocular pain may be a significant side effect, but rarely an indication for discontinuing the drug. To date, the local anesthetic effect of this drug has not been reported in humans. Theoretically, all of the side effects reported with timolol could be seen with carteolol. However, it is apparent from controlled trials that there seem to be fewer systemic side effects with this agent than with timolol. While this agent can reduce the mean heart rate and possibly the mean blood pressure, these have been insignificant clinically. There have been cases in the literature and reported to the Registry of asthma, decompensated heart failure, headaches, asthenopsia, and dizziness, but these are in a much smaller proportion than seen with other nonselective beta blockers. There are two cases in the Registry, both with challenge and rechallenge, of a bleeding diathesis with nosebleeds and easy bruisability while taking this drug. This has not been reported with the other beta blockers, and while interesting, this is difficult to understand from a pharmacologic standpoint. *(see timolol)*

References:
Brazier, D.J., and Smith, S.E.: Ocular and cardiovascular response to topical carteolol 2% and timolol 0.5% in healthy volunteers. Br. J. Ophthalmol. 72:101–103, 1988.
Chrisp, P., and Sorkin, E.M.: Ocular carteolol—A review of its pharmacological properties, and therapeutic use in glaucoma and ocular hypertension. Drugs and Aging. 2:58–77, 1992.
Freedman, S.F., et al.: Effects of ocular carteolol and timolol on plasma high-density lipoprotein cholesterol level. Am. J. Ophthalmol. *116*:600–611, 1993.
Grunwald, J.E., and Delehanty, J.: Effect of topical carteolol on the normal human retinal circulation. Inv. Ophthalmol. & Vis. Sci. *33*:1853–1863, 1992.
Hoh, H.: Surface anesthetic effect and subjective compatibility of 2% carteolol and 0.6% metipranolol in eye-healthy people. Lens and Eye Toxicity Res. 7:347–352, 1990.

Kitazawa, Y., Horie, T., and Shirato, S.: Efficacy and safety of carteolol hydrochloride: a new beta-blocking agent for the treatment of glaucoma. Int. Cong. Ophthalmol. *1*:683–685, 1983.

LeJeune, C., Munera, Y., and Hughes, F.: Systemic effects of three beta-blocker eyedrops: comparison in healthy volunteers of beta1- and beta2-adrenoreceptor inhibition. Clin. Pharmacol. and Ther. *47*:578–583, 1990.

Rolando, M., et al.: New beta blockers: comparison of efficacy versus timolol maleate. Glaucoma. *11*:27–30, 1989.

Scoville, B., et al.: Double-masked comparison of carteolol and timolol in ocular hypertension. Am. J. Ophthalmol. *105*:150–154, 1988.

Ueda, C.N.S., et al.: Effects of beta-blocking agent carteolol on healthy volunteers and glaucoma patients. Jpn. J. Ophthalmol. *113*:57–66, 1980

Generic Name: Dipivefrin, DPE

Proprietary Name: d Epifrin (Germ.), Diopine (Neth., Span., Switz.), Diphemin (Switz.), Glaucothil (Germ.), Propine (Austral., Canad., G.B., Ire., Ital., Mon., Swed.)

Primary Use: This sympathomimetic is indicated as initial therapy for the control of intraocular pressure in chronic open-angle glaucoma.

Ocular Side Effects:
   A. Local Ophthalmic Use or Exposure
      1. Decreased intraocular pressure
      2. Irritation
         a. Lacrimation
         b. Hyperemia
         c. Ocular pain
         d. Burning sensation
      3. Eyelids or conjunctiva
         a. Allergic reactions
         b. Blepharoconjunctivitis—follicular
         c. Pemphigoid lesion with symblepharon
      4. Decreased vision
      5. Mydriasis—may precipitate narrow-angle glaucoma
      6. Photophobia
      7. Cornea
         a. Keratitis
         b. Intraepithelial vesicles
      8. Cystoid macular edema

Systemic Side Effects:
   A. Local Ophthalmic Use or Exposure
      1. Tachycardia

2. Cardiac arrhythmia
3. Hypertension
4. Headache
5. Asthma

Clinical Significance: Dipivefrin is a prodrug that is biotransformed to epinephrine inside the eye. This drug is better tolerated than standard epinephrine preparations, but at concentrations greater than 0.1%, there are increased epinephrine-like side effects. Dipivefrin is a medication surprisingly free of major ocular adverse effects. It does not show the epinephrine effects of contact lens discoloration or conjunctival pigment deposits. Upper and lower palpebral conjunctival follicles are common in patients taking long-term dipivefrin, with perilimbal, bulbar, or plica follicular reactions occurring rarely. Petersen, et al. have individually tested each component of commercial preparations and found dipivefrin the cause for each of the external ocular findings. Conjunctival shrinkage and symblepharon have also been related to chronic dipivefrin usage. Although the Registry has received cases of maculopathy in aphakic eyes and cystoid macular edema in phakic glaucomatous eyes after treatment with dipivefrin, these may be chance occurrences. The potential for systemic adverse reactions similar to those seen with topical ophthalmic epinephrine also exists for dipivefrin administration, although probably with a much lower frequency. Clinicians need to be aware of potential sensitivity in patients taking this agent who complain of respiratory difficulties, because some of these medications contain sulfites.

References:

Boerner, C.F.: Dipivefrine. Total punctate keratopathy due to dipivefrin. Arch. Ophthalmol. *106*:171, 1988.

Cebon, L., West, R.H., and Gillies, W.E.: Experience with dipivalyl epinephrine. Its effectiveness, alone or in combination, and its side effects. Aust. J. Ophthalmol. *11*:159, 1983.

Coleiro, J.A., Sigurdsson, H., and Lockyer, J.A.: Follicular conjunctivitis on dipivefrin therapy for glaucoma. Eye 2:440–442, 1988.

Duffey, R.J., and Ferguson, J.G., Jr.: Interaction of dipivefrin and epinephrine with the pilocarpine ocular therapeutic system (Ocusert). Arch. Ophthalmol. *104*:1135, 1986.

Fledelius, H.C.: Central vein thrombosis and topical dipivalyl epinephrine. Acta Ophthalmol. *68*:491–492, 1990.

Kerr, C.R., et al.: Cardiovascular effects of epinephrine and dipivalyl epinephrine applied topically to the eye in patients with glaucoma. Br. J. Ophthalmol. *66*:109, 1982.

Liesegang, T.J.: Bulbar conjunctival follicles associated with dipivefrin therapy. Ophthalmology *92*:228, 1985.

Mehelas, T.J., Kollarits, C.R., and Martin, W.G.: Cystoid macular edema presumably induced by dipivefrin hydrochloride (Propine). Am. J. Ophthalmol. *94*:682, 1982.

Petersen, P.E., et al.: Evaluation of ocular hypersensitivity to dipivalyl epinephrine by component eye-drop testing. J. Allergy Clin. Immunol. *85*:954–958, 1990.

Satterfield, D., Mannis, M.J., and Glover, A.T.: Unilateral corneal vesicles secondary to dipivefrin therapy. Am. J. Ophthalmol. *113(3)*:339–340, 1992.

Schwab, I.R., et al: Foreshortening of the inferior conjunctival fornix associated with chronic glaucoma medications. Ophthalmology *99(2)*:197–202, 1992.

Schwartz, H.J., and Sher, T.H.: Bisulfite intolerance manifest as bronchospasm following topical dipivefrin hydrochloride therapy for glaucoma. Arch. Ophthalmol. *103*: 14, 1985.

Wandel, T., and Spinak, M.: Toxicity of dipivalyl epinephrine. Ophthalmology *88*: 259, 1981.

West, R.H., Cebon, L., and Gillies, W.E.: Drop attack in glaucoma. The Melbourne experience with topical miotics, adrenergic and neuronal blocking drops. Aust. J. Ophthalmol. *11*:149, 1983

Generic Name: Metipranolol

Proprietary Name: Betanol (Mon.), Beta-Ophthiole (S. Afr., Neth.), Disorat (Germ.), Glauline (G.B.), **Optipranolol**

Primary Use: *Systemic*: Used in the management of cardiac disorders and hypertension. *Ophthalmic*: This noncardioselective beta blocker is used to reduce intraocular pressure associated with open-angle glaucoma.

Ocular Side Effects:
  A. Local Ophthalmic Use or Exposure
    1. Decreased intraocular pressure
    2. Irritation
       a. Hyperemia
       b. Photophobia
       c. Ocular pain
       d. Burning sensation
    3. Decreased vision
    4. Anterior uveitis
    5. Punctate keratitis
    6. Eyelids or conjunctiva
       a. Allergic reactions
       b. Erythema
       c. Blepharoconjunctivitis
    7. Corneal anesthesia
    8. Contact lens intolerance
       a. Corneal erosion
       b. Unable to wear
    9. Tear film break-up time—decreased
    10. Conjunctival keratinization

Systemic Side Effects:
   (Basically similar to timolol)

Clinical Significance: While there is still limited experience with this drug in the United States, it has been used for well over a decade in Europe. Metipranolol has been popular because of its lower cost, a lower concentration of preservatives, possibly fewer CNS side effects, and, possibly, less corneal anesthesia than seen with other beta blockers. Regardless, since it is a nonselective beta blocker, it has the potential to cause any of the local or systemic side effects seen with other nonselective beta blockers. What is unique about this agent is that it may cause an anterior uveitis. While it seems apparent, based on a comparison of the German and British data that this may be, in part, due to the vehicle. Uveitis is characterized by large anterior chamber keratic precipitates with cells and flare. On topical ocular steroids, the uveitis usually subsides within 4 to 6 weeks. There seems to be a dose-response curve that shows significantly less incidence and less severe uveitis with the 0.1% and 0.3% when compared with the 0.06% solution. There has been excellent challenge/rechallenge data to show that this is clearly a drug or drug-vehicle response. In some cases, a marked elevation of intraocular pressure, blepharoconjunctivitis, and periorbital dermatitis is associated with this uveitis. In the United States, both Schultz, Hoenig, and Charles as well as Melles and Wong have reported granulomatous iritis secondary to this drug.

References:
Akingbehin, T., and Villada, J.R.: Metipranolol-associated granulomatous anterior uveitis. Br. J. Ophthalmol. 75:519, 1991.
Cervantes, R., Hernandez, H.H., and Frati, A.: Pulmonary and heart rate changes associated with nonselective beta-blocker glaucoma therapy. J. Toxicol. Cut. Ocular Toxicol. 5:185–193, 1986.
Derous, D., et al.: Conjunctival keratinization, an abnormal reaction to an ocular beta-blocker. Acta Ophthalmol. 67:333–338, 1989.
Drager, J., and Winter, R.: Corneal sensitivity and intraocular pressure. Glaucoma Update II, Krieglstein and Leydhecker (Eds). Springer-Verlag, 1983. pp. 63–70.
Flaxel, C., and Samples, J.R.: Metipranolol. J. Toxicol. Cut. Ocular Toxicol. 10: 171–174, 1991.
Hoh, H.: Surface anesthetic effect and subjective compatibility of 2% carteolol and 0.6% m metipranolol in eye-healthy people. Lens and Eye Toxic. Res. 7:347–352, 1990.
Kessler, C. and Christ, T.: Incidence of Uveitis in glaucoma patients using metipranolol. J. Glaucoma 2:166–170, 1993.
Melles, R.B., and Wong, I.G.: Metipranolol-associated granulomatous iritis. Am. J. Ophthalmol. 118:712–715, 1994.
Schultz, J.S., Hoenig, J.A., and Charles, H.: Possible bilateral anterior uveitis secondary to metipranolol (OptiPranolol) therapy. Arch. Ophthalmol. 111:1607–1607, 1993.
Serle, J.B., Lustgarten, J.S., and Podos, S.M.: A clinical trial of metipranolol, a non-

cardioselective beta-adrenergic antagonist, in ocular hypertension. Am. J. Ophthalmol. *112*:302–307, 1991.

Stempel, I.: Different beta-blockers and their short-time effect on break-up time. Ophthalmologica *192*:11, 1986.

Class: Antibacterial Agents

Generic Name: 1. Colloidal Silver (Argentum Colloidal); 2. Silver Nitrate (Argentum Nitrate); 3. Silver Protein (Argentum Protein)

Proprietary Name: 1. None; 2. Argenpal (Span.), Howe's Solution (Austral.), Mova Nitrat (Germ.), Pluralane (Germ.), Quit (Austral.); 3. Stillargol (Fr.), Vitargénol (Fr.)

Primary Use: These topical ocular antibacterial agents are effective in the treatment of conjunctivitis and in the prophylaxis of ophthalmia neonatorum.

Ocular Side Effects:
    A. Local Ophthalmic Use or Exposure
        1. Silver deposits
            a. Cornea
            b. Conjunctiva
            c. Eyelids
            d. Lens
            e. Lacrimal sac
        2. Irritation
            a. Hyperemia
            b. Photophobia
            c. Ocular pain
            d. Edema
        3. Eyelids or conjunctiva
            a. Allergic reactions
            b. Conjunctivitis—nonspecific
            c. Edema
            d. Discoloration
            e. Photosensitivity
            f. Symblepharon
        4. Scarring or opacities of any ocular structure (silver nitrate—when exposed to caustic concentrations)
        5. Decreased vision
        6. Problems with color vision—objects have yellow tinge
        7. Decreased dark adaptation
        8. Dark episcleral mass (silver clips)
    B. Inadvertent Systemic Exposure

1. Silver deposits
   a. Cornea
   b. Conjunctiva
   c. Lens
2. Eyelids or conjunctiva
   a. Discoloration
   b. Photosensitivity

Clinical Significance: The overall use of silver-containing medication has been decreasing; however, in some countries it is still commonly prescribed. Ocular side effects other than with silver nitrate in caustic concentrations (silver nitrate sticks or concentrated solutions) seldom cause serious adverse reactions. Conjunctivitis is probably the most common side effect from topical ocular solutions, but rarely requires discontinuation of the medication. Topical ocular silver application for even a few months may cause conjunctival silver deposition. Long-term dosage may cause corneal, lens, eyelid, or lacrimal sac silver deposition. Silver deposits in the cornea or lens rarely interfere with vision. Ocular and periocular silver deposits over many years are absorbed if the drug is discontinued. Silver clips used decades ago for strabismus surgery have caused episcleral melanoma-like masses.

References:

Bartley, G.B.: Argyrosis secondary to a silver extraocular muscle clip. Arch. Ophthalmol. *110*:596, 1992.

Burstein, N.L.: Corneal cytotoxicity of topically applied drugs, vehicles and preservatives. Surv. Ophthalmol. *25*:15, 1980.

Cohen, S.Y., et al.: The dark choroid in systemic argyrosis. Retina *13(4)*:312–316, 1993.

Granstein, R.D., and Sober, A.J.: Drug- and heavy metal-induced hyperpigmentation. J. Am. Acad. Dermatol. *5*:1, 1981.

Rich, L.F.: Toxic drug effects on the cornea. J. Toxicol. Cut. Ocular Toxicol. *1*:267, 1982–1983.

Sandstrom, I., et al.: Toxic effects cf silver nitrate prophylaxis on corneal epithelium. Int. Cong. Ophthalmol. *2*:1090, 1983.

Smith, S.Z., et al.: Argyria. Arch. Dermatol. *117*:595, 1981.

Spencer, W.H., et al.: Endogenous and exogenous ocular and systemic silver deposition. Trans. Ophthalmol. Soc. UK *100*:171, 1980.

Stokinger, H.E.: The metals. *In* Clayton, G.D., and Clayton, F.E. (Eds.): Patty's Industrial Hygiene and Toxicology. New York, John Wiley & Sons, Vol. 2A, 1981, pp. 1881–1894.

Sziklai, I., et al.: New results on the experimental investigation of argyrosis. *In* Trace Element—Analytical Chemistry in Medicine and Biology. New York, Walter de Gruyter & Co., 1983, pp. 363–370.

Weiler, H.H., et al.: Argyria of the cornea due to self-administration of eyelash dye. Ann. Ophthalmol. *14*:822, 1982.

Class: Antiviral Agents

Generic Name: Acyclovir

Proprietary Name: *Systemic*: Acicloftal (Ital.), Acyvir (Ital.), Clovix (Ital.), Cusiviral (Span.), Cycloviran (Ital.), Maynar (Span.), Milavir (Span.), Sifiviral (Ital.), Vipral (Span.), Virherpes (Span.), Virmcn (Span.), **Zovirax** (Austral., Canad., Fr., G.B., Germ., Ire., Ital., Neth., S. Afr., Span., Swed., Switz.) *Ophthalmic*: Zovirax (Austral., G.B., Germ., Neth., Span., Switz.) *Topical*: Virherpes (Span.), **Zovirax** (Canad., G.B., Germ., Neth., Span., Switz.)

Primary Use: This purine nucleoside is used in the treatment and management of herpes simplex infections.

Ocular Side Effects:
- A. Systemic Administration
  - 1. Decreased vision
  - 2. Visual hallucinations
  - 3. Eyelids
    - a. Erythema
    - b. Urticaria
    - c. Edema
  - 4. Keratoconjunctivitis sicca—aggravates
  - 5. Subconjunctival or retinal hemorrhages secondary to drug-induced anemia
- B. Local Ophthalmic Use or Exposure
  - 1. Irritation
    - a. Lacrimation
    - b. Hyperemia
    - c. Ocular pain
    - d. Edema
    - e. Burning sensation
  - 2. Superficial punctate keratitis
  - 3. Eyelids or conjunctiva
    - a. Allergic reaction
    - b. Blepharitis
    - c. Conjunctivitis—follicular
  - 4. Narrowing or occlusion of lacrimal puncta

Clinical Significance: Oral acyclovir has very few ocular side effects. The most common is probably periocular edema with or without perioral numbness. Since the drug is secreted in human tears, ocular sicca may be aggravated in rare instances. Visual hallucinations have been reported secondary to systemic acyclovir therapy. Topical ophthalmic acyclovir is generally well tolerated, although mild transient burning or a stinging sensation (apparently caused by delayed solubilization of the ointment in the precorneal tear film) have been reported immediately following application of the drug. Punctate epithelial staining of the inferior bulbar conjunctiva and limbus is reversible with discontinuation of the agent. Punctal stenosis or occlusion, follicular conjunctivitis, contact blepharoconjunctivitis, palpebral allergy, or other signs of hypersensitivity have also occurred occasionally. Acyclovir does not appear to interfere significantly with the healing of stromal wounds.

References:

Auwerx, J., Knockaert, D., and Hofkens, P.: Acyclovir and neurologic manifestations. Ann. Intern. Med. *99*:882, 1983.

Collum, L.M.T., Logan, P., and Ravenscroft, T.: Acyclovir (Zovirax) in herpetic disciform keratitis. Br. J. Ophthalmol. *67*:115, 1983.

de Koning, E.W.J., van Bijsterveld, O.P., and Cantell, K.: Combination therapy for dendritic keratitis with acyclovir and a-interferon. Arch. Ophthalmol. *101*:1866, 1983.

Jones, P.G., and Beier-Hanratty, S.A.: Acyclovir: Neurologic and renal toxicity. Ann. Intern. Med. *104*:892, 1986.

Koliopoulos, J.: Acyclovir—A promising antiviral agent: A review of the preclinical and clinical data in ocular herpes simplex management. Ann. Ophthalmol. *16*:19, 1984.

Richards, D.M., et al.: Acyclovir. A review of its pharmacodynamic properties and therapeutic efficacy. Drugs *26*:378, 1983

Generic Name: 1. Idoxuridine (IDU); 2. Trifluridine (F_3T, Trifluorothymidine); 3. Vidarabine (Adenine Arabinoside, Ara-A)

Proprietary Name: *Systemic*: 3. **Vira-A** (Austral., Canad., Fr., Span.) *Ophthalmic*: 1. Cheratil (Ital.), Gel V (Fr.), Herpidu (Switz.), Herplex Liquifilm (Austral., Canad.), Herplex-D Liquifilm (Austral., Canad.), Idoxene (G.B.), Iducher 2M (Ital.), Iduviran (Fr.), Stoxil (Austral., Canad., S. Afr.), Synmiol (Germ.), Virexen (Span.), Virunguent (Germ.); 2. Aflomin (Span.), TFT (Germ., Neth., S. Afr.), Triherpine (Switz.), Viromidin (Span.), Virophta (Mon.), **Viroptic** (Canad.); 3. **Vira-A** (Canad.) *Topical*: Antizona (Span.), Herpid (G.B.), Herplex D (Ire., S. Afr.), Iducutit (Germ.), Iduridin (G.B.), Idustatin (Ital.), Virexen (Switz.), Virpex (Neth.), Virudox (G.B.), Virunguent (Switz.), Zostrum (Germ.)

Primary Use: *Systemic*: Vidarabine, a purine nucleoside, is used in the treatment of herpes simplex encephalitis and herpes zoster due to reactivated varicella-zoster virus infections in immunosuppressed patients. *Ophthalmic*: Idoxuridine, trifluridine, and vidarabine are used in the treatment of herpes simplex keratitis.

Ocular Side Effects:
A. Systemic Administration
   1. Visual hallucinations
   2. Blepharospasm
   3. Ocular flutter
   4. Subconjunctival or retinal hemorrhages secondary to drug-induced anemia
B. Local Ophthalmic Use or Exposure
   1. Irritation
      a. Lacrimation
      b. Hyperemia
      c. Photophobia
      d. Ocular pain
      e. Edema
   2. Cornea
      a. Superficial punctate keratitis
      b. Edema
      c. Filaments
      d. Delayed wound healing
      e. Erosions or indolent ulceration
      f. Stromal opacities
      g. Superficial vascularization (late)
      h. Epithellal dysplasia (chronic therapy)
   3. Eyelids or conjunctiva
      a. Allergic reactions
      b. Hyperemia
      c. Blepharitis
      d. Conjunctivitis—follicular
      e. Edema
      f. Pemphigoid lesion with symblepharon
      g. Perilimbal filaments
      h. Conjunctival punctate staining
      i. Conjunctival scarring
      j. Ischemia (trifluridine)
   4. Lacrimal system
      a. Canaliculitis
      b. Stenosis
      c. Occlusion
   5. Ptosis
   6. Anterior segment ischemia (trifluridine)

Clinical Significance: Systemic vidarabine-induced neurotoxic effects may include ocular symptoms of visual hallucinations and blepharospasm. Gizzi, Rudolph, and Perakis described saccadic ocular movements in rapid sequence without an intersaccadic interval occurring after intravenous vidarabine. This abnormality ceased after the drug was discontinued. Adverse ocular reactions to topical ophthalmic antivirals are often overlooked and frequently assumed to be a worsening of the clinical disease. Ocular side effects seem to occur most frequently in eyes with decreased tear production. The occasional appearance of corneal clouding, stippling, and small punctate defects in the corneal epithelium is common. These corneal changes can be painful, even in these partial anesthetic corneas, but may significantly decrease after the drug has been discontinued. Not all ocular side effects are reversible after discontinuing use of these drugs, because in some cases ptosis and occlusion of the lacrimal punctum have been permanent. Ischemic changes, especially with ocular sicca, have been reported in the conjunctiva and anterior segment, possibly secondary to trifluridine. Idoxuridine seems to have the highest degree of local irritation and toxicity, followed by vidarabine and trifluridine. There is evidence of cross reactivity with other pyrimidine analogues, not only ocular but cutaneous as well. Although several instances of premalignant changes have occurred after topical application of idoxuridine or trifluridine, the causal relationship has not been proven, in part since herpes type II has also been associated with malignant changes. There is a case in the Registry of a 38-year-old woman who developed conjunctival intraepithelial neoplasia inferonasally at the limbus after 3 years of idoxuridine use.

References:

Burdge, D.R., Chow A.W, and Sacks, S.L.: Neurotoxic effects during vidarabine therapy for herpes zoster. Can. Med. Assoc. J. *132*:392, 1985.

Cullis, P.A., and Cushing, R.: Vidarabine encephalopathy. J. Neurol. Neurosurg. Psychiatry *47*:1351, 1984.

Gizzi, M., Rudolph, S., and Perakis, A.: Ocular flutter in vidarabine toxicity. Am. J. Ophthalmol. *109*:105, 1990.

Kaufman, H.E.: Chemical bleplaritis following drug treatment. Am. J. Ophthalmol. *95*:703, 1983.

Kremer, I., Rozenbaum, D., and Aviel, E.: Immunofluorescence findings in pseudopemphigoid induced by short-term idoxuridine administration. Am. J. Ophthalmol. *111(3)*:375–377, 1991.

Lass, J.H., Troft, R.A., and Dohlman, C.H.: Idoxuridine-induced conjunctival cicatrization. Arch. Ophthalmol. *101*:747, 1983.

Maudgal, P.C., Van Damme, B., and Missotten, L.: Corneal epithelial dysplasia after trifluridine use. Graefes Arch. Clin. Exp. Ophthalmol. *220*:6, 1983.

Shearer, D.R., and Bourne, W.M.: Severe ocular anterior segment ischemia after long-term trifluridine treatment for presumed herpetic keratitis. Am. J. Ophthalmol. *109(3)*:346–347, 1990.

Udell, I.J.: Trifluridine-associated conjunctival cicatrization. Am. J. Ophthalmol. *99*:363, 1985.

Class: Carbonic Anhydrase Inhibitors

Generic Name: 1. Acetazolamide; 2. Dichlorphenamide; 3. Ethoxzolamide; 4. Methazolamide

Proprietary Name: 1. Défiltran (Fr.), **Diamox** (Austral., Canad., Fr., G.B., Germ., Ital., Neth., S. Afr., Span., Swed., Switz.), Edemox (Span.), Glaupax (Germ., Neth., Swed., Switz.), **Storzolamide**; 2. Antidrasi (Ital.), **Daranide** (Austral., G.B.), Fenamide (Ital.), Glauconide (Span.), Glaumid (Ital.), Oralcon (Swed.), Oratrol (Span., Switz.), Tensodilen (Span.); 3. None; 4. **Neptazane** (Canad.), Neptazine (Austral.)

Primary Use: These enzyme inhibitors are effective in the treatment of all forms of glaucoma. Some of these drugs have also been used to treat edema due to congestive heart failure, drug-induced edema, and centrencephalic epilepsies.

Ocular Side Effects:
  A. Systemic Administration
      1. Decreased intraocular pressure
      2. Decreased vision
      3. Myopia
      4. Decreased accommodation
      5. Forward displacement of lens
      6. Eyelids or conjunctiva
          a. Allergic reactions
          b. Erythema
          c. Photosensitivity
          d. Urticaria
          e. Purpura
          f. Erythema multiforme
          g. Stevens-Johnson Syndrome
          h. Lyell's syndrome
          i. Loss of eyelashes or eyebrows
      7. Retinal or macular edema
      8. Iritis
      9. Ocular signs of gout
      10. Globus hystericus
      11. Subconjunctival or retinal hemorrhages secondary to drug-induced anemia
      12. Problems with color vision (methazolamide)
          a. Color vision defect
          b. Objects have yellow tinge

Systemic Side Effects:
  A. Systemic Administration
      1. Paresthesia
      2. Malaise syndrome
          a. Acidosis
          b. Asthenia

       c. Anorexia
       d. Weight loss
       e. Depression
       f. Somnolence
       g. Confusion
       h. Impotence
       i. Decreased libido
  3. Gastrointestinal disorder
       a. Nausea
       b. Vomiting
  4. Renal disorder
       a. Urolithiasis
       b. Polyuria
       c. Hematuria
       d. Glycosuria
  5. Blood dyscrasia
       a. Aplastic anemia
       b. Thrombocytopenia
       c. Agranulocytosis
       d. Hypochromic anemia
  6. Convulsion

Clinical Significance: Ocular side effects due to carbonic anhydrase inhibitors are transient and usually insignificant. The most common significant ocular side effect of this group of drugs is probably the acute transient myopia. It appeared most commonly in the nonglaucomatous woman, especially in the last months of pregnancy when the drug was given for water retention without toxemia. There are, however, many well-documented cases of from 1 to 8 diopters of myopia, usually occurring within hours to days after starting the drug. There are also numerous reports of deepening of the anterior chamber and alterations in the hydration of the lens. One of the more unusual side effects, however, is reported by Vela and Campbell, in which the drug induced a cilio-choroidal detachment after glaucoma surgery. There are well-documented cases of both anterior and forward displacement of the lens. Other ocular side effects are usually of minimal importance and do not appear to be dose related. Areas of greatest concern with this agent are systemic side effects. The most complete review is Grant and Schuman's current edition of *Toxicology of the Eye*. Probably the most common systemic side effects are the paresthesias, but these generally are not long lasting and seldom cause the patient to stop therapy. Malaise can be a major problem; patients often do not associate it with the use of this drug and just believe that they are getting older. Some of the happiest patients I have encountered are those who have stopped taking carbonic anhydrase inhibitors—they did not realize how good they could feel until this medication was ceased. Cases of gout have been induced by carbonic anhydrase inhibitors because it may elevate serum uric acid. Urolithiasis is rare but can be a major problem with some patients. Respiratory difficulties can occur in patients, especially those with chronic lung disease. Osteomalacia has been reported in patients taking anticonvulsive medications. These agents can also increase CNS salicylate toxicity. Metabolic acidosis can occasionally cause a coma to occur. Patients with renal insufficiency are especially susceptible to high blood levels of carbonic anhydrase inhibitors, and serious acidoses have been reported. Diabetic patients with nephropathy may have the same problem. Cirrhosis of the liver is a contraindication to the use of carbonic anhydrase inhibitors because ammonia poisoning may result. Patients taking other potassium-lowering agents, such as some of the hypertensive medications, may require potassium supplements. The most serious, however, are the blood dyscrasias that have been well documented with all carbonic anhydrase inhibitors. This is a source of significant controversy not as to causation, but as to the need for periodic blood testing and the importance of early recognition. My opinion is that before using these agents, a baseline CBC and platelet count should be done along with obtaining informed consent.

References:

Epstein, R.J., Allen, R.C., and Lunde, M.W.: Organic impotence associated with carbonic anhydrase inhibitor therapy for glaucoma. Ann. Ophthalmol. *19*:48, 1987.

Fraunfelder, F.T., et al.: Hematologic reactions to carbonic anhydrase inhibitors. Am. J. Ophthalmol. *100*:79, 1985.

Grant, W.M., and Schuman, J.S.: Toxicology of the Eye. 4th Ed., Charles C. Thomas, Springfield, Illinois. 1993, pp. 43, 542, 658, 951.

Lichter, P.R.: Reducing side effects of carbonic anhydrase inhibitors. Ophthalmology *88*:266, 1981.

Margo, C.E.: Acetazolamide and advanced liver disease. Am. J. Ophthalmol. *100*:611, 1986.

Niven, B.I., and Manoharan, A.: Acetazolamide-induced anaemia. Med. J. Aust. *142*: 120, 1985.

Shuster, J.N.: Side effects of commonly used glaucoma medications. Geriatr. Ophthalmol. *2*:30, 1986.

Vela, M.A., and Campbell, D.G.: Hypotony and ciliochoroidal detachment following pharmacologic aqueous suppressant therapy in previously filtered patients. Ophthalmology *92*:50–57, 1985.

White, G.L., Pribble, J.P., and Murdock, R.T.: Acetazolamide and the sulfonamide-sensitive patient. Ophthalmol. Times *10*:15, 1985.

Class: Decongestants

Generic Name: 1. Naphazoline; 2. Tetrahydrozoline

Proprietary Name: 1. Ak-Con (Canad.), Albalon (Ire., S. Afr., Switz.), Albalon Liquifilm (Austral., Canad., Neth.), Alfa (Ital., Span.), Allergy Drops

(Canad.), **Clear Eyes** (Austral., Canad.), Degest 2 (Canad.), Desamin Same (Ital.), Imidazyl (Ital.), Imizol (Ital.), Iridina Due (Ital.), Minha (Switz.), Murine (G.B.), Murine Clear Eyes (S. Afr.), Naftazolina (Ital.), Naphcon Forte (Canad.), Opcon (Canad.), Optazine (Austral., Switz.), Piniol (Germ.), Privin (Germ.), Privina (Span.), **Privine** (Canad.), Ran (Ital.), Rhino-Mex-N (Canad.), Rimidol (Swed.), Rinazina (Ital.), Rino Naftazolina (Ital.), Rinoftal (Ital.), Transpulmina Rino (Ital.), Vasocon (Canad.), Vasoconstrictor Pensa (Span.), Virginiana (Ital.), Vistalbalon (Germ.), 2. Cleer (Germ.), Constrilia (Fr., Neth., Switz.), Demetil (Ital.), **Eyesine**, Octilia (Ital.), Rhinopront (Germ.), Rinobios (Ital.), Stilla (Ital.), Tyzine (Germ., Switz.), Vasorinil (Ital.), Visine (Austral., Ital., Neth., Switz.), Yxin (Germ.)

Primary Use: These sympathomimetic amines are effective in the symptomatic relief of ophthalmic congestion of allergic or inflammatory origin.

Ocular Side Effects:
    A. Local Ophthalmic Use or Exposure
        1. Conjunctival Vasoconstriction
        2. Irritation
            a. Lacrimation
            b. Reactive hyperemia
            c. Ocular pain
            d. Burning sensation
        3. Mydriasis—may precipitate narrow-angle glaucoma
        4. Decreased intraocular pressure
        5. Decreased vision
        6. Punctate keratitis
        7. Eyelids or conjunctiva
            a. Allergic reactions
            b. Blepharoconjunctivitis
        8. Increased pigment granules in anterior chamber
        9. Decreased tolerance to contact lenses
      10. Increased width of palpebral fissures

Systemic Side Effects:
    A. Local Ophthalmic Use or Exposure
        1. Headache
        2. Hypertension
        3. Nervousness
        4. Nausea
        5. Dizziness
        6. Asthenia
        7. Somnolence
        8. Cardiac arrhythmia
        9. Hyperglycemia

10. Hypothermia
11. Anaphylaxis

Clinical Significance: Ocular side effects due to these ocular decongestants are seldom significant, except with frequent or long-term use. The conjunctival vasculature may fail to respond to the vasoconstrictive properties when these agents are used excessively or for prolonged periods. Adverse ocular reactions secondary to these drugs are almost always reversible with discontinuation of the drug; however, keratitis requiring months to resolve has been reported. In addition, the Registry has received reports of a possible association between acute central retinal artery occlusion and topical ocular naphazoline. Two cases of probable bilateral acute narrow-angle glaucoma secondary to tetrahydrozoline use have been reported to the Registry. Eleven cases of mydriasis have been associated with this agent as well. Major systemic adverse reactions following use of ocular decongestants are rare and occur primarily when these drugs are used more frequently than recommended by the manufacturer.

References:
Abelson, M.B., Allansmith, M.R., and Friedlaender, M.H.: Effects of topically applied ocular decongestant and antihistamine. Am. J. Ophthalmol, 90:254, 1980.
Abelson, M .B., et al.: Tolerance and absence of rebound vasodilation following topical ocular decongestant usage. Ophthalmology 91:1364, 1984.
Abelson, M.B., Yamamoto, G.K., and Allansmith, M.R.: Effects of ocular decongestants. Arch. Ophthalmol. 98:856, 1980.
Gandolfi, C.: Therapeutic ocular application of sympathomimetic substances. Boll Oculist 26:397–400, 1947.
Grossmann, E.E., and Lehman, R.H.: Ophthalmic use of Tyzine. Am. J. Ophthalmol. 42:121, 1956.
Lisch, K.: Conjunctival alterations by sympathomimetic drugs. Klin. Mbl. Augenheilk. 173:404–406, 1973.
Menger, H.C.: New ophthalmic decongestant, tetrahydrozoline hydrochloride. JAMA 170:178, 1959.
Rich, L.F.: Toxic drug effects on the cornea. J. Toxicol. Cut. Ocular Toxicol. 1:267, 1982–1983.

Class: Miotics

Generic Name: Aceclidine

Proprietary Name: Glaucostat (Fr., Neth., Span., Switz.), Glaucotat (Germ.), Glaunorm (Ital.)

Primary Use: This topical parasympathomimetic agent is used to lower intraocular pressure in the treatment of open-angle glaucoma.

Ocular Side Effects:
  A. Local Ophthalmic Use or Exposure
    1. Miosis
    2. Decreased intraocular pressure
    3. Accommodative spasm
    4. Decreased vision
    5. Irritation
      a. Lacrimation
      b. Hyperemia
      c. Burning sensation
      d. Browache
    6. Problems with color vision—color vision defect
    7. Retinal detachment

Clinical Significance: Although the miotic effect of aceclidine may be slightly greater than that of other miotics in comparable concentrations, the degree of accommodative spasm has been reportedly less. Irritation does not appear to be a common problem with 2% to 4% solutions.

References:

Crandall, D.C., and Leopold, I.H.: The influence of systemic drugs on tear constituents. Ophthalmology 86:115, 1979.

Fechner, P.U., Teichmann, K.D., and Weyrauch, W.: Accommodative effects of aceclidine in the treatment of glaucoma. Am. J. Ophthalmol. 79:104, 1975.

Laroche, J., and Laroche, C.: Nouvelles recherches sur la modification de la vision des couleurs sous l'action des médicaments à dose thérapeutique. Ann. Pharm. Fr. 35:173, 1977.

Lieberman, T.W., and Leopold, I.H.: The use of aceclydine in the treatment of glaucoma. Its effect on intraocular pressure and facility of aqueous humor outflow as compared to that of pilocarpine. Am. J. Ophthalmol. 64:405, 1967.

Romano, J.H.: Double-blind cross-over comparison of aceclidine and pilocarpine in open-angle glaucoma. Br. J. Ophthalmol. 54:510, 1970

Generic Name: Acetylcholine

Proprietary Name: Covochol (S. Afr.), **Miochol** (Austral., Canad., G.B., Swed.)

Primary Use: This intraocular quaternary ammonium parasympathomimetic agent is used to produce prompt, short-term miosis.

Ocular Side Effects:
  A. Local Ophthalmic Use or Exposure—Subconjunctival or Intracameral Injection
    1. Miosis

2. Decreased intraocular pressure
3. Conjunctival hyperemia
4. Accommodative spasm
5. Iris atrophy
6. Blepharoclonus
7. Lacrimation
8. Retinal hemorrhages
9. Paradoxical mydriasis
10. Decreased anterior chamber depth
11. Cataract—transient
12. Corneal edema
13. Corneal opacities

Systemic Side Effects:
A. Local Ophthalmic Use or Exposure—Subconjunctival or Intracameral Injection
   1. Bradycardia
   2. Hypotension
   3. Vasodilation
   4. Dyspnea
   5. Perspiration

Clinical Significance: Few ocular side effects due to acetylcholine are seen. Although miosis is the primary ophthalmic effect, mydriasis may occur on rare occasions. Ocular side effects are rarely of clinical significance; however, a few cases of corneal edema have been reported to the Registry, but it is difficult to distinguish the drug's effects from surgical trauma. Transient lens opacities have been reported, probably on the basis of an osmotic effect. To date, no long-term effect on the lens has been seen due to this drug. If acetylcholine is administered intraocularly, it may cause lacrimation. Bradycardia and hypotension have been seen following irrigation of the anterior chamber with acetylcholine.

References:
Brinkley, J.R., Jr., and Henrick, A.: Vascular hypotension and bradycardia following intraocular injection of acetylcholine during cataract surgery. Am. J. Ophthalmol. 97:40, 1984.

Fraunfelder, F.T.: Corneal edema after use of carbachol. Arch. Ophthalmol. 97:975, 1979.

Fraunfelder, F.T.: Recent advances in ocular toxicology. In Srinivasan, B.D. (Ed.): Ocular Therapeutics. New York, Masson, 1980, pp. 123–126.

Gombos, G.M.: Systemic reactions following intraocular acetylcholine instillation. Ann. Ophthalmol. 14:529, 1982.

Hagan, J.: Severe bradycardia and hypotension following intraocular acetylcholine in patients who previously tolerated the medication. Missouri Med. 87:4, 1990.

Lazar, M., Rosen, N., and Nemet, P.: Miochol-induced transient cataract. Ann. Ophthalmol. 9:1142, 1977.
Leopold, I.H.: The use and side effects of cholinergic agents in the management of intraocular pressure. In Drance, S.M., and Neufeld, A.H. (Eds.): Glaucoma: Applied Pharmacology in Medical Treatment. New York, Grune & Stratton, 1984, pp. 357–393.
Rasch, D., et al.: Bronchospasm following intraocular injection of acetylcholine in a patient taking metoprolol. Anesthesiology 59:583, 1983

Generic Name: Dapiprazole

Proprietary Name: Glamidolo (Ital.), **Rev-Eyes**

Primary Use: To reverse iatrogenically induced mydriasis.

Ocular Side Effects:
A. Local Ophthalmic Use or Exposure
   1. Miosis
   2. Conjunctiva
      a. Injection
      b. Chemosis
   3. Eyelids
      a. Ptosis
      b. Erythema
      c. Edema
   4. Symptoms
      a. Burning
      b. Tearing
      c. Itching
      d. Dryness
      e. Brow ache
      f. Pain
   5. Cornea
      a. Superficial punctate keratitis
      b. Edema
      c. Infiltration
   6. Miosis
   7. Increased accommodation
   8. Allergic reactions
      a. Chemosis
      b. Keratitis
      c. Grayish corneal infiltrates

Clinical Significance: Dapiprazole's primary action is reversing drug-induced mydriasis. While rapid miosis occurs, the primary benefit may be the more rapid recovery of accommodation. The most common side effect is palpebral and bulbar conjunctival injection. This may occur in close to 100% of patients. This is transitory and of little practical importance. Ptosis may occur in up to 10% of patients, but this also is transitory. Symptoms such as burning are common and may, in rare instances, last up to 20 minutes. Rarely, gray corneal infiltrates adjacent to the limbus may occur. This is believed to be an allergic effect. Corneal edema and sicca have been reported, but these, as well as most other side effects, are transitory and of little clinical importance. Dapiprazole has been used to treat narrow-angle glaucoma because it can induce miosis with little effect on peripheral iris vasculature.

References:

Allinson, R.W., et al.: Reversal of mydriasis by dapiprazole. Ann. Ophthalmol. *22*: 131–138, 1990.

Bonomi, L., Marchini, G., and De Gregorio, M.: Ultrasonographic study of the ocular effects of topical dapiprazole. Glaucoma *8*:30–31, 1986.

Cheeks, L., Chapman, J.M., and Green, K.: Corneal endothelial toxicity of dapiprazole hydrochloride. Lens and Eye Tox. Res. *9(2)*:79–84, 1992.

Iuglio, N.: Ocular effects of topical application of dapiprazole in man. Glaucoma *6*: 110–116, 1984.

Paggiarino, D.A., Brancato, L.J., and Newton, R.E.: The effects on pupil size and accommodation of sympathetic and parasympatholytic agents. Ann. Ophthalmol. *25*:244–253, 1993.

Rev-Eyes (Dapiprazole HCL) ophthalmic eyedrops. A clinical and safety profile. Storz Ophthalmics, Inc., St. Louis, MO, 1991

Generic Name: 1. Demecarium; 2. Echothiophate; 3. Isoflurophate (DFP)

Proprietary Name: 1. **Humorsol**, Tosmilen (G.B.); 2. Phospholine (Switz.), **Phospholine Iodide** (Austral., Canad., Fr., G.B., Ital., Neth.), Phospholin-jodid (Germ.); 3. Diflupyl (Fr.), **Floropryl**

Primary Use: These topical anticholinesterases are used in the management of open-angle glaucoma, conditions in which movement or constriction of the pupil is desired, and accommodative esotropia. Demecarium is also used in the early management of ocular myasthenia gravis, and isoflurophate is used in periocular louse infestations.

Ocular Side Effects:

A. Local Ophthalmic Use or Exposure
1. Miosis
2. Decreased vision
3. Accommodative spasm
4. Irritation

      a. Lacrimation
      b. Hyperemia
      c. Photophobia
      d. Ocular pain
      e. Edema
      f. Burning sensation

5. Cataracts
      a. Anterior or posterior subcapsular

6. Eyelids or conjunctiva
      a. Allergic reactions
      b. Conjunctivitis—follicular
      c. Edema
      d. Pemphigoid lesion with symblepharon
      e. Depigmentation (isoflurophate)

7. Blepharoclonus

8. Myopia

9. Iris or ciliary body cysts—especially in children

10. Intraocular pressure
      a. Increased—initial
      b. Decreased

11. Iritis
      a. Occasionally fine (keratic precipitates)
      b. Activation of latent iritis or uveitis
      c. Formation of anterior or posterior synechiae

12. Decreased scleral rigidity

13. Occlusion of lacrimal canaliculi

14. Decreased anterior chamber depth

15. Hyphema—during surgery

16. Vitreous hemorrhages

17. Decreased size of filtering bleb

18. Corneal deposits (echothiophate)

19. Retinal detachment

20. May aggravate myasthenia gravis

Systemic Side Effects:

A. Local Ophthalmic Use or Exposure

1. Gastrointestinal disorders
      a. Nausea
      b. Vomit
      c. Abdominal pain
      d. Diarrhea

2. Urinary incontinence

3. Increased saliva

4. Dyspnea

5. Bradycardia

6. Cardiac arrhythmia
7. Perspiration
8. Asthenia

Clinical Significance: Ocular side effects are most common with isofluro-phate followed by echothiophate and demecarium. Visual complaints with or without accommodative spasm are the most frequent adverse ocular reactions. Drug-induced lens changes are well documented and are primarily seen in the older age group. In shallow anterior chamber angles, these agents are contraindicated because they may precipitate narrow-angle glaucoma. This is probably due to peripheral vascular congestion of the iris, which may further aggravate an already compromised angle. Also, the parasympathomimetic agents allow the iris lens diaphragm to come forward and, under certain circumstances, to induce a relative pupillary block. While irritative conjunctival changes are common with long-term use, allergic reactions are rare. These strong miotics, primarily in diseased retinas, may cause retinal detachments by exerting traction on the peripheral retina. *See* pilocarpine for a more-detailed explanation of possible cause. Cases of irreversible miosis due to long-term therapy have been reported. An atypical band-shaped keratopathy has been said to be due to long-term miotic therapy; however, others suggest this is due to long-term elevation of intraocular pressure and is not drug induced. A slowly progressive drug-related cicatricial process of the conjunctiva that may be clinically indistinguishable from ocular cicatricial pemphigoid may occur with these drugs. Patients receiving topical ocular anticholinesterases and those being treated for myasthenia may have increased systemic and ocular side effect risks if exposed to organic phosphorous insecticides. Topical demecarium may have the greatest risk because it has the highest degree of penetrability of the blood-cerebrospinal fluid barrier. This combination has resulted in cardiac arrest, hypotension, gastrointestinal effects, and respiratory failure. In addition, anesthetic deaths have been reported in patients receiving topical ocular anticholinesterases after receiving succinylcholine. This effect is due to the lowered blood cholinesterase from the topical ocular anticholinesterase agents.

References:

Adams, S.L., Mathews, J., and Grammer, L.C.: Drugs that may exacerbate myasthenia gravis. Ann. Emerg. Med. *13*:532, 1984.

Adler, A.G., et al.: Systemic effects of eye drops. Arch. Intern. Med. *142*:2293, 1982.

Eggers, H.M.: Toxicity of drugs used in diagnosis and treatment of strabismus. *In* Srinivasan, D.: Ocular Therapeutics. New York, Masson, 1980, pp. 115–122.

Eshagian, J.: Human posterior subcapsular cataracts. Trans. Ophthalmol. Soc. UK *102*: 364, 1982.

Hirst, L.W., et al.: Drug-induced cicatrizing conjunctivitis simulating ocular pemphigoid. Cornea *1*:121, 1982.

Tseng, S.C.G., et al.: Topical retinoid treatment for various dry-eye disorders. Ophthalmology 92:717, 1985.
West, R.H., Cebon, L., and Gillies, W.E.: Drop attack in glaucoma. The Melbourne
experience with topical miotics, adrenergic and neuronal blocking drops. Aust. J.
Ophthalmol. 11:149, 1983.
Wood, J.R., Anderson, R.L., and Edwards, J.J.: Phospholine iodide toxicity and Jones'
tubes. Ophthalmology 87:346, 1980

Generic Name: 1. Neostigmine; 2. Physostigmine

Proprietary Name: *Systemic*: 1. Intrastigmina (Ital.), **Prostigmin** (Austral.,
Canad., G.B., Germ., Ire., Neth., S. Afr.), Prostigmina (Ital.), Prostigmine
(Fr., Span., Switz.); 2. Anticholium (Germ.), **Antilirium** (Canad.) *Ophthal-
mic*: 1. Prostigmin (Germ.); 2. **Eserine, Eserine Salicylate, Isopto Eserine**

Primary Use: *Systemic*: Neostigmine is used in the treatment of myasthenia
gravis. Physostigmine is used to reverse the CNS effects caused by clinical
or toxic dosages of drugs capable of producing an anticholinergic syndrome.
Ophthalmic: These topical parasympathomimetic agents are used in the
management of narrow-angle and open-angle glaucoma.

Ocular Side Effects:
   A. Systemic Administration
      1. Miosis
      2. Decreased vision
      3. Eyelids or conjunctiva
         a. Allergic reactions
         b. Erythema
         c. Urticaria
      4. Lacrimation—toxic states
      5. Visual hallucinations—toxic states
   B. Local Ophthalmic Use or Exposure
      1. Miosis
      2. Decreased intraocular pressure
      3. Irritation
         a. Lacrimation
         b. Hyperemia
         c. Photophobia
         d. Ocular pain
      4. Accommodative spasm
      5. Decreased vision
      6. Eyelids or conjunctiva
         a. Allergic reactions
         b. Conjunctivitis—follicular
         c. Blepharoconjunctivitis

      d. Depigmentation
      e. Blepharoclonus
  7. Myopia
  8. Iritis
  9. Iris cysts
10. Decreased anterior chamber depth
11. Vitreous hemorrhages
12. Cataracts
13. Occlusion of lacrimal punctum
14. Retinal detachment
15. Atypical band keratopathy (physostigmine)

Clinical Significance: Ocular side effects due to these anticholinesterases are usually reversible with discontinued drug use. These agents should be used with caution since peripheral vascular congestion of the iris may precipitate narrow-angle glaucoma. Long-term use of these drugs is seldom possible because allergic or irritative conjunctivitis occurs frequently. An allergic blepharitis may cause skin depigmentation. The normal coloration usually returns after discontinuance of the drug. An atypical band keratopathy has been said to be due to long-term miotic therapy; however, others suggest it is due to long-term elevation of intraocular pressure and is not drug-induced. Physostigmine is sensitive to heat and light; discolored solutions are irritating and clinically ineffective. As with any miotic, the potential of a pull on an already diseased retina may precipitate a retinal detachment. (See *pilocarpine* for a more-detailed explanation of possible cause.)

References:

Apt, L., and Gaffney, W.L.: Toxic effects of topical eye medication in infants and children. *In* Duane, T.D., and Jaeger, E.A. (Eds.): Biomedical Foundations of Ophthalmology. Philadelphia, J.B. Lippincott, 1982, Vol. 3, pp. 43:1–13.

Crandall, D.C., and Leopold, I.H.; The influence of systemic drugs on tear constituents. Ophthalmology *86*:115, 1979.

Leopold, I.H.: The use and side effects of cholinergic agents in the management of intraocular pressure. *In* Drance, S.M., and Neufeld, A.H. (Eds.): Glaucoma: Applied Pharmacology in Medical Treatment. New York, Grune & Stratton, 1984, pp. 357–393.

Sugar, H.S.: Pitfalls in glaucoma treatment. Ann. Ophthalmol. *11*:1043, 1979

Generic Name: Pilocarpine

Proprietary Name: Akarpine, Asthenopin (Germ.), Chibro-Pilocarpin (Germ.), Dropil (Ital.), Isopto Carpina (Span.), **Isopto Carpine** (Austral., Canad., G.B., Neth., S. Afr., Switz.), Licarpin (Swed.), Liocarpina (Ital.), Miocarpine (Canad.), **Ocu-Carpine, Ocusert** (Austral., Canad., G.B.), **Pilagan Liquifilm**, Pilo (Fr., Switz.), **Pilocar**, Pilocarp (Span.), Pilocarpol

(Germ.), Pilogel (Germ., Ital., Neth., S. Afr.), Pilogel HS (Switz.), Pilomann (Germ.), Pilomann-Öl (Germ.), **Pilopine HS** (Canad.), Pilopos (Germ.), Pilopt (Austral.), **Pilostat** (Canad.), Pilotonina (Ital.), P.V. Carpine (Austral., Ire., S. Afr., Switz.), Sno Pilo (G.B.), Spersacarpin (Germ.), Spersacarpine (Canad., Swed., Switz.), Vistacarpin (Germ.), Vitacarpine (Fr.)

Primary Use: This topical ocular parasympathomimetic agent is used in the management of glaucoma and in conditions in which constriction of the pupil is desired.

Ocular Side Effects:
   A. Local Ophthalmic Use or Exposure
       1. Pupils
           a. Miosis
           b. Mydriasis—rare
       2. Decreased vision (light hunger)
       3. Paralysis or spasm of accommodation
       4. Intraocular pressure
           a. Increased—initial
           b. Decreased
           c. No effect
       5. Decreased anterior chamber depth
       6. Eyelids or conjunctiva
           a. Allergic reactions
           b. Hyperemia
           c. Conjunctivitis—follicular
           d. Muscle spasms
           e. Angioneurotic edema
           f. Pseudomembrane
           g. Pseudo-ocular pemphigoid
           h. Cicatricial shortening of fornices
           i. Conjunctival dysplasia or epithelial proliferation
           j. Conjunctival hemorrhage
       7. Irritation
           a. Lacrimation
           b. Burning sensation
       8. Myopia—transient
       9. Retina
           a. Bleeds
           b. Detachment
           c. Macular hole
       10. Cornea
           a. Punctate keratitis
           b. Edema
           c. Epithelial microcysts

      d. Atypical band keratopathy
      e. Dysplasia or epithelial proliferation
  11. Decreased dark adaptation
  12. Blepharoclonus
  13. Iris cysts
  14. Increased axial lens diameter
  15. Decreased scleral rigidity
  16. Cataracts
  17. Problems with color vision—color vision defect
  18. Iritis
  19. Malignant glaucoma
  20. Vitreous hemorrhage
  21. Punctal or canalicular stenosis

Systemic Side Effects:
  A. Local Ophthalmic Use or Exposure
    1. Headache, browache
    2. Perspiration
    3. Gastrointestinal disorder
      a. Nausea
      b. Vomiting
      c. Diarrhea
    4. Saliva increased
    5. Tremor
    6. Bradycardia
    7. Hypotension
    8. Bronchospasm
    9. Pulmonary edema
    10. Mental status changes
      a. Confusion
      b. Short-term memory loss
      c. Depression
      d. Aggravation of Alzheimer's syndrome
      e. Aggravation of Parkinson's syndrome
    11. Epistaxis
    12. Rhinorrhea
    13. Voice changes including hoarseness
    14. Abdominal spasms
    15. Tenesmus

Clinical Significance: Side effects from pilocarpine can be divided into short-term and long-term exposure. The most frequent short-term effects are those that affect the pupil, i.e., miosis that causes "light hunger," effects on accommodation, transient myopia, and periocular muscle spasms. Acute toxic or allergic reactions of the anterior segment are infrequent. The most bothersome are superficial punctate keratitis and, rarely, corneal edema. Cases of edema are primarily seen with a poor corneal epithelium, possibly allowing a direct effect on the endothelium. The most serious side effects, however, are retinal detachments and malignant glaucoma. Retinal detachments or macular holes may well be caused by drug-induced accommodation with the forward displacement of the posterior lens surface and elongation of the eye. This causes a more anterior position of the vitreous face and body. This forward movement may cause traction in areas where the vitreous is attached to the retina. A partial macular hole (Stage 1-A) that resolved on discontinuation of the miotic has also been reported (Benedict and Shami). Animal data show that a miotic can cause a pull on the peripheral retina by constriction of the ciliary body. Either of these mechanisms, i.e., forward vitreous displacement or accommodation in already diseased retinas, may precipitate a retinal hole or tear. Vitreous hemorrhages have been reported secondary to this process involving a retinal vessel. Pilocarpine's ability to increase the A-P diameter of the lens and decrease the depth of the anterior chamber may also play a prominent role in some forms of malignant glaucoma. Fraunfelder and Morgan reported bizarre behavior after topical ocular pilocarpine was administered to elderly patients. This is possibly due to miosis causing "light hunger," thereby causing a decrease in sensory input that may be enough to cause confusion to occur in some patients. Reyes, et al. believe that this is most common in subclinical Alzheimer syndrome patients. They postulated that this may be a direct pilocarpine effect on the CNS and noted an increase of symptomatology in patients with Parkinson's disease after taking topical ocular pilocarpine. Ocular changes secondary to the long-term use of pilocarpine may be divided into those specifically due to the drug itself or various combinations of the drug, preservatives, or vehicles. Clearly, iris cysts are due to the miosis induced by this drug. Pilocarpine may well be a weak cataractogenic agent. It is likely that most of the other side effects are due to repeated exposure of the drug and its preservatives over a period of months to years. This includes conjunctival, corneal and lacrimal outflow system changes. Epithelial microcysts are similar in appearance to Cogan's microcystic dystrophy but are often smaller and usually clear. Corneal and conjunctival dysplasia or hyperplasia occur most often on the inferior nasal limbus. Chronic topical ocular drug exposure has been implicated in changes in the conjunctiva and Tenon's capsule to the extent that they may adversely influence the success of filtration procedures for glaucoma. While rare, this has clearly been found with any long-term topical ocular medication. The above can also cause cicatricial shortening in the fornices and lacrimal outflow system and even pseudo-ocular pemphigoid. The most frequent finding in the FDA spontaneous reporting system includes literally hundreds of reports of pilocarpine of various concentrations having no effect on intraocular pressure. Even today with improved manufacturing, there are still occasional reports of pilocarpine causing mydriasis and cycloplegia. This may be due to an impurity of the stereo-isomer of pilocarpine, jaborine, an atropine-like side effect. There have been numerous reports of an atypical band keratopathy caused by phenylmercuric nitrate, a preservative no longer in use with pilocarpine. However, rare reports still are received by the Registry of peripheral, white, subepithelial deposits occurring with pilocarpine use. This seems to occur more frequently in eyes with pre-existing band keratopathy. Iritis has been reported secondary to pilocarpine use. Human data support that pilocarpine increases the blood-aqueous barrier permeability to plasma protein in a dose-dependent manner. In some individuals, this will give cells and flare on slit lamp examination. Mothers receiving topical ocular pilocarpine giving birth may have infants with signs mimicking neonatal meningitis—hyperthermia, restlessness, convulsions, and diaphoresis. Pediatricians should be made aware of this syndrome so unnecessary tests and manipulations are avoided. Although it is not known whether pilocarpine is excreted in human milk, caution should be advised when miotics are administered to nursing mothers.

References:

Abramson, D.H., MacKay, C., and Coleman, J.: Pilocarpine-induced retinal tear: An ultrasonic evaluation of lens movements. Glaucoma *3*:9, 1981.

Beasley, H., and Fraunfelder, F.T.: Retinal detachments and topical ocular miotics. Ophthalmology *86(1)*:95–98, 1979.

Benedict, W.L. and Shami, M.: Impending macular hole associated with topical pilocarpine. Am. J. Ophthalmol. *114(6)*:765–766, 1992.

Crandall, A.S., et al.: Characterization of subtle corneal deposits. J. Toxicol. Cut. Ocular Toxicol. *3*:263, 1984.

Duffey, R.J., and Ferguson, J.G., Jr.: Interaction of dipivefrin and epinephrine with the pilocarpine ocular therapeutic system (Ocusert). Arch. Ophthalmol. *104*:1135, 1986.

Flore, P.M., Jacobs, I.H. and Goldberg, D.B.: Drug-induced pemphigoid. Arch. Ophthalmol. *105*:1660–1663, 1987.

Fraunfelder, F.T., and Morgan, R.: The aggravation of dementia by pilocarpine. JAMA *271(22)*:1742–1743, 1994.

Johnson, D.H., et al.: A one-year multicenter clinical trial of pilocarpine gel. Am. J. Ophthalmol. *97*:723,1984.

Kastl, P.R.: Inadvertent systemic injection of pilocarpine. Arch. Ophthalmol. *105*:28, 1987.

Levine, R.Z.: Uniocular miotic therapy. Trans. Am. Acad. Ophthalmol. Otolaryngol. *79*:376–380, 1975.

Littman, L., et al.: Severe symptomatic atrioventricular block induced by pilocarpine eye drops. Arch. Intern. Med. *147*:586, 1987.

Merritt, J.C.: Malignant glaucoma induced by miotics postoperatively in open-angle glaucoma. Arch. Ophthalmol. *95*:1988–1989, 1977.

Mishra, P., et al.: Intraoperative bradycardia and hypotension associated with timolol and pilocarpine eyedrops. Br. J. Anaesthesiol. *55*:897, 1983.

Mori, M., et al.: Effects of pilocarpine and tropicamide on blood-aqueous barrier permeability in man. Invest. Ophthalmol. Vis. Sci. *33(2)*:416–423, 1992.

Naveh-Floman, N., Stahl, V., and Korczyn, A.D.: Effect of pilocarpine on intraocular pressure in ocular hypertensive subjects. Ophthalmic Res. *18*:34, 1986.

Pouliquen, Y., et al.: Drug-induced cicatricial pemphigoid affecting the conjunctiva. Ophthalmology *93(6)*:775–783, 1986.

Reyes, P.F., et al.: Mental status changes induced by eyedrops in dementia of the Alzheimer type. J. Neurol. Neurosurg. Psychiatry *50*:113, 1987.

Samples, J.R. and Meyer, S.M.: Use of ophthalmic medications in pregnant and nursing women. Am. J. Ophthalmol. *106(5)*: 616–623, 1988.

Schuman, J.S., Hersh, P., and Kylstra, J.: Vitreous hemorrhage associated with pilocarpine. Am. J. Ophthalmol. *108(3)*:333–334, 1989.

Schwab, I.R., et al.: Foreshortening of the inferior conjunctival fornix associated with chronic glaucoma medications. Ophthalmology *99(2)*:197–202, 1992.

Sherwood, M.B., et al.: Long-term morphologic effects of antiglaucoma drugs on the conjunctiva and Tenon's capsule in glaucomatous patients. Ophthalmology *96(3)*: 327–335, 1989.

Wright, P.: Squamous metaplasia or epidermalization of the conjunctiva as an adverse reaction to topical medication. Trans. Ophthalmol. Soc. UK *99*:244–246, 1979.

Zimmerman, T.J., and Wheeler, T.M.: Miotics. Side effects and ways to avoid them. Ophthalmology *89*:76, 1982.

Class: Mydriatics and Cycloplegics

Generic Name: 1. Cyclopentolate; 2. Tropicamide

Proprietary Name: 1. Ak-Pentolate (Canad.), Alnide (G.B.), Ciclolux (Ital.), Ciclopleg (Span.), Cicloplegico (Span.), Cicloplejico (Span.), Cyclogyl (Austral., Canad., Neth., S. Afr., Swed., Switz.), Cyclomydri (Neth.), Mydrilate (G.B.), Ophtomydrol (Germ.), Skiacol (Fr.), Zykolat (Germ.); 2. Mydriacyl (Austral., Canad., G.B., S. Afr., Swed.), Mydriaticum (Fr., Germ., Neth., S. Afr., Switz.), Tropicacyl (Canad.), Tropimil (Ital.), Visumidriatic (Ital.)

Primary Use: These topical ocular short-acting anticholinergic mydriatic and cycloplegic agents are used in refractions and fundus examination.

Ocular Side Effects:
    A. Local Ophthalmic Use or Exposure
        1. Decreased vision
        2. Mydriasis—may precipitate narrow-angle glaucoma
        3. Irritation
            a. Hyperemia
            b. Photophobia
            c. Ocular pain
            d. Burning sensation
        4. Decrease or paralysis of accommodation
        5. Increased intraocular pressure

   6. Eyelids or conjunctiva
      a. Allergic reactions
      b. Blepharoconjunctivitis
   7. Visual hallucinations
   8. Synechiae
   9. Keratitis

Systemic Side Effects:
   A. Local Ophthalmic Use or Exposure
      1. CNS effects
         a. Personality disorders
         b. Psychosis
         c. Ataxia
         d. Speech disorder
         e. Agitation
         f. Hallucinations
         g. Confusion
         h. Convulsion
      2. Tachycardia
      3. Fever
      4. Vasodilation
      5. Urinary retention
      6. Gastrointestinal disorder
      7. Dry mouth
      8. Paresthesia

Clinical Significance: Major ocular side effects due to these drugs are quite rare. Both cyclopentolate and tropicamide can elevate intraocular pressure in open-angle glaucoma and precipitate narrow-angle glaucoma; cycloplegics have been shown to decrease the coefficient outflow. Some have suggested that the use of these agents may cause an instability of vitreous face, which could aggravate cystoid macular edema. This, however, is debatable. Visual hallucinations or psychotic reactions after topical applications are primarily seen with cyclopentolate. Systemic adverse reactions from these agents are common, especially in children. Disorientation, somnolence, hyperactivity, vasomotor collapse, tachycardia, seizures, and even death have been reported. There have also been cases of addiction to topical ocular application of these drugs because some patients get a CNS "high" from their use. Sato, de Freitas, and Foster reaffirmed this in two patients. Mori, et al., recently showed tropicamide reduces aqueous barrier permeability. McCormack showed reduced mydriasis from either of these drugs with repeat dosage. He recommended that they not be used the day before surgery if one wants to achieve maximum dilation.

References:

Brooks, A.M.V., West, R.H., and Gillies, W.E.: The risks of precipitating acute angle-closure glaucoma with the clinical use of mydriatic agents. Med. J. Aust. *145*:34, 1986.

Eggers, M.H.: Toxicity of drugs used in diagnosis and treatment of strabismus. *In* Srinivasan, D.: Ocular Therapeutics. Masson, New York, 1980, pp. 115–122.

Fitzgerald, D.A., et al.: Seizures associated with 1% cyclopentolate eyedrops. J. Paediatr. Child Health. *26*:106–107, 1990.

Hermansen, M.C., and Sullivan, L.S.: Feeding intolerance following ophthalmologic examination. Am. J. Dis. Child. *139*:367, 1985.

Isenberg, S.J., Abrams, C., and Hyman, P.E.: Effects of cyclopentolate eyedrops on gastric secretory function in pre-term infants. Ophthalmology *92*:698, 1985.

Jones, L.W.J., and Hodes, D.T.: Cyclopentolate. First report of hypersensitivity in children: 2 case reports. Ophthalmic Physiol. Opt. *11*:16–20, 1991.

McCormack, D.L.: Reduced mydriasis from repeated doses of tropicamide and cyclopentolate. Ophthal. Surg. *21(7)*:508–512, 1990.

Mori, M., et al.: Effects of pilocarpine and tropicamide on blood-aqueous barrier permeability in man. Invest. Ophthalmol. Vis. Sci. *33(2)*:416–423, 1992.

Rosales, T., et al.: Systemic effects of mydriatrics in low weight infants. J. Pediatr. Ophthalmol. *18*:42 1981.

Sato, E.H., de Freitas, D., and Foster, C.S.: Abuse of cyclopentolate hydrochloride (Cyclogyl) drops. N. Engl. J. Med. *326*:1363–1364, 1992.

Shihab, Z.M.: Psychotic reaction in an adult after topical cyclopentolate. Ophthalmologica *181*:228, 1980.

Class: Neurotoxins

Generic Name: Botulinum A Toxin

Proprietary Name: Dysport (G.B.), **Oculinum**

Primary Use: This neurotoxin is used primarily to treat blepharospasm, hemifacial spasms, and Meige's syndrome. It has also been used in selected strabismus and various neuromuscular disorders of the head and neck.

Ocular Side Effects:

    A. Periocular Injection
        1. Ptosis
        2. Sicca
        3. Extraocular muscles
            a. Paresis (in muscles other than those intended)
            b. Hemorrhage
            c. Diplopia
            d. Hyperdeviation
        4. Eyelids
            a. Hemorrhage

       b. Lagophthalmos
       c. Edema
       d. Pruritis
       e. Paralytic ectropion
       f. Paralytic entropion
  5. Cornea—exposure keratitis
  6. Pupil
       a. Mydriasis
       b. Acute glaucoma
  7. Photophobia
  8. Facial weakness or numbness
  9. Blurred vision
10. Brow droop
11. Epiphora

Clinical Significance: There have been no proven systemic side effects from periocular injections of botulinum toxin. Ocular side effects are transitory and are usually gone by 2 weeks; however, they can last up to 6 weeks. The most frequently encountered side effect is ptosis with or without lagophthalmos and decreased blink rate. Sicca is the second most commonly seen, but it is unclear if this is due to exposure or a decrease in tear production. The incidence of both ptosis and dry eyes is roughly between 6% and 8%. The next most common side effect is diplopia, which occurs in approximately 3% of patients. The inferior oblique is the most commonly involved extraocular muscle. This side effect is surprisingly well tolerated by most patients. It has been suggested that diplopia will be decreased by avoiding treatment of the medial two-thirds of the lower eyelids and keeping the injection superficial when treating blepharospasm. There have been reports of injection around eyelids for blepharospasm in which mydriasis with secondary acute glaucoma occurred. A report of possible enhancement of anterior segment ischemia following vertical muscle transposition after botulinum injection is reported by Keech, et al. They recommended injection of the botulinum toxin several days after strabismus surgery rather than intraoperatively. A questionable case of the toxin causing transitory paresis of an arm after periocular injection was reported by Sanders, Massey, and Buckley. Histologic features have shown no persistent toxic changes to the muscle, although there were some changes into the nerve fiber endings. Attempts to find antibody production secondary to botulinum toxin have been negative in humans thus far.

References:
Biglan, A.W., et al.: Absence of antibody production in patients treated with botulinum A toxin. Am. J. Ophthalmol. *101*:232–235, 1986.
Burns, C.L., Gammon, A., and Gemmill, M.C.: Ptosis associated with botulinum toxin

treatment of strabismus and blepharospasm. Ophthalmology *93(12)*:1621–1627, 1986.

Corridan, P., et al.: Acute angle-closure glaucoma following botulinum toxin injection for blepharospasm. Br. J. Ophthalmol. *74*:309–310, 1990.

Dunlop, D., Pittar, G., and Dunlop, C.: Botulinum toxin in ophthalmology. Aust. N. Z. J. Ophthalmol. *16*:15–20, 1988.

Dutton, J.J., and Buckley, E.G.: Long-term results and complications of botulinum A toxin in the treatment of blepharospasm. Ophthalmology *95(11)*:1529–1534, 1988.

Engstrom, P.F., et al.: Effectiveness of botulinum toxin therapy for essential blepharospasm. Ophthalmology *94(8)*:971–975, 1987.

Frueh, B.R., et al.: The effect of omitting botulinum toxin from the lower eyelid in blepharospasm treatment. Am. J. Ophthalmol. *106*:45–47, 1988; *106*:765–766, 1988.

Harris, C.P., et al.: Histologic features of human orbicularis oculi treated with botulinum A toxin. Arch. Ophthalmol. *109*:393–395, 1991.

Huges, A.J.: Botulinum toxin in clinical practice. Practical Therapeutics. Drugs *48(6)*: 888–893, 1994.

Kalra, H.K., and Magoon, E.H.: Side effects of the use of botulinum toxin for treatment of benign essential blepharospasm and hemifacial spasm. Ophthal. Surg. *21(5)*: 335–338, 1990.

Keech, R.V., et al.: Anterior segment ischemia following vertical muscle transposition and botulinum toxin injection. Arch Ophthalmol. *108*:176, 1990.

Magoon, E.H.: Chemodenervation of strabismic children. Ophthalmology *96(7)*: 931–934, 1989.

Mauriello, J.A., Coniaris, H., and Haupt, E.J.: Use of botulinum toxin in the treatment of one hundred patients with facial dyskinesias. Ophthalmology *94(8)*:976–979, 1987.

Sanders, D.B., Massey, E.W., and Buckley, E.G.: Botulinum toxin for blepharospasm. Neurology *36*:545–547, 1986.

Class: Ophthalmic Dyes

Generic Name: 1. Alcian Blue; 2. Fluorescein; 3. Rose Bengal; 4. Trypan Blue

Proprietary Name: *Systemic*: 2. **Ak-Fluor** (Canad.), **Fluorescite**, Funduscein (Canad.), **Funduscein-10, Funduscein-25, Ophthifluor** *Ophthalmic*: 2. Disclo-Plaque (Austral.), Fluores (S. Afr.), **Fluorescein HCL**, Fluorescite (Austral., Canad., S. Afr.), **Fluorets** (G.B., S. Afr.), **Fluor-I-Strip, Fluor-I-Strip A.T.** (Canad.), **Ful-Glo** (Austral.); 3. Ak-Rose (Canad.), **Rose Bengal Solution, Rose Bengal Strips, Rosets**

Primary Use: *Systemic*: Fluorescein is used to study the aqueous secretion of the ciliary body; as an aid in the diagnosis of internal carotid artery insufficiency; to document perfusion of blood vessels, i.e., skin grafts; and to locate cerebral spinal fluid leakage when given intrathecally. *Ophthalmic*: These topical dyes are used in various ocular diagnostic tests.

Ocular Side Effects:
 A. Systemic Administration—Fluorescein
  1. Stains ocular fluids and tissues yellow-green
  2. Eyelids or conjunctiva
   a. Allergic reactions
   b. Hyperemia
   c. Yellow-orange discoloration
   d. Angioneurotic edema
   e. Urticaria
   f. Eczema
 B. Local Ophthalmic Use or Exposure
  1. Stains mucus and connective tissue blue (alcian blue) (stains mucus rose bengal)
  2. Stains ocular fluids and tissues yellow-green (fluorescein)
  3. Stains epithelium not adequately covered by periocular tear film (rose bengal)
  4. Stains degenerated epithelial cells and mucus blue (trypan blue)
  5. Irritation
   a. Ocular pain
   b. Burning sensation
  6. Eyelids or conjunctivitis
   a. Blue discoloration (alcian blue, trypan blue)
   b. Yellow-orange discoloration (fluorescein)
   c. Red discoloration (rose bengal)
   d. Photosensitizer (rose bengal greater than fluorescein)
  7. Tears and/or contact lenses stained
  8. Iritis (fluorescein—radial keratotomy)

Systemic Side Effects:
 A. Systemic Administration—Fluorescein (Intravenous)
  1. Nausea
  2. Vomiting
  3. Urine discolor
  4. Headache
  5. Dizziness
  6. Fever
  7. Syncope
  8. Hypotension
  9. Dyspnea
  10. Shock
  11. Thrombophlebitis
  12. Skin necrosis
  13. Cardiac arrest
  14. Myocardial infarction

15. Anaphylaxis
16. Generalized seizure
B. Intrathecal Injection—Fluorescein
  1. Lower extremity weakness
  2. Numbness
  3. Generalized seizures
  4. Opisthotonos
  5. Cranial nerve paralysis
  6. Paralysis lower extremities

Clinical Significance: Mild adverse systemic reactions (nausea, vomiting) in fluorescein angiography are common and transient; moderate and severe adverse reactions are rare. Because of the risk of subretinal hemorrhages, some physicians elect to give an antiemetic before administration of the agent in patients with choroidal neovascular membranes undergoing fluorescein angiography. Ocular side effects due to these ophthalmic dyes are rare and transient. Brodsky, Bauerberg, and Sterzovsky reported that if microperforations occur following radial keratotomy incisions, topical ocular fluorescein may cause an acute iritis with an inflammatory membrane. Corneal transplant surgeries commonly use topical ocular fluorescein and have not reported this problem. Solutions of fluorescein can readily become contaminated with *Pseudomonas* because fluorescein inactivates the preservatives found in most ophthalmic solutions. Rose bengal, especially in concentrations above 1%, may occasionally cause significant ocular irritation after topical ocular instillation. It was thought that rose bengal was a vital dye; however, it has recently been shown that it stains primarily epithelium not adequately covered by the periocular tear film. If the corneal or conjunctival epithelium is not intact, the topical application of alcian blue or rose bengal may cause long-term or even permanent stromal deposits of the dye.

References:

Antoszyk, A.N., et al.: Subretinal hemorrhages during fluorescein angiography. Am. J. Ophthalmol. *103*:111, 1987.

Brodsky, M.E., Bauerberg, J.M., and Sterzovsky, A.: Case report: Probable fluorescein-induced uveitis following radial keratotomy. J. Refract. Surg. *3(1)*:29, 1987.

Chishti, M.I.: Adverse reactions to intravenous fluorescein. Pak. J. Ophthalmol. *2*:19, 1986.

Chodosh, J., Banks, M.C., and Stroop, W.G.: Rose bengal inhibits herpes simplex virus replication in vero and human corneal epithelial cells in vitro. Invest. Ophthalmol. Vis. Sci. *33(8)*:2520–2527, 1992.

Feenstra, R.P.G., and Tseng, S.C.G.: What is actually stained by rose bengal? Arch. Ophthalmol. *110*:984–993, 1992.

Karhunen, U., Raitta, C., and Kala, R.: Adverse reactions to fluorescein angiography. Acta Ophthalmol. *64*:282, 1986.

Menon, I.A., et al.: Reactive oxygen species in the photosensitization of retinal pigment epithelial cells by rose bengal. J. Toxicol. Cut. Ocular Toxicol. *11(4)*:269–283, 1992.

Spaeth, G.L., Nelson, L.B., and Beaudoin, A.R.: Ocular teratology. *In* Jakobiec, F.A. (Ed.): Ocular Anatomy, Embryology and Teratology. Philadelphia, J.B. Lippincott, 1982, pp. 955–975.

Yannuzzi, L.A., et al.: Fluorescein angiography complication survey. Ophthalmology *93*:611 1986

Generic Name: Indocyanine Green

Proprietary Name: Cardio Green (CG) (Canad.)

Primary Use: This tricarbocyanine dye is given intravenously to measure hepatic function, liver blood flow, and cardiac output as well as for ocular angiography.

Ocular Side Effects:
None reported

Systemic Side Effects:
1. Nausea and vomiting
2. Urticaria
3. Vasovagal episodes
4. Cardiorespiratory arrest
5. Hypotension
6. Urge to defecate

Clinical Significance: Indocyanine green dye has been used for more than 30 years in other areas of medicine and only recently has gained popularity in ophthalmology. The side effects of this drug are less frequent than with fluorescein. Mild adverse reactions to fluorescein were between 1% and 10%, while mild adverse reactions to this dye were approximately 0.15%. The rate of moderate reactions to fluorescein was 1.6% compared with 0.2% for indocyanine green dye. Severe reactions were 0.05% with indocyanine green, which was similar to that with fluorescein (Hope-Ross, et al.). Since indocyanine green is an established iodine allergen, is metabolized in the liver, and will cross the placental barrier, its use is contraindicated in patients with iodine allergies, who are pregnant, or who have liver or kidney disease. Patients with uremia have a higher incidence of significant adverse systemic reactions to indocyanine green than normal. The reason for this is unknown but may be due to an allergic hypersensitivity reaction. Deaths have been reported with this agent, as with fluorescein, probably due to an anaphylactic reaction and cardiorespiratory arrest. There may well be an increased incidence of reactions with repeat administration, but this has not been proven.

References:

Benya, R., Quintana, J., and Brundage, B.: Adverse reactions to indocyanine green: a case report and a review of the literature. Cathet. Cardiovasc. Diagn. *17*:231–233, 1989.

Guyer, D.R., et al.: Digital indocyanine-green angiography in chorioretinal disorders. Ophthalmology *99*:287–291, 1992.

Hope-Ross, M., et al.: Adverse reactions due to indocyanine green. Ophthalmology *101(3)*:529–533, 1994.

Kogure, K., et al.: Infrared absorption angiography of the fundus circulation. Arch. Ophthalmol. *83*:209–214, 1970.

Nanikawa, R., et al.: A case of fatal shock induced by indocyanine green (ICG) test. Jpn. J. Leg. Med. *32*:209–214, 1978.

Obana, A., et al.: Survey of complications of indocyanine green angiography in Japan. Am. J. Ophthalmol. *118*:749–753, 1994.

Schatz, H.: Sloughing of skin following fluorescein extravasation. Ann. Ophthalmol. *10*:625, 1978.

Wolf, S., et al.: Severe anaphylactic reaction after indocyanine green fluorescence angiography (letter). Am. J. Ophthalmol. *114*:638–639, 1992.

Yannuzzi, L.A., et al.: Fluorescein angiography complication survey. Ophthalmology *93*:611–617, 1986.

Yannuzzi, L.A., et al.: Digital indocyanine green videoangiography and choroidal neovascularization. Retina *12*:191–223, 1992.

Class: Ophthalmic Implants

Generic Name: Silicone

Proprietary Name: None

Primary Use: Silicone polymers of various viscosities or solids are used in ophthalmology as lubricants, implants, and volume expanders.

Ocular Side Effects:
    A. Local Ophthalmic Use or Exposure
        1. Conjunctiva
            a. Irritation
            b. Burning sensation
    B. Intraocular—Oil
        1. Cornea
            a. Edema
            b. Opacity
            c. Vascularization
            d. Thinning
            e. Vacuoles (silicone)
            f. Keratopathy—bullous and/or band
        2. Chamber angle

      a. Glaucoma
      b. Vacuoles (silicone)
   3. Iris—vacuoles (silicone)
   4. Retina—vacuoles (silicone)
   5. Optic nerve
      a. Vacuoles (silicone)
      b. Atrophy
 C. Implants—Silicone
      a. Granulomatous reactions
      b. Increase in infections

Clinical Significance: Silicone solutions or solids rarely cause adverse ocular reactions; however, significant side effects may occur under certain circumstances. Like any foreign body buried within tissue, the implant, even if inert, will be encased by scar tissue or granulomatous tissue. Postoperative infection rates are also higher if an implant is included in the procedure. As with silicone liquids placed in other areas of the body, the solution within the eye may migrate to new locations with time. Since the usual site of injection is intravitreal, occasionally the solution may come in contact with the lens or enter the anterior chamber, with the potential to affect the outflow channels, lens, or cornea. Shields, et al. have also shown its potential to migrate posteriorly to affect glaucomatous optic nerves and enhance atrophy, probably on a mechanical basis. Corneal changes are probably not a toxic process, but rather, as pointed out by Norman, et al., act as a nutritional barrier. Silicone oils may increase permeability by dissolving substances such as cholesterol and other lipophilic substances out of membranes in the corneal endothelium and retina.

References:

Ando, F.: Intraocular hypertension resulting from pupillary block by silicone oil. Am. J. Ophthalmol. *99*:87, 1985.

Beekhuis, W.H., van Rij, G., and Zivojnovic, R.: Silicone oil keratopathy: Indication for keratoplasty. Br. J. Ophthalmol. *69*:247, 1985.

Bennett, S.R., and Abrams, G.W.: Band keratopathy from emulsified silicone oil. Arch Ophthalmol. *108*:1387, 1990.

Chuo, N., et al.: Intravitreous silicone injection. Histopathologic findings in a human eye after 12 years. Arch. Ophthalmol. *101*:1399, 1983.

Foulks, G.N., et al.: Histopathology of silicone oil keratopathy in humans. Cornea *10*: 29–37, 1991.

Friberg, T.R., Verstraeten, T.C., and Wilcox, D.K.: Effects of emulsification, purity, and fluorination of silicone oil on human retinal pigment epithelial cells. Invest. Ophthalmol. Vis. Sci. *32*:2030–2034, 1991.

Jalkh, A.E., et al.: Silicone oil retinopathy. Arch. Ophthalmol. *104*:178, 1986.

Laroche, L., et al.: Ocular findings following intravitreal silicone injection. Arch. Ophthalmol. *101*:1422, 1983.

Norman, B.C., et al.: Corneal endothelial permeability after anterior chamber silicone oil. Ophthalmology *97(12)*:1671–1677, 1990.

Parmley, V.C., et al.: Foreign-body giant cell reaction to liquid silicone. Am. J. Ophthalmol. *101*:680 1986.
Shields, C.L., et al.: Silicone oil. Optic atrophy: case report. Arch. Ophthalmol. *107*: 683–686, 714–717, 1989.

Class: Ophthalmic Preservatives

Generic Name: Benzalkonium

Proprietary Name: 3D Tipo P-Disinfettante (Ital.), Armil (Span.), Baktonium (Germ.), Benzalc (Span.), Benzaltex (Switz.), Bluesteril (Ital.), Bradosol (G.B.), Capitol (G.B.), Cetal Concentrate (Austral.), Citrosil Spray (Ital.), Comprimés Gynécologiques Pharmatex (Fr.), Crème Pharmatex (Fr.), Crema Contracep Lanzas (Span.), Dermo-Sterol (Canad.), Detergil (Ital.), Di-Mill (Ital.), D-Pronto-Disinfettante Analcolico (Ital.), Elialconio (Ital.), Esoform Deterferri (Ital.), Esoform Sanacasa (Ital.), Esosan (Ital.), Euronormol-Disinfettante Concentrato Profumato (Ital.), Germicidin (Ital.), Germiphene (Canad.), Germozero (Ital.), Geyderm Disinfettante (Ital.), Helis (Ital.), Killavon (Germ.), Laudamonium (Germ.), Lozione Vittoria (Ital.), Mini Ovulo Lanzas (Span.), Mini-Ovule Pharmatex (Fr.), Neo-Desogen (Ital.), Norica (Ital.), Oraldettes (S. Afr.), Ovules Pharmatex (Fr.), Pharmatex (Canad.), Quack (Ital.), Quartamon (Germ.), Roccal (G.B., Ire.), Sanaform (Ital.), Sapocitrosil (Ital.), Sebogel (Ital.), Solution Gynécologique Pharmatex (Fr.), Steramina G (Ital.), Tearisol (Span.), Zefirol (Ital.), Zensyls (G.B.), Zephiran (Canad.), Zephirol (Germ.)

Primary Use: This topical ocular quaternary ammonium agent is used as a preservative in ophthalmic solutions and as a germicidal cleaning solution for contact lenses.

Ocular Side Effects:
    A. Local Ophthalmic Use or Exposure
        1. Irritation
            a. Lacrimation
            b. Hyperemia
            c. Photophobia
            d. Ocular pain
            e. Burning sensation
        2. Eyelids or conjunctiva
            a. Allergic reactions
            b. Hyperemia
            c. Erythema
            d. Blepharitis
            e. Conjunctivitis—papillary

  f. Edema
  g. Pemphigoid lesion with symblepharon
 3. Cornea
  a. Punctate keratitis
  b. Edema
  c. Pseudomembrane formation
  d. Decreased epithelial microvilli
  e. Vascularization
  f. Scarring
  g. Delayed wound healing
  h. Increased transcorneal permeability
 4. Decreased lacrimation
 5. Aggravate keratoconjunctivitis sicca

Clinical Significance: Adverse ocular reactions to benzalkonium are common, even at exceedingly low concentrations. Concentrations as low as 0.01% may cause cell damage by emulsification of the cell wall lipids. Almost all ocular side effects are reversible after use of the drug is discontinued, and most of the damage is fairly superficial. However, long-term use has caused extensive corneal damage requiring corneal transplantation. A case report to the Registry showed irreversible corneal damage with vascularization when 1·1000 benzalkonium was inadvertently placed on both eyes and not irrigated out until 20 minutes later. Benzalkonium may also destroy the corneal epithelial microvilli, and thereby possibly prevent adherence of the mucoid layer of the tear film to the cornea. This drug allows for an increased penetration of some drugs through the corneal epithelium and is added to some commercial ophthalmic preparations for this reason. Topical epithelial cell sensitization to benzalkonium chloride has been postulated to cause increased fibrosis and inflammation, decreasing the success of glaucoma filtration procedures. Benzalkonium binds to soft and hard contact lenses, and the use of this preservative may cause increased epithelial breakdown. This agent is clearly toxic to the corneal endothelium and even in the small amounts used in ophthalmic solutions may cause problems in denuded corneas that receive multiple topical ocular applications daily. Benzalkonium used in solutions introduced within the eye are equally damaging to the corneal endothelium.

References:

Baudouin, C., et al.: Expression of inflammatory membrane markers by conjunctival cells in chronically treated patients with glaucoma. Ophthalmology *101(3)*: 454–460, 1994.

Bernal, D.L., and Ubels, J.L.: Quantitative evaluation of the corneal epithelial barrier: effect of artificial tears and preservatives. Curr. Eye Res. *10*:645–656, 1991.

Burstein, N.L.: Corneal cytotoxicity of topically applied drugs, vehicles and preservatives. Surv. Ophthalmol. *25*:15, 1980.

Chapman, J.M., Cheeks, L., and Green, K.: Interactions of benzalkonium chloride with soft and hard contact lenses. Arch Ophthalmol. *108*:244–246, 1990.

Dormans, J.A.M.A., and van Logten, M.J.: The effects of ophthalmic preservatives on corneal epithelium of the rabbit: A scanning electron microscopical study. Toxicol. Appl. Pharmacol. *62*:251, 1982.

Keller, N., et al.: Increased corneal permeability induced by the dual effects of transient tear film acidification and exposure to benzalkonium chloride. Exp. Eye Res. *30*: 203, 1980.

Kilp, H., et al.: Acute and chronic influence of benzalkonium chloride as a preservative. *In* Homburger, F. (Ed.): Concepts in Toxicology. Basel, Karger, Vol. 4, 1987, pp. 59–63.

Lavine, J.B., Binder, P.S., and Wickham, M.G.: Antimicrobials and the corneal endothelium. Ann. Ophthalmol. *11*:1517, 1979.

Lens solution preservatives may be incompatible with new lenses. Ophthalmol. Times *10*:80,1985.

Maudgal, P.C., Cornelis, H., and Missotten, L.: Effects of commercial ophthalmic drugs on rabbit corneal epithelium. A scanning electron-microscopic study. Graefes Arch. Clin. Exp. Ophthalmol. *216*:191, 1981.

Means, T.L., et al.: Corneal edema from an intraocular irrigating solution containing benzalkonium chloride. J. Toxicol. Cut. Ocular Toxicol. *13(1)*:67–81, 1994.

Samples, J.R., Binder, P.S., and Nayak, S.: The effect of epinephrine and benzalkonium chloride on cultured corneal endothelial and trabecular meshwork cells. Exp. Eye Res. *49*:1–12, 1989

Generic Name: Chlorhexidine

Proprietary Name: *Topical*: Acriflex (G.B.), Anti-Plaque Chewing Gum (Austral.), Aseptil Liquido (Ital.), Bacticlens (G.B.), Bactigras (Austral., Canad., G.B., Germ., S. Afr.), Baxedin (Canad.), Bush Formula (Austral.), Cefasept (Neth.), Cepton (G.B.), Cetal Aerosol (Austral.), Chlorasept (G.B.), Chlorhexamed (Germ.), Chlorhex-a-myl (Fr.), Chlorohex (Austral., Switz.), Chlorohex-U (Switz.), Clorhexitulle (Austral., G.B.), Corsodyl (G.B., Germ., Ire., Ital., Switz.), Cristalmina (Span.), CX Powder (G.B.), Cyteal (Ital.), Dentohexine (Switz.), Deratin (Span.), Descutan (Swed.), Effetre (Ital.), Ekuba (Ital.), Elgydium (G.B., Span.), Eurosan-Antisettico Battericida (Ital.), **Exidine Skin**, Frubilurgyl (Germ.), Hansamed (Germ.), Hexophene (Austral.), **Hibiclens** (Austral., Germ.), Hibident (Fr., Neth., S. Afr.), Hibidil (Canad., Fr., Ire., Ital., S. Afr.), Hibigel (Neth.), Hibiscrub (Fr., G.B., Ire., Ital., Neth., S. Afr., Span., Swed., Switz.), Hibisprint (Fr.), **Hibistat**, Hibitane (Austral., Canad., Fr., G.B., Ire., Ital., Neth., S. Afr., Span., Swed., Switz.), Lemocin (Germ.), Lenixil (Ital.), **Luroscrub**, Neoxene (Ital.), Odontoxina (Ital.), Orosept (S. Afr.), Percyl (Ital.), **Peridex**, pHiso-MED (G.B.), Plak Out (Ital.), Plurexid (Fr.), Rhino-Blache (Fr.), Rimargen (Ital.), Rotersept (G.B., Germ.), Rouhex-G (Canad.), Savacol Mouth and Throat Rinse (Austral.), Savacol Throat Lozenges (Austral.), Savlon Medicated Powder (Austral.), Septeal (Fr.), Serotulle (G.B.), Spotoway (G.B.), Sterexidine (G.B.), Sterilon (Neth.), Uniscrub (G.B.), Unisept

(G.B.), Urgospray (Fr.), Uriflex C (G.B.), Urogliss-S (Neth.) *Ophthalmic*: Chlorhexidine is an ingredient in: **Bausch & Lomb Disinfectant Solution, Flex-Care, Soft Mate**

Primary Use: *Topical*: This disinfectant is used as an antiseptic wound and general skin cleanser for preoperative preparation of the patient, as a surgical scrub, and as a handwash for health-care personnel. *Ophthalmic*: Chlorhexidine is a topical antiseptic and surfactant commonly used in contact lens solutions.

Ocular Side Effects:
 A. Inadvertent Ocular Exposure
    1. Cornea
       a. Punctate keratitis
       b. Edema (including bullous)
       c. Opacification (all layers)
       d. Vascularization (all layers)
       e. Decreased endothelial counts
    2. Conjunctiva
       a. Hyperemia
       b. Lacrimation
       c. Photophobia
       d. Ocular pain
       e. Burning sensation
    3. Decreased tolerance to contact lenses

Clinical Significance: Serious and permanent eye injury may occur during inadvertent ocular exposure mainly from preoperative scrub of the head with accidental ocular exposure. Most severe injuries in the Registry's experience are in cases of head surgeries where this agent was used as a disinfectant on a patient under general anesthesia. Usually the head is turned and gravity allows the chemical to enter the dependent eye. The head drape covered this area; therefore, a significant delay occurred before recognition of the problem and ocular irrigation. Almost total destruction of the corneal endothelium can occur, with only variable success gained from corneal grafting. In general, with immediate irrigation, only superficial punctate keratitis, mild corneal edema with a conjunctivitis lasting 7 to 10 days occurs. The role of the detergent with this chemical is unclear; however, it has been suggested that this enhances the penetration of chlorhexidine, allowing for greater stromal concentration and possible toxicity to the corneal endothelium. Although concentrations of 0.002% to 0.005% chlorhexidine used as a chemical disinfectant of soft contact lenses may present problems of toxic irritation, adverse ocular reactions with proper use of this agent are rare. Transitory corneal edema and a ''chlorhexidine conjunctivitis'' can occur.

References:

Apt L., Isenberg S.J.: Hibiclens keratitis. Am. J. Ophthalmol. *104*:670, 1987.

Hamed, L.M., et al.: Hibiclens keratitis. Am. J. Ophthalmol. *104*:50, 1987.

Khurana, A.K., Ahluwalie, B.K., and Sood S.: Savlon keratopathy, a clinical profile. Acta. Ophthalmol. *67*:465–466, 1989.

MacRae, S.M., Brown, B., and Edelhauser, H.F.: The corneal toxicity of presurgical skin antiseptics. Am. J. Ophthalmol. *97*:221, 1984.

Morgan, J.F.: Complications associated with contact lens solutions. Ophthalmology *86*:1107, 1979.

Paugh, J.R., Caywood, T.G., and Peterson, S.D.: Toxic reactions associated with chemical disinfection of soft contact lenses. Int. Contact Lens Clin. *11*:680, 1984.

Rich, L.F.: Toxic drug effects on the cornea. J. Toxicol. Cut. Ocular Toxicol. *1*:267, 1982–1983.

Tabor, E., Bostwick, D.C., and Evans, C.C.: Corneal damage due to eye contact with chlorhexidine gluconate. JAMA *261*:557–558, 1989

Generic Name: 1. Mercuric Oxide (Hydrargyric Oxide Flavum); 2. Nitromersol; 3. Phenylmercuric Acetate; 4. Phenylmercuric Nitrate (Phenylhydrargyric Nitrate); 5. Thimerosal

Proprietary Name: 1. Golden Eye Ointment (Austral.), Pomada Mercurial (Span.); 2. Metaphen (Austral.); 3. Aderman (Germ.), Merfen-Orange N (Germ.); 4. Hemofibrine Spugna (Ital.); 5. **Aeroaid,** Merseptyl (Fr.), Merthiolate (Ital., S. Afr., Span.), Topicaldermo (Span.), Vitaseptol (Fr.)

Primary Use: These topical ocular organomercurials are used as antiseptics, preservatives, and antibacterial or antifungal agents in ophthalmic solutions and ointments.

Ocular Side Effects:

    A. Local Ophthalmic Use or Exposure

        1. Irritation

           a. Lacrimation

           b. Hyperemia

           c. Photophobia

           d. Ocular pain

           e. Burning sensation

        2. Eyelids or conjunctiva

           a. Allergic reactions

           b. Hyperemia

           c. Erythema

           d. Blepharitis

           e. Conjunctivitis—follicular

           f. Edema

           g. Urticaria

           h. Eczema

3. Bluish-gray mercury deposits (mercuric oxide, phenylmercuric nitrate, thimerosal)
   a. Eyelids
   b. Conjunctiva
   c. Cornea
   d. Lens
4. Cornea (thimerosal)
   a. Punctate keratitis
   b. Opacities
   c. Edema
   d. Subepithelial infiltrates
   e. Vascularization
   f. Band keratopathy (mercuric oxide, phenylmercuric nitrate, thimerosal)
   g. Hypersensitivity reactions
5. Decreased tolerance to contact lenses (thimerosal)

Clinical Significance: Adverse ocular side effects due to these organomercurials are rare and seldom of significance. The most striking side effect is mercurial deposits in various ocular and periocular tissues. This is an apparently harmless side effect because it is asymptomatic and no visual impairments due to it have been found. Conjunctival mercurial deposits are seen around blood vessels near the cornea, corneal deposits are in the peripheral Descemet's membrane, and lens deposits are mainly in the pupillary area. No deposits have been reported in any ocular tissue with the topical ocular use of thimerosal. Thimerosal is now a commonly used preservative in many ophthalmic contact lens solutions. Mercurialentis has not been seen with thimerosal at concentrations of 0.005%, the concentration used as a preservative in some ophthalmic solutions. There are a surprisingly large number of people allergic to thimerosal. In a Japanese series, up to 50% of eye patients became hypersensitive, while in the United States this rate was about 10%. To evaluate this agent as a factor for ocular intolerance, thimerosal skin testing can be performed. Soft contact lenses cleaned and stored in thimerosal-containing solution may produce an ocular inflammation process similar to superior limbic keratoconjunctivitis. The corneal changes are transient and range from faint epithelial opacities to a coarse, punctate epithelial keratopathy.

References:

Binder, P.S,, Rasmussen, D.M., and Gordon, M.: Keratoconjunctivitis and soft contact lens solutions. Arch. Ophthalmol. 99:87, 1981.

Brazier, D.J., and Hitchings, R.A.: Atypical band keratopathy following long-term pilocarpine treatment. Br. J. Ophthal. 73:294–296, 1989.

de la Cuadra, J., Pujol, C., and Aliagia, A.: Clinical evidence of cross-sensitivity between thiosalicylic acid, a contact allergen, and piroxicam, a photoallergen. Cont. Dermatol. 21:349–351, 1989.

Gero, G.: Superficial punctate keratitis with CSI contact lenses dispensed with the Allergan Hydrocare cold kit. Int. Contact Lens Clin. *11*:674, 1984.

Mondino, B.J., Salamon, S.M. and Zaidman, G.W.: Allergic and toxic reactions in soft contact lens wearers. Surv. Ophthalmol. *26*:337, 1982.

Rietschel, R.L., and Wilson, L.A.: Ocular inflammation in patients using soft contact lenses. Arch. Dermtol. *118*:147, 1982.

Wilson, L.A., McNatt, J., and Reitschel, R.: Delayed hypersensitivity to thimerosal in soft contact lens wearers. Ophthalmology *88*:804, 1981.

Wilsonholt, N., and Dart, J.K.G.: Thiomersal keratoconjunctivitis, frequency, clinical spectrum and diagnosis. Eye *3*:581–587, 1989.

Wright, P., and Mackie, I.: Preservative-related problems in soft contact lens wearers. Trans. Ophthalmol. Soc. UK *102*:3, 1982.

Class: Proteolytic Enzymes

Generic Name: Urokinase

Proprietary Name: Abbokinase (Canad., Germ., Span., Swed.), Actosolv (Fr., Germ.), Alphakinase (Germ.), Kisolv (Ital.), Natel (Span.), Persolv Richter (Ital.), Purochin (Ital.), Ukidan (Austral., G.B., Germ., Ital., Neth., Swed., Switz.), Uroquidan (Span.), Uroquinasa (Span.)

Primary Use: This proteolytic enzyme is injected into the anterior chamber or vitreous to possibly aid in the removal of blood.

Ocular Side Effects:
  A. Ophthalmic—Intravitreal
     1. Hypopyon
     2. Uveitis
     3. Intraocular pressure
        a. Increased
        b. Decreased
     4. Abnormal ERG
     5. Cornea
        a. Edema
        b. Fold in Descemet's membrane

Clinical Significance: After intravitreal injections of urokinase, as high as a 50% incidence of sterile hypopyon has occurred. This is thought to be cellular debris in the anterior chamber that usually absorbs within 5 days. Uveitis is usually mild, although severe cases have been reported. A transient decrease in the b-wave of the ERG, corneal edema, and folds in Descemet's membrane have been reported following intravitreal injection of urokinase for treatment of vitreous hemorrhage. In addition, one patient developed a discrete posterior subcapsular opacity 2 months after the third injection of 15,000 units of urokinase. Fourteen months after urokinase treatment, the posterior lens capsule ruptured.

References:

Berman, M., et al.: Plasminogen activator (urokinase) causes vascularization of the cornea. Invest. Ophthalmol. Vis. Sci. *22*:191, 1982.

Bramsen, T.: The effect of urokinase on central corneal thickness and vitreous hemorrhage. Acta Ophthalmol. *56*:1006, 1978.

Higuchi, M., and Hinokuma, R.: The effect of intravitreal injection of urokinase on longstanding vitreous hemorrhage. Folia Ophthalmol. Jpn. *32*:316, 1981.

Hull, D.S., and Green, K.: Effect of urokinase on corneal endothelium. Arch. Ophthalmol. *98*:1285, 1980.

Koch, H.R.: Experimental approaches to elucidate clinical cataract problems. *In* Regnault, F.: Symposium on the Lens. Amsterdam, Elsevier, 1981, pp. 5–12.

Textorius, O., and Stenkula, S.: Toxic ocular effects of two fibrinolytic drugs. An experimental electroretinographic study on albino rabbits. Acta Ophthalmol. *61*: 322, 1983.

Class: Topical Local Anesthetics

Generic Name: 1. Benoxinate; 2. Butacaine; 3. Dibucaine (Cinchocaine); 4. Dyclonine; 5. Phenacaine; 6. Piperocaine; 7. Proparacaine (Proxymetacaine); 8. Tetracaine

Proprietary Name: *Ophthalmic*: 1. Benoxinato (Span.), Cébésine (Fr.), Conjuncain (Germ.), Novesin (Canad., S. Afr., Switz.), Novesina (Ital.), Novésine (Fr., Switz.), Novesine (Germ., Neth.), Prescaina (Span.), Vesiform S (Germ.); 7. **Ak-Taine** (Canad.), **Alcaine** (Austral., Canad., Switz.), Chibro-Kerakain (Germ.), **Kainair, Ocu-caine**, Ophthaine (Austral., Canad., G.B., Ire.), **Ophthetic** (Austral., Canad., Germ., S. Afr.), Proparakain-POS (Germ.); 8. Anethaine (G.B., S. Afr.), Covostet (S. Afr.), Lubricante Urol (Span.), Pontocaine (Canad.) *Topical*: **Cincain**, Nupercainal (Switz.), **Nupercainal** (Canad., G.B.); 4. **Dyclone**

Primary Use: *Ophthalmic*: These topical local anesthetics are used in diagnostic and surgical procedures.

Ocular Side Effects:

    A. Local Ophthalmic Use or Exposure
        1. Corneal epithelium
            a. Punctate keratitis
            b. Gray, ground glass appearance
            c. Edema
            d. Softening, erosions, and sloughing
            e. Filaments
            f. Ulceration

2. Corneal stroma
   a. Yellow-white opacities
   b. Vascularization
   c. Scarring
   d. Ulceration
   e. Crystalline keratopathy
   f. Perforation
   g. Increased incidences of Acanthamoeba
3. Corneal endothelium
   a. Loss of cells
   b. Variation in cell size
4. Uveitis
   a. Plastic
   b. Fibrinous
   c. Hypopyon
5. Irritation
   a. Lacrimation
   b. Hyperemia
   c. Ocular pain
   d. Burning sensation
6. Delayed wound healing
7. Eyelids or conjunctiva
   a. Allergic reactions
   b. Blepharoconjunctivitis
   c. Stevens-Johnson syndrome (proparacaine)
8. Decreased stability of corneal tear film
9. Subconjunctival hemorrhages
10. Decreased blink reflex
11. Inhibits fluorescence of fluorescein
12. Decreased vision

Systemic Side Effects:
   A. Local Ophthalmic Use or Exposure
      1. Nervousness
      2. Tremors
      3. Convulsion
      4. Bradycardia
      5. Asthma
      6. Apnea

Clinical Significance: Few significant ocular side effects are seen with these agents if they are given topically for short periods; however, prolonged use will inevitably cause severe and permanent corneal damage, including visual loss. Local anesthetics inhibit the rate of corneal epithelial cell migration by disruption of cytoplasmic action in filaments and destruction of superficial corneal epithelial microvilli. This allows for permanent epithelial defects and disruption of the corneal tear film with continued drug use. Chronic use of local anesthetics causes denuding of corneal epithelium, which may cause dense yellow-white rings in the corneal stroma. This may occur as early as the sixth or as late as the sixtieth day after initial use. The ring resembles a Wessely ring and often resolves once the local anesthetic is discontinued. Secondary infection is common, and an increase in the frequency of Acanthamoeba may be seen. Infectious crystalline keratopathy has been reported due to topical local anesthetic abuse (Kintner, et al.). With time, from one-third to two-thirds of the endothelial loss may occur. Various degrees of uveitis have been reported, including plastic and fibrinous forms. An excellent review of this subject, including cases of ocular perforation requiring enucleation, has been reported by Rosenwasser, et al. Numerous systemic reactions from topical ocular applications of local anesthetics have been reported. Many of these occur, in part, from the fear of the impending procedure or possibly an oculocardiac reflex. Side effects include syncope, convulsions, and anaphylactic shock.

References:

Burns, R.P., and Gipson, I: Toxic effects of local anesthetics. JAMA *240*:347, 1978.

Duffin, R.M., and Olson, R.J.: Tetracaine toxicity. Ann. Ophthamol. *16*:836, 1984.

Fraunfelder, F.T., Sharp, J.D., and Silver, B.E.: Possible adverse effects from topical ocular anesthetics. Doc. Ophthalmol. *18*:341, 1979.

Gild, W.M., et al.: Eye injuries associated with anesthesia. Anesthesiology 76:204-208, 1992.

Grant, W.M., and Schuman, J.S.: Toxicology of the Eye. 4th Ed., Springfield, Ill., Charles C. Thomas, 1993, pp. 144-157.

Haddad, R.: Fibrinous iritis due to oxybuprocaine. Br. J. Ophthalmol. *73*:76-77, 1989.

Kintner, J.C., et al.: Infectious crystalline keratopathy associated with topical anesthetic abuse. Cornea *9(1)*:77-80, 1990.

Lemagne, J.-M., et al.: Purtscher-like retinopathy after retrobulbar anesthesia. Ophthalmology *97(7)*:859-861, 1990.

Rosenwasser, G.O.D., et al.: Topical anesthetic abuse. Ophthalmology *97(8)*:967-972, 1990

Generic Name: Cocaine

Proprietary Name: None

Street Name: *Nasal, Oral*: Base, Bernice, Bernies, Blow, C, Coke, Crack, Flake, Freebase, Girl, Gold Dust, Happy Dust, Heaven Dust, Pearl, Rock, Snow, Toot

Primary Use: *Injection*: Intravenous cocaine may be used by drug abusers. *Nasal, Oral*: Cocaine is a potent CNS stimulant that is commonly available on the illicit drug market. *Ophthalmic*: This topical local anesthetic is used in diagnostic and surgical procedures.

Ocular Side Effects:
A. Systemic Administration—Nasal or Oral
1. Decreased vision
2. Visual hallucinations
3. Photosensitivity
4. Pupils
    a. Mydriasis
    b. Absence of reaction to light—toxic states
5. Paralysis of accommodation
6. Exophthalmos
7. Secondary optic nerve involvement (sinusitis)
    a. Optic neuritis
    b. Optic atrophy
8. Madarosis
9. Iritis

B. Local Ophthalmic Use or Exposure
1. Corneal epithelium
    a. Punctate keratitis
    b. Gray, ground glass appearance
    c. Edema
    d. Softening, erosions, and sloughing
    e. Filaments
    f. Ulceration
2. Corneal stroma
    a. Yellow-white opacities
    b. Vascularization
    c. Scarring
3. Iritis
4. Irritation
    a. Lacrimation
    b. Hyperemia
    c. Ocular pain
    d. Burning sensation
5. Delayed corneal wound healing
6. Eyelids or conjunctiva
    a. Allergic reactions
    b. Blepharoconjunctivitis
    c. Widening of palpebral aperture
7. Decreased stability of corneal tear film
8. Subconjunctival hemorrhages
9. Decreased blink reflex
10. Hypopyon

11. Inhibits bacterial growth
12. Inhibits fluorescence of fluorescein
13. Decreased vision
14. Conjunctival vasoconstriction
15. Mydriasis—may precipitate narrow-angle glaucoma
16. Paralysis of accommodation
17. Visual hallucinations—especially Lilliputian

Systemic Side Effects:
  A. Local Ophthalmic Use or Exposure
    1. Nervousness
    2. Tremors
    3. Convulsion
    4. Bradycardia
    5. Asthma
    6. Apnea

Clinical Significance: There has been a marked increase in the illicit use of cocaine with new and more potent drugs available. One of the most common methods of using this drug systemically is by applying it to the nasal mucosa. There has been a large number of cases of optic neuropathies associated with chronic sinusitis and orbital inflammation secondary to chronic co-caine-induced nasal pathology. This has included optic neuritis, optic atrophy, and blindness. Intracranial hemorrhages have occurred secondary to cocaine use, including bilateral and unilateral intranuclear ophthalmoplegia secondary to micro-infarcts in the medial longitudinal vesiculous. Vascular strokes with secondary visual field changes and various infarcts have caused extraocular muscle dysfunction. Mydriasis can occur, and there have been reports of precipitation of narrow-angle glaucoma. The question of ocular teratogenic effects secondary to cocaine administration is not clear. Dominguez, et al. reported that nine infants had ophthalmic abnormalities, including strabismus, nystagmus, and hypoplastic optic discs. Good, et al. reported 13 cocaine-exposed infants who had optic nerve abnormalities, delayed visual maturation, and prolonged eyelid edema. There have also been reports of abnormal visual evoked potentials in 11 of 12 neonates with cocaine present in their urine. Stafford, et al., however, showed no significant effects of prenatal cocaine exposure on the infant eye, with axial lengths agreeing to the statistical norm, along with other parameters that were normal for fetal growth. It is apparent, however, that many of the infants who have cocaine in their urine at birth may show increased congestion, engorgements, and bleeding of their retinal and iris vessels. Another form of cocaine use is crack cocaine, in which the fumes from the cocaine cause significant ocular irritation, dryness, and loss of eyebrows. It has become advisable to consider crack cocaine on the differential diagnosis if a young patient comes in with corneal ulcers or epithelial defects and no related medical or traumatic cause. Various bacterial and fungal organisms have been identified in these ulcers. McHenry, et al., have reported central retinal artery occlusions, unilateral mydriasis, cranial nerve palsies, and optic neuropathies with crack cocaine use. They also believe that crack cocaine babies have an increased incidence of strabismus and nystagmus. Topical ocular cocaine can cause all the side effects that one sees from the topical abuse of local anesthetics. It differs, however, from other local anesthetics in that it causes conjunctival vasoconstriction, may cause mydriasis precipitating narrow-angle glaucoma, and may affect accommodation. In rare patients, visual hallucinations, especially Lilliputian, may occur. A potential problem is that a detectable level of cocaine may be present in the urine for 72 hours after the application of topical ocular cocaine use by ophthalmologists, either to denude the cornea or as a local anesthetic.

References:

Cruz, O.A., et al.: Urine drug screening for cocaine after lacrimal surgery. Am. J. Ophthalmol. *111*:703–705, 1991.

Dominguez, A.A., et al.: Brain and ocular abnormalities in infants with in utero exposure to cocaine and other street drugs. Am. J. Dis. Child. *145*:688–695, 1991.

Goldberg, R.A., et al.: Orbital inflammation and optic neuropathies associated with chronic sinusitis of intranasal cocaine abuse. Arch. Ophthalmol. *107*:831–835, 1989.

Good, W.V., et al.: Abnormalities of the visual system in infants exposed to cocaine. Ophthalmology *99(3)*:341–346, 1992.

McHenry, J.G., et al.: Ophthalmic complications of crack cocaine (letter). Ophthalmology *100(12)*:1747, 1993.

Munden, P.M., et al.: Palpebral fissure responses to topical adrenergic drugs. Am. J. Ophthalmol. *111*:706–710, 1991.

Perinatal toxicity of cocaine. Medical Newsletter. *30*:59–60, June 1988.

Sachs, R., Zagelbaum, B.M., and Hersh, P.S.: Corneal complications associated with the use of crack cocaine. Ophthalmology *100(2)*:187–191, 1993.

Stafford, J.R., Jr., et al.: Prenatal cocaine exposure and the development of the human eye. Ophthalmology *101(2)*:301–308, 1994.

Strominger, M.B., Sachs, R., and Hersh, P.S.: Microbial keratitis with crack cocaine. Arch. Ophthalmol. *108*:1672, 1990.

Tames, S.M., and Goldenring, J.M.: Madarosis from cocaine use. N. Engl. J. Med. May 15:1324, 1986.

Zagelbaum, B.M., Tannenbaum, M.H., and Hersh, P.S.: *Candida albicans* corneal ulcer associated with crack cocaine. Am. J. Ophthalmol. *111(2)*:248–249, 1991.

Zeiter, J.H., et al.: Sudden retinal manifestations of intranasal cocaine and methamphetamine abuse (letter). Am. J. Ophthalmol. *114*:780–781, 1992.

Zeiter, J.H., McHenry, J.G., and McDermott, M.L.: Unilateral pharmacologic mydriasis secondary to crack cocaine (letter). Am. J. Emerg. Med. *8*:568, 1990.

Class: Topical Ocular, Nonsteroidal Anti-inflammatory Drugs

Generic Name: 1. Diclofenac; 2. Ketorolac Tromethamine

Proprietary Name: 1. Allvoran (Germ.), Anfenax (S. Afr.), Apo-Diclo (Canad.), Arcanafenac (S. Afr.), Benfofen (Germ.), Cataflam (Neth.), Delphinac (Germ.), Diclac (Germ.), diclo-basan (Switz.), Diclo-OPT (Germ.), Diclophlogont (Germ.), Diclo-Puren (Germ.), Diclo-rektal (Germ.), Dicloreum (Ital.), Diclo-Spondyril (Germ.), Diclo-Tablinen (Germ.), Diclo-Wolff (Germ.), Diclozip (G.B.), Difenac (S. Afr.), Dignofenac (Germ.), dolobasan (Germ.), Dolotren (Span.), DoloVisano Diclo (Germ.), duravolten (Germ.), Ecofénac (Switz.), Effekton (Germ.), Flector (Switz.), Flogofenac (Ital.), Forgenac (Ital.), Inflamac (Switz.), Liberalgium (Span.), Monoflam (Germ.), Myogit (Germ.), Naclof (S. Afr.), Novapirina (Ital.), Novodifenac (Canad.), Olfen (Switz.), Panamor (S. Afr.), Primofénac (Switz.), Rheumasan D (Germ.), Rhumalgan (G.B.), Silino (Germ.), Toryxil (Germ.), Valenac (G.B.), Veltex (S. Afr.), Voldal (Fr.), Volraman (G.B.), **Voltaren** (Austral., Canad., Germ., Ital., Neth., S. Afr., Span., Swed.), Voltaren Emulgel (Germ., S. Afr.), Voltaren Ophtha (Switz.), Voltaren T (Swed.), Voltarène (Fr., Switz.), Voltarène Emulgel (Fr., Switz.), Voltarène Rapide (Switz.), Voltarol (G.B., Ire.), Voltarol Emulgel (G.B., Ire.), Xenid (Fr.); 2. **Toradol** (G.B., Swed.)

Primary Use: These topical ocular nonsteroidal anti-inflammatory agents are used in the management of postoperative inflammation, after cataract surgery (diclofenac), and for relief of ocular itching due to seasonal allergies (ketorolac tromethamine).

Ocular Side Effects:
   A. Topical Ocular
      1. Irritation
         a. Burning
         b. Stinging
      2. Keratitis—superficial punctate
      3. Conjunctivitis
      4. Corneal anesthesia
      5. Inhibits surgically induced miosis (diclofenac)
      6. Delayed corneal epithelial wound healing
      7. Potentiates ocular bleeding
      8. Post-surgical atonic mydriasis (diclofenac)

Clinical Significance: These nonsteroidal anti-inflammatory agents cause surprisingly few serious topical ocular side effects. The most common ocular side effect is transitory irritation, which may be present in up to 40% of patients. This is seldom an indication for not using the drug. Szerenyi, et al. have documented that diclofenac can cause a significant decrease in corneal sensitivity. Superficial keratitis can be found with both drugs; however, this resolves once the drug is discontinued. Neither of these agents has been shown to cause elevation in intraocular pressure, nor is there data to show that either delays stromal wound healing. Both have cross sensitivity with other nonsteroidal anti-inflammatory agents, including acetylsalicylic acid, and have the potential to increase bleeding time. This is especially true if they are used in conjunction with other systemic drugs that cause this side effect as well. It is believed that this is probably due to inhibition of platelet aggregation. Because of this, in some people's opinion, there may well be a higher incidence of postoperative hyphemas if these drugs are used. Nonsteroidal anti-inflammatory agents, in general, have not been shown to enhance viral infections, such as herpes simplex, in animal models. Diclofenac has significant analgesic activity, reduces the occurrences and severity of cystoid macular edema, and may release surgically induced miosis.

References:
Buckley, M.M.T., and Brogden, R.N.: Ketorolac: A review of its pharmacodynamic and pharmacokinetic properties, and therapeutic potential. Drugs *39*:86–109, 1990.

Buckley, D.C., Caldwell, D.R., and Reaves, T.A., Jr.: Treatment of vernal conjunctivitis with suprofen, a topical nonsteroidal anti-inflammatory agent. Invest. Ophthalmol. Vis. Sci. *27*:29, 1986.

Eiferman, R.A., Hoffman, R.S., and Sher, N.A.: Topical diclofenac reduces pain following photorefractive keratectomy. Arch. Ophthalmol. *111*:1022, 1993.

Jampol, L.M., et al.: Nonsteroidal anti-inflammatory drugs and cataract surgery. Arch. Ophthalmol. *112*:891–893, 1994.

Flach, A.J.: Cyclo-oxygenase inhibitors in ophthalmology. Surv. Ophthalmol. *36*: 259–285, 1992.

Flach, A.J., et al.: Quantitative assessment of postsurgical breakdown of the blood-aqueous barrier following administration of 0.5% ketorolac tromethamine solution. Arch. Ophthalmol. *106*:344–347, 1988.

Hersh, P.S., et al.: Topical nonsteroidal agents and corneal wound healing. Arch. Ophthalmol. *108*:577–583, 1990.

Kraff, M.C., et al.: Inhibition of blood-aqueous humor barrier breakdown with diclofenac. Arch. Ophthalmol. *108*:380–383, 1990.

Noonan, W.D., and Samples, J.R.: New drugs in ophthalmology—Diclofenac sodium. J. Toxicol. Cut. Ocular Toxicol. *12(4)*:265–272, 1993.

Strelow, S.A., Sherwood, M.B., Broncata, L.J., et al.: The effect of diclofenac sodium ophthalmic solution on intraocular pressure following cataract extraction. Ophthalmic Surg. *23*:170–175, 1992.

Szerenyi, K., et al.: Decrease in normal human corneal sensitivity with topical diclofenac sodium. Am. J. Ophthalmol. *118(3)*:312–315, 1994.

Class: Topical Osmotic Agents

Generic Name: Sodium Chloride

Proprietary Name: Adsorbonac (Germ., Ital.), Amuchina (Switz.), Biosteril (Germ.), Cordema (Canad.), Larmes Artificielles (Fr.), Lisal (Swed.), Muro-128 (Canad.), Naaprep (Switz.), **NaSal**, Normasol (G.B.), Physiologica Gifrer (Switz.), Salinex (Canad.), Sérophy (Fr.), Slow-Sodium (G.B., Ire.), Sterac (G.B.), Topiclens (G.B.), Tresal (Swed.), Uriflex S (G.B.), Uro-Pract

N (Germ.), Uro-Tainer M (G.B.), Vésirig (Fr.) Sodium Chloride is also used as an ingredient in Darrow's Solution.

Primary Use: This topical ocular hypertonic salt solution is used to reduce corneal edema.

Ocular Side Effects:
  A. Local Ophthalmic Use or Exposure—Topical Application
    1. Irritation
      a. Hyperemia
      b. Ocular pain
      c. Burning sensation
    2. Corneal dehydration
    3. Subconjunctival hemorrhages
  B. Local Ophthalmic Use or Exposure—Subconjunctival Injection
    1. Conjunctival hyperemia
    2. Increased intraocular pressure

Clinical Significance: Few significant adverse ocular reactions are seen with commercial topical sodium chloride solutions. The most frequent ocular side effects are irritation and discomfort, which are primarily related to the frequency of application. At suggested dosages, all ocular side effects are reversible and transient. Kushner reported that nose bleeds may occur after use of topical ocular hypertonic salt solutions or ointment; two cases in the Registry support this. This is not unexpected because subconjunctival hemorrhages are seen as well. Numerous patients experience ocular irritation and keratitis induced by preserved saline solution used in soft contact lens wear; however, the symptoms are usually alleviated with the use of preservative-free saline.

References:
Kushner, F.H.: Sodium chloride eye drops as a cause of epistaxis. Arch. Ophthalmol. *105*:1643, 1987.
Shapiro, A., et al.: The effect of salt loading diet on the intraocular pressure. Acta Ophthalmol. *60*:35, 1982.
Shaw, E.L.: Allergies induced by contact lens solution. Contact Lens *6*:273, 1980.
Spizziri, L.J .: Stromal corneal changes due to preserved saline solution used in soft contact lens wear: Report of a case. Ann. Ophthalmol. *13*:1277, 1981.

Class: Viscoelastics

Generic Name: 1. Sodium Hyaluronate; 2. Hyaluronic Acid; 3. Chondroitin Sulfate; 4. Hydroxypropyl Methylcellulose

Proprietary Name: 1. Amvisc (Canad., Swed.), Connettivina (Ital.), Healon (Austral., Canad., Germ., Ital., Neth., S. Afr., Swed.), Hyalgan (Ital.), Ial

(Ital.), Ialugen (Switz.), Jossalind (Germ.), Pandermin Cicatrizante (Span.)
Vitrax; 2. None; 3. None; 4. BJ6 (G.B.), Hymecel (Canad.), Isopto Alkaline
(G.B.), Isopto Fluid (Germ.), Isopto Plain (G.B., S. Afr., Swed.), Isopto
Tears (Austral., Canad., Switz.), Lacril (Austral., Canad.), Lacrimill (Ital.),
Lacrisifi (Ital.), M C (Canad.), Methocel (Canad., Germ., S. Afr.), Methopt
(Austral.), Spersatear (S. Afr.), Ultra-Tears (Switz.), Viscotraan (S. Afr.)

Primary Use: Viscoelastic material in ophthalmic surgery.

Ocular Side Effects:
  A. Systemic Administration
     1. Elevated intraocular pressure
     2. Uveitis—transient
     3. Opacities (corneal injection)
     4. Crystalline deposition on intraocular lenses (high molecular
        weight sodium hyaluronate)

Clinical Significance: Improvements have been made in the manufacture of
  viscoelastics since the 1970s, so that many of the initial adverse events,
  such as uveitis or precipitation of calcium salts due to excessive phosphate
  in the buffer, have now been eliminated. The sodium salt of hyaluronic acid
  is sodium hyaluronate, which is one of the more commonly used viscoelastics. All of the viscoelastics can cause transitory elevations in pressure,
  usually peaking between 6 and 12 hours and returning to normal within 24
  hours. This pressure elevation seems to be more acute and lasting in patients
  with glaucoma. There is some evidence that lower molecular weight viscoelastics do not produce as great a pressure elevation as those with higher
  molecular weights. Since postoperative uveitis is common, it is difficult
  to determine a true incidence of inflammation attributed to these agents.
  Regardless, this was more of a problem initially than it is currently. Studies
  by Storr-Paulsen and Larsen show little difference in the severity of iritis
  among the various viscoelastics. In general, these products seldom cause a
  significant inflammatory response. Jensen et al. recently described a series
  of patients with visually significant deposition of a high molecular weight
  sodium hyaluronate (Healon GV®). These deposits may remain up to 6
  months and decrease vision to 20/40 or worse. Isolated cases have been
  reported of corneal opacities occurring after inadvertent corneal injection
  of viscoelastics; however, they seem to absorb and resolve in a matter of
  months. There is little evidence that the viscoelastics bind with drugs to
  significantly inhibit their action in the eye.

References:
Alpar, J.J.: Comparison of healon and amvisc. Ann. Ophthalmol. *17*:647–651, 1985.
Daily, L.: Caution on sodium hyaluronate (Healon) syringe. Am. J. Ophthalmol. *94(4)*:
    559, 1982.

Glasser, D.B., Matsuda, M., and Edelhauser, H.F.: A comparison of the efficacy and toxicity of and intraocular pressure response to viscous solutions in the anterior chamber. Arch. Ophthalmol. *104*:1819–1824, 1986.

Goa, K.L., and Benfield, P.: Hyaluronic acid: A review of its pharmacology and use as a surgical aid in ophthalmology, and its therapeutic potential in joint disease and wound healing. Drugs *47(3)*:536–566, 1994.

Hoover, D.L., Giangiacomo, J., and Benson, R.L.: Descemet's membrane detachment by sodium hyaluronate. Arch. Ophthalmol. *103*:805–808, 1985.

Jensen, M.K., et al.: Crystallization on intraocular lens surfaces associated with the use of Healon GV. Arch. Ophthalmology *112*:1037–1042, 1994.

MacRae, S.M., et al.: The effects of sodium hyaluronate, chondroitin sulfate, and methylcellulose on the corneal endothelium and intraocular pressure. Am. J. Ophthalmol. *95*:332–341, 1983.

McDermott, M.L., and Edelhauser, H.F.: Drug binding of ophthalmic viscoelastic agents. Arch. Ophthalmol. *107*:261–263, 1989.

Pape, L.G., and Balazs, E.A.: The use of sodium hyaluronate (Healon®)in human anterior segment surgery. Ophthalmology *87(7)*:699–705, 1980.

Passo, M.S., Ernest, J.T., and Goldstick, T.K.: Hyaluronate increases intraocular pressure when used in cataract extraction. Br. J. Ophthalmol. *69(8)*:572–575, 1985.

Storr-Paulsen, A.: Analysis of the short-term effect of two viscoelastic agents on the intraocular pressure after extracapsular cataract extraction. Acta Ophthalmologica *71*:173–176, 1993.

Storr-Paulsen, A., and Larsen, M.: Long-term results of extracapsular cataract extraction with posterior chamber lens implantation. Acta Ophthalmologica *69*.766–769, 1991.

Index of Side Effects

*Lists of drugs causing the following side effects appear on page **486** and following pages.*

Abnormal Conjugate Deviations
Abnormal ERG, EOG, VEP or Critical Flicker Fusion
Abnormal Visual Sensations
Absence of Foveal Reflex. See *Decreased or Absent Foveal Reflex*
Absence of Pupillary Reaction to Light. See *Decreased or Absent Pupillary Reaction to Light*
Accommodative Spasm
Anisocoria
Blepharitis. See also *Blepharoconjunctivitis*
Blepharoclonus
Blepharoconjunctivitis. See also *Blepharitis; Conjunctivitis—Follicular; Conjunctivitis—Nonspecific*
Blepharospasm
Cataracts
Colored Haloes around Lights
Color Vision Defect
Conjunctival Deposits. See *Eyelids or Conjunctiva—Deposits*
Conjunctival—Edema. See *Eyelids or Conjunctiva—Edema*
Conjunctival Hyperemia. See also *Ocular Exposure—Irritation and Systemic Administration—Nonspecific Ocular Irritation*
Conjunctivitis. See also *Blepharoconjunctivitis*

Follicular
Nonspecific
Constriction of Visual Fields. See *Visual Field Defects*
Corneal Deposits
Corneal Discoloration
Corneal Edema
Corneal Opacities
Corneal Scarring
Corneal Ulceration
Corneal Vascularization
Cortical Blindness
Decreased Accommodation. See *Decreased or Paralysis of Accommodation*
Decreased Anterior Chamber Depth
Decreased Convergence
Decreased Corneal Reflex
Decreased Dark Adaptation
Decreased Dark Perception
Decreased Foveal Reflex. See *Decreased or Absent Foveal Reflex*
Decreased Intraocular Pressure
Decreased Lacrimation
Decreased or Absent Foveal Reflex
Decreased or Absent Pupillary Reaction to Light
Decreased or Paralysis of Accommodation
Decreased Resistance to Infection
Decreased Spontaneous Eye Movements

484

Abnormal Conjugate Deviations

Alseroxylon
Alprazolam
Amitriptyline
Amoxapine
Carbon Dioxide
Chlordiazepoxide

Clonazepam
Clorazepate
Deserpidine
Desipramine
Diazepam
Flurazepam
Halazepam
Imipramine
Ketamine
Lithium Carbonate
Lorazepam
Midazolam
Nitrazepam
Nortriptyline
Oxazepam
Prazepam
Protriptyline
Rauwolfia Serpentina
Rescinnamine
Reserpine
Syrosingopine
Temazepam
Triazolam

Abnormal ERG, EOG, VEP or Critical Flicker Fusion

Acetophenazine
Acetyldigitoxin
Adrenal Cortex Injection
Alcohol
Aldosterone
Allobarbital
Amobarbital
Amodiaquine
Aprobarbital
Barbital
Beclomethasone
Betamethasone
Butabarbital
Butalbital
Butallylonal
Butaperazine
Butethal
Carphenazine
Chloroquine
Chlorpromazine
Ciprofloxacin
Cisplatin
Clonidine

Cortisone
Cyclobarbital
Cyclopentobarbital
Deferoxamine
Deslanoside
Desoxycorticosterone
Dexamethasone
Diazepam
Diethazine
Digitalis
Digitoxin
Digoxin
Ethambutol
Ethopropazine
Etretinate
Fludrocortisone
Fluphenazine
Fluprednisolone
Gitalin
Glycine
Heptabarbital
Hexethal
Hexobarbital
Hydrocortisone
Hydroxychloroquine
Ibuprofen
Indomethacin
Interferon
Isotretinoin
Lanatoside C
Lidocaine
Lithium Carbonate
LSD
Lysergide
Mephobarbital
Meprednisone
Mescaline
Mesoridazine
Metharbital
Methdilazine
Methitural
Methohexital
Methotrimepazine
Methylprednisolone
Nitrous Oxide
Ouabain
Oxygen
Paramethasone
Pentobarbital

Perazine
Periciazine
Perphenazine
Phenobarbital
Piperacetazine
Prednisolone
Prednisone
Primidone
Probarbital
Prochlorperazine
Promazine
Promethazine
Propiomazine
Psilocybin
Quinine
Secobarbital
Talbutal
Thiamylal
Thiethylperazine
Thiopental
Thiopropazate
Thioproperazine
Thioridazine
Triamcinolone
Trifluoperazine
Triflupromazine
Trimeprazine
Triprolidine
Urokinase
Vinbarbital
Vincristine

Abnormal Visual Sensations

Acetyldigitoxin
Amodiaquine
Aspirin
Bromide
Capreomycin
Chloroquine
Clomiphene
Clonidine
Cycloserine
Deslanoside
Digitalis
Digitoxin
Digoxin
Dronabinol
Gitalin
Guanethidine

Hashish
Hydralazine
Hydroxychloroquine
Ibuprofen
Iophendylate
Lanatoside C
LSD
Lysergide
Marihuana
Mecamylamine
Mescaline
Nalidixic Acid
Ouabain
Paramethadione
Phenytoin
Piperazine
Piperidolate
Propantheline
Psilocybin
Quinine
Sodium Salicylate
Streptomycin
Tetrahydrocannabinol
THC
Thiabendazole
Trimethadione
Tryparsamide

Accommodative Spasm

Aceclidine
Acetylcholine
Carbachol
Demecarium
DFP
Digitalis
Echothiophate
Guanethidine
Isoflurophate
Methylene Blue
Morphine
Neostigmine
Opium
Physostigmine
Pilocarpine

Anisocoria

Alcohol
Antazoline

Bromide
Bromisovalum
Brompheniramine
Bupivacaine
Carbinoxamine
Carbromal
Chloroprocaine
Chlorpheniramine
Clemastine
Contraceptives
Dexbrompheniramine
Dexchlorpheniramine
Diacetylmorphine
Dimethindene
Diphenhydramine
Diphenylpyraline
Doxylamine
Dronabinol
Ethchlorvynol
Etidocaine
Hashish
Isocarboxazid
Lidocaine
LSD
Lysergide
Marihuana
Mepivacaine
Mescaline
Methaqualone
Nialamide
Phenelzine
Pheniramine
Phenylpropanolamine
Prilocaine
Procaine
Propoxycaine
Psilocybin
Pyrilamine
Scopolamine
Tetrahydrocannabinol
THC
Tranylcypromine
Trichloroethylene
Tripelennamine
Tripolidine

Blepharitis

Acyclovir
Benzalkonium

F₃T
Idoxuridine
IDU
Meperidine
Mercuric Oxide
Mitomycin
Nitromersol
Phenylmercuric Acetate
Phenylmercuric Nitrate
Thimerosal
Trifluridine
Vidarabine

Blepharoclonus

Acetylcholine
Allobarbital
Ambenonium
Amobarbital
Amodiaquine
Aprobarbital
Barbital
Bupivacaine
Butabarbital
Butalbital
Butallylonal
Butethal
Carbachol
Carbamazepine
Chloroprocaine
Chloroquine
Clofibrate
Cyclobarbital
Cyclopentobarbital
Demecarium
DFP
Dibucaine
Echothiophate
Edrophonium
Etidocaine
Heptabarbital
Hexethal
Hexobarbital
Hydroxychloroquine
Isoflurophate
Levodopa
Lidocaine
Mephobarbital
Mepivacaine
Methacholine

Metharbital
Methitural
Methohexital
Methylphenidate
Neostigmine
Pentobarbital
Phenobarbital
Physostigmine
Pilocarpine
Piperocaine
Prilocaine
Primidone
Probarbital
Procaine
Propoxycaine
Pyridostigmine
Secobarbital
Talbutal
Tetracaine
Thiamylal
Thiopental
Vinbarbital

Blepharoconjunctivitis

Albuterol
Amiodarone
Amoxicillin
Ampicillin
Atropine
Auranofin
Aurothioglucose
Aurothioglycanide
Bacitracin
Benoxinate
Benzathine Penicillin G
Betaxolol
Bromide
Bupivacaine
Butacaine
Captopril
Carbenicillin
Carteolol
Chloroprocaine
Cloxacillin
Cocaine
Cyclopentolate
Cyclophosphamide
Dibucaine
Dicloxacillin

Dipivefrin
DPE
Dyclonine
Enalapril
Epinephrine
Etidocaine
Etretinate
Floxuridine
Fluorouracil
Framycetin
Gentamicin
Gold Au^{198}
Gold Sodium Thiomalate
Gold Sodium Thiosulfate
Hetacillin
Homatropine
Hydrabamine Penicillin V
Indomethacin
Influenza Virus Vaccine
Insulin
Iodine Solution
Isotretinoin
Levobunolol
Lidocaine
Mechlorethamine
Melphalan
Mepivacaine
Methicillin
Methotrexate
Metipranolol
Metoprolol
Nafcillin
Naphazoline
Neomycin
Neostigmine
Oxacillin
Penicillamine
Phenacaine
Physostigmine
Piperocaine
Potassium Penicillin G
Potassium Penicillin V
Potassium Phenethicillin
Prilocaine
Procaine
Procaine Penicillin G
Proparacaine
Propoxycaine
Rifampin

Smallpox Vaccine
Sulindac
Tetracaine
Tetrahydrozoline
Thiacetazone
Thimerosal
Timolol
Trazodone
Tropicamide

Blepharospasm

Acetaphenazine
Amitriptyline
Amodiaquine
Amoxapine
Amphetamine
Anatazoline
Brompheniramine
Butaperazine
Carbinoxamine
Carphenazine
Chloroquine
Chlorpheniramine
Chlorpromazine
Clemastine
Clomipramine
Desipramine
Dexbrompheniramine
Dexchlorpheniramine
Dextroamphetamine
Dextrothyroxine
Diethazine
Dimercaprol
Dimethindene
Diphenhydramine
Diphenylpyraline
Doxepin
Doxylamine
Dronabinol
Droperidol
Emetine
Ethopropazine
Floxuridine
Fluorouracil
Fluphenazine
Haloperidol
Hashish
Hydroxychloroquine
Imipramine

Levodopa
Levothyroxine
Liothyronine
Liotrix
Lorazepam
Marihuana
Mesoridazine
Methamphetamine
Methdilazine
Methotrimeprazine
Nortriptyline
Perazine
Periciazine
Perphenazine
Pheniramine
Phenmetrazine
Phenylephrine
Piperacetazine
Prochlorperazine
Promazine
Promethazine
Propiomazine
Protriptyline
Pyrilamine
Selegiline
Tetrahydrocannabinol
THC
Thiethylperazine
Thiopropazate
Thioproperazine
Thioridazine
Thyroglobulin
Thyroid
Trifluoperazine
Trifluperidol
Triflupromazine
Trimeprazine
Trimipramine
Tripelennamine
Triprolidine
Vidarabine
Vinblastine

Cataracts

Acetohexamide
Acetophenazine
Acetylcholine
Adrenal Cortex Injection
Alcohol

Aldosterone
Allopurinol
Amiodarone
Beclomethasone
Benoxinate
Betamethasone
Bleomycin
Bupivacaine
Busulfan
Butacaine
Butaperazine
Cactinomycin
Carphenazine
Chloroprocaine
Chlorpromazine
Chlorpropamide
Chlorprothixene
Cortisone
Dactinomycin
Daunorubicin
Demecarium
Desoxycorticosterone
Dexamethasone
DFP
Dibucaine
Diethazine
Doxorubicin
Droperidol
Dyclonine
Echothiophate
Ergot
Ethopropazine
Etidocaine
Fludrocortisone
Fluorometholone
Fluphenazine
Fluprednisolone
Glyburide
Haloperidol
Hydrocortisone
Isofluorophate
Lidocaine
Medrysone
Mepivacaine
Meprednisone
Mesoridazine
Methdilazine
Methotrimeprazine
Methoxsalen

Methylprednisolone
Mitomycin
Mitotane
Neostigmine
Oxygen
Paramethasone
Perazine
Periciazine
Perphenazine
Phenacaine
Phenmetrazine
Phenytoin
Physostigmine
Pilocarpine
Piperacetazine
Piperocaine
Prednisolone
Prednisone
Prilocaine
Procaine
Prochlorperazine
Promazine
Promethazine
Proparacaine
Propiomazine
Propoxycaine
Tetracaine
Thiethylperazine
Thiopropazate
Thioproperazine
Thioridazine
Thiothixene
Tolazamide
Tolbutamide
Triamcinolone
Trifluoperazine
Trifluperidol
Triflupromazine
Trimeprazine
Trioxsalen

Colored Haloes Around Lights

Acetophenazine
Acetyldigitoxin
Adrenal Cortex Injection
Aldosterone
Amiodarone
Amodiaquine
Amyl Nitrite

Beclomethasone
Betamethasone
Butaperazine
Carphenazine
Chloroquine
Chlorpromazine
Contraceptives
Cortisone
Deslanoside
Desoxycorticosterone
Dexamethasone
Diethazine
Digitalis
Digitoxin
Digoxin
Ethopropazine
Fludrocortisone
Fluorometholone
Fluphenazine
Fluprednisolone
Gitalin
Hydrocortisone
Hydroxychloroquine
Lanatoside C
Medrysone
Meprednisone
Mesoridazine
Methdilazine
Methotrimeprazine
Methylprednisolone
Nitroglycerin
Ouabain
Paramethadione
Paramethasone
Perazine
Periciazine
Perphenazine
Piperacetazine
Prednisolone
Prednisone
Prochlorperazine
Promazine
Promethazine
Propiomazine
Quinacrine
Thiethylperazine
Thiopropazate
Thioproperazine
Thioridazine

Triamcinolone
Trifluoperazine
Triflupromazine
Trimeprazine
Trimethadione

Color Vision Defect

Aceclidine
Acenocoumarol
Acetohexamide
Acetophenazine
Acetyldigitoxin
Adrenal Cortex Injection
Alcohol
Aldosterone
Allobarbital
Alseroxylon
Amiodarone
Amobarbital
Amodiaquine
Aprobarbital
Aspirin
Atropine
Barbital
Beclomethasone
Belladonna
Betamethasone
Bromide
Broxyquinoline
Butabarbital
Butalbital
Butallylonal
Butaperazine
Butethal
Carbon Dioxide
Carphenazine
Cephaloridine
Chloramphenicol
Chloroquine
Chlorpromazine
Chlorpropamide
Chlortetracycline
Cisplatin
Cortisone
Cyclobarbital
Cyclopentobarbital
Deferoxamine
Deserpidine
Deslanoside

Promazine
Promethazine
Propiomazine
Psilocybin
Quinacrine
Quinidine
Quinine
Radioactive Iodides
Rauwolfia Serpentina
Ranitidine
Rescinnamine
Reserpine
Rifampin
Secobarbital
Selegiline
Sodium Salicylate
Streptomycin
Sulfacetamide
Sulfachlorpyridazine
Sulfacytine
Sulfadiazine
Sulfadimethoxine
Sulfamerazine
Sulfameter
Sulfamethazine
Sulfamethizole
Sulfamethoxazole
Sulfamethoxypyridazine
Sulfanilamide
Sulfaphenazole
Sulfapyridine
Sulfasalazine
Sulfathiazole
Sulfisoxazole
Sulthiame
Syrosingopine
Talbutal
Tetrahydrocannabinol
THC
Thiabendazole
Thiamylal
Thiethylperazine
Thioguanine
Thiopental
Thiopropazate
Thioproperazine
Thioridazine
Tobramycin
Tolazamide

Tolbutamide
Tranylcypromine
Triamcinolone
Trichloroethylene
Trifluoperazine
Triflupromazine
Trimeprazine
Trimethadione
Vinbarbital
Vincristine

Conjunctival Hyperemia

Acetohexamide
Acetylcholine
Adrenal Cortex Injection
Aldosterone
Alseroxylon
Auranofin
Aurothioglucose
Aurothioglycanide
BCNU
Benzalkonium
Betamethasone
Bupivacaine
Carbachol
Carmustine
Chloral Hydrate
Chlorhexidine
Chloroprocaine
Chlorpropamide
Chrysarobin
Cimetidine
Ciprofloxacin
Clindamycin
Colchicine
Cortisone
Cyclosporine
Deferoxamine
Deserpidine
Desoxycorticosterone
Dexamethasone
Dextrothyroxine
Diacetylmorphine
Diatrizoate Meglumine and Sodium
Disodium Clodronate
Disodium Etidronate
Disodium Pamidronate
Erythromycin
Ether

Etidocaine
Fludrocortisone
Fluorescein
Fluprednisolone
F_3T
Gentamicin
Glyburide
Gold Au^{198}
Gold Sodium Thiomalate
Gold Sodium Thiosulfate
Griseofulvin
Hydrocortisone
Idoxuridine
IDU
Iodide and Iodine Solutions and
    Compounds
Levothyroxine
Lidocaine
Lincomycin
Liothyronine
Liotrix
Measles and Rubella Virus Vaccine
    Live
Measles, Mumps, and Rubella Virus
    Vaccine Live
Measles Virus Vaccine Live
Mepivacaine
Meprednisone
Mercuric Oxide
Methacholine
Methyldopa
Methylprednisolone
Metoprolol
Minoxidil
Mumps Virus Vaccine Live
Nitromersol
Norepinephrine
Norfloxacin
Oxprenolol
Oxyphenbutazone
Paramethasone
Phenoxybenzamine
Phenylbutazone
Phenylmercuric Acetate
Phenylmercuric Nitrate
Pilocarpine
Practolol
Prednisolone
Prednisone

Prilocaine
Procaine
Propoxycaine
Radioactive Iodides
Rauwolfia Serpentina
Rescinnamine
Reserpine
Rifampin
Rubella and Mumps Virus Vaccine
    Live
Rubella Virus Vaccine Live
Sodium Chloride
Syrosingopine
Thiabendazole
Thiacetazone
Thimerosal
Thyroglobulin
Thyroid
Tolazamide
Tolazoline
Tolbutamide
Triamcinolone
Trifluridine
Vancomycin
Vidarabine

Conjunctivitis—Follicular

Acyclovir
Amphotericin B
Apraclonidine
Carbachol
Demecarium
DFP
Diatrizoate Meglumine and Sodium
Diclofenac
Dipivefrin
DPE
Echothiophate
Framycetin
F_3T
Hyaluronidase
Idoxuridine
IDU
Isoflurophate
Mefanamic Acid
Neomycin
Neostigmine
Physostigmine
Pilocarpine

Scopolamine
Sulfacetamide
Sulfamethizole
Sulfisoxazole
Trifluridine
Vidarabine

Conjunctivitis—Nonspecific

Acenocoumarol
Acetaminophen
Acetanilid
Acetohexamide
Allobarbital
Allopurinol
Alprazolam
Amobarbital
Anisindione
Antazoline
Antipyrine
Aprobarbital
Aspirin
Barbital
Bendroflumethiazide
Benzalkonium
Benzthiazide
Butabarbital
Butalbital
Butallylonal
Butethal
Carbamazepine
Carbimazole
Cefaclor
Cefadroxil
Cefamandole
Cefazolin
Cefonicid
Cefoperazone
Ceforanide
Cefotaxime
Cefotetan
Cefoxitin
Cefsulodin
Ceftazidime
Ceftizoxime
Ceftriaxone
Cefuroxime
Cephalexin
Cephaloglycin
Cephaloridine

Cephalothin
Cephapirin
Cephradine
Chloramphenicol
Chlordiazepoxide
Chlorothiazide
Chlorpropamide
Chlortetracycline
Chlorthalidone
Chrysarobin
Cimetidine
Cisplatin
Clofibrate
Clonazepam
Clorazepate
Colloidal Silver
Cyclobarbital
Cyclopentobarbital
Cycloserine
Cyclosporine
Cyclothiazide
Cytarabine
Dextran
Diazepam
Dicumarol
Diethylcarbamazine
Diltiazem
Dimercaprol
Diphenadione
Diphtheria and Tetani s Toxoids and
    Pertussis Vaccine Adsorbed
Disopyramide
DPT Vaccine
Emetine
Ephedrine
Ethotoin
Ethyl Biscoumacetate
Fenoprofen
Flurazepam
Flurbiprofen
Halazepam
Heparin
Heptabarbital
Hexethal
Hexobarbital
Hydralazine
Hydrochlorothiazide
Hydroflumethiazide
Ibuprofen

Tolbutamide
Triazolam
Trichlormethiazide
Trichloroethylene
Verapamil
Vinbarbital
Vitamin A
Warfarin

Corneal Deposits

Acetophenazine
Acid Bismuth Sodium Tartrate
Adrenal Cortex Injection
Alcohol
Aldosterone
Amantadine
Amiodarone
Amodiaquine
Auranofin
Aurothioglucose
Aurothioglycanide
Beclomethasone
Betamethasone
Bismuth Oxychloride
Bismuth Sodium Tartrate
Bismuth Sodium Thioglycollate
Bismuth Sodium Triglycollamate
Bismuth Subcarbonate
Bismuth Subsalicylate
Butaperazine
Calcitriol
Carphenazine
Chloroquine
Chlorpromazine
Chlorprothixene
Cholecalciferol
Clofazimine
Colloidal Silver
Cortisone
Desoxycorticosterone
   (Desoxycortone)
Dexamethasone
Diethazine
Echothiophate
Epinephrine
Ergocalciferol
Ethopropazine
Ferrocholinate
Ferrous Fumarate

Ferrous Gluconate
Ferrous Succinate
Ferrous Sulfate
Flecainide
Fludrocortisone
Fluorometholone
Fluphenazine
Fluprednisolone
Gold Au^{198}
Gold Sodium Thiomalate
Gold Sodium Thiosulfate
Hydrocortisone
Hydroxychloroquine
Indomethacin
Iron Dextran
Iron Sorbitex
Medrysone
Meprednisone
Mercuric Oxide
Mesoridazine
Methdilazine
Methotrimeprazine
Methylprednisolone
Mitomycin
Paramethasone
Perazine
Periciazine
Perphenazine
Phenylmercuric Nitrat
Piperacetazine
Polysaccharide-Iron Complex
Prednisolone
Prednisone
Prochlorperazine
Promazine
Promethazine
Propiomazine
Quinacrine
Quinidine
Silver Nitrate
Silver Protein
Suramin
Thiethylperazine
Thimerosal
Thiopropazate
Thioproperazine
Thioridazine
Thiothixene
Triamcinolone

Trifluoperazine
Triflupromazine
Trimeprazine
Vitamin D2
Vitamin D3

Corneal Discoloration

Chlortetracycline
Ferrocholinate
Ferrous Fumarate
Ferrous Gluconate
Ferrous Succinate
Ferrous Sulfate
Iodine Solution
Iron Dextran
Iron Sorbitex
Methylene Blue
Polysaccharide-Iron Complex
Quinacrine
Tetracycline

Corneal Edema

Acetophenazine
Acetylcholine
Acetyldigitoxin
Amantadine
Amodiaquine
Amphotericin B
Bacitracin
Benoxinate
Benzalkonium
Benzathine Penicillin G
Bupivacaine
Butacaine
Butaperazine
Carbachol
Carphenazine
Cefaclor
Chloramphenicol
Chlorhexidine
Chloroprocaine
Chloroquine
Chlorpromazine
Chlortetracycline
Cocaine
Colistin
Deslanoside
Dibucaine

Diethazine
Digitoxin
Digoxin
Dyclonine
Epinephrine
Erythromycin
Ethopropazine
Etidocaine
Fluphenazine
F₃T
Gitalin
Hexachlorophene
Hydrabamine Penicillin V
Hydroxychloroquine
Idoxuridine
IDU
Lanatoside C
Lidocaine
Melphalan
Mepivacaine
Mesoridazine
Methdilazine
Methicillin
Methotrimeprazine
Mitomycin
Neomycin
Ouabain
Perazine
Periciazine
Perphenazine
Phenacaine
Phenylephrine
Pilocarpine
Piperacetazine
Piperocaine
Polymyxin B
Potassium Penicillin G
Potassium Penicillin V
Potassium Phenethicillin
Prilocaine
Procaine
Procaine Penicillin G
Prochlorperazine
Promazine
Promethazine
Proparacaine
Propiomazine
Propoxycaine
Quinacrine

Silicone
Streptomycin
Tetracaine
Tetracycline
Thiethylperazine
Thimerosal
Thiopropazate
Thioproperazine
Thioridazine
Thiotepa
Trifluoperazine
Triflupromazine
Trifluridine
Trimeprazine
Urokinase
Vidarabine
Vinblastine

Corneal Opacities

Acetylcholine
Alcohol
Amantadine
Amodiaquine
Benoxinate
Butacaine
Chlorhexidine
Chloroform
Chloroquine
Chrysarobin
Cloxacillin
Cocaine
Cytarabine
Dibucaine
Diethylcarbamazepine
Dyclonine
Emetine
Ether
Etretinate
F$_3$T
Floxuridine
Fluorouracil (5-FU)
Hydroxychloroquine
Idoxuridine
IDU
Isotretinoin
Naproxen
Oxyphenbutazone
Phenacaine
Phenylbutazone

Piperocaine
Practolol
Proparacaine
Protriptyline
Silicone
Silver Nitrate
Tamoxifen
Tetracaine
Thimerosal
Tretinoin
Trichloroethylene
Trifluridine
Vidarabine
Vinblastine

Corneal Scarring

Benoxinate
Benzalkonium
Butacaine
Cocaine
Dibucaine
Dyclonine
Iodine Solution
Oxyphenbutazone
Phenacaine
Phenylbutazone
Piperocaine
Proparacaine
Silver Nitrate
Smallpox Vaccine
Tetracaine
Tretinoin

Corneal Ulceration

Alcohol
Aspirin
Auranofin
Aurothioglucose
Aurothioglycanide
Benoxinate
Butacaine
Chloroform
Cocaine
Cytarabine
Dibucaine
Dyclonine
Emetine
Etretinate

Ferrocholinate
Ferrous Fumarate
Ferrous Gluconate
Ferrous Succinate
Ferrous Sulfate
Floxuridine
Fluorouracil
F_3T
Gentamicin
Gold Au[198]
Gold Sodium Thiomalate
Gold Sodium Thiosulfate
Idoxuridine
IDU
Iron Dextran
Iron Sorbitex
Isotretinoin
Oxyphenbutazone
Phenacaine
Phenylbutazone
Piperocaine
Polysaccharide-Iron Complex
Practolol
Proparacaine
Sodium Salicylate
Tetracaine
Thiotepa
Trichloroethylene
Trifluridine
Vidarabine
Vinblastine

Corneal Vascularization

Benoxinate
Benzalkonium
Butacaine
Chlorhexidine
Cocaine
Dibucaine
Dyclonine
F_3T
Idoxuridine
IDU
Iodine Solution
Oxyphenbutazone
Phenacaine
Phenylbutazone
Piperocaine
Proparacaine

Silicone
Tetracaine
Thimerosal
Tretinoin
Trifluridine
Vidarabine

Cortical Blindness

Cisplatin
Cyclosporine
Diatrizoate Meglumine and/or
    Sodium
Glycine
Iopamidol
Iothalamate Meglumine and/or
    Sodium
Iothalamic Acid
Metrizamide
Sulfacetamide
Sulfachlorpyridazine
Sulfacytine
Sulfadiazine
Sulfadimethoxine
Sulfamerazine
Sulfameter
Sulfamethazine
Sulfamethizole
Sulfamethoxazole
Sulfamethoxypyridazine
Sulfanilamide
Sulfaphenazole
Sulfapyridine
Sulfasalazine
Sulfathiazole
Sulfisoxazole
Thiopental
Vincristine

Decreased Anterior Chamber Depth

Acetylcholine
Demecarium
DFP
Echothiophate
Edrophonium
Isoflurophate
Neostigmine
Physostigmine

Pilocarpine
Sulfacetamide
Sulfachlorpyridazine
Sulfadiazine
Sulfadimethoxine
Sulfamerazine
Sulfameter
Sulfamethazine
Sulfamethizole
Sulfamethoxazole
Sulfamethoxypyridazine
Sulfanilamide
Sulfaphenazole
Sulfapyridine
Sulfasalazine
Sulfathiazole
Sulfisoxazole

Decreased Convergence

Alcohol
Allobarbital
Amobarbital
Amphetamine
Aprobarbital
Barbital
Bromide
Bromisovalum
Butabarbital
Butalbital
Butallylonal
Butethal
Carbon Dioxide
Chloral Hydrate
Cyclobarbital
Cyclopentobarbital
Dextroamphetamine
Floxuridine
Fluorouracil
Heptabarbital
Hexethal
Hexobarbital
Mephobarbital
Methamphetamine
Metharbital
Methitural
Methohexital
Metocurine Iodide
Morphine
Opium

Penicillamine
Pentobarbital
Phenmetrazine
Phenobarbital
Phenytoin
Primidone
Probarbital
Secobarbital
Talbutal
Thiamylal
Thiopental
Tubocurarine
Vinbarbital

Decreased Corneal Reflex

Acebutolol
Amiodarone
Amitriptyline
Atenolol
Betaxolol
Bromide
Carbon Dioxide
Carisoprodol
Chloroquine
Clorazepate
Desipramine
Diazepam
Glutethimide
Imipramine
Labetolol
Levobunolol
Meprobamate
Methyprylon
Metoprolol
Nadolol
Nortriptyline
Phencyclidine
Pindolol
Propranolol
Protriptyline
Timolol
Trichloroethylene
Vinblastine
Vincristine

Decreased Dark Adaptation

Alcohol
Amodiaquine

Canthaxanthin
Carbon Dioxide
Chloroquine
Colloidal Silver
Deferoxamine
Dronabinol
Ergonovine
Ergotamine
Etretinate
Hashish
Hydroxychloroquine
Isotretinoin
Lithium Carbonate
LSD
Lysergide
Marihuana
Mescaline
Methylergonovine
Methysergide
Nilutamide
Oxygen
Pilocarpine
Psilocybin
Silver Nitrate
Silver Protein
Tetrahydrocannabinol
THC
Vincristine

Decreased Depth Perception

Alcohol
Chlordiazepoxide
Clonazepam
Clorazepate
Diazepam
Flurazepam
Lorazepam
Nitrazepam
Oxazepam
Prazepam
Sulfacetamide
Sulfachlorpyridazine
Sulfacytine
Sulfadiazine
Sulfadimethoxine
Sulfamerazine
Sulfameter
Sulfamethazine
Sulfamethizole

Sulfamethoxazole
Sulfamethoxypyridazine
Sulfanilamide
Sulfaphenazole
Sulfapyridine
Sulfasalazine
Sulfathiazole
Sulfisoxazole

Decreased Intraocular Pressure

Acebutolol
Aceclidine
Acetazolamide
Acetylcholine
Acetyldigitoxin
Adrenal Cortex Injection
Albuterol
Alcohol
Aldosterone
Allobarbital
Alseroxylon
Amobarbital
Amyl Nitrate
Antazoline
Aprobarbital
Aspirin
Atenolol
Barbital
Beclomethasone
Bendroflumethiazide
Benzthiazide
Betamethasone
Betaxolol
Bupivacaine
Butabarbital
Butalbital
Butallylonal
Butethal
Carbachol
Carteolol
Chloroform
Chlorothiazide
Chlorthalidone
Clofibrate
Clonidine
Cortisone
Cyclobarbital
Cyclopentobarbital
Cyclothiazide

Probarbital
Procaine
Propranolol
Protriptyline
Quinethazone
Rauwolfia Serpentina
Rescinnamine
Reserpine
Secobarbital
Sodium Salicylate
Spironolactone
Succinylcholine
Syrosingopine
Talbutal
Tetraethylammonium
Tetrahydrocannabinol
Tetrahydrozoline
THC
Thiamylal
Thiopental
Timolol
Tolazoline
Triamcinolone
Trichlormethiazide
Trichloroethylene
Trifluperidol
Trimethaphan
Trimethidinium
Trolnitrate
Tubocurarine
Urokinase
Vinbarbital
Vitamin A

Decreased Lacrimation

Acebutolol
Acetophenazine
Albuterol
Aluminum Nicotinate
Amitriptyline
Antazoline
Atenolol
Atropine
Azatadine
Belladonna
Bendroflumethiazide
Benzalkonium
Benzthiazide
Brompheniramine

Busulfan
Butaperazine
Carbinoxamine
Carphenazine
Chlorisondamine
Chlorothiazide
Chlorpheniramine
Chlorpromazine
Chlorthalidone
Clemastine
Clonidine
Cyclothiazide
Cyproheptadine
Desipramine
Dexbrompheniramine
Dexchlorpheniramine
Diethazine
Dimethindene
Diphenhydramine
Diphenylpyraline
Disopyramide
Doxylamine
Dronabinol
Ether
Ethopropazine
Etretinate
Fluphenazine
Hashish
Hexamethonium
Homatropine
Hydrochlorothiazide
Hydroflumethiazide
Imipramine
Indapamide
Isotretinoin
Labetolol
Lithium Carbonate
Marihuana
Mesoridazine
Methdilazine
Methotrexate
Methotrimeprazine
Methoxsalen
Methscopolamine
Methyclothiazide
Methylthiouracil
Metolazone
Metoprolol
Morphine

Nadolol
Niacin
Niacinamide
Nicotinyl Alcohol
Nitrous Oxide
Nortriptyline
Opium
Oxprenolol
Perazine
Periciazine
Perphenazine
Pheniramine
Pimozide
Pindolol
Piperacetazine
Polythiazide
Practolol
Prochlorperazine
Promazine
Promethazine
Propiomazine
Propranolol
Protriptyline
Pyrilamine
Quinethazone
Scopolamine
Tetrahydrocannabinol
THC
Thiethylperazine
Thiopropazate
Thioproperazine
Thioridazine
Timolol
Trichlormethiazide
Trichloroethylene
Trifluoperazine
Triflupromazine
Trimeprazine
Trioxsalen
Tripelennamine
Triprolidine

Decreased or Absent Foveal Reflex

Amodiaquine
Broxyquinoline
Chloroquine
Hydroxychloroquine
Iodochlorhydroxyquin

Iodoquinol
Quinine

Decreased or Absent Pupillary Reaction to Light

Acetaminophen
Acetanilid
Acetophenazine
Alcohol
Allobarbital
Alprazolam
Amitriptyline
Amobarbital
Amoxapine
Amphetamine
Antazoline
Aprobarbital
Aspirin
Atropine
Baclofen
Barbital
Belladonna
Benztropine
Biperiden
Bromide
Bromisovalum
Brompheniramine
Butabarbital
Butalbital
Butallylonal
Butaperazine
Butethal
Calcitriol
Carbinoxamine
Carbon Dioxide
Carbromal
Carisoprodol
Carmustine
Carphenazine
Chloramphenicol
Chlorcyclizine
Chlordiazepoxide
Chlorpheniramine
Chlorphenoxamine
Chlorpromazine
Chlorprothixene
Cholecalciferol
Cimetidine
Clemastine

Tetanus Immune Globulin
Tetanus Toxoid
Thiamylal
Thiethylperazine
Thiopental
Thiopropazate
Thioproperazine
Thioridazine
Thiothixene
Tranylcypromine
Triazolam
Trichloroethylene
Trifluoperazine
Triflupromazine
Trihexyphenidyl
Trimeprazine
Trimipramine
Tripelennamine
Triprolidine
Urethan
Vinbarbital
Vitamin D2
Vitamin D3

Decreased or Paralysis of Accommodation

Acetazolamide
Acetophenazine
Adiphenine
Adrenal Cortex Injection
Alcohol
Aldosterone
Alprazolam
Ambutonium
Amitriptyline
Amodiaquine
Amoxapine
Amphetamine
Anisindione
Anisotropine
Antazoline
Atropine
Baclofen
Beclomethasone
Belladonna
Bendroflumethiazide
Benzathine Penicillin G
Benzphetamine
Benzthiazide

Benztropine
Betamethasone
Bethanechol
Biperiden
Bromide
Butaperazine
Caramiphen
Carbachol
Carbamazepine
Carbinoxamine
Carbon Dioxide
Carisoprodol
Carphenazine
Chloramphenicol
Chlordiazepoxide
Chloroquine
Chlorothiazide
Chlorphenoxamine
Chlorphentermine
Chlorpromazine
Chlorprothixene
Chlorthalidone
Cimetidine
Clemastine
Clidinium
Clomipramine
Clonazepam
Clorazepate
Cocaine
Cortisone
Cyclopentolate
Cycloserine
Cyclothiazide
Cycrimine
Desipramine
Desoxycorticosterone
Dexamethasone
Dextroamphetamine
Diacetylmorphine
Diazepam
Dichlorphenamide
Dicyclomine
Diethazine
Diethylpropion
Diphemanil
Diphenadione
Diphenhydramine
Diphenylpyraline

Phendimetrazine
Phenindione
Phenmetrazine
Phentermine
Phenytoin
Pilocarpine
Pimozide
Pipenzolate
Piperacetazine
Piperazine
Piperidolate
Piroxicam
Poldine
Polythiazide
Potassium Penicillin G
Potassium Penicillin V
Potassium Phenethicillin
Pralidoxime
Prazepam
Prednisolone
Prednisone
Primidone
Procaine Penicillin G
Procarbazine
Prochlorperazine
Procyclidine
Promazine
Promethazine
Propantheline
Propiomazine
Propranolol
Protriptyline
Psilocybin
Pyrilamine
Quinethazone
Radioactive Iodides
Scopolamine
Streptomycin
Temazepam
Tetanus Immune Globulin
Tetanus Toxoid
Tetraethylammonium
Tetrahydrocannabinol
THC
Thiethylperazine
Thiopropazate
Thioproperazine
Thioridazine
Thiothixene

Tocainide
Triamcinolone
Triazolam
Trichlormethiazide
Trichloroethylene
Tridihexethyl
Trifluoperazine
Trifluperidol
Triflupromazine
Trihexyphenidyl
Trimeprazine
Trimethaphan
Trimethidinium
Trimipramine
Tripelennamine
Tropicamide
Vincristine

Decreased Resistance to Infection

Adrenal Cortex Injection
Aldosterone
Azathioprine
Beclomethasone
Betamethasone
Cortisone
Cytarabine
Desoxycorticosterone
Dexamethasone
Fludrocortisone
Fluorometholone
Fluprednisolone
Hydrocortisone
Medrysone
Meprednisone
Methylprednisolone
Paramethasone
Prednisolone
Prednisone
Triamcinolone

Decreased Spontaneous Eye Movements

Alcohol
Alprazolam
Alseroxylon
Amitriptyline
Bromide
Carbamazepine

Chlordiazepoxide
Clonazepam
Clorazepate
Deserpidine
Desipramine
Diazepam
Flurazepam
Halazepam
Imipramine
Lithium Carbonate
Lorazepam
Methadone
Midazolam
Nitrazepam
Nortriptyline
Oxazepam
Pentazocine
Prazepam
Protriptyline
Rauwolfia Serpentine
Rescinnamine
Reserpine
Syrosingopine
Temazepam
Triazolam

Decreased Tear Lysozymes

Adrenal Cortex Injection
Aldosterone
Beclomethasone
Betamethasone
Cortisone
Desoxycorticosterone
Dexamethasone
Fludrocortisone
Fluprednisolone
Hydrocortisone
Insulin
Meprednisone
Methscopolamine
Methylprednisolone
Paramethasone
Practolol
Prednisolone
Prednisone
Scopolamine
Triamcinolone

Decreased Tolerance to Contact Lenses

Antazoline
Azatadine
Brompheniramine
Carbinoxamine
Chlorcyclizine
Chlorhexidine
Chlorpheniramine
Clemastine
Clomiphene
Cyclizine
Cyproheptadine
Dexbrompheniramine
Dexchlorpheniramine
Dimethindene
Diphenhydramine
Diphenylpyraline
Doxylamine
Etretinate
Furosemide
Isotretinoin
Meclizine
Naphazoline
Oral Contraceptives
Orphenadrine
Pheniramine
Pyrilamine
Tetrahydrozoline
Thimerosal
Tripelennamine
Triprolidine

Decreased Vision

Acebutolol
Aceclidine
Acetaminophen
Acetanilid
Acetazolamide
Acetohexamide
Acetophenazine
Acetyldigitoxin
Acyclovir
Adiphenine
Adrenal Cortex Injection
Albuterol
Alcohol
Aldosterone

THC
Thiabendazole
Thiacetazone
Thiamylal
Thiethylperazine
Thiopental
Thiopropazate
Thioproperazine
Thioridazine
Thiothixene
Thyroglobulin
Thyroid
Timolol
Tobramycin
Tocainide
Tolazamide
Tolbutamide
Tranylcypromine
Trazodone
Triamcinolone
Triazolam
Trichlormethiazide
Trichloroethylene
Tridihexethyl
Triethylenemelamine
Trifluoperazine
Trifluperidol
Triflupromazine
Trihexyphenidyl
Trimeprazine
Trimethaphan
Trimethidinium
Trimipramine
Tripelennamine
Triprolidine
Trolnitrate
Tropicamide
Tryparsamide
Uracil Mustard
Urethan
Verapamil
Veratrum Viride Alkaloids
Vinbarbital
Vinblastine
Warfarin

Amphotericin B
Azathioprine
Bacitracin
Beclomethasone
Benoxinate
Benzalkonium
Betamethasone
Butacaine
Cocaine
Colchicine
Cortisone
Cytarabine
Desoxycorticosterone
Dexamethasone
Dibucaine
Dyclonine
Fludrocortisone
Fluorometholone
Fluorouracil
Fluprednisolone
Flurbiprofen
F_3T
Gentamicin
Hydrocortisone
Idoxuridine
IDU
Iodine Solution
Medrysone
Meprednisone
Methylprednisolone
Mitomycin
Paramethasone
Phenacaine
Piperocaine
Prednisolone
Prednisone
Proparacaine
Sulfacetamide
Sulfamethizole
Sulfisoxazole
Tetracaine
Thiotepa
Triamcinolone
Trifluridine
Vidarabine

Delayed Corneal Wound Healing

Adrenal Cortex Injection
Aldosterone

Diplopia

Acetohexamide
Acetyldigitoxin

Phensuximide
Phentermine
Phenylbutazone
Pipenzolate
Piperidolate
Piperocaine
Piroxicam
Poldine
Polymyxin B
Potassium Penicillin G
Potassium Penicillin V
Potassium Phenethicillin
Pralidoxime
Prazepam
Prednisolone
Prednisone
Prilocaine
Primidone
Probarbital
Procaine
Procaine Penicillin G
Procarbazine
Propantheline
Propofol
Propoxycaine
Propranolol
Protriptyline
Pyridostigmine
Pyrilamine
Quinidine
Rabies Immune Globulin
Rabies Vaccine
Secobarbital
Sodium Salicylate
Succinylcholine
Sulindac
Sulthiame
Talbutal
Temazepam
Tetracaine
Tetracycline
Tetrahydrocannabinol
THC
Thiamylal
Thiopental
Thiothixene
Tocainide
Tolazamide
Tolbutamide

Tranylcypromine
Trazodone
Triamcinolone
Triazolam
Trichloroethylene
Tridihexethyl
Tripelennamine
Triprolidine
Tubocurarine
Valproate Sodium
Valproic Acid
Vinbarbital
Vincristine
Vitamin A
Zidovudine

Drug Found in Tears

Alcian Blue
Aspirin
Fenoprofen
Flurbiprofen
Fluorescein
Ibuprofen
Indomethacin
Indometacin
Ketoprofen
Methotrexate
Naproxen
Oxyphenbutazone
Phenylbutazone
Piroxicam
Rose Bengal
Sodium Salicylate
Sulindac
Trypan Blue
Vitamin A

Exophthalmos

Adrenal Cortex Injection
Aldosterone
Beclomethasone
Betamethasone
Carbimazole
Cocaine
Contraceptives
Cortisone
Desoxycorticosterone
Dexamethasone

Dextrothyroxine
Fludrocortisone
Fluprednisolone
Hydrocortisone
Iodide and Iodine Solutions and
    Compounds
Levothyroxine
Liothyronine
Liotrix
Lithium Carbonate
Meprednisone
Methimazole
Methylprednisolone
Methylthiouracil
Paramethasone
Poliovirus Vaccine
Prednisolone
Prednisone
Propranolol
Propylthiouracil
Radioactive Iodides
Thyroglobulin
Thyroid
Triamcinolone
Vitamin A

Eyelashes—Increased (Hypertrichosis)

Cycloserine
Cyclosporine
Diazoxide
Methoxsalen
Minoxidil
Penicillamine
Phenytoin
Psoralens
Steroids
Streptomycin
Thiacetazone
Trioxsalen
Zidovudine

Eyelids—Depigmentation

Adrenal Cortex Injection
Aldosterone
Amodiaquine
Beclomethasone
Betamethasone

Carbimazole
Chloramphenicol
Chloroquine
Cortisone
Desoxycorticosterone
Dexamethasone
Fludrocortisone
Fluorometholone
Fluprednisolone
Gentamicin
Hydrocortisone
Hydroxychloroquine
Isoflurophate
Medrysone
Meprednisone
Methimazone
Methotrexate
Methylprednisolone
Methylthiouracil
Neostigmine
Paramethasone
Physostigmine
Prednisolone
Prednisone
Propylthiouracil
Thiotepa
Triamcinolone

Eyelids—Eczema

Amantadine
BCG Vaccine
Captopril ·
Diphtheria and Tetanus Toxoids
    Adsorbed
Emetine
Enalapril
Fluorescein
Ketoprofen
Measles and Rubella Virus Vaccine
    Live
Measles, Mumps, and Rubella Virus
    Vaccine Live
Measles Virus Vaccine Live
Mercuric Oxide
Methyldopa
Metoprolol
Mumps Virus Vaccine Live
Nitromersol
Phenylephrine

Phenylmercuric Acetate
Phenylmercuric Nitrate
Piperazine
Piroxicam
Practolol
Quinacrine
Rubella and Mumps Virus Vaccine
  Live
Rubella Virus Vaccine Live
Scopolamine
Smallpox Vaccine
Thimerosal

Eyelids—Erythema

Acebutolol
Acetaminophen
Acetanilid
Acetazolamide
Acyclovir
Adrenal Cortex Injection
Aldosterone
Albuterol
Allopurinol
Alprazolam
Amitriptyline
Amoxapine
Antazoline
Atenolol
Auranofin
Aurothioglucose
Aurothioglycanide
Azatadine
BCG Vaccine
BCNU
Beclomethasone
Benzalkonium
Benzathine Penicillin G
Benzphetamine
Betamethasone
Betaxolol
Bleomycin
Bromide
Brompheniramine
Busulfan
Cactinomycin
Captopril
Carbinoxamine
Carmustine
Carteolol

CCNU
Cefaclor
Cefadroxil
Cefamandole
Cefazolin
Cefonicid
Cefoperazone
Ceforanide
Cefotaxime
Cefotetan
Cefoxitin
Cefsulodin
Ceftazidime
Ceftizoxime
Ceftriaxone
Cefuroxime
Cephalexin
Cephaloglycin
Cephaloridine
Cephalothin
Cephapirin
Cephradine
Chlorambucil
Clordiazepoxide
Chlorpheniramine
Chlorphentermin
Chlortetracycline
Cimetidine
Ciprofloxacin
Cisplatin
Clemastine
Clofibrate
Clomipramine
Clonazepam
Clorazepate
Cortisone
Cyclophosphamide
Cyclosporine
Cyproheptadine
Cytarabine
Dacarbazine
Danazol
Dactinomycin
Daunorubicin
Deferoxamine
Demeclocycline
Desipramine
Desoxycorticosterone
Dexamethasone

Midazolam
Minocycline
Minoxidil
Mitotane
Mitomycin
Moxalactam
Mumps Virus Vaccine Live
Nadolol
Nalorphine
Naloxone
Naltrexone
Naproxen
Neomycin
Neostigmine
Nifedipine
Nitrazepam
Nitromersol
Nortriptyline
Oxazepam
Oxprenolol
Oxytetracycline
Paramethasone
Pentazocine
Phenacetin
Phendimetrazine
Pheniramine
Phentermine
Phenylephrine
Phenylmercuric Acetate
Phenylmercuric Nitrate
Pindolol
Piroxicam
Poliovirus Vaccine
Potassium Penicillin G
Potassium Penicillin V
Potassium Phenethicillin
Practolol
Prazepam
Prazosin
Prednisolone
Prednisone
Procaine Penicillin G
Procarbazine
Propranolol
Protriptyline
Pyrilamine
Rabies Immune Globulin
Rabies Vaccine
Ranitidine

Rifampin
Rubella and Mumps Virus Vaccine
   Live
Rubella Virus Vaccine Live
Semustine
Smallpox Vaccine
Spironolactone
Streptomycin
Streptozocin
Succinylcholine
Sulindac
Temazapam
Tetanus Immune Globulin
Tetanus Toxoid
Tetracycline
Thimerosal
Thiotepa
Timolol
Tocainide
Trazodone
Triamcinolone
Triazolam
Triethylenemelamine
Trimipramine
Trioxsalen
Tripelennamine
Triprolidine
Tubocurarine
Uracil Mustard
Verapamil

Eyelids—Exfoliative Dermatitis

Acetohexamide
Acetophenazine
Acid Bismuth Sodiun Tartrate
Adiphenine
Allobarbital
Allopurinol
Ambutonium
Amobarbital
Amodiaquine
Amoxicillin
Ampicillin
Anisindione
Anisotropine
Aprobarbital
Auranofin
Aurothioglucose
Aurothioglycanide

Mannitol Hexanitrate
Mechlorethamine
Mepenzolate
Mephenytoin
Mephobarbital
Mepivacaine
Meprobamate
Mesoridazine
Methantheline
Metharbital
Methdilazine
Methicillin
Methimazole
Methitural
Methixene
Methohexital
Methotrimeprazine
Methsuximide
Methylatropine Nitrate
Methylphenidate
Methylthiouracil
Methyprylon
Moxalactam
Nafcillin
Naltrexone
Naproxen
Nitroglycerin
Oxacillin
Oxyphenbutazone
Oxyphencyclimine
Oxyphenonium
Paramethadione
Pentaerythritol Tetranitrate
Pentobarbital
Perazine
Periciazine
Perphenazine
Phenindione
Phenobarbital
Phensuximide
Phenylbutazone
Phenytoin
Pimozide
Pipenzolate
Piperacetazine
Piperidolate
Piroxicam
Poldine
Practolol

Prilocaine
Primidone
Probarbital
Procaine
Procarbazine
Prochlorperazine
Promazine
Promethazine
Propantheline
Propiomazine
Propoxycaine
Propranolol
Propylthiouracil
Quinacrine
Quinidine
Radio Iodides
Rifampin
Secobarbital
Streptomycin
Sulfacetamide
Sulfachlorpyridazine
Sulfacytine
Sulfadiazine
Sulfadimethoxine
Sulfamerazine
Sulfameter
Sulfamethazine
Sulfamethizole
Sulfamethoxazole
Sulfamethoxypyridazine
Sulfanilamide
Sulfaphenazole
Sulfapyridine
Sulfasalazine
Sulfathiazole
Sulfisoxazole
Sulindac
Talbutal
Thiabendazole
Thiacetazone
Thiamylal
Thiethylperazine
Thiopental
Thiopropzate
Thioproperazine
Thioridazine
Thiothixene
Tolazamide
Tolbutamide

Trichloroethylene
Tridihexethyl
Trifluoperazine
Trifluperidol
Triflupromazine
Trimeprazine
Trimethadione
Trolnitrate
Vancomycin
Vinbarbital
Vitamin A

Eyelids—Urticaria

Acenocoumarol
Acetaminophen
Acetanilid
Acetazolamide
Acyclovir
Adrenal Cortex Injection
Albuterol
Aldosterone
Allobarbital
Allopurinol
Alprazolam
Aluminum Nicotinate
Amikacin
Amiodarone
Amitriptyline
Amobarbital
Amoxapine
Amoxicillin
Ampicillin
Anisindione
Antazoline
Antipyrine
Aprobarbital
Aspirin
Auranofin
Aurothioglucose
Aurothioglycanide
Azatadine
Bacitracin
Barbital
BCG Vaccine
Beclomethasone
Bendroflumethiazide
Benzathine Penicillin G
Benzphetamine
Benzthiazide

Bethamethasone
Betaxolol
Bleomycin
Brompheniramine
Bupivacaine
Busulfan
Butabarbital
Butalbital
Butallylonal
Cactinomycin
Capreomyin
Captopril
Carbamazepine
Carbenicillin
Carbimazole
Carbinoxamine
Carisoprodol
Cefaclor
Cefadroxil
Cefamandole
Cefazolin
Cefonicid
Cefoperazone
Ceforanide
Cefotaxime
Cefotetan
Cefoxitin
Cefsulodin
Ceftazidime
Ceftizoxime
Ceftriaxone
Cefuroxime
Cephalexm
Cephaloglycin
Cephaloridine
Cephalothin
Cephapirin
Cephradine
Chlorambucil
Chloramphenicol
Chlordiazepoxide
Chloroprocaine
Chlorothiazide
Chlorpheniramine
Chlorphentermine
Chlorprothixene
Chlortetracycline
Chlorthalidone
Cimetidine

Triprolidine
Tubocurarine
Vancomycin
Verapamil
Vinbarbital
Warfarin
Zidovudine

Eyelids or Conjunctiva—Allergic Reactions

Acenocoumarol
Acetaminophen
Acetanilid
Acetazolamide
Acetohexamide
Acetophenazine
Acetyldigitoxin
Acyclovir
Adiphenine
Adrenal Cortex Injection
Aldosterone
Allobarbital
Allopurinol
Alprazolam
Aluminum Nicotinate
Ambutonium
Amobarbital
Amodiaquine
Amoxicillin
Amphotericin B
Ampicillin
Amyl Nitrite
Anisindione
Anisotropine
Antazoline
Antipyrine
Apraclonidine
Aprobarbital
Aspirin
Atropine
Auranofin
Aurothioglucose
Aurothioglycanide
Bacitracin
Barbital
BCNU
Beclomethasone
Belladonna
Bendroflumethiazide

Benoxinate
Benzalkonium
Benzathine Penicillin G
Benzphetamine
Benzthiazide
Betamethasone
Betaxolol
Bleomycin
Bromide
Bupivacaine
Busulfan
Butabarbital
Butacaine
Butalbital
Butallylonal
Butaperazine
Butethal
Cactinomycin
Carbachol
Carbamazepine
Carbenicillin
Carbimazole
Carisoprodol
Carmustine
Carphenazine
Carteolol
CCNU
Cefaclor
Cefadroxil
Cefamandole
Cefazolin
Cefonicid
Cefoperazone
Ceforanide
Cefotaxime
Cefotetan
Cefoxitin
Cefsulodin
Ceftazidime
Ceftizoxime
Ceftriaxone
Cefuroxime
Cephalexin
Cephapirin
Cephaloglycin
Cephaloridine
Cephalothin
Cephradine
Chlorae Hydrate

Sulfameter
Sulfamethazine
Sulfamethizole
Sulfamethoxazole
Sulfamethoxypyridazine
Sulfanilamide
Sulfaphenazole
Sulfapyridine
Sulfasalazine
Sulfathiazole
Sulfisoxazole
Talbutal
Temazepam
Tetanus Immune Globulin
Tetanus Toxoid
Tetracaine
Tetracycline
Tetrahydrozoline
Thiabendazole
Thiacetazone
Thiamylal
Thiethylperazine
Thimerosal
Thiopental
Thiopropazate
Thioproperazine
Thioridazine
Thiotepa
Thiothixene
Timolol
Tolazamide
Tolbutamide
Trazodone
Triamcinolone
Triazolam
Trichlormethiazide
Tridihexethyl
Triethylenemelamine
Trifluoperazine
Trifluperidol
Triflupromazine
Trifluridine
Trimeprazine
Trimethadione
Tropicamide
Uracil Mustard
Vancomycin
Vidarabine
Vinbarbital

Warfarin
Zidovudine

Eyelids or Conjunctiva— Angioneurotic Edema

Acetaminophen
Acetanilid
Acetophenazine
Acetyldigitoxin
Adrenal Cortex Injection
Albuterol
Aldosterone
Allobarbital
Alprazolam
Aluminum Nicotinate
Amobarbital
Amoxicillin
Ampicillin
Aprobarbital
Aspirin
Auranofin
Aurothioglucose
Aurothioglycanide
Bacitracin
Barbital
Beclomethasone
Benzathine Pencillin G
Betamethasone
Bleomycin
Butabarbital
Butalbital
Butallylonal
Butaperazine
Butethal
Cactinomycin
Capreomycin
Captopril
Carbenicillin
Carisoprodol
Carphenazine
Cefaclor
Cefadroxil
Cefamandole
Cefazolin
Cefonicid
Cefoperazone
Ceforanide
Cefotaxime
Cefotetan

Thiothixene
Tocainide
Triamcinolone
Triazolam
Trifluoperazine
Trifluperidol
Triflupromazine
Trimeprazine
Trimethadione
Vancomycin
Verapamil
Vinbarbital

Eyelids or Conjunctiva—Deposits

Amiodarone
Auranofin
Aurothioglucose
Aurothioglycanide
Calcitriol
Cholecalciferol
Clofazimine
Colloidal Silver
Epinephrine
Ergocalciferol
Ferrocholinate
Ferrous Fumarate
Ferrous Gluconate
Ferrous Succinate
Ferrous Sulfate
Gold Au^{198}
Gold Sodium Thiomalate
Gold Sodium Thiosulfate
Iron Dextran
Iron Sorbitex
Mercuric Oxide
Nitromersol
Phenylmercuric Acetate
Phenylmercuric Nitrate
Polysaccharide-Iron Complex
Quinacrine
Silver Nitrate
Silver Protein
Sulfacetamide
Sulfamethizole
Sulfisoxazole
Thimerosal
Vitamin D2
Vitamin D3

Eyelids or Conjunctiva—Discoloration

Acid Bismuth Sodium Tartrate
Alcian Blue
Amiodarone
Amodiaquine
Amphotericin B
Antipyrine
Bismuth Oxychloride
Bismuth Sodium Tartrate
Bismuth Sodium Thioglycollate
Bismuth Sodium Triglycollamate
Bismuth Subcarbonate
Bismuth Subsalicylate
Captopril
Chloroquine
Chlortetracycline
Chrysarobin
Clofazimine
Colloidal Silver
Demeclocycline
Diethazine
Doxycycline
Enalapril
Ethopropazine
Ferrocholinate
Ferrous Fumarate
Ferrous Gluconate
Ferrous Succinate
Ferrous Sulfate
Fluorescem
Hydroxychloroquine
Iron Dextran
Iron Sorbitex
Ketoprofen
Methacycline
Methylene Blue
Minocycline
Minoxidil
Oxytetracycline
Penicillamine
Polysaccharide-Iron Complex
Quinacrine
Rifabutin
Rifampin
Rose Bengal
Silver Nitrate
Silver Protein

Tetracycline
Trypan Blue
Vitamin A

Eyelids or Conjunctiva—Edema

Acetaminophen
Acetanilid
Acetohexamide
Acetophenazine
Acyclovir
Adrenal Cortex Injection
Albuterol
Aldosterone
Allobarbital
Allopurinol
Aluminum Nicotinate
Amitriptyline
Amobarbital
Amoxapine
Amoxicillin
Ampicillin
Antipyrine
Apraclonidine
Aprobarbital
Aspirin
Auranofin
Aurothioglucose
Aurothioglycanide
Azatadine
Bacitracin
Barbital
Beclomethasone
Benzalkonium
Benzathine Penicillin G
Betamethasone
Bleomycin
Botulinum A Toxin
Bupivacaine
Butabarbital
Butalbital
Butallylonal
Butaperazine
Butethal
Cactinomycin
Captopril
Carbamazepine
Carbenicillin
Carphenazine
Cefaclor

Cefadroxil
Cefamandole
Cefazolin
Cefonicid
Celoperazone
Ceforanide
Cefotaxime
Cefotetan
Cefoxitin
Cefsulodin
Ceftazidime
Ceftizoxime
Ceftriaxone
Cefuroxime
Cephalexin
Cephaloglycin
Cephaloridime
Cephalothin
Cephapirin
Cephradine
Chloral Hydrate
Chlorambucil
Chloroprocaine
Chlorpromazine
Chlorpropamide
Chlortetracycline
Chrysarobin
Ciprofloxacin
Cisplatin
Clofibrate
Clomipramine
Cloxacillin
Colloidal Silver
Cortisone
Cyclobarbital
Cyclopentobarbital
Cyclosporine
Cyproheptadine
Dactinomycin
Danazol
Dapsone
Daunorubicin
Demecarium
Demeclocycline
Desipramine
Desoxycorticosterone
Dexamethasone
Dextrothyroxine
DFP

Oxyphenbutazone
Oxytetracycline
Paramethasone
Pentazocine
Pentobarbital
Pentolinium
Perazine
Periciazine
Perphenazine
Phenacetin
Phenobarbital
Phenylbutazone
Phenylmercuric Acetate
Phenylmercuric Nitrate
Pimozide
Piperacetazine
Piperazine
Poliovirus Vaccine
Potassium Penicillin G
Potassium Penicillin V
Potassium Phenethicillin
Practolol
Prazosin
Prednisolone
Prednisone
Prilocaine
Primidone
Probarbital
Procaine
Procaine Penicillin G
Prochlorperazine
Promazine
Promethazine
Propiomazine
Propofol
Propoxycaine
Protriptyline
Quinacrine
Quinine
Radioactive Iodides
Rifampin
Rubella Virus Vaccine Live
Secobarbital
Silver Nitrate
Silver Protein
Smallpox Vaccine
Sodium Salicylate
Streptomycin
Succinylcholine

Sulindac
Sulthiame
Suramin
Talbutal
Tetracycline
Tetraethylammonium
Thiamylal
Thiethylperazine
Thimerosal
Thiopental
Thiopropazate
Thioproperazine
Thioridazine
Thyroglobulin
Thyroid
Tolazamide
Tolbutamide
Tretinoin
Triamcinolone
Trifluoperazine
Triflupromazine
Trifluridine
Trimeprazine
Trimethaphan
Trimethidinium
Trimipramine
Vidarabine
Vinbarbital

Eyelids or Conjunctiva— Erythema Multiforme

Acetaminophen
Acetanilid
Acetazolamide
Acetohexamide
Allobarbital
Allopurinol
Alprazolam
Amobarbital
Amodiaquine
Amoxicillin
Ampicillin
Antipyrine
Aprobarbital
Aspirin
Auranofin
Aurothioglucose
Aurothioglycanide

Metharbital
Methazolamide
Methicillin
Methitural
Methohexital
Methotrexate
Methsuximide
Methyclothiazide
Methylphenidate
Metolazone
Mianserin
Midazolam
Minocycline
Mitomycin
Moxalactam
Nafcillin
Naloxone
Naproxen
Nifedipine
Nitrazepam
Nitrofurantoin
Oxacillin
Oxazepam
Oxyphenbutazone
Oxytetracycline
Paramethadione
Pentobarbital
Phenacetin
Phenobarbital
Phensuximide
Phenylbutazone
Phenytoin
Piperazine
Piroxicam
Polythiazide
Prazepam
Primidone
Probarbital
Propranolol
Quinethazone
Quinine
Secobarbital
Smallpox Vaccine
Sodium Salicylate
Sulfacetamide
Sulfachlorpyridazine
Sulfacytine
Sulfadiazine
Sulfadimethoxine

Sulfamerazine
Sulfameter
Sulfamethazine
Sulfamethizole
Sulfamethoxazole
Sulfamethoxypyridazine
Sulfanilamide
Sulfaphenazole
Sulfapyridine
Sulfasalazine
Sulfathiazole
Sulfisoxazole
Sulindac
Talbutal
Temazepam
Tetracycline
Thiabendazole
Thiacetazone
Thiamylal
Thiopental
Timolol
Tolazamide
Tolbutamide
Trazodone
Triazolam
Trichlormethiazide
Trimethadione
Verapamil
Vinbarbital

Eyelids or Conjunctiva—Hyperpigmentation

Acetophenazine
Aluminum Nicotinate
Amodiaquine
Bleomycin
Busulfan
Butaperazine
Cactinomycin
Carmustine
Carphenazine
Chlorambucil
Chloroquine
Chlorpromazine
Ciprofloxacin
Cyclophosphamide
Cytarabine
Dactinomycin
Dapsone

Daunorubicin
Diethazine
Doxorubicin
Doxycycline
Ethopropazine
Etretinate
Floxuridine
Fluorouracil
Fluphenazine
Hydroxychloroquine
Hydroxyurea
Isotretinoin
Lidocaine with Sodium Bicarbonate
Loxapine
Mechlorethamine
Mercaptopurine
Mesoridazine
Methacycline
Methdilazine
Methotrexate
Methotrimeprazine
Methoxsalen
Minocycline
Minoxidil
Mitomycin
Mitotane
Niacin
Niacinamide
Nicotinyl Alcohol
Oral Contraceptives
Oxprenolol
Perazine
Periciazine
Perphenazine
Piperacetazine
Practolol
Procarbazine
Prochlorperazine
Promazine
Promethazine
Propiomazine
Quinacrine
Quinidine
Tetracycline
Thiethylperazine
Thioguanine
Thiopropazate
Thioproperazine
Thioridazine

Thiotepa
Timolol
Tretinoin
Trifluoperazine
Triflupromazine
Trimeprazine
Trioxsalen
Uracil Mustard
Zidovudine

Eyelids or Conjunctiva—Lupoid Syndrome

Acebutolol
Acetophenazine
Allobarbital
Allopurinol
Alseroxylon
Amobarbital
Aprobarbital
Auranofin
Aurothioglucose
Aurothioglycanide
Barbital
BCG Vaccine
Bendroflumethiazide
Benzathine Penicillin G
Benzthiazide
Butabarbital
Butalbital
Butallylonal
Butaperazine
Butethal
Captopril
Carbamazepine
Carbimazole
Carphenazine
Chlorothiazide
Chlorpromazine
Chlorprothixene
Chlortetracycline
Chlorthalidone
Clofibrate
Cyclobarbital
Cyclopentobarbital
Cyclothiazide
Demeclocycline
Deserpidine
Diethazine
Digitalis

Doxycycline
Enalapril
Ergonovine
Ergotamine
Ethopropazine
Ethosuximide
Ethotoin
Flecainide
Fluphenazine
Furosemide
Gold Au[198]
Gold Sodium Thiomalate
Gold Sodium Thiosulfate
Griseofulvin
Heptabarbital
Hexethal
Hexobarbital
Hydrabamine Penicillin
Hydralazine
Hydrochlorothiazide
Hydroflumethiazide
Ibuprofen
Indapamide
Indomethacin
Isocarboxazid
Isoniazid
Labetolol
Levodopa
Mephenytoin
Mephobarbital
Mesoridazine
Methacycline
Metharbital
Methdilazine
Methimazole
Methitural
Methohexital
Methotrimeprazine
Methsuximide
Methyclothiazide
Methyldopa
Methylergonovine
Methylthiouracil
Methysergide
Metolazone
Mexiletine
Minocycline
Nalidixic Acid
Nialamide

Nitrofurantoin
Oral Contraceptives
Oxyphenbutazone
Oxytetracycline
Paramethadione
Penicillamine
Pentobarbital
Perazine
Periciazine
Perphenazine
Phenelzine
Phenobarbital
Phensuximide
Phenylbutazone
Phenytoin
Piperacetazine
Polythiazide
Potassium Penicillin G
Potassium Penicillin V
Potassium Phenethicillin
Practolol
Primidone
Probarbital
Procaine Penicillin G
Prochlorperazine
Promazine
Promethazine
Propiomazine
Propranolol
Propylthiouracil
Quinethazone
Quinidine
Rauwolfia Serpentina
Rescinnamine
Reserpine
Rifampin
Secobarbital
Spironolactone
Streptomycin
Sulfacetamide
Sulfachlorpyridazine
Sulfacytine
Sulfadiazine
Sulfadimethoxine
Sulfamerazine
Sulfameter
Sulfamethazine
Sulfamethizole
Sulfamethoxazole

Sulfamethoxypyridazine
Sulfanilamide
Sulfaphenazole
Sulfapyridine
Sulfasalazine
Sulfathiazole
Sulfisoxazole
Sulindac
Syrosingopine
Talbutal
Tetracycline
Thiamylal
Thiethylperazine
Thiopental
Thiopropazate
Thioproperazine
Thioridazine
Thiothixene
Tocainide
Tolazamide
Tranylcypromine
Trichlormethiazide
Trifluoperazine
Triflupromazine
Trimeprazine
Trimethadione
Vinbarbital

Eyelids or Conjunctiva—Lyell's Syndrome

Acetaminophen
Acetanilid
Acetazolamide
Acid Bismuth Sodium Tartrate
Adrenal Cortex Injection
Aldosterone
Allobarbital
Allopurinol
Amiodarone
Amobarbital
Amoxapine
Amoxicillin
Ampicillin
Antipyrine
Aprobarbital
Aspirin
Auranofin
Aurothioglucose
Aurothioglycanide

Barbital
Beclomethasone
Bendroflumethiazide
Benzthiazide
Benzathine Penicillin G
Betamethasone
Bismuth Oxychloride
Bismuth Sodium Tartrate
Bismuth Sodium Thioglycollate
Bismuth Sodium Triglycollamate
Bismuth Subcarbonate
Bismuth Subsalicylate
Butabarbital
Butalbital
Butallylonal
Butethal
Carbamazepine
Carbenicillin
Carbimazole
Chlorothiazide
Chlortetracycline
Chlorthalidone
Ciprofloxacin
Clomipramine
Cloxacillin
Cortisone
Cyclobarbital
Cyclopentobarbital
Cyclothiazide
Dapsone
Demeclocycline
Desoxycorticosterone
Dexamethasone
Dichlorphenamide
Dicloxacillin
Diltiazem
Doxepin
Doxycycline
Erythromycin
Ethambutol
Ethotoin
Ethoxzolamide
Fludrocortisone
Fluprednisolone
Gold Au[198]
Gold Sodium Thiomalate
Gold Sodium Thiosulfate
Heparin
Heptabarbital

Hetacillin
Hexethal
Hexobarbital
Hydrabamine Penicillin V
Hydrochlorothiazide
Hydroflumethiazide
Hydrocortisone
Ibuprofen
Indapamide
Indomethacin
Isoniazid
Kanamycin
Mephenytoin
Mephobarbital
Meprednisone
Methacycline
Metharbital
Methazolamide
Methicillin
Methitural
Methohexital
Methotrexate
Methyclothiazide
Methylprednisolone
Metolazone
Minocycline
Nafcillin
Naproxen
Nitrofurantoin
Oxacillin
Oxyphenbutazone
Oxytetracycline
Paramethadione
Paramethasone
Penicillamine
Pentobarbital
Phenacetin
Phenobarbital
Phenylbutazone
Phenytoin
Piroxicam
Poliovirus Vaccine
Polythiazide
Potassium Penicillin G
Potassium Penicillin V
Potassium Phenethicillin
Prednisolone
Prednisone
Primidone

Probarbital
Procaine Penicillin G
Procarbazine
Quinethazone
Secobarbital
Smallpox Vaccine
Sodium Salicylate
Streptomycin
Sulfacetamide
Sulfachlorpyridazine
Sulfacytine
Sulfadiazine
Sulfadimethoxine
Sulfamerazine
Sulfameter
Sulfamethazine
Sulfamethizole
Sulfamethoxazole
Sulfamethoxypyridazine
Sulfanilamide
Sulfaphenazole
Sulfapyridine
Sulfasalazine
Sulfathiazole
Sulfisoxazole
Sulindac
Talbutal
Tetracycline
Thiabendazole
Thiamylal
Thiopental
Triamcinolone
Trichlormethiazide
Trimethadione
Trimipramine
Vinbarbital

Eyelids or Conjunctiva—Necrosis

Acenocoumarol
Amphotericin B
Anisindione
Dicumarol
Diphenadione
Ethyl Biscoumacetate
Nafcillin
Phenindione
Phenprocoumon
Tobramycin
Warfarin

Eyelids or Conjunctiva—Purpura

Acetazolamide
Acetohexamide
Adrenal Cortex Injection
Aldosterone
Allopurinol
Alprazolam
Amantadine
Amikacin
Amitriptyline
Aspirin
Auranofin
Aurothioglucose
Aurothioglycanide
BCG Vaccine
Beclomethasone
Bendroflumethiazide
Benzthiazide
Betamethasone
Betaxolol
Carbamazepine
Chlordiazepoxide
Chlorothiazide
Chlorpropamide
Chlorthalidone
Cimetidine
Clofibrate
Clonazepam
Clorazepate
Cortisone
Cyclothiazide
Cytarabine
Danazol
Dapsone
Desipramine
Desoxycorticosterone
Dexamethasone
Diazepam
Dichlorphenamide
Diltiazem
Emetine
Ethoxzolamide
Fludrocortisone
Fluorometholone
Fluprednisolone
Flurazepam
Furosemide
Glutethimide

Glyburide
Gold Au^{198}
Gold Sodium Thiomalate
Gold Sodium Thiosulfate
Halazepam
Hydrochlorothiazide
Hydrocortisone
Hydroflumethiazide
Ibuprofen
Imipramine
Indapamide
Indomethacin
Influenza Virus Vaccine
Interferon
Ketoprofen
Levobunolol
Lorazepam
Measles and Rubella Virus Vaccine
    Live
Measles, Mumps, and Rubella Virus
    Vaccine Live
Measles Virus Vaccine Live
Medrysone
Meprednisone
Methaqualone
Methazolamide
Methyclothiazide
Methylprednisolone
Methyprylon
Metolazone
Metoprolol
Midazolam
Mumps Virus Vaccine Live
Naproxen
Nifedipine
Nitrazepam
Nortriptyline
Oxazepam
Oxprenolol
Paramethasone
Phenytoin
Piperazine
Piroxicam
Polythiazide
Prazepam
Prednisolone
Prednisone
Procarbazine
Propranolol

Protriptyline
Quinethazone
Quinine
Rifampin
Rubella and Mumps Virus Vaccine
 Live
Rubella Virus Vaccine Live
Smallpox Vaccine
Sodium Salicylate
Sulfacetamide
Sulfachlorpyridazine
Sulfacytine
Sulfadiazine
Sulfadimethoxine
Sulfamerazine
Sulfameter
Sulfamethazine
Sulfamethizole
Sulfamethoxazole
Sulfimethoxypyridazine
Sulfanilamide
Sulfaphenazole
Sulfapyridine
Sulfasalazine
Sulfathiazole
Sulfisoxazole
Temazepam
Tetanus Immune Globulin
Tetanus Toxoid
Timolol
Tolazamide
Tolbutamide
Triamcinolone
Triazolam
Trichlormethiazide
Verapamil

Eyelids or Conjunctiva— Stevens-Johnson Syndrome

Acetaminophen
Acetanilid
Acetazolamide
Acetohexamide
Acetophenazine
Allobarbital
Allopurinol
Amiodarone
Amobarbital
Amodiaquine

Amoxicillin
Ampicillin
Antipyrine
Aprobarbital
Aspirin
Auranofin
Aurothioglucose
Aurothioglycanide
Barbital
Belladonna
Bendroflumethiazide
Benzathine Penicillin G
Benzthiazide
Bromide
Bromisovalum
Butabarbital
Butalbital
Butallylonal
Butaperazine
Butethal
Captopril
Carbamazepine
Carbenicillin
Carbromal
Carisoprodol
Carphenazine
Cefaclor
Cefadroxil
Cefamandole
Cefazolin
Cefonicid
Cefoperazone
Ceforanide
Cefotaxime
Cefotetan
Cefoxitin
Cefsulodin
Ceftazidime
Ceftizoxime
Ceftriaxone
Cefuroxime
Cephalexin
Cephaloglycin
Cephaloridine
Cephalothin
Cephapirin
Cephradine
Chloroquine
Chlorothiazide

Secobarbital
Smallpox Vaccine
Sodium Salicylate
Sulfacetamide
Sulfachlorpyridazine
Sulfacytine
Sulfadiazine
Sulfadimethoxine
Sulfamerazine
Sulfameter
Sulfamethazine
Sulfamethizole
Sulfamethoxazole
Sulfamethoxypyridazine
Sulfanilamide
Sulfaphenazole
Sulfapyridine
Sulfasalazine
Sulfathiazole
Sulfisoxazole
Sulindac
Sulthiame
Talbutal
Tetracycline
Thiabendazole
Thiacetazone
Thiamylal
Thiethylperazine
Thiopental
Thiopropazate
Thioproperazine
Thioridazine
Tolazamide
Tolbutamide
Trichlormethiazide
Trifluoperazine
Triflupromazine
Trimeprazine
Trimethadione
Vancomycin
Vinbarbital

Eyelids or Conjunctiva—Ulceration

Allopurinol
Amphotericin B
Ferrocholinate
Ferrous Fumarate
Ferrous Gluconate

Ferrous Succinate
Ferrous Sulfate
Floxuridine
Fluorouracil
Gentamicin
Iron Dextran
Iron Sorbitex
Phenytoin
Polysaccharide-Iron Complex

Heightened Color Perception

Dronabinol
Ethionamide
Hashish
LSD
Lysergide
Marihuana
Mescaline
Oxygen
Psilocybin
Tetrahydrocannabinol
THC

Hippus

Allobarbital
Amobarbital
Aprobarbital
Barbital
Butabarbital
Butalbital
Butallylonal
Butethal
Cyclobarbital
Cyclopentobarbital
Heptabarbital
Hexethal
Hexobarbital
Mephobarbital
Metharbital
Methitural
Methohexital
Pentobarbital
Phenobarbital
Primidone
Probarbital
Secobarbital
Talbutal
Thiamylal

Thiopental
Vinbarbital

Horner's Syndrome

Acetophenazine
Alseroxylon
Bupivacaine
Butaperazine
Carphenazine
Chloroprocaine
Chlorpromazine
Deserpidine
Diacetylmorphine
Diethazine
Ethopropazine
Etidocaine
Fluphenazine
Guanethidine
Influenza Virus Vaccine
Levodopa
Lidocaine
Mepivacaine
Mesoridazine
Methdilazine
Methotrimeprazine
Perazine
Periciazine
Perphenazine
Piperacetazine
Prilocaine
Procaine
Prochlorperazine
Promazine
Promethazine
Propiomazine
Propoxycaine
Rauwolfla Serpentina
Rescinnamine
Reserpine
Syrosingopine
Thiethylperazine
Thiopropazate
Thioproperazine
Thioridazine
Trifluoperazine
Triflupromazine
Trimeprazine

Hypermetropia

Ergot
Penicillamine

Hypopyon

Benoxinate
Cocaine
Dibucaine
Dyclonine
Ferrocholinate
Ferrous Fumarate
Ferrous Gluconate
Ferrous Succinate
Ferrous Sulfate
Iodide and Iodine Solutions and
    Compounds
Iron Dextran
Iron Sorbitex
Phenacaine
Piperocaine
Polysaccharide-Iron Complex
Proparacaine
Radioactive Iodides
Rifabutin
Tetracaine
Urokinase

Impaired Oculomotor Coordination

Alcohol
Dronabinol
Hashish
Marihuana
Tetrahydrocannabinol
THC

Increased Intraocular Pressure

Adrenal Cortex Injection
Aldosterone
Beclomethasone
Atropine
Benoxinate
Betamethasone
Butacaine
Carbon Dioxide
Carmustine
Chondroitin Sulfate
Cortisone

Cyclopentolate
Demecarium
Desoxycorticosterone
Dexamethasone
DFP
Dibucaine
Diltiazem
Dyclonine
Echothiophate
Fludrocortisone
Fluorometholone
Fluprednisolone
Homatropine
Hyaluronic Acid
Hydrocortisone
Hydroxypropylmethylcellulose
Insulin
Isoflurophate
Ketamine
Medrysone
Meprednisone
Methoxsalen
Methylprednisolone
Nifedipine
Nitrous Oxide
Oxyphenonium
Paramethasone
Phenacaine
Phencyclidine
Pilocarpine
Piperocaine
Prednisolone
Prednisone
Proparacaine
Scopolamine
Sodium Chloride
Sodium Hyaluronate
Succinylcholine
Tetracaine
Tolazoline
Triamcinolone
Trioxsalen
Tropicamide
Urokinase
Verapamil

Iris or Ciliary Body Cysts

Adrenal Cortex Injection
Aldosterone

Betamethasone
Cortisone
Demecarium
Desoxycorticosterone
Dexamethasone
DFP
Echothiophate
Edrophonium
Epinephrine
Fludrocortisone
Fluprednisolone
Hydrocortisone
Isoflurophate
Meprednisone
Methylprednisolone
Neostigmine
Paramethasone
Physostigmine
Pilocarpine
Prednisolone
Prednisone
Triamcinolone

Iritis

Acetazolamide
Auranofin
Aurothioglucose
Aurothioglycanide
Cocaine
Cytarabine
Demecarium
DFP
Dichlorphenamide
Echothiophate
Emetine
Epinephrine
Ethoxzolamide
Gold Au[198]
Gold Sodium Thiomalate
Gold Sodium Thiosulfate
Iodide and Iodine Solutions and
    Compounds
Isoflurophate
Methazolamide
Neostigmine
Physostigmine
Pralidoxime
Radioactive Iodides
Suramin

Jerky Pursuit Movements

Acetophenazine
Alcohol
Allobarbital
Alprazolam
Alseroxylon
Amitriptyline
Amobarbital
Aprobarbital
Barbital
Bromide
Bupivacaine
Butabarbital
Butalbital
Butallylonal
Butaperazine
Butethal
Carphenazine
Chloral Hydrate
Chlordiazepoxide
Chloroprocaine
Chlorpromazine
Clonazepam
Clorazepate
Cyclobarbital
Cyclopentobarbital
Deserpidine
Desipramine
Diazepam
Diethazine
Ethopropazine
Etidocaine
Fluphenazine
Flurazepam
Halazepam
Heptabarbital
Hexethal
Hexobarbital
Imipramine
Lidocaine
Lithium Carbonate
Lorazepam
Mephobarbital
Mepivacaine
Mesoridazine
Metharbital
Methdilazine
Methitural

Methohexital
Methotrimeprazine
Midazolam
Nitrazepam
Nortriptyline
Oxazepam
Pentobarbital
Perazine
Periciazine
Perphenazine
Phencyclidine
Phenobarbital
Piperacetazine
Prazepam
Prilocaine
Primidone
Probarbital
Procaine
Prochlorperazine
Promazine
Promethazine
Propiomazine
Propoxycaine
Protriptyline
Rauwolfia Serpentina
Rescinnamine
Reserpine
Secobarbital
Syrosingopine
Talbutal
Temazepam
Thiamylal
Thiethylperazine
Thiopental
Thiopropazate
Thioproperazine
Thioridazine
Triazolam
Trifluoperazine
Triflupromazine
Trimeprazine
Vinbarbital

Keratitis

Acetophenazine
Acetyldigitoxin
Acyclovir
Adrenal Cortex Injection
Aldosterone

Minoxidil
Nadolol
Naphazoline
Neomycin
Niacin
Ouabain
Oxprenolol
Oxyphenbutazone
Paramethasone
Perazine
Periciazine
Perphenazine
Phenacaine
Pheniramine
Phenylbutazone
Phenylephrine
Pilocarpine
Pindolol
Piperacetazine
Piperocaine
Prednisolone
Prednisone
Prochlorperazine
Promazine
Promethazine
Proparacaine
Propiomazine
Propofol
Propylthiouracil
Quinacrine
Radioactive Iodides
Rubella Virus Vaccine Live
Smallpox Vaccine
Sodium Salicylate
Sulfacetamide
Sulfachlorpyridazine
Sulfacytine
Sulfadiazine
Sulfadimethoxine
Sulfamerazine
Sulfameter
Sulfamethazine
Sulfamethizole
Sulfamethoxazole
Sulfamethoxypyridazine
Sulfanilamide
Sulfaphenazole
Sulfapyridine
Sulfasalazine

Sulfathiazole
Sulfisoxazole
Sulindac
Suramin
Tetracaine
Tetracycline
Tetrahydrozoline
Thiethylperazine
Thimerosal
Thiopropazate
Thioproperazine
Thioridazine
Thiotepa
Thiothixene
Timolol
Tobramycin
Triamcinolone
Trichloroethylene
Trifluoperazine
Triflupromazine
Trifluridine
Trimeprazine
Trioxsalen
Triprolidine
Tropicamide
Vinblastine
Vidarabine

Keratoconjunctivitis

Chrysarobin
Floxuridine
Fluorouracil
Morphine
Opium
Vinblastine

Keratoconjunctivitis Sicca

Acebutolol
Acyclovir
Amiodarone
Atenolol
Benzalkonium
Betaxolol
Busulfan
Chlorambucil
Cyclophosphamide
Ibuprofen
Indomethacin

Iodide and Iodine
Solutions and Compounds
Labetolol
Levobunolol
Methyldopa
Metoprolol
Nadolol
Naproxen
Pindolol
Practolol
Primidone
Propoxyphene
Quinidine
Radioactive Iodides
Sulindac
Thiabendazole
Timolol

Lacrimation

Acetophenazine
Acetylcholine
Adrenal Cortex Injection
Alcohol
Aldosterone
Ambenonium
Beclomethasone
Betamethasone
Bleomycin
Butaperazine
Cactinomycin
Carphenazine
Chloral Hydrate
Chlorpromazine
Ciprofloxacin
Cocaine
Codeine
Cortisone
Dactinomycin
Dantrolene
Daunorubicin
Desoxycorticosterone
Dexamethasone
Diazoxide
Dicumarol
Diethazine
Disodium pamidronate
Doxorubicin
Edrophonium
Epinephrine

Ether
Ethopropazine
Fludrocortisone
Fluorometholone
Fluphenazine
Fluprednisolone
Heparin
Hydrocortisone
Ketamine
Levallorphan
Medrysone
Meprednisone
Mesoridazine
Methacholine
Methaqualone
Methdilazine
Methotrimeprazine
Methylprednisolone
Mitomycin
Morphine
Nalorphine
Naloxone
Naltrexone
Neostigmine
Opium
Paramethasone
Pentazocine
Perazine
Periciazine
Perphenazine
Piperacetazine
Piperazine
Prednisolone
Prednisone
Prochlorperazine
Promazine
Promethazine
Propiomazine
Propoxyphene
Pyridostigmine
Rifampin
Thiethylperazine
Thiopropazate
Thioproperazine
Thioridazine
Triamcinolone
Trifluoperazine
Triflupromazine
Trimeprazine

Vinblastine
Warfarin

Lens Deposits

Amiodarone
Auranofin
Aurothioglucose
Aurothioglycanide
Chlorprothixene
Colloidal Silver
Gold Au^{198}
Gold Sodium Thiomalate
Gold Sodium Thiosulfate
Mercuric Oxide
Phenylmercuric Nitrate
Silver Nitrate
Silver Protein
Thiothixene

Loss of Eyelashes or Eyebrows

Acetazolamide
Allopurinol
Aluminum Nicotinate
Amantadine
Amiodarone
Amodiaquine
BCNU
Betaxolol
Bleomycin
Busulfan
Cactinomycin
Carmustine
CCNU
Chlorambucil
Chloroquine
Cisplatin
Clofibrate
Clomiphene
Clonazepam
Cyclophosphamide
Dacarbazine
Dactinomycin
Daunorubicin
DIC
Dichlorphenamide
Diethylcarbamazine
Diltiazem
Doxorubicin

Epinephrine
Flecainide
Floxuridine
Fluorouracil
Gentamicin
Hydroxychloroquine
Levobunolol
Lithium Carbonate
Lomustine
Mechlorethamine
Melphalan
Methazolamide
Methotrexate
Mexiletine
Mitomycin
Niacin
Niacinamide
Nicotinyl Alcohol
Nifedipine
Nitrofurantoin
Piroxicam
Semustine
Streptozocin
Sulfacetamide
Sulfachlorpyridazine
Sulfacytine
Sulfadiazine
Sulfadimethoxine
Sulfamerazine
Sulfameter
Sulfamethazine
Sulfamethizole
Sulfamethoxazole
Sulfamethoxypyridazine
Sulfanilamide
Sulfaphenazole
Sulfapyridine
Sulfasalazine
Sulfathiazole
Sulfisoxazole
Thiotepa
Timolol
Tocainide
Triethylenemelamine
Uracil Mustard
Verapamil
Vincristine
Vitamin A

Macular Edema

Acetazolamide
Aluminum Nicotinate
Benoxinate
Betaxolol
Broxyquinoline
Bupivacaine
Butacaine
Chloroprocaine
Dibucaine
Diclorphenamide
Dipivefrin
DPE
Dyclonine
Epinephrine
Ethoxzolamide
Etidocaine
Hexamethonium
Indomethacin
Iodide and Iodine Solutions and
    Compounds
Iodochlorhydroxyquin
Iodoquinol
Iothalamate Meglumine and Sodium
Iothalamic Acid
Lidocaine
Mepivacaine
Methazolamide
Niacin
Niacinamide
Nicotinyl Alcohol
Phenacaine
Piperocaine
Prilocaine
Procaine
Proparacaine
Propoxycaine
Quinine
Radioactive Iodides
Sulindac
Tamoxifen
Tetracaine
Zidovudine

Macular or Paramacular Degeneration

Amodiaquine
Broxyquinoline

Chloroquine
Hydroxychloroquine
Indomethacin
Iodochlorhydroxyquin
Iodoquinol
Quinine

Miosis

Aceclidine
Acetophenazine
Acetylcholine
Alcohol
Allobarbital
Ambenonium
Amobarbital
Aprobarbital
Baclofen
Barbital
Bethanechol
Bromide
Bromisovalum
Bupivacaine
Butabarbital
Butalbital
Butallylonal
Butaperazine
Butethal
Carbachol
Carbromal
Carisoprodol
Carphenazine
Chloral Hydrate
Chloroform
Chloroprocaine
Chlorpromazine
Chlorprothixene
Clonidine
Codeine
Cyclobarbital
Cyclopentobarbital
Demecarium
DFP
Diacetylmorphine
Dibucaine
Diethazine
Dronabinol
Droperidol
Echothiophate
Edrophonium

Ergot
Ergotamine
Ether
Ethopropazine
Etidocaine
Fluphenazine
Haloperidol
Hashish
Heptabarbital
Hexachlorophene
Hexethal
Hexobarbital
Hydromorphone
Indomethacin
Isocarboxazid
Isoflurophate
Levallorphan
Levodopa
Lidocaine
Marihuana
Meperidine
Mephobarbital
Mepivacaine
Meprobamate
Mesoridazine
Methacholine
Methadone
Metharbital
Methdilazine
Metitural
Methohexital
Methotrimeprazine
Methyprylon
Midazolam
Morphine
Nalorphine
Naloxone
Naltrexone
Neostigmine
Nialamide
Nitrous Oxide
Opium
Oxprenolol
Oxymorphone
Pentazocine
Pentobarbital
Perazine
Periciazine
Perphenazine

Phencyclidine
Phenelzine
Phenobarbital
Phenoxybenzamine
Phenylephrine
Physostigmine
Pilocarpine
Piperacetazine
Piperazine
Piperocaine
Prilocaine
Primidone
Probarbital
Procaine
Prochlorperazine
Promazine
Promethazine
Propiomazine
Propoxycaine
Propoxyphene
Propranolol
Pyridostigmine
Secobarbital
Sulindac
Talbutal
Tetracaine
Tetrahydrocannabinol
THC
Thiamylal
Thiethylperazine
Thiopental
Thiopropazate
Thioproperazine
Thioridazine
Thiothixene
Tolazoline
Tranylcypromine
Trifluoperazine
Trifluperidol
Triflupromazine
Trimeprazine
Vinbarbital
Vitamin A

Myasthenic Neuromuscular Blocking Effect

Acebutolol
Acetophenazine
Adrenal Cortex Injection

Aldosterone
Amodiaquine
Amoxicillin
Ampicillin
Atenolol
Auranofin
Aurothioglucose
Aurothioglycanide
Azlocillin
Bacampicillin
Bacitracin
Beclomethasone
Betamethasone
Betaxolol
Butaperazine
Carbenicillin
Carphenazine
Chloroquine
Chlorpromazine
Chlortetracycline
Ciprofloracin
Cisplatin
Clindamycin
Cloxacillin
Colistimethate
Colistin
Cortisone
Cyclacillin
Demeclocycline
Desoxycorticosterone
Dexamethasone
Dextrothyroxine
Dicloxacillin
Diethazine
Doxycycline
Erythromycin
Ethopropazine
Fludrocortisone
Fluphenazine
Fluprednisolone
Gentamicin
Gold Au[198]
Gold Sodium Thiomalate
Gold Sodium Thiosulfate
Hetacillin
Hydrocortisone
Hydroxychloroquine
Iothalamate Meglumine and Sodium
Iothalamic Acid

Isocarboxazid
Kanamycin
Labetolol
Levobunolol
Levothyroxine
Lincomycin
Liothyronine
Liotrix
Lithium Carbonate
Meprednisone
Mesoridazine
Methacillin
Methacycline
Methdilazine
Methotrimeprazine
Methoxyflurane
Methylprednisolone
Metoprolol
Mezlocillin
Minocycline
Nadolol
Nafcillin
Neomycin
Nialamide
Oxacillin
Oxprenolol
Oxytetracycline
Paramethadione
Paramethasone
Penicillamine
Perazine
Periciazine
Perphenazine
Phenelzine
Phenytoin
Pindolol
Piperacetazine
Piperacillin
Polymyxin B
Practolol
Prednisolone
Prednisone
Prochlorperazine
Promazine
Promethazine
Propiomazine
Propranolol
Quinidine
Quinine

Streptomycin
Sulfacetamide
Sulfachlorpyridazine
Sulfacytine
Sulfadiazine
Sulfadimethoxine
Sulfamerazine
Sulfameter
Sulfamethazine
Sulfamethizole
Sulfamethoxazole
Sulfamethoxypyridazine
Sulfanilamide
Sulfaphenazole
Sulfapyridine
Sulfasalazine
Sulfathiazole
Sulfisoxazole
Tetracycline
Tetraethylammonium
Thiethylperazine
Thiopropazate
Thioproperazine
Thioridazine
Thyroglobulin
Thyroid
Ticarcillin
Timolol
Tobramycin
Tranylcypromine
Triamcinolone
Trifluoperazine
Triflupromazine
Trimeprazine
Trimethadione
Trimethaphan

Mydriasis

Acetaminophen
Acetanilid
Acetophenazine
Acetylcholine
Adiphenine
Adrenal Cortex Injection
Albuterol
Alcohol
Aldosterone
Alkavervir
Allobarbital

Alprazolam
Alseroxylon
Amantadine
Ambutonium
Amitriptyline
Amobarbital
Amoxapine
Amphetamine
Amyl Nitrite
Anisotropine
Antazoline
Apraclonidine
Aprobarbital
Aspirin
Atropine
Azatadine
Baclofen
Barbital
Beclomethasone
Belladonna
Benzathine Penicillin G
Benzphetamine
Benztropine
Betamethasone
Biperiden
Botulinum A Toxin
Bromide
Bromisovalum
Brompheniramine
Bupivacaine
Butabarbital
Butalbital
Butallylonal
Butaperazine
Butethal
Caramiphen
Carbamazepine
Carbinoxamine
Carbon Dioxide
Carbromal
Carisoprodol
Carphenazine
Chloral Hydrate
Chloramphenicol
Chlorcyclizine
Chlordiazepoxide
Chloroform
Chloroprocaine
Chlorpheniramine

Protoveratrines A and B
Protriptyline
Psilocybin
Pyrilamine
Quinidine
Quinine
Radioactive Iodides
Rauwolfia Serpentina
Rescinnamine
Reserpine
Rubella and Mumps Virus Vaccine
    Live
Rubella Virus Vaccine Live
Scopolamine
Secobarbital
Sodium Salicylate
Syrosingopine
Talbutal
Temazepam
Tetraethylammonium
Tetrahydrozoline
Thiamylal
Thiethylperazine
Thiopental
Thiopropazate
Thioproperazine
Thioridazine
Thiothixene
Tranylcypromine
Trazodone
Triamcinolone
Triazolam
Tridihexethyl
Trifluoperazine
Trifluperidol
Triflupromazine
Trihexyphenidyl
Trimeprazine
Trimethaphan
Trimethidinium
Trimipramine
Tripelennamine
Triprolidine
Tropicamide
Urethan
Veratrum Viride Alkaloids
Vinbarbital

Myopia

Acetazolamide
Acetophenazine
Adrenal Cortex Injection
Alcohol
Aldosterone
Aspirin
Beclomethasone
Bendroflumethiazide
Benzthiazide
Betamethasone
Betaxolol
Butaperazine
Carbachol
Carphenazine
Chlorothiazide
Chlorpromazine
Chlortetracycline
Chlorthalidone
Clofibrate
Codeine
Contraceptives
Cortisone
Cyclophosphamide
Cyclothiazide
Demecarium
Demeclocycline
Desoxycorticosterone
Dexamethasone
DFP
Dichlorphenamide
Diethazine
Doxycycline
Echothiophate
Ethopropazine
Ethosuximide
Ethoxzolamide
Etretinate
Fludrocortisone
Fluphenazine
Fluprednisolone
Glibenclamide
Haloperidol
Hyaluronidase
Hydrochlorothiazide
Hydrocortisone
Hydroflumethiazide
Ibuprofen

Indapamide
Isoflurophate
Isosorbide Dinitrate
Isotretinoin
Levobunolol
Meprednisone
Mesoridazine
Methacholine
Methacycline
Methazolamide
Methdilazine
Methotrimeprazine
Methsuximide
Methyclothiazide
Methylprednisolone
Metolazone
Metronidazole
Minocycline
Morphine
Neostigmine
Opium
Oxygen
Oxytetracycline
Paramethasone
Penicillamine
Perazine
Periciazine
Perphenazine
Phensuximide
Physostigmine
Pilocarpine
Piperacetazine
Polythiazide
Prednisolone
Prednisone
Prochlorperazine
Promazine
Promethazine
Propiomazine
Quinethazone
Quinine
Sodium Salicylate
Spironolactone
Sulfacetamide
Sulfachlorpyridazine
Sulfacytine
Sulfadiazine
Sulfadimethoxine
Sulfamerazine

Sulfameter
Sulfamethazine
Sulfamethizole
Sulfamethoxazole
Sulfamethoxypyridazine
Sulfanilamide
Sulfaphenazole
Sulfapyridine
Sulfasalazine
Sulfathiazole
Sulfisoxazole
Tetracycline
Thiethylperazine
Thiopropazate
Thioproperazine
Thioridazine
Timolol
Triamcinolone
Trichlormethiazide
Trifluoperazine
Triflupromazine
Trimeprazine

Narrowing or Occlusion of Lacrimal Canaliculi or Puncta

Acyclovir
Colloidal Silver
Demecarium
DFP
Echothiophate
Epinephrine
Floxuridine
Fluorouracil
F_3T
Idoxuridine
IDU
Isoflurophate
Neostigmine
Physostigmine
Quinacrine
Silver Nitrate
Silver Protein
Thiotepa
Trifluridine
Vidarabine

Night Blindness

Acetophenazine
Butaperazine

Carphenazine
Chlorpromazine
Diethazine
Ethopropazine
Fluphenazine
Mesoridazine
Methdilazine
Methotrimeprazine
Paramethadione
Perazine
Periciazine
Perphenazine
Piperacetazine
Prochlorperazine
Promazine
Promethazine
Propiomazine
Quinidine
Quinine
Thiethylperazine
Thiopropazate
Thioproperazine
Thioridazine
Trifluoperazine
Triflupromazine
Trimeprazine
Trimethadione

Nystagmus

Acetophenazine
Alcohol
Allobarbital
Alprazolam
Amiodarone
Amitriptyline
Amobarbital
Amodiaquine
Amoxapine
Aprobarbital
Aspirin
Auranofin
Aurothioglucose
Aurothioglycanide
Baclofen
Barbital
Bromide
Bromisovalum
Broxyquinoline
Bupivacaine

Butabarbital
Butalbital
Butallylonal
Butaperazine
Butethal
Calcitriol
Carbamazepine
Carbinoxamine
Carbromal
Carisoprodol
Carphenazine
Cefaclor
Cefadroxil
Cefaniandole
Cefazolin
Cefonicid
Cefoperazone
Ceforanide
Cefotaxime
Cefotetan
Cefoxitin
Cefsulodin
Ceftazidime
Ceftizoxime
Ceftriaxone
Cefuroxime
Cephalexin
Cephaloglycin
Cephaloridine
Cephalothin
Cephapirin
Cephradine
Chloral Hydrate
Chlordiazepoxide
Chloroform
Chloroprocaine
Chloroquine
Chlorpromazine
Cholecalciferol
Ciprofloxacin
Clemastine
Clomiphene
Clomipramine
Clonazepam
Clorazepate
Colistimethate
Colistin
Contraceptives
Cyclobarbital

Polymyxin B
Prazepam
Prilocaine
Primidone
Probarbital
Procaine
Procarbazine
Prochlorperazine
Promazine
Promethazine
Propiomazine
Propoxycaine
Protriptyline
Quinine
Scopolamine
Secobarbital
Sodium Salicylate
Streptomycin
Talbutal
Temazcpam
Tetanus Immune Globulin
Tetanus Toxoid
Tetrahydrocannabinol
THC
Thiamylal
Thiethylperazine
Thiopental
Thioperazine
Thiopropazate
Thioproperazine
Thioridazine
Tobramycin
Tocainide
Tranylcypromine
Triazolam
Trichloroethylene
Trifluoperazine
Triflupromazine
Trimeprazine
Thrimethadione
Trimipramine
Tripelennamine
Tubocurarine
Urethan
Valproate Sodium
Valproic Acid
Verapamil
Vinbarbital
Vincristine

Vitamin A
Vitamin D2
Vitamin D3
Zidovudine

Objects Have Blue Tinge

Acetyldigitoxin
Alcohol
Amodiaquine
Amphetamine
Chloroquine
Deslanoside
Digitalis
Digitoxin
Digoxin
Gitalin
Hydroxyamphetamine
Hydroxychloroquine
Lanatoside C
Methylene Blue
Nalidixic Acid
Oral Contraceptives
Ouabain
Quinacrine

Objects Have Brown Tinge

Acetophenazine
Butaperazine
Carphenazine
Chlorpromazine
Diethazine
Ethopropazine
Fluphenazine
Mesoridazine
Methdilazine
Methotrimeprazine
Perazine
Periciazine
Perphenazine
Piperacetazine
Prochlorperazine
Promazine
Promethazine
Propiomazine
Thiethylperazine
Thiopropazate
Thioproperazine
Thioridazine

Trifluoperazine
Triflupromazine
Trimeprazine

Objects Have Green Tinge

Acetyldigitoxin
Allobarbital
Amobarbital
Amodiaquine
Aprobarbital
Barbital
Butabarbital
Butalbital
Butallylonal
Butethal
Chloroquine
Cyclobarbital
Cyclopentobarbital
Deslanoside
Digitalis
Digitoxin
Digoxin
Epinephrine
Gitalin
Griseofulvin
Heptabarbital
Hexethal
Hexobarbital
Hydroxychloroquine
Iodide and Iodine Solutions and
    Compounds
Lanatoside C
Mephobarbital
Metharbital
Methitural
Methohexital
Nalidixic Acid
Ouabain
Pentobarbital
Phenobarbital
Primidone
Probarbital
Quinacrine
Quinine
Radioactive Iodides
Secobarbital
Talbutal
Thiamylal

Thiopental
Vinbarbital

Objects Have Red Tinge

Acetyldigitoxin
Atropine
Belladonna
Deslanoside
Digitalis
Digitoxin
Digoxin
Ergonovine
Ergotamine
Gitalin
Homatropine
Lanatoside C
Methylergonovine
Methysergide
Ouabain
Quinine
Sulfacetamide
Sulfachlorpyridazine
Sulfacytine
Sulfadiazine
Sulfadimethoxine
Sulfamerazine
Sulfameter
Sulfamethazine
Sulfamethizole
Sulfamethoxazole
Sulfamethoxypyridazine
Sulfanilamide
Sulfaphenazole
Sulfapyridine
Sulfasalazine
Sulfathiazole
Sulfisoxazole
Sulthiame

Objects Have Violet Tinge

Dronabinol
Hashish
Marihuana
Nalidixic Acid
Quinacrine
Tetrahydrocannabinol
THC

Objects Have White Tinge

Capreomycin
Paramethadione
Phenytoin
Trimethadione

Objects Have Yellow Tinge

Acetaminophen
Acetophenazine
Acetyldigitoxin
Allobarbital
Alseroxylon
Amobarbital
Amodiaquine
Amyl Nitrite
Aprobarbital
Aspirin
Barbital
Butabarbital
Butalbital
Butallylonal
Butaperazine
Butethal
Carbachol
Carbon Dioxide
Carphenazine
Chloramphenicol
Chloroquine
Chlorothiazide
Chlorpromazine
Chlortetracycline
Colloidal Silver
Cyclobarbital
Cyclopentobarbital
Deserpidine
Deslanoside
Diethazine
Digitalis
Digitoxin
Digoxin
Dronabinol
Ethchlorvynol
Ethopropazine
Fluorescein
Fluphenazine
Furosemide
Gitalin
Hashish

Heptabarbital
Hexethal
Hexobarbital
Hydroxychloroquine
Lanatoside C
Marihuana
Mephobarbital
Mesoridazine
Methaqualone
Metharbital
Methazolamide
Methdilazine
Methitural
Methohexital
Methotrimeprazine
Nalidixic Acid
Nitrofurantoin
Ouabain
Pentobarbital
Perazine
Periciazine
Perphenazine
Phenacetin
Phenobarbital
Piperacetazine
Primidone
Probarbital
Prochlorperazine
Promazine
Promethazine
Propiomazine
Quinacrine
Rauwolfia Serpentina
Rescinnamine
Reserpine
Secobarbital
Silver Nitrate
Silver Protein
Sodium Salicylate
Streptomycin
Sulfacetamide
Sulfachlorpyridazine
Sulfacytine
Sulfadiazine
Sulfadimethoxine
Sulfamerazine
Sulfameter
Sulfamethazine
Sulfamethizole

Sulfamethoxazole
Sulfamethoxypyridazine
Sulfanilamide
Sulfaphenazole
Sulfapyridine
Sulfasalazine
Sulfathiazole
Sulfisoxazole
Syrosingopine
Talbutal
Tetrahydrocannabinol
THC
Thiabendazole
Thiamylal
Thiethylperazine
Thiopental
Thiopropazate
Thioproperazine
Thioridazine
Trifluoperazine
Triflupromazine
Trimeprazine
Vinbarbital
Vitamin A

Ocular Exposure—Irritation

Aceclidine
Acyclovir
Adrenal Cortex Injection
Alcian Blue
Alcohol
Aldosterone
Amoxicillin
Amphotericin B
Ampicillin
Antazoline
Atenolol
Atropine
Auranofin
Aurothioglucose
Aurothioglycanide
Bacitracin
Beclomethasone
Benoxinate
Benzalkonium
Benzathine Penicillin G
Betamethasone
Betaxolol
Butacaine

Carbachol
Carbenicillin
Carteolol
Cefaclor
Cefadroxil
Cefamandole
Cefazolin
Cefonicid
Cefoperazone
Ceforanide
Cefotaxime
Cefotetan
Cefoxitin
Cefsulodin
Ceftazidime
Ceftizoxime
Ceftriaxone
Cefuroxime
Cephalexin
Cephaloglycin
Cephaloridine
Cephalothin
Cephapirin
Cephradine
Chloramphenicol
Chloroform
Chlortetracycline
Chrysarobin
Ciprofloxacin
Clindamycin
Cloxacillin
Cocaine
Colistin
Colloidal Silver
Cortisone
Cyclopentolate
Cyclosporine
Cytarabine
Demecarium
Desoxycorticosterone
Dexamethasone
DFP
Dibucaine
Diclofenac
Dicloxacillin
Diethylcarbamazine
Dimercaprol
Dimethyl Sulfoxide
Dipivefrin

Thimerosal
Thiotepa
Timolol
Tobramycin
Triamcinolone
Trichloroethylene
Trifluridine
Tropicamide
Trypan Blue
Vidarabine
Vinblastine

Ocular Teratogenic Effects

Acetophenazine
Adrenal Cortex Injection
Alcohol
Aldosterone
Azathioprine
Beclomethasone
Betamethasone
Bleomycin
Butaperazine
Cactinomycin
Carphenazine
Chlorpromazine
Clomiphene
Cortisone
Dactinomycin
Daunorubicin
Desoxycorticosterone
Dexamethasone
Diethazine
Doxorubicin
Ethopropazine
Etretinate
Floxuridine
Fludrocortisone
Fluorometholone
Fluorouracil
Fluphenazine
Fluprednisolone
Hydrocortisone
Isotretinoin
LSD
Lysergide
Medrysone
Meprednisone
Mescaline
Mesoridazine

Methamphetamine
Methdilazine
Methotrimeprazine
Methylprednisolone
Mitomycin
Paramethasone
Perazine
Periciazine
Perphenazine
Phenytoin
Piperacetazine
Prednisolone
Prednisone
Primidone
Prochlorperazine
Promazine
Promethazine
Propiomazine
Psilocybin
Quinine
Radioactive Iodides
Thiethylperazine
Thiopropazate
Thioproperazine
Thioridazine
Triamcinolone
Trifluoperazine
Triflupromazine
Trimeprazine
Trimethadione
Warfarin

Oculogyric Crises

Acetophenazine
Alprazolam
Alseroxylon
Amantadine
Amitriptyline
Amodiaquine
Butaperazine
Carbamazepine
Carphenazine
Chlordiazepoxide
Chloroquine
Chlorpromazine
Chlorprothixene
Cisplatin
Clonazepam

Clorazepate
Deserpidine
Desipramine
Diazepam
Diazoxide
Diethazine
Doxepin
Droperidol
Edrophonium HCL
Ethopropazine
Fluphenazine
Flurazepam
Halazepam
Haloperidol
Hydroxychloroquine
Imipramine
Influenza Virus Vaccine
Levodopa
Lithium Carbonate
Lorazepam
Loxapine
Mesoridazine
Methdilazine
Methotrimeprazine
Metoclopramide
Metronidazole
Midazolam
Nitrazepam
Nortriptyline
Oxazepam
Pemoline
Perazine
Periciazine
Perphenazine
Phencyclidine
Pimozide
Piperacetazine
Prazepam
Prochlorperazine
Promazine
Promethazine
Propiomazine
Protriptyline
Rauwolfia Serpentina
Rescinnamine
Reserpine
Syrosingopine
Temazepam
Thiethylperazine

Thiopropazate
Thioproperazine
Thioridazine
Thiothixene
Triazolam
Trifluoperazine
Trifluperidol
Triflupromazine
Trimeprazine

Optic Atrophy

Acetophenazine
Adrenal Cortex Injection
Allobarbital
Amobarbital
Amodiaquine
Aprobarbital
Aspirin
Barbital
Beclomethasone
Betamethasone
Bromisovalum
Broxyquinoline
Butabarbital
Butalbital
Butallylonal
Butaperazine
Butethal
Calcitriol
Carbromal
Carphenazine
Chloramphenicol
Chloroquine
Chlorpromazine
Cholecalciferol
Clindamycin
Cocaine
Cortisone
Cyclobarbital
Cyclopentobarbital
Dapsone
Desoxycorticosterone
Dexamethasone
Dideoxyinosine
Diethazine
Ergocalciferol
Ethambutol
Ethopropazine
Fludrocortisone

Fluorometholone
Fluphenazine
Fluprednisolone
Gentamicin
Heptabarbital
Hexachlorophene
Hexamethonium
Hexethal
Hexobarbital
Hydrocortisone
Hydroxychloroquine
Iodide and Iodine Solutions and
    Compounds
Iodochlorhydroxyquin
Iodoquinol
Isoniazid
Medrysone
Mephobarbital
Meprednisone
Mesoridazine
Metharbital
Methdilazine
Methitural
Methohexital
Methotrexate
Methotrimeprazine
Methyl Alcohol
Methylene Blue
Methylprednisolone
Oxyphenbutazone
Paramethasone
Pentobarbital
Perazine
Periciazine
Perphenazine
Phenobarbital
Phenylbutazone
Piperacetazine
Prednisolone
Prednisone
Primidone
Probarbital
Prochlorperazine
Promazine
Promethazine
Propiomazine
Propoxyphene
Quinine
Radioactive Iodides

Secobarbital
Silicone
Sodium Salicylate
Streptomycin
Suramin
Talbutal
Thiamylal
Thiethylperazine
Thiopental
Thiopropazate
Thioproperazine
Thioridazine
Tobramycin
Triamcinolone
Trichloroethylene
Trifluoperazine
Triflupromazine
Trimeprazine
Tryparsamide
Vinbarbital
Vincristine
Vitamin A
Vitamin D2
Vitamin D3

Oscillopsia

Alcohol
Allobarbital
Amobarbital
Aprobarbital
Barbital
Butabarbital
Butalbital
Butallylonal
Butethal
Cyclobarbital
Cyclopentobarbital
Divalproex Sodium
Heptabarbital
Hexethal
Hexobarbital
Lithium Carbonate
Mephobarbital
Metharbital
Methitural
Methohexital
Pentobarbital
Phenobarbital
Primidone

Probarbital
Secobarbital
Talbutal
Thiamylal
Thiopental
Valproate Sodium
Valproic Acid
Vinbarbital

Papilledema

Acetophenazine
Allobarbital
Amobarbital
Aprobarbital
Aspirin
Barbital
Butabarbital
Butalbital
Butallylonal
Butaperazine
Butethal
Calcitriol
Carbamazepine
Carbon Dioxide
Carphenazine
Chlorpromazine
Cholecalciferol
Ciprofloxacin
Cisplatin
Colchicine
Cortisone
Cyclobarbital
Cyclopentobarbital
Diethazine
Ergocalciferol
Ethambutol
Ethopropazine
Fluorometholone
Fluphenazine
Glutethimide
Heptabarbital
Hexethal
Hexobarbital
Indomethacin
Influenza Virus Vaccine
Interferon
Isoniazid
Levonorgestrel

Measles and Rubella Virus Vaccine
  Live
Measles, Mumps, and Rubella Virus
  Vaccine Live
Measles Virus Vaccine Live
Mephobarbital
Mesoridazine
Metharbital
Methdilazine
Methitural
Methohexital
Methotrimeprazine
Methyl Alcohol
Methylene Blue
Methyprylon
Mitotane
Mumps Virus Vaccine Live
Naproxen
Pentobarbital
Perazine
Periciazine
Perphenazine
Phenobarbital
Piperacetazine
Primidone
Probarbital
Procarbazine
Prochlorperazine
Promazine
Promethazine
Propiomazine
Quinine
Rubella and Mumps Virus Vaccine
  Live
Rubella Virus Vaccine Live
Secobarbital
Sodium Salicylate
Sulfacetamide
Sulfachlorpyridazine
Sulfacytine
Sulfadiazine
Sulfadimethoxine
Sulfamerazine
Sulfameter
Sulfamethazine
Sulfamethizole
Sulfamethoxazole
Sulfamethoxypyridazine
Sulfanilamide

Sulfaphenazole
Sulfapyridine
Sulfasalazine
Sulfathiazole
Sulindac
Sulfisoxazole
Sulthiame
Talbutal
Tamoxifen
Thiamylal
Thiethylperazine
Thiopental
Thiopropazate
Thioproperazine
Thioridazine
Trifluoperazine
Triflupromazine
Trimeprazine
Vinbarbital
Vitamin D2
Vitamin D9

Papilledema Secondary to Pseudotumor Cerebri

Adrenal Cortex Injection
Aldosterone
Amiodarone
Beclomethasone
Benzathine Penicillin G
Betamethasone
Chlorambucil
Chlortetracycline
Ciprofloxacin
Contraceptives
Cortisone
Danazol
Demeclocycline
Desoxycorticosterone
Dexamethasone
Diphtheria and Tetanus Toxoids and
    Pertussis (DPT) Vaccine
    Adsorbed
Doxycycline
DPT Vaccine
Etretinate
Fludrocortisone
Fluprednisolone
Gentamicin
Griseofulvin

Hexachlorophene
Hydrabamine Penicillin V
Hydrocortisone
Ibuprofen
Indomethacin
Isotretinoin
Leuprolide Acetate
Levothyroxine
Lithium Carbonate
Meprednisone
Methacycline
Methylprednisolone
Minocycline
Nalidixic Acid
Naproxen
Nitrofurantoin
Nitroglycerin
Norfloxacin
Ofloxacin
Oxytetracycline
Paramethasone
Perhexilene
Phenylpropanolamine
Phenytoin
Potassium Penicillin G
Potassium Penicillin V
Potassium Phenethicillin
Prednisolone
Prednisone
Procaine Penicillin G
Tetracycline
Triamcinolone
Vitamin A

Paresis or Paralysis of Extraocular Muscles

Acetohexamide
Alcohol
Allobarbital
Alprazolam
Amitriptyline
Amobarbital
Amoxapine
Amphotericin B
Aprobarbital
Aspirin
Barbital
Beclomethasone
Botulinum-A Toxin

Sulindac
Succinylcholine
Talbutal
Temazepam
Thiamylal
Thiopental
Tolazamide
Tolbutamide
Triazolam
Trichloroethylene
Trimipramine
Tubocurarine
Vinbarbital
Vincristine
Vitamin A

Pemphigoid Lesion

Aspirin
Benzalkonium
Captopril
Carbachol
Demecarium
DFP
Dipivefrin
DPE
Echothiophate
Enalapril
Epinephrine
Fluorouracil
F3T
Furosemide
Idoxuridine
IDU
Indomethacin
Isoflurophate
Penicillamine
Phenacetin
Phenylbutazone
Pilocarpine
Piroxicam
Practolol
Propranolol
Rifampin
Sodium Salicylate
Sulfacetamide
Sulfachlorpyridazine
Sulfacytine
Sulfadiazine
Sulfadimethoxine

Sulfamerazine
Sulfameter
Sulfamethazine
Sulfamethizole
Sulfamethoxazole
Sulfamethoxypyridazine
Sulfanilamide
Sulfaphenazole
Sulfapyridine
Sulfasalazine
Sulfathiazole
Sulfisoxazole
Timolol
Trifluridine
Vidarabine

Periorbital Edema

Epinephrine
Ethosuximide
Fluorouracil
Hydralazine
Methotrexate
Methsuximide
Nifedipine
Phensuximide
Sulfacetamide
Sulfachlorpyridazine
Sulfacytine
Sulfadiazine
Sulfadimethoxine
Sulfamerazine
Sulfameter
Sulfamethazine
Sulfamethizole
Sulfamethoxazole
Sulfamethoxypyridazine
Sulfanilamide
Sulfaphenazole
Sulfapyridine
Sulfasalazine
Sulfathiazole
Sulfisoxazole

Photophobia

Acetohexamide
Acetophenazine
Adiphenine
Adrenal Cortex Injection

Aldosterone
Ambutonium
Amiodarone
Amitriptyline
Anisotropine
Apraclonidine
Atropine
Auranofin
Aurothioglucose
Aurothioglycanide
Beclomethasone
Belladonna
Betamethasone
Botulinum A Toxin
Bromide
Butaperazine
Carbon Dioxide
Carphenazine
Carteolol
Chlorpromazine
Chlorpropamide
Chlortetracycline
Cimetidine
Ciprofloxacin
Clidinium
Clomiphene
Cortisone
Deferoxamine
Demeclocycline
Desipramine
Desoxycorticosterone
Dexamethasone
Dextrothyroxine
Dicyclomine
Diethazine
Digitalis
Digitoxin
Dimethyl Sulfoxide
Diphemanil
Dipivefrin
Disopyramide
DMSO
Doxycycline
DPE
Ethambutol
Ethionamide
Ethopropazine
Ethosuximide
Ethotoin

Fludrocortisone
Fluorometholone
Fluoxetine Hydrochloride
Fluphenazine
Fluprednisolone
Fluvoxamine Maleate
Glyburide
Glycopyrrolate
Gold Au^{198}
Gold Sodium Thiomalate
Gold Sodium Thiosulfate
Hexocyclium
Homatropine
Hydrocortisone
Ibuprofen
Imipramine
Indomethacin
Iopamidol
Isocarboxazid
Isoniazid
Isopropamide
Levothyroxine
Liothyronine
Liotrix
Medrysone
Mepenzolate
Mephenytoin
Meprednisone
Mesoridazine
Methacycline
Methantheline
Methdilazine
Methixene
Methotrimeprazine
Methoxsalen
Methsuximide
Methyl Alcohol
Methylatropine Nitrate
Methyldopa
Methylprednisolone
Metipranolol
Metoclopramide
Metoprolol
Metrizamide
Metronidazole
Minocycline
Mitomycin
Nalidixic Acid
Naproxen

Nialamide
Nifedipine
Norepinephrine
Norfloxacin
Nortriptyline
Oxyphenbutazone
Oxyphencyclimine
Oxyphenonium
Oxytetracycline
Paramethadione
Paramethasone
Perazine
Periciazine
Perphenazine
Phenelzine
Phensuximide
Phenylbutazone
Phenytoin
Pipenzolate
Piperacetazine
Piperidolate
Poldine
Prednisolone
Prednisone
Procarbazine
Prochlorperazine
Promazine
Promethazine
Propantheline
Propiomazine
Protriptyline
Quinacrine
Quinidine
Quinine
Rabies Immune Globulin
Rabies Vaccine
Selegiline
Streptomycin
Tetanus Immune Globulin
Tetracycline
Thiacetazone
Thiethylperazine
Thiopropazate
Thioproperazine
Thioridazine
Thyroglobulin
Thyroid
Tobramycin
Tolazamide

Tolbutamide
Tranylcypromine
Triamcinolone
Trichloroethylene
Tridihexethyl
Trifluoperazine
Triflupromazine
Trimeprazine
Trimethadione
Trioxsalen
Vinblastine
Vincristine

Photosensitivity

Acetazolamide
Acetohexamide
Acetophenazine
Adrenal Cortex Injection
Alcian Blue
Aldosterone
Allobarbital
Allopurinol
Alprazolam
Amantadine
Amiodarone
Amitriptyline
Amobarbital
Amodiaquine
Amoxapine
Amoxicillin
Ampicillin
Antazoline
Aprobarbital
Auranofin
Aurothioglucose
Aurothioglycanide
Azatadine
Barbital
Beclomethasone
Bendroflumethiazide
Benzthiazide
Betamethasone
Brompheniramine
Butabarbital
Butalbital
Butallylonal
Butaperazine
Butethal
Captopril

Thiopropazate
Thioproperazine
Thioridazine
Thiothixene
Tolazamide
Tolbutamide
Tranylcypromine
Trazodone
Triamcinolone
Triazolam
Trichlormethiazide
Trifluoperazine
Trifluperidol
Triflupromazine
Trimeprazine
Trimethadione
Trimipramine
Trioxsalen
Tripelennamine
Triprolidine
Trypan Blue
Vancomycin
Verapamil
Vinbarbital
Vincristine

Poliosis

Adrenal Cortex Injection
Aldosterone
Amodiaquine
Beclomethasone
Betamethasone
Chloroquine
Cortisone
Desoxycorticosterone
Dexamethasone
Epinephrine
Fludrocortisone
Fluorometholone
Fluprednisolone
Hydrocortisone
Hydroxychloroquine
Medrysone
Meprednisone
Methylprednisolone
Paramethasone
Prednisolone
Prednisone

Thiotepa
Triamcinolone

Ptosis

Alcohol
Allobarbital
Amobarbital
Aprobarbital
Barbital
Beclomethasone
Betamethasone
Botulinum A Toxin
Bupivacaine
Butabarbital
Butalbital
Butallylonal
Butethal
Carbon Dioxide
Carbromal
Chloral Hydrate
Chloroprocaine
Contraceptives
Cortisone
Cyclobarbital
Cyclopentobarbital
Dexamethasone
Digitalis
Diphtheria and Tetanus Toxoids and
    Pertussis (DPT) Vaccine
    Adsorbed
DPT Vaccine
Etidocaine
Fluorometholone
Fluoxetine Hydrochloride
Fluvoxamine Maleate
F3T
Heptabarbital
Hexethal
Hexobarbital
Hydrocortisone
Idoxuridine
IDU
Lidocaine
Loxapine
Measles Virus Vaccine Live
Medrysone
Mephenesin
Mephobarbital
Mepivacaine

Metharbital
Methitural
Methohexital
Methyl Alcohol
Metocurine Iodide
Opium
Pentobarbital
Phencyclidine
Phenobarbital
Phenoxybenzamine
Prednisolone
Prilocaine
Primidone
Probarbital
Procaine
Propoxycaine
Secobarbital
Succinylcholine
Sulthiame
Talbutal
Thiamylal
Thiopental
Tolazoline
Trichloroethylene
Trifluridine
Tubocurarine
Vidarabine
Vinbarbital
Vincristine

Random Ocular Movements

Allobarbital
Amobarbital
Aprobarbital
Barbital
Butabarbital
Butalbital
Butallylonal
Butethal
Carisoprodol
Cyclobarbital
Cyclopentobarbital
Heptabarbital
Hexethal
Hexobarbital
Ketamine
Mephobarbital
Meprobamate
Metharbital

Methitural
Methohexital
Pentobarbital
Phenobarbital
Primidone
Probarbital
Secobarbital
Talbutal
Thiamylal
Thiopental
Vinbarbital

Retinal Degeneration

Adrenal Cortex Injection
Aldosterone
Amodiaquine
Beclomethasone
Betamethasone
Chloroquine
Cortisone
Deferoxamine
Desoxycorticosterone
Dexamethasone
Ferrocholinate
Ferrous Fumarate
Ferrous Gluconate
Ferrous Succinate
Ferrous Sulfate
Fludrocortisone
Fluorometholone
Fluprednisolone
Gentamicin
Hydrocortisone
Hydroxychloroquine
Indomethacin
Iodide and Iodine Solutions and
    Compounds
Iron Dextran
Iron Sorbitex
Medrysone
Meprednisone
Methylprednisolone
Paramethasone
Polysaccharide-Iron Complex
Prednisolone
Prednisone
Quinine
Radioactive Iodides
Sulindac

Tamoxifen
Tobramycin
Triamcinolone

Retinal Detachment

Aceclidine
Adrenal Cortex Injection
Aldosterone
Beclomethasone
Betamethasone
Carbachol
Cortisone
Demecarium
Desoxycorticosterone
Dexamethasone
DFP
Echothiophate
Fludrocortisone
Fluorometholone
Fluprednisolone
Hydrocortisone
Isoflurophate
Medrysone
Meprednisone
Methylphenidate
Methylprednisolone
Neostigmine
Oxygen
Paramethasone
Penicillamine
Physostigmine
Pilocarpine
Prednisolone
Prednisone
Triamcinolone

Retinal Edema

Acetazolamide
Acetophenazine
Adrenal Cortex Injection
Aldosterone
Amodiaquine
Aspirin
Beclomethasone
Bendroflumethiazide
Benzthiazide
Betamethasone
Butaperazine

Carbromal
Carphenazine
Chloramphenicol
Chloroquine
Chlorothiazide
Chlorpromazine
Chlorthalidone
Cortisone
Cyclothiazide
Desoxycorticosterone
Dexamethasone
Dichlorphenamide
Diethazine
Ergot
Ethambutol
Ethopropazine
Ethoxzolamide
Fludrocortisone
Fluphenazine
Fluprednisolone
Hydrochlorothiazide
Hydrocortisone
Hydroflumethiazide
Hydroxychloroquine
Indapamide
Indomethacin
Iodide and Iodine Solutions and
    Compounds
Iothalamate Meglumine and Sodium
Iothalamic Acid
Meprednisone
Mesoridazine
Methazolamide
Methdilazine
Methotrimeprazine
Methyclothiazide
Methylprednisolone
Metolazone
Paramethasone
Perazine
Periciazine
Perphenazine
Piperacetazine
Polythiazide
Prednisolone
Prednisone
Prochlorperazine
Promazine
Promethazine

Propiomazine
Quinethazone
Quinine
Radioactive Iodides
Sodium Salicylate
Sulindac
Tamoxifen
Thiacetazone
Thiethylperazine
Thiopropazate
Thioproperazine
Thioridazine
Triamcinolone
Trichlormethiazide
Trichloroethylene
Trifluoperazine
Triflupromazine
Trimeprazine

Retinal or Macular Pigmentary Changes or Deposits

Acetophenazine
Amiodarone
Amodiaquine
Azathioprine
Butaperazine
Carbamazepine
Carphenazine
Chloramphenicol
Chloroquine
Chlorpromazine
Chlorprothixene
Cisplatin
Deferoxamine
Didanosine
Diethazine
Diethylcarbamazine
Ethambutol
Ethopropazine
Fluphenazine
Hydroxychloroquine
Mesoridazine
Methdilazine
Methotrexate
Methotrimeprazine
Mitotane
Penicillamine
Perazine
Periciazine

Perphenazine
Piperacetazine
Prochlorperazine
Promazine
Promethazine
Propiomazine
Quinine
Tamoxifen
Thiethylperazine
Thiopropazate
Thioproperazine
Thioridazine
Thiothixene
Trifluoperazine
Triflupromazine
Trimeprazine

Retinal Vascular Disorders

Acetaminophen
Acetanilid
Adrenal Cortex Injection
Aldosterone
Allobarbital
Amobarbital
Amodiaquine
Amyl Nitrite
Aprobarbital
Barbital
Betamethasone
Butabarbital
Butalbital
Butallylonal
Butethal
Carbon Dioxide
Carmustine
Chloroquine
Contraceptives
Cortisone
Cyclobarbital
Cyclopentobarbital
Desoxycorticosterone
Dexamethasone
Diatrizoate Meglumine and Sodium
Diltiazem
Ergonovine
Ergot
Ergotamine
Ethambutol
Fludrocortisone

Fluprednisolone
Gentamicin
Heptabarbital
Hexamethonium
Hexethal
Hexobarbital
Hydrocortisone
Hydroxychloroquine
Indomethacin
Iodide and Iodine Solutions and
    Compounds
Mephobarbital
Meprednisone
Metharbital
Methitural
Methohexital
Methyl Alcohol
Methylergonovine
Methylprednisolone
Methysergide
Nifedipine
Nitroglycerin
Oxygen
Paramethasone
Pentobarbital
Perhexilene
Phenacetin
Phenmetrazine
Phenobarbital
Phenylpropanolamine
Prednisolone
Prednisone
Primidone
Probarbital
Quinine
Radioactive Iodides
Secobarbital
Streptomycin
Sulfacetamide
Sulfachlorpyridazine
Sulfacytine
Sulfadiazine
Sulfadimethoxine
Sulfamerazine
Sulfameter
Sulfamethazine
Sulfamethizole
Sulfamethoxazole
Sulfamethoxypyridazine

Sulfanilamide
Sulfaphenazole
Sulfapyridine
Sulfasalazine
Sulfathiazole
Sulfisoxazole
Talbutal
Thiamylal
Thiopental
Triamcinolone
Trichloroethylene
Vinbarbital

Retrobulbar or Optic Neuritis

Acetohexamide
Acetyldigitoxin
Alcohol
Allobarbital
Amitriptyline
Amobarbital
Aprobarbital
Barbital
Bromisovalum
Broxyquinoline
Butabarbital
Butalbital
Butallylonal
Butethal
Caramiphen
Carbromal
Carmustine
Chloramphenicol
Chlorpropamide
Ciprofloxacin
Cisplatin
Clindamycin
Cocaine
Contraceptives
Cyclobarbital
Cyclopentobarbital
Dapsone
Deferoxamine
Desipramine
Deslanoside
Dideoxyinosine
Digitalis
Digitoxin
Digoxin

Diphtheria and Tetanus Toxoids
  Adsorbed
Diphtheria and Tetanus Toxoids and
  Pertussis (DPT) Vaccine
  Adsorbed
Diphtheria Toxoid Adsorbed
Disulfiram
DPT Vaccine
Ethambutol
Ethchlorvynol
Etretinate
Floxuridine
Fluorouracil
Gitalin
Glyburide
Heptabarbital
Hexethal
Hexobarbital
Ibuprofen
Imipramine
Indomethacin
Influenza Virus Vaccine
Iodide and Iodine Solutions and
  Compounds
Iodochlorhydroxyquin
Iodoquinol
Isoniazid
Isotretinoin
Lanatoside C
Measles and Rubella Virus Vaccine
  Live
Measles, Mumps, and Rubella Virus
  Vaccine Live
Measles Virus Vaccine Live
Mephobarbital
Metharbital
Methitural
Methohexital
Methyl Alcohol
Metronidazole
Minoxidil
Mumps Virus Vaccine Live
Naproxen
Nortriptyline
Nystatin
Ofloxacin
Ouabain
Oxyphenbutazone
Penicillamine

Pentobarbital
Phenobarbital
Phenylbutazone
Piroxicam
Primidone
Probarbital
Protriptyline
Quinacrine
Quinidine
Rabies Immune Globulin
Rabies Vaccine
Radioactive Iodides
Rubella and Mumps Virus Vaccine
  Live
Rubella Virus Vaccine Live
Secobarbital
Smallpox Vaccine
Streptomycin
Sulfacetamide
Sulfachlorpyridazine
Sulfacytine
Sulfadiazine
Sulfadimethoxine
Sulfamerazine
Sulfameter
Sulfamethazine
Sulfamethizole
Sulfamethoxazole
Sulfamethoxypyridazine
Sulfanilamide
Sulfaphenazole
Sulfapyridine
Sulfasalazine
Sulfathiazole
Sulfisoxazole
Sulindac
Talbutal
Tamoxifen
Thiamylal
Thiopental
Tolazamide
Tolbutamide
Trichloroethylene
Tryparsamide
Vinbarbital
Vincristine

Strabismus

Alcohol
Baclofen

Calcitriol
Chloroform
Cholecalciferol
Diazepam
Ergocalciferol
Insulin
Iopamidol
Iothalamate Meglumine and Sodium
Iothalamic Acid
Isocarboxazid
Measles and Rubella Virus Vaccine
    Live
Measles, Mumps, and Rubella Virus
    Vaccine Live
Measles Virus Vaccine Live
Metoclopramide
Metrizamide
Mumps Virus Vaccine Live
Nialamide
Pemoline
Phenelzine
Rubella and Mumps Virus Vaccine
    Live
Rubella Virus Vaccine Live
Tranylcypromine
Tripelennamine
Vitamin A
Vitamin D2
Vitamin D3

Subconjunctival or Retinal Hemorrhages

Acetylcholine
Acid Bismuth Sodium Tartrate
Adrenal Cortex Injection
Aldosterone
Allopurinol
Alseroxylon
Aspirin
Beclomethasone
Benoxinate
Betamethasone
Bismuth Oxychloride
Bismuth Sodium Tartrate
Bismuth Sodium Thioglycollate
Bismuth Sodium Triglycollamate
Bismuth Subcarbonate
Bismuth Subsalicylate
Butacaine

Cocaine
Cortisone
Deserpidine
Desoxycorticosterone
Dexamethasone
Dibucaine
Dyclonine
Epinephrine
Fludrocortisone
Fluorouracil
Fluprednisolone
Glycerin
Hexachlorophene
Hydrocortisone
Indomethacin
Isosorbide
Lincomycin
Mannitol
Meprednisone
Methaqualone
Methylphenidate
Methylprednisolone
Mithramycin
Mitotane
Oxyphenbutazone
Paramethasone
Penicillamine
Phenacaine
Phenylbutazone
Piperocaine
Plicamycin
Pralidoxime
Prednisolone
Prednisone
Proparacaine
Rauwolfia Serpentina
Rescinnamine
Reserpine
Sodium Chloride
Sodium Salicylate
Sulfacetamide
Sulfachlorpyridazine
Sulfacytine
Sulfadiazine
Sulfadimethoxine
Sulfamerazine
Sulfameter
Sulfamethazine
Sulfamethizole

Sulfamethoxazole
Sulfamethoxypyridazine
Sulfanilamide
Sulfaphenazole
Sulfapyridine
Sulfasalazine
Sulfathiazole
Sulfisoxazole
Sulindac
Syrosingopine
Tamoxifen
Tetracaine
Triamcinolone
Trichloroethylene
Vitamin A

Subconjunctival or Retinal Hemorrhages Secondary to Drug-Induced Anemia

Acebutolol
Acenocoumarol
Acetaminophen
Acetanilid
Acetazolamide
Acetohexamide
Acetophenazine
Acyclovir
Allobarbital
Allopurinol
Alprazolam
Amitriptyline
Amobarbital
Amodiaquine
Amoxicillin
Amphotericin B
Ampicillin
Anisindione
Antazoline
Antipyrine
Aprobarbital
Atenolol
Auranofin
Aurothioglucose
Aurothioglycanide
Azatadine
Azathioprine
Barbital
BCG Vaccine
BCNU

Bendroflumethiazide
Benzathine Penicillin G
Benzthiazide
Bleomycin
Brompheniramine
Busulfan
Butabarbital
Butalbital
Butallylonal
Butaperazine
Butethal
Cactinomycin
Calcitriol
Captopril
Carbamazepine
Carbenicillin
Carbimazole
Carbinoxamine
Carisoprodol
Carmustine
Carphenazine
CCNU
Cefaclor
Cefadroxil
Cefamandole
Cefazolin
Cefonicid
Cefoperazone
Ceforanide
Cefotaxime
Cefotetan
Cefoxitin
Cefsulodin
Ceftazidime
Ceftizoxime
Ceftriaxone
Cefuroxime
Cephalexin
Cephaloglycin
Cephaloridine
Cephalothin
Cephapirin
Cephradine
Chlorambucil
Chloramphenicol
Chlordiazepoxide
Chloroquine
Chlorothiazide
Chlorpheniramine

Protriptyline
Pyrilamine
Quinacrine
Quinethazone
Quinidine
Quinine
Ranitidine
Rifampin
Rubella and Mumps Virus Vaccine
   Live
Rubella Virus Vaccine Live
Secobarbital
Semustine
Streptomycin
Streptozocin
Suramin
Talbutal
Temazepam
Tetracycline
Thiabendazole
Thiacetazone
Thiamylal
Thiethylperazine
Thioguanine
Thiopental
Thiopropazate
Thioproperazine
Thioridazine
Thiotepa
Thiothixene
Tocainide
Tolazamide
Tolazoline
Tolbutamide
Tranylcypromine
Trazodone
Triazolam
Trichlormethiazide
Triethylenemelamine
Trifluoperazine
Trifluperidol
Triflupromazine
Trimeprazine
Trimethadione
Tripelennamine
Triprolidine
Uracil Mustard
Urethan
Vancomycin

Verapamil
Vidarabine
Vinbarbital
Vincristine
Vitamin D2
Vitamin D3
Warfarin

Symblepharon

Amobarbital
Aprobarbital
Auranofin
Aurothioglucose
Aurothioglycanide
Barbital
Benzalkonium
Butabarbital
Butalbital
Butethal
Carbachol
Colloidal Silver
Cyclobarbital
Demecarium
Dipivefrin
DFP
DPE
Echothiophate
Epinephrine
F3T
Gold Au[198]
Gold Sodium Thiomalate
Gold Sodium Thiosulfate
Hexobarbital
Idoxuridine
IDU
Isoflurophate
Mephobarbital
   (Methylphenobarbital)
Metharbital
Methohexital
Mitomycin
Penicillamine
Pentobarbital
Phenobarbital
Phenylbutazone
Pilocarpine
Primadone
Secobarbital
Silver Nitrate

Silver Protein
Sulfacetamide
Sulfachlorpyridazine
Sulfacytine
Sulfadiazine
Sulfadimethoxine
Sulfamerazine
Sulfameter
Sulfamethazine
Sulfamethizole
Sulfamethoxazole
Sulfamethoxypyridazine
Sulfanilamide
Sulfaphenazole
Sulfapyridine
Sulfasalazine
Sulfathiazole
Sulfisoxazole
Talbutal
Thiamylal
Thiopental
Timolol
Trifluridine
Vidarabine

Systemic Administration—Nonspecific Ocular Irritation

Alprazolam
Alseroxylon
Benzphetamine
Bethanechol
Brompheniramine
Carisoprodol
Clofazimine
Chloral Hydrate
Chlordiazepoxide
Chlorpheniramine
Chlorphentermine
Clofazimine
Clonazepam
Clonidine
Clorazepate
Cyclophosphamide
Cytarabine
Deserpidine
Dexbrompheniramine
Dexchlorpheniramine
Dextran

Diacetylmorphine
Diatrizoate Meglumine and Sodium
Diazepam
Diethylpropion
Diltiazem
Dimercaprol
Dimethindene
Dronabinol
Emetine
Ether
Fenfluramine
Flecainide
Floxuridine
Fluorouracil
Flurazepam
Guanethidine
Halazepam
Hashish
Hydralazine
Influenza Virus Vaccine
Iodide and Iodine Solutions and
    Compounds
Iophendylate
Iothalamate Meglumine and Sodium
Iothalamic Acid
Ketoprofen
Labetolol
Lithium Carbonate
Lorazepam
Marihuana
Measles and Rubella Virus Vaccine
    Live
Measles, Mumps, and Rubella Virus
    Vaccine Live
Measles Virus Vaccine Live
Mefenamic Acid
Meprobamate
Methotrexate
Metoprolol
Midazolam
Mumps Virus Vaccine Live
Naltrexone
Nifedipine
Nitrazepam
Nitrofurantoin
Oxazepam
Oxprenolol
Penicillamine
Phendimetrazine

Pheniramine
Phentermine
Piroxicam
Practolol
Prazepam
Propranolol
Radioactive Iodides
Rauwolfia Serpentina
Rescinnamine
Reserpine
Rubella and Mumps Virus Vaccine
  Live
Rubella Virus Vaccine Live
Sulfacetamide
Sulfachlorpyridazine
Sulfacytine
Sulfadiazine
Sulfadimethoxine
Sulfamerazine
Sulfameter
Sulfamethazine
Sulfamethizole
Sulfamethoxazole
Sulfamethoxypyridazine
Sulfanilamide
Sulfaphenazole
Sulfapyridine
Sulfasalazine
Sulfathiazole
Sulfisoxazole
Suramin
Syrosingopine
Temazepam
Tetrahydrocannabinol
THC
Thiacetazone
Trazodone
Triazolam
Triprolidine
Verapamil

Toxic Amblyopia

Acetophenazine
Adrenal Cortex Injection
Alcohol
Aldosterone
Allobarbital
Amitriptyline
Amobarbital

Antipyrine
Aprobarbital
Aspirin
Barbital
Beclomethasone
Betamethasone
Broxyquinoline
Butabarbital
Butalbital
Butallylonal
Butaperazine
Butethal
Carphenazine
Chloramphenicol
Chlorpromazine
Cortisone
Cyclobarbital
Cyclopentobarbital
Desipramine
Desoxycorticosterone
Dexamethasone
Diethazine
Diethylcarbamazine
Digitalis
Disulfiram
Ergot
Ethambutol
Ethchlorvynol
Ethopropazine
Fludrocortisone
Fluorometholone
Fluphenazine
Fluprednisolone
Heptabarbital
Hexachlorophene
Hexamethonium
Hexethal
Hexobarbital
Hydrocortisone
Ibuprofen
Imipramine
Indomethacin
Iodide and Iodine Solutions and
  Compounds
Iodochlorhydroxyquin
Iodoquinol
Isoniazid
Medrysone
Mephobarbital

Meprednisone
Mesoridazine
Metharbital
Methdilazine
Methitural
Methohexital
Methotrimeprazine
Methyl Alcohol
Methylprednisolone
Nortriptyline
Paramethasone
Pentobarbital
Perazine
Periciazine
Perphenazine
Phenobarbital
Piperacetazine
Prednisolone
Prednisone
Primidone
Probarbital
Prochlorperazine
Promazine
Promethazine
Proparacaine
Propiomazine
Protriptyline
Quinidine
Quinine
Radioactive Iodides
Secobarbital
Sodium Salicylate
Streptomycin
Talbutal
Thiamylal
Thiethylperazine
Thiopental
Thiopropazate
Thioproperazine
Thioridazine
Triamcinolone
Trichloroethylene
Trifluoperazine
Triflupromazine
Trimeprazine
Tryparsamide
Vinbarbital

Uveitis

Amphotericin B
Bacitracin
BCG Vaccine
Benoxinate
Benzathine Penicillin G
Bupivacaine
Butacaine
Chloramphenicol
Chloroprocaine
Chlortetracycline
Chondroitin Sulfate
Cobalt
Colistin
Contraceptives
Demecarium
DFP
Dibucaine
Diethylcarbamazine
Diphtheria and Tetanus Toxoids and
    Pertussis (DPT) Vaccine
    Adsorbed
Disodium Clodronate
Disodium Etidronate
Disodium Pamidronate
DPT Vaccine
Dyclonine
Echothiophate
Erythromycin
Etidocaine
Hyaluronate Acid
Hydrabamine Penicillin V
Hydroxypropylmethylcellulose
Isoflurophate
Lidocaine
Mepivacaine
Methicillin
Metipranolol
Neomycin
Phenacaine
Piperocaine
Polymyxin B
Potassium Penicillin G
Potassium Penicillin V
Potassium Phenethicillin
Prilocaine
Procaine
Procaine Penicillin G

Propoxycaine
Quinidine
Rifabutin
Rifampin
Smallpox Vaccine
Sodium Hyaluronate
Streptokinase
Streptomycin
Sulfacetamide
Sulfachlorpyridazine
Sulfacytine
Sulfadiazine
Sulfadimethoxine
Sulfamerazine
Sulfameter
Sulfamethazine
Sulfamethizole
Sulfamethoxazole
Sulfamethoxypyridazine
Sulfanilamide
Sulfaphenazole
Sulfapyridine
Sulfasalazine
Sulfathiazole
Sulfisoxazole
Tetracaine
Tetracycline
Thiotepa
Urokinase

Visual Agnosia

Benzathine Penicillin G
Hydrabamine Penicillin G
Potassium Penicillin G
Potassium Penicillin V
Potassium Phenethicillin
Procaine Penicillin G

Visual Field Defects

Acetophenazine
Acetyldigitoxin
Adrenal Cortex Injection
Alcohol
Aldosterone
Allobarbital
Amiodarone
Amobarbital
Amodiaquine

Antazoline
Aprobarbital
Aspirin
Barbital
Beclomethasone
Betamethasone
Bromide
Bromisovalum
Brompheniramine
Butabarbital
Butalbital
Butallylonal
Butaperazine
Butethal
Caramiphen
Carbinoxamine
Carbon Dioxide
Carbromal
Carisoprodol
Carphenazine
Chloramphenicol
Chloroquine
Chlopheniramine
Chlorpromazine
Chlorpropamide
Chlortetracycline
Ciprofloxacin
Cisplatin
Clemastine
Clomiphene
Contraceptives
Cortisone
Cyclobarbital
Cyclopentobarbital
Danazol
Deferoxamine
Demeclocycline
Deslanoside
Desoxycorticosterone
Dexamethasone
Dexbrompheniramine
Dexchlorpheniramine
Diatrizoate Meglumine and Sodium
Diazoxide
Didanosine
Dideoxyinosine
Diethazine
Diethylcarbamazine
Digitalis

Sulfacetamide
Sulfachlorpyridazine
Sulfacytine
Sulfadiazine
Sulfadimethoxine
Sulfamerazine
Sulfameter
Sulfamethazine
Sulfamethizole
Sulfamethoxazole
Sulfamethoxypyridazine
Sulfanilamide
Sulfaphenazole
Sulfapyridine
Sulfasalazine
Sulfathiazole
Sulfisoxazole
Sulindac
Talbutal
Tamoxifen
Tetracycline
Thiamylal
Thiethylperazine
Thiopental
Thiopropazate
Thioproperazine
Thioridazine
Tolbutamide
Tranylcypromine
Triamcinolone
Trichloroethylene
Trifluoperazine
Triflupromazine
Trimeprazine
Trimethadione
Tripelennamme
Triprolidine
Tryparsamide
Vinbarbital
Vincristine
Vitamin A

Visual Hallucinations

Acebutolol
Acetaminophen
Acetanilid
Acetophenazine
Acid Bismuth Sodium Tartrate
Acyclovir

Adrenal Cortex Injection
Albuterol
Alcohol
Aldosterone
Allobarbital
Alprazolam
Amantadine
Amitriptyline
Amobarbital
Amodiaquine
Amoxapine
Amphetamine
Amyl Nitrite
Antazoline
Aprobarbital
Aspirin
Atenolol
Atropine
Azatadine
Baclofen
Barbital
Beclomethasone
Bendroflumethiazide
Benzthiazide
Belladonna
Benzathine Penicillin G
Benzphetamine
Benztropine
Betamethasone
Betaxolol
Biperiden
Bismuth Oxychloride
Bismuth Sodium Tartrate
Bismuth Sodium Thioglycollate
Bismuth Sodium Triglycollamate
Bismuth Subcarbonate
Bismuth Subsalicylate
Bromide
Brompheniramine
Butabarbital
Butalbital
Butallylonal
Butaperazine
Butethal
Calcitriol
Captopril
Carbamazepine
Carbinoxamine
Carbon Dioxide

Carphenazine
Cefaclor
Cefadroxil
Cefamandole
Cefazolin
Cefonicid
Cefoperazone
Ceforanide
Cefotaxime
Cefotetan
Cefoxitin
Cefsulodin
Ceftazidime
Ceftizoxime
Ceftriaxone
Cefuroxime
Cephalexin
Cephaloglycin
Cephaloridine
Cephalothin
Cephapirin
Cephradine
Chloral Hydrate
Chlorambucil
Chlorcyclizine
Chlordiazepoxide
Chloroquine
Chlorothiazide
Chlorpheniramine
Chlorphenoxamine
Chlorphentermine
Chlorpromazine
Chlortetracycline
Chlorthalidone
Cholecalciferol
Cimetidine
Ciprofloxacin
Clemastine
Clomipramine
Clonazepam
Clonidine
Clorazepate
Cocaine
Codeine
Cortisone
Cyclizine
Cyclobarbital
Cyclopentobarbital
Cyclopentolate

Cycloserine
Cyclosporine
Cyclothiazide
Cycrimine
Cyproheptadine
Dantrolene
Dapsone
Demeclocycline
Desipramine
Desoxycorticosterone
Dexamethasone
Dexbrompheniramine
Dexchlorpheniramine
Dextroamphetamine
Dextrothyroxine
Diazepam
Diethazine
Diethylpropion
Digitalis
Digoxin
Diltiazem
Dimethindene
Diphenhydramine
Diphenylpyraline
Disopyridamide
Disulfiram
Divalproex Sodium
Doxepin
Doxycycline
Doxylamine
Dronabinol
Droperidol
Enalapril
Ephedrine
Ergocalciferol
Erythropoietin
Ethchlorvynol
Ethionamide
Ethosuximide
Ethopropazine
Fenfluramine
Flecainide
Fludrocortisone
Fluphenazine
Fluprednisolone
Flurazepam
Furosemide
Gentamicin
Glutethimide

Index